Metabolic Brain Dysfunction in Systemic Disorders

Metabolic Brain Dysfunction in Systemic Disorders

Edited by

Allen I. Arieff, M.D.
Professor of Medicine, University of California, San Francisco, School of Medicine; Chief, Geriatrics Research, Veterans Affairs Medical Center, San Francisco, California

Robert C. Griggs, M.D.
Edward and Alma Vollertsen Professor of Neurophysiology, Chairman, Department of Neurology, and Professor of Neurology, Medicine, Pathology, and Pediatrics, University of Rochester School of Medicine and Dentistry, Rochester, New York

Little, Brown and Company
Boston/Toronto/London

First Edition

Library of Congress Cataloging-in-Publication Data
Metabolic brain dysfunction in systemic disorders / edited by
Allen I. Arieff, Robert C. Griggs.
p. cm.
Includes bibliographical references and index.
ISBN 0-316-05067-9 (cloth)
1. Neurologic manifestations of general diseases. I. Arieff, Allen I. (Allen Ives), 1938- . II. Griggs, Robert C., 1939- .
[DNLM: 1. Neurologic Manifestations. WL 340 N49272]
RC346.M43 1992
616.8′4—dc20
DNLM/DLC
for Library of Congress 91-43882
CIP

Printed in the United States of America

MV-NY

Contents

Contributing Authors

Britt Anderson, M.D.
Assistant Professor of Neurology, University of Alabama School of Medicine, Birmingham, Alabama

Allen I. Arieff, M.D.
Professor of Medicine, University of California, San Francisco, School of Medicine; Chief, Geriatrics Research, Veterans Affairs Medical Center, San Francisco, California

Juan Carlos Ayus, M.D.
Professor of Medicine, Baylor College of Medicine, Houston, Texas

Neal L. Benowitz, M.D.
Professor of Medicine and Chief, Division of Clinical Pharmacology and Experimental Therapeutics, University of California, San Francisco, School of Medicine; Attending Physician, San Francisco General Hospital, San Francisco, California

Stephen Brennan, M.D.
Assistant Professor of Medicine, Baylor College of Medicine, Houston, Texas

Hugh J. Carroll, M.D.
Professor of Medicine, State University of New York Health Science Center at Brooklyn College of Medicine; Attending Physician, University Hospital of Brooklyn, Brooklyn, New York

David A. Chad, M.D.
Professor of Neurology, University of Massachusetts Medical School; Attending Neurologist, University of Massachusetts Medical Center, Worcester, Massachusetts

David M. Dawson, M.D.
Associate Professor of Neurology, Harvard Medical School, Boston; Chief, Neurology Service, West Roxbury Veterans Administration Medical Center, West Roxbury, Massachusetts

John R. Fike, Ph.D.
Assistant Professor, Departments of Neurological Surgery, Radiation Oncology, Radiology, and the Brain Tumor Research Center, University of California, San Francisco, School of Medicine, San Francisco, California

Cosmo Lyle Fraser, M.D.
Assistant Professor of Medicine in Residence, University of California, San Francisco, School of Medicine; Chief, Inpatient Dialysis, and Research Associate, Veterans Affairs Medical Center, San Francisco, California

Daniel W. Giang, M.D.
Assistant Professor of Neurology, University of Rochester School of Medicine and Dentistry; Attending Neurologist, University of Rochester Medical Center, Rochester, New York

John E. Greenlee, M.D.
Professor of Neurology, University of Utah School of Medicine; Chief, Neurology Service, Veterans Affairs Medical Center, Salt Lake City, Utah

Robert C. Griggs, M.D.
Edward and Alma Vollertsen Professor of Neurophysiology, Chairman, Department of Neurology, and Professor of Neurology, Medicine, Pathology, and Pediatrics, University of Rochester School of Medicine and Dentistry, Rochester, New York

David M. Holtzman, M.D.
Assistant Adjunct Professor of Neurology, University of California, San Francisco, School of Medicine, San Francisco, California

James P. Knochel, M.D.
Professor of Internal Medicine, University of Texas Southwestern Medical Center at Dallas Southwestern Medical School; Chairman, Department of Internal Medicine, Presbyterian Hospital of Dallas, Dallas, Texas

John Kucharczyk, Ph.D.
Associate Professor of Radiology, University of California, San Francisco, School of Medicine; Director, Neuroradiology Research, The Medical Center at the University of California, San Francisco, San Francisco, California

David A. Larson, M.D., Ph.D.
Associate Professor and Vice Chairman, Department of Radiation Oncology, University of California, San Francisco, School of Medicine, San Francisco, California

David E. Levy, M.D.
Associate Professor of Neurology, Cornell University Medical College; Associate Attending Neurologist, New York Hospital, New York, New York

Alan H. Lockwood, M.D
Professor of Neurology and Nuclear Medicine, State University of New York at Buffalo School of Medicine and Biomedical Sciences; Attending Neurologist, Veterans Administration Medical Center, Buffalo, New York

David W. McCandless, Ph.D.
John Sheinen Professor, Department of Cell Biology and Anatomy, Chicago Medical School, North Chicago, Illinois

Alberto Montanari, M.D.
Riceratore, Istituto di Semeiotica Medica, Università di Parma, Parma, Italy

L. Creed Pettigrew, M.D.
Assistant Professor of Neurology, University of Kentucky College of Medicine; Attending Neurologist, Veterans Administration Medical Center, Lexington, Kentucky

Keith R. Powell, M.D.
George Washington Goler Professor of Pediatrics, and Chief, Division of Infectious Diseases, University of Rochester School of Medicine and Dentistry; Associate Chairman for Clinical Affairs, Department of Pediatrics, Strong Memorial Hospital, Rochester, New York

Lawrence D. Recht, M.D.
Associate Professor of Neurology, University of Massachusetts Medical School; Attending Neurologist, University of Massachusetts Medical Center, Worcester, Massachusetts

Roger N. Rosenberg, M.D.
Abe (Brunky), William, and Morris Zale Distinguished Professor, Department of Neurology, University of Texas Southwestern Medical Center at Dallas Southwestern Medical School; Chief, Neurological Services, Parkland Hospital and Zale/Lipshy University Hospital, Dallas, Texas

Randolph B. Schiffer, M.D.
Associate Professor of Neurology and Psychiatry, and Associate Chairman, Department of Neurology, University of Rochester School of Medicine and Dentistry, Rochester, New York

Steven A. Schonfeld, M.D.
Assistant Professor of Medicine, Division of Pulmonary and Critical Care Medicine, Johns Hopkins University School of Medicine; Associate Director, Pulmonary Division, Sinai Hospital of Baltimore, Baltimore, Maryland

Roger P. Simon, M.D.
Professor of Neurology, University of California, San Francisco, School of Medicine; Chair, Neurology Service, San Francisco General Hospital, San Francisco, California

Neal A. Snyder, M.D.
Clinical Instructor, Department of Medicine, University of California, San Francisco, School of Medicine, San Francisco; Medical Director, Home Health Department, Permanente Medical Group, Redwood City, California

Barney J. Stern, M.D.
Associate Professor of Neurology, Johns Hopkins University School of Medicine; Director, Division of Neurology, Sinai Hospital of Baltimore, Baltimore, Maryland

John R. Sutton, M.D.
Deputy Principal and Professor of Medicine, Cumberland College of Health Sciences, University of Sydney, Sydney, Australia

Jaime Uribarri, M.D.
Assistant Professor of Medicine, Mount Sinai School of Medicine of the City University of New York; Attending Physician, The Mount Sinai Hospital, New York, New York

Robert M. Wachter, M.D.
Assistant Professor of Medicine and Epidemiology, University of California, San Francisco, School of Medicine; Attending Physician, Division of General Internal Medicine, San Francisco General Hospital, San Francisco, California

William M. Wara, M.D.
Professor and Executive Vice Chairman, Department of Radiation Oncology, University of California, San Francisco, School of Medicine, San Francisco, California

Preface

There are many systemic medical illnesses that can affect the central nervous system. These include such common afflictions as diabetes, heart failure, cirrhosis of the liver, and chronic obstructive pulmonary disease. There is, however, a subgroup of medical illness that has major and important systemic manifestations in the central nervous system. These disorders can and most certainly do affect other bodily systems, but the central nervous system manifestations are such that serious injury, disability, or even death can result. In particular, metabolic encephalopathies have their most important effects on the central nervous system. Metabolic encephalopathies include those central nervous system disorders that are not primarily caused by structural abnormalities—not only such obvious disorders as phosphate depletion and hypernatremia but also the sequelae of less obvious insults, such as head trauma and hypoxia/ischemia. Furthermore, metabolic encephalopathies can result in secondary structural damage to the central nervous system, as can occur with hepatic encephalopathy, hyponatremia, and hypoxemia.

Other systemic disorders may have pervasive effects on various systems in the body, including the central nervous system. In the 1990s, AIDS is one of the newer and most widespread and dangerous disorders that can affect the body. AIDS has effects on many body systems, including the brain. Although encephalopathy is not among the major causes of death in AIDS patients, it is a poorly understood and devastating complication. It may well be that AIDS dementia is a direct consequence of central nervous system infection with the AIDS virus, but recent evidence suggests a possible alternate pathomechanism. In rat nervous tissue, a protein from the human immunodeficiency virus may increase intracellular calcium in nerve cells in the hippocampus. Although such studies are preliminary, they provide evidence that an increase of intracellular calcium may be important in the neurotoxicity of AIDS, and thus AIDS encephalopathy may indeed be a form of metabolic encephalopathy.

Hyponatremia is the most common electrolyte abnormality seen in a general hospital population. It is associated with a plethora of systemic disease states, including heart failure, nephrotic syndrome, diabetic coma, liver failure, stroke, and psychogenic polydipsia. Hyponatremia has some effect on many different systems, but its effects on the nervous system are those that are commonly associated with morbidity or mortality. In a similar manner, such diverse disorders as hypoglycemia, alcoholism, sarcoid, and hypoxemia can affect many body systems, but their effects on the central nervous system most frequently result in morbidity and/or mortality.

As an internist and a neurologist, we both have a long-standing and wide-ranging interest in disorders that affect the nervous system. In this volume, we have assembled an international cast of specialists in neurology and internal medicine. The contributing authors have been asked to write their chapters with an eye toward both internal medicine and neurology, and many of the chapters are in fact collaborative efforts. The general purpose of the book, of course, is to aid physicians from both specialties in the diagnosis and therapy of medical disorders that can affect the nervous system. This book is dedicated to the contributors, as it is certainly theirs.

A.I.A.
R.C.G.

Metabolic Brain Dysfunction in Systemic Disorders

Notice

1 General Considerations in Metabolic Encephalopathies and Systemic Disorders Affecting the Nervous System

Allen I. Arieff and Robert C. Griggs

Metabolic encephalopathies are by definition those disorders of the central nervous system that are not due primarily to structural abnormalities (Table 1-1). These include not only such obvious disorders as phosphate depletion and hypernatremia, but the sequelae of less obvious insults, such as closed head trauma and hypoxia/ischemia. Furthermore, metabolic encephalopathies can result in secondary structural damage to the central nervous system, as can occur with phosphate depletion [92], Wernicke's encephalopathy [139], hepatic encephalopathy [161], hyponatremia [63], or hypernatremia [55,148].

This introductory chapter first considers the approach to neurologic diagnosis in the patient with a systemic disease or a metabolic encephalopathy, outlining the approach to clinical evaluation of the patient. Secondly, it considers the metabolism of brain in general terms and the mechanisms of neurologic dysfunction produced by metabolic disorders.

Supported in part by the Research Service of the Veterans Affairs Medical Center, San Francisco, California, and NIH grant RR 00044 from the Division of Research Resources.

RECOGNIZING THE NEUROLOGIC COMPLICATIONS OF SYSTEMIC DISEASE

When a patient with a known, major systemic illness such as systemic lupus erythematosus or sarcoidosis develops neurologic symptoms and signs, it is a relatively straightforward matter to consider the catalogue of neurologic complications of the underlying disease. Arriving at a diagnosis is often easy, and if the neurologic problem is dire, maximal therapy consists of administering for the disease in question. However, there are two common situations in which diagnosis is difficult: (1) The neurologic manifestation precedes the diagnosis of the sys-

Table 1-1. Metabolic encephalopathies

Hyponatremia
Hypernatremia
Phosphate depletion
Uremia
Uremic encephalopathy
Dialysis disequilibrium syndrome
Dialysis dementia
Hepatic coma
Hypocalcemia
Hypercalcemia
Hyperparathyroidism
Hypoparathyroidism
Metabolic alkalosis
Wernicke's encephalopathy
Diabetic ketoacidosis
Nonketotic hyperosmolar coma
Phosphate depletion
Hypoglycemia
Ethanol intoxication
Hypoxemia
Hypercapnia
Exogenous intoxications
Salicylate
Paraldehyde
Heroin
Amphetamine
Cocaine
Phencyclidine (angel dust)
Barbiturates
Trace metals
Tin
Aluminum
Lead

temic disease; and (2) the neurologic disorder is *not* the result of the underlying disease but rather an unrelated, coincidental disease. The chapters in this volume that consider specific disorders such as systemic lupus and sarcoidosis address the first issue. The second is much more difficult and demands that the clinician be aware of all of the permutations and combinations of abnormalities produced by the systemic disease.

CLINICAL PICTURE OF METABOLIC ENCEPHALOPATHY

The brain responds to metabolic disorders with a limited array of symptoms and signs. Most causes of metabolic encephalopathy (Table 1-1) produce a relatively stereotyped constellation of findings on neurologic examination [73]. Three broad mechanisms account for the clinical findings. The first, generalized depression of brain function, is the most frequently encountered situation, with cerebral hemispheres being more susceptible to such depression. Thus, consciousness is depressed, respirations are normal or diminished, and pupils small but reactive. Reflex eye movements become disinhibited and motor tone diminished. Asterixis, one of the hallmarks of metabolic encephalopathy, may also relate to intermittent depression of motor function. Secondly, the findings in certain types of metabolic encephalopathy can be understood in terms of heightened excitability of neural tissue resulting from a direct lowering of threshold for neuronal excitability or because of a selective depression of inhibitory influences on neuronal function. Thus, Cheyne-Stokes respiration may result from the loss of bihemispheric inhibition of brain stem respiratory control, and most types of seizures from heightened neuronal excitability. Finally, in certain metabolic encephalopathies, selective vulnerability of a specific brain region may result in focal alterations in neurologic function. The vulnerability of the cerebellum in the alcoholic person may relate to a relatively high level of an enzyme for which thiamine is a cofactor. Regional differences in tissue metabolic requirements for oxygen, glucose, or amino acids may similarly underlie the selective vulnerability of an area of brain to a systemic metabolic insult. The blood flow to an area of brain or the characteristics of vascular response to exogenous hormones may also influence the response of the tissue to metabolic perturbations.

Respiratory Abnormalities

Metabolic encephalopathies cause a variety of respiratory abnormalities: hypopnea, hyperpnea, ataxic respirations, and Cheyne-Stokes respirations. Respiratory depression resulting in hypopnea is the most frequently encountered abnormality seen in metabolic encephalopathy and is associated with overdosage of most exogenous sedatives and with some endogenous disorders. A sequentially worsening decrease in the tidal volume heralds a decrease in the rate of respirations and culminates in apnea. In contrast, many endogenous metabolic encephalopathies such as uremia, hypoxia, and hepatic encephalopathy result in hyperventilation. In patients with metabolic acidosis, the extent of hyperventilation correlates with the degree of acidosis and reflects a compensatory ventilatory drive that operates to maintain normal brain pH. In acidotic patients with hyperventilation, the differential diagnosis includes uremia, diabetic ketoacidosis, alcoholic ketoacidosis, hypoxia, and exogenous toxins such as ethylene glycol. Blood pH is often acidotic and blood PCO_2 lowered. Studies of blood for lactate, pyruvate, beta-hydroxybutyrate, acetoacetate, sulfate, phosphate, or exogenous anions usually establish the cause. In certain patients with hyperventilation, however, the blood PCO_2 is low but the blood pH is alkalotic and no increase in blood anion accounts for the hyperventilation. Examples include patients after cardiac arrest, in whom an inappropriate hyperventilation is often present even after lactic acidosis has been reversed. Similarly in hepatic encephalopathy, salicylate toxicity, gram-negative sepsis, and occasional other settings, blood pH is alkalotic and no clear etiology for hyperventilation can be established. Various endogenous and exogenous metabolites have been implicated in this hyperventilation. For example, an increase in blood short-chain fatty acids has been found in hepatic encephalopathy and can induce hyperventilation in experimental animals [158].

Ataxic respirations usually suggest pontine damage or compression [134]. Patients with meningitis, however, who have no evidence of brain stem structural disease by either physical examination or by computed tomography (CT) or magnetic resonance imaging (MRI) studies, frequently have either short-cycle Cheyne-Stokes respirations or ataxic respirations [134]. This respiratory pattern was initially described by Biot [134]. As in patients with structural pontine disease, such ataxic respirations are often the prelude to respiratory arrest.

Cheyne-Stokes respirations result from bilateral hemispheric dysfunction but are frequently encountered in elderly patients without established neurologic disease [33]. In this setting the respiratory abnormalities are often attributed to congestive heart failure or chronic lung disease. In fact, the respiratory abnormalities are invariably associated with either bilateral hemispheric disease or a metabolic abnormality such as hypoxia [52]. Cheyne-Stokes respirations improve when hypoxia is reversed [77]. A variety of other metabolic encephalopathies from exogenous or endogenous toxins are also associated with Cheyne-Stokes respirations. Such patients may have a normal respiratory pattern when awake and develop hypopnea-hyperpnea cycles when asleep. Post-hyperventilation apnea is often elicitable in such patients while they are awake.

Pupils

The pupillary responses to light and pain are usually preserved in the patient with metabolic encephalopathy. If the level of consciousness is depressed, the pupils are typically small, much as they are in normal subjects during slow-wave sleep. In the patient with a depressed level of consciousness from a metabolic encephalopathy, the pupils typically are 2 to 4 mm in diameter and briskly reactive. It is characteristic of the pupillary responses in patients with moderate generalized metabolic depression of the nervous system that repeated stimulation will result in the arousal of the patient and associated enlargement of the pupils. Interestingly, patients with Cheyne-Stokes respirations or milder hypopnea-hyperpnea cycles often have pupils that are small when the patient is hypopneic or apneic and increase in size when the patient is hyperpneic. The level of consciousness also fluctuates with the hypopnea-hyperpnea cycles. In such patients, arousal produced by vigorous stimuli results in rapid enlargement of pupils from 2 or 3 mm to as large as 6 or 7 mm (this arousal is often useful in examining the optic fundi in the stuporous patient). Pupils are equal in size in metabolic encephalopathy as a rule, but pupillary inequalities of a millimeter or more are common in the normal population (approximately 10%) and subtler abnormalities are detectable in up to 25 percent of the normal population [155]. Minor differences in pupillary diameter are therefore not unexpected in patients with metabolic encephalopathy.

Abnormal Pupils from Metabolic Encephalopathy

Certain metabolic encephalopathies are characterized by distinctive abnormalities in the pupils. Fixed and dilated pupils can often result from hypoxia, ischemia, or local or systemic sympathometics. Less commonly, phenothiazine overdosage, hypothermia, or high-dose intravenous lidocaine produces large, unreactive pupils. Pupils that are unequal, abnormal in shape, and eccentric in position may result from glutethimide overdosage [133]. Miotic pupils are common with opiates and related agents, and anisocoria is often noted in patients withdrawing from opiates [42].

Ocular Motility

Voluntary eye movements, eye position, and spontaneous involuntary eye movements are all useful in characterizing metabolic encephalopathy. In the unconscious patient, ocular motility is tested by examining oculovestibular reflexes and caloric reflexes. Interobserver variability in the assessment of eye movements is high, lessening their value in following patients [30]. Ocular motility is typically normal in patients with mild metabolic encephalopathy, but in the markedly obtunded patient, particularly those with barbituate and tricyclic antidepressant overdosage, oculocephalic and caloric responses are often lost [134]. Patients with sedative overdosage not uncommonly lose oculocephalic responses even while respirations are maintained. Occasional patients lose caloric and oculovestibular responses while preserving normal ventilation and remaining responsive. A direct and disproportionate effect of exogenous or endogenous toxins on the vestibular nuclei may account for the abnormalities [159].

The eyes are typically midposition with most metabolic encephalopathies, but hepatic encephalopathy is frequently associated with conjugate downward deviation of the eyes [36]. The eyes are midposition when the patient is unconscious, but with arousal, sustained downward gaze is elicited. Skew deviation, ocular bobbing, and convergence spasm also occur with hepatic encephalopathy [36,134,147]. Dysconjugate eye movements or skew deviation also occurs in bromism and in phenytoin, carbamazepine, and tricyclic antidepressant drug overdosage. Patients with sedative overdosage typically lose the rapid, cortical phase of caloric testing [50]. Forced downward deviation of the eyes as a reaction to unilateral cold water irrigation is frequently seen [149]. All of the aforementioned abnormalities of ocular motility are reversible when the encephalopathy improves. Other ocular motility disturbances have been identified in metabolic encephalopathies but may relate to focal, permanent damage produced by the metabolic disorder. Thus, ocular dipping has been observed in patients with anoxic coma [143], and downbeating nystagmus has been noted in vitamin B_{12} deficiency [111] and with lithium toxicity [41].

Eyelid position and eye opening response to arousal are occasionally helpful in the diagnosis of metabolic encephalopathies. The eyelids are closed and the patient appears asleep in most severe metabolic encephalopathy, which alters consciousness. Efforts at arousing the patient will often result in eye opening and other signs of returning consciousness. Following severe hypoxic-ischemic injury, forced eyelid opening and associated frontalis muscle myoclonus are common [166]. Following severe metabolic insults such as hypoxia, hypoglycemia, and carbon monoxide poisoning, the persistent vegetative state may develop and patients will develop sleep-wake cycles with both spontaneous eye openings and eye openings in response to external stimuli. In all such patients there is evidence of severe bihemispheric destruction [166].

Motor Examination

Generalized flaccidity is the characteristic motor finding in acute, severe metabolic encephalopathy, but a number of other responses can be seen. Decerebrate posturing, ordinarily a harbinger of cerebral herniation with reticular formation compression, is frequent in hepatic encephalopathy [40], in hypoglycemia, and with many drug ingestions. Decorticate posturing also occurs. Following hypoxic-ischemic damage decorticate or decerebrate posturing are often present, and although in many instances irreversible brain damage has occurred, recovering patients may evolve from decerebrate posturing to decorticate posturing and return to apparently normal mentation [99]. Conscious patients with mild metabolic encephalopathy have a spectrum of motor abnormalities of both a generalized and focal nature related to the cause of the encephalopathy.

Asterixis

This motor abnormality results from the loss of postural tone in voluntary muscles of the limbs, trunk, head, or tongue. The demonstration of asterixis requires that the patient be sufficiently conscious to maintain a sustained posture of the limbs or trunk. Severe asterixis can result in loss of body tone and lead to drop attacks. Bilateral asterixis of the arms, initially described as "liver flap" [1] is frequent in uremia, hypercapnea, sedative intoxication, subarachnoid hemorrhage, salicylate toxicity [6], and many other settings. Unilateral asterixis can also occur and usually implies a focal lesion in either the thalamus or midbrain [153], but it may also indicate the superimposition of a metabolic insult on an underlying structural abnormality [48]. Thus, a patient with subarachnoid hemorrhage and a mild hemiparesis often has asterixis in the hemiparetic limb. Patients with focal cerebral disease treated with phenytoin or carbamazepine often show asterixis on the hemiparetic side. Asterixis can occur without metabolic abnormalities. A lesion in the ventrolateral nucleus of the thalamus is present in some patients with unilateral asterixis [51].

Myoclonus

Multifocal myoclonus and focal seizures are common in many metabolic disturbances, particularly uremia, respiratory alkalosis, and with toxic levels of a number of drugs including many of the penicillins, meperidine, and theophylline. Periodic and stereotyped synchronous myoclonus involving the levator palpebrae superioris, tongue, and limbs is frequent in patients who have sustained hypoxic brain damage [166].

Focal Seizures and Weakness

Hyperglycemia is associated with focal seizures, particularly in elderly patients [32,104]. In patients with hyperosmotic states the degree of osmolar abnormality is more important than the level of blood glucose. Focal ischemia of brain may be responsible for the seizures [53]. Focal findings such as hemiparesis are remarkably frequent in metabolic encephalopathies including uremia, hepatic encephalopathy, hypoglycemia, and hypercalcemia. Although the basis for the focal findings is often unclear, a reversible vasospasm has been demonstrated in patients with hypercalcemia [102,160,169]. Metabolic abnormalities such as hypoglycemia may also cause focal signs by producing a so-called anamnestic response of a previously damaged area of brain [118].

BRAIN METABOLISM: GENERAL

The average weight of the human brain is about 1300 gm, which represents less than 2 percent of body mass. However, for such a small organ, the brain is a disproportionate consumer of resources, receiving about 20 percent of cardiac output, consuming about 65 percent of the glucose used by the body, and utilizing about 20 percent of the body's oxygen supply [26,79]. In addition, about 75 percent of oxygen used by the brain is utilized by cortical gray matter neurons, which constitute only about 20 percent of brain mass. Thus, the brain has enormous needs in terms of substrate and blood flow. About 85 percent of all glucose used by the brain is aerobically metabolized, and about half of the energy produced is utilized to maintain normal ionic gradients across brain cell membranes. The most important of these ionic gradients include those for sodium, potassium, hydrogen ion, and calcium. It is these ionic gradients that are needed to generate action potentials and conduct nerve impulses. If there is a deficiency of oxygen, adequate glucose cannot be oxidized aerobically, resulting in a shift to anaerobic energy production by the brain. No measurable cerebral dysfunction occurs when cerebral oxygen utilization is maintained at a level of 50 percent of normal, which corresponds to an arterial $PO_2(PaO_2)$ of about 50 mm Hg. When PaO_2 is below such levels, anaerobic metabolism is present, which cannot supply enough energy for the brain to function very long. When PaO_2 declines below about 30 mm Hg, there is usually some depression of sensorium. A recent study of well-conditioned individuals at altitudes of up to 8848 meters demonstrated steady-state arterial PO_2 of about 30 mm Hg at rest [82] and about 28 mm Hg with exercise. Individuals with such a degree of systemic hypoxemia for several days were found to have developed permanent brain damage when subjected to a sophisticated battery of motor, intellectual, and psychological tests [82]. The PaO_2 level of 30 mm Hg or less corresponds quite well to the minimum level in laboratory animals that is compatible with survival [12,47]. In addition, when hypoxia is combined with another metabolic insult, the net effects are substantially more than that associated with either entity alone. The combination of hypoxia plus hyponatremia is far more deleterious than either entity by itself [8,25,78].

Brain Ionic Composition

The chemical constituents of the brain are generally quite different from those of other tissues. The differences become particularly important in situations where there is a disturbance of osmotic equilibrium. The brain adapts differently to osmotic disturbances than does any other tissue in the body, and this is largely because of differences in intracellular electrolyte content and the control systems that regulate their concentrations. The principal osmotically active constituents of brain consist of both organic and inorganic solutes. The major inorganic constituents of the brain and their approximate concentrations (mmol/kg wet weight) in the cerebral cortex of mammalian species (rat, cat, dog, human) are Na^+ (50–60 mmol/kg), K^+ (85–100 mmol/kg), Cl^- (35–45 mmol/kg), Ca^{+2} (1.0–2.8 mmol/kg), Mg^{+2} (5–6 mmol/kg), and bicarbonate (10–12 mmol/kg) [16,87].

The total brain cation concentration is thus about 170 mmol/kg wet weight, while anions, including Cl^-, bicarbonate, sulfates, phosphates, and organic acid anions (such as lactate, glutamine, glutamate, and *N*-acetylaspartate) are at most about 90 mmol/kg wet weight [87,156]. The remaining brain intracellular anions are probably polyionic lipids and proteins. Since most brain Cl^- is extracellular, the bulk of intracellular anions are organic and macromolecular [88]. Additionally, there are also minute quantities in the brain of certain trace metals, such as copper, manganese, zinc, iron, tin, aluminum, and rubidium [83,112,123,164].

The actual osmotic activity of any of the constituents mentioned above is not entirely clear. Most Ca^{+2} and Mg^{+2} are probably bound and not osmotically active. Unlike most other tissues in the body, the primary intracellular cations in brain consist of both sodium and potassium, with a substantial portion of intracellular sodium being osmotically active [116]. The osmotic activity in brain of amino acids and other organic acids is uncertain, although they appear to play a major role in osmotic adaptation in the cells of many invertebrates and amphibians [57,59,107]. Glutamate, glutamine, aspartate, taurine, lysine, threonine, inositol, lactate, and alanine are organic intracellular metabolites for which the osmotic activity has not been determined [27,38,126,157,167].

Adaptation to Osmotic Imbalance

There is a substantial quantity of evidence, both in humans and experimental animals, that there may be changes in plasma osmolality where the apparent net loss or gain of cellular water and solute does not account for the change in tissue osmolality [17,18,22,116,162]. In these instances there may be apparent inactivation of intracellular solute or a gain in solute that is not due to commonly measured substances [19,37,38,56,113,115,146]. This undetermined solute has been called idiogenic osmoles [19,56,113]. Furthermore, there is a substantial body of evidence that suggests the brain undergoes osmotic adaptation to hyperosmolar states in a manner that is distinctly different from other tissues. For example, in birds and mammals, muscle and nucleated red blood cells may adapt to hyperosmolar states by loss of water and gain in cation [58,74,75,93], while brain adapts primarily by de novo generation of solute by yet unexplained mechanisms [14,19,38,101,113]. These mechanisms apparently are not activated immediately, and as a result, overly rapid induction of either hyperosmolality or hypo-osmolality may result in permanent brain damage [13,14,20,55]. Abrupt shrinkage of the brain could lead to tearing of cerebral vessels and meninges, with subsequent subdural hemorrhage, as has been described in humans and animals with acute hypernatremia [56]. Thus, from a clinical standpoint, the ability of the brain to generate idiogenic osmoles to maintain cellular volume intact is crucial to survival. In this sense, it is of interest that the brains of some vertebrates who live parts of their lives in both saltwater and freshwater environments appear to have the ability to adapt to the changing osmotic environment by altering intracellular content of amino acids and other organic molecules.

CHARACTERISTICS OF THE BLOOD-BRAIN BARRIER

Brain Extracellular Space

In general, extracellular space (ECS) is thought of as that fluid compartment that is outside of cells. In practice, the ECS is defined as that fluid compartment that is available for the distribution of a particular marker. It is determined as the ratio of distribution of the marker in the tissue to its distribution in a reference fluid that is considered to represent extracellular fluid [45]. If plasma is used as the extracellular fluid, it must be corrected for the Donnan effect. There is a dual circulation of fluids about the brain (both blood and cerebrospinal fluid [CSF]). The vast bulk of evidence suggests that the CSF is identical to and is a continuation of the extracellular fluid of the brain [45,88,97]. The measurement of ECS assumes that the marker has equilibrated between tissue and extracellular fluid. In the case of the brain, there is a tendency for any substance entering the brain via the blood or CSF to be siphoned off, so that equilibration may not be reached. This tendency is known as the "sink action" of CSF [97,124]. Several different in vivo techniques and markers have been employed to measure brain ECS. These include estimation by electron microscopy, tissue diffusion profiles, and measurement of cortical electrical impedance. When brain ECS is appropriately determined in mammalian cerebral cortex by any of these techniques, the range is from 15 to 25 percent, with a mean value of about 20 percent.

Anatomy of the Blood-Brain Barrier

When a nonmetabolizable, nontoxic substance is administered via the bloodstream such that steady-state conditions are maintained for several hours, it will achieve a similar volume of distribution throughout most cell systems. Such substances include inulin, sulfate, salicylic acid, antipyrine, and urea. However, for a given time interval, none will achieve a concentration in the brain that is as high as its concentration in other tissues such as liver or muscle. This selective behavior of the brain, whereby passage of certain substances out of the blood is restricted, has been called the blood-brain barrier [29,31,141]. The anatomic delineation of the blood-brain barrier is complex, with the principal components being the astrocytic processes (end-feet processes), the thick basement membrane of the brain capillaries, and the thick wall of the neuronal cells [46]. In contrast to capillaries elsewhere in the body, the brain capillary basement membranes function as an epithelial sheet. Brain capillaries are made of a single layer of endothelial cells, with a dense cytoplasm containing few vesicles. In contrast to other capillaries, brain endothelial cells are connected by tight junctions that act to form a continuous cell layer [91]. A basement membrane surrounds the cells, and this is in turn covered by the glial cells, whose astrocytic processes cover about 85 percent of the capillary surface. The intracerebral arterioles and venules are also covered by continuous endothelial cell layers with tight junctions. Both the astrocytic end-feet processes that surround the capillaries and the unfenestrated endothelial cells with their complex tight junctions, as well as the thick neuronal cell walls, probably constitute the bulk of the blood-brain barrier.

ACID-BASE REGULATION IN THE CENTRAL NERVOUS SYSTEM

The regulation of acid-base balance in the central nervous system is distinctly different from that of other organs in the body. Regulation of acid-base balance in the CSF is reasonably straightforward and less controversial because of the ready applicability of common techniques used for measurement of blood gases to measure gases in CSF directly. Lumbar CSF is commonly obtained for analysis by lumbar puncture. The bicarbonate concentration is similar in cisternal versus lumbar CSF [136]. The pH in lumbar CSF is about 0.04 pH units less than that of cisternal CSF because the PCO_2 is about 4 mm Hg higher [136]. Neither of these differences are normally of clinical importance.

By contrast, the techniques for evaluation of intracellular pH (pHi) in brain have generally involved the use of indirect measurements. Such techniques have generally employed either the creatine phosphate equilibrium in brain, brain carbon dioxide content, or isotope techniques, such as ^{14}C-labeled dimethadione [72,142]. The intracellular PCO_2 in brain is generally assumed to be represented by the PCO_2 in cortical CSF [72,84]. All of these techniques have the major drawback that brain tissue biopsy is required by invasive techniques [15]. Representing a major but very expensive methodologic advance, at this time pHi in brain is generally measured by use of magnetic resonance spectroscopy (MRS), a technique that allows serial measurements of brain pHi without invasive interventions [24,81]. None of the other invasive techniques is suitable for evaluation of brain pHi in vivo in humans. Currently, MRS can be used to evaluate pHi in vivo in humans, and it is expected that such techniques will rapidly expand our knowledge base in this area in the 1990s [119].

Many physicians have traditionally assumed that the pH of CSF reflects the pHi of brain better than does arterial pH. In fact, this is generally incorrect. The CSF is more of a passive "sink" for both blood and brain. In many clinical circum-

Fig. 1-1. Relationship between the acid-base balance in arterial blood versus cisternal cerebrospinal fluid (CSF) in human subjects. (From A. I. Arieff, [7].)

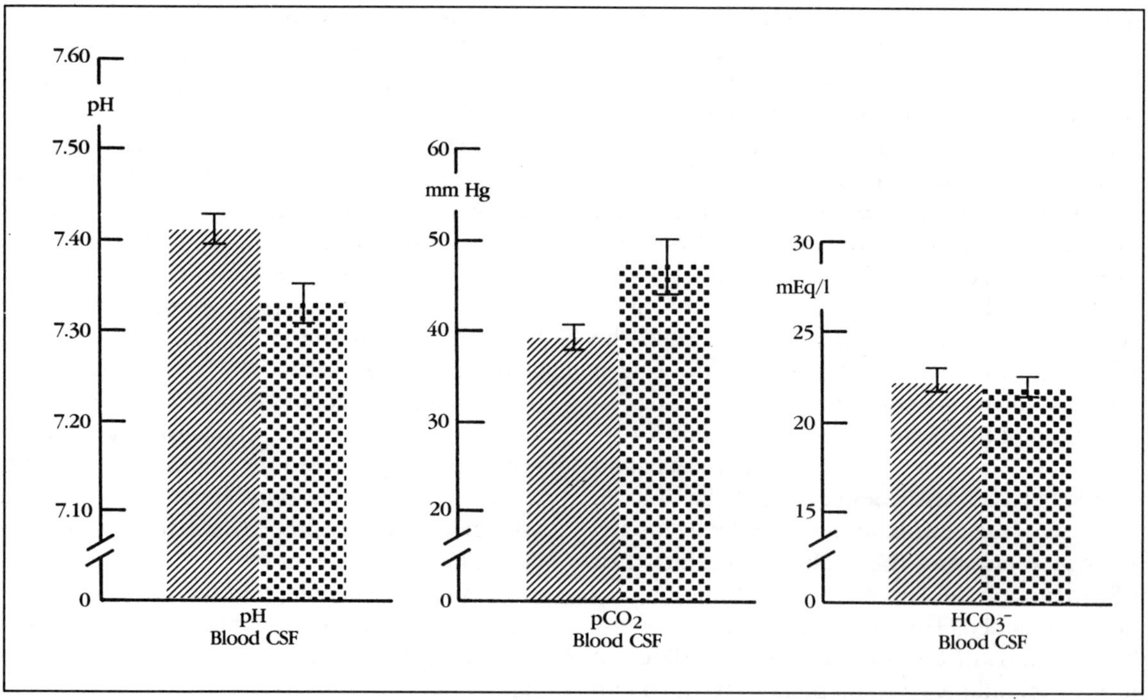

stances, brain pHi is often closer to arterial pH than to that of CSF. Actually, there are three separate compartments in the central nervous system—blood, brain, and CSF—which are separated by the blood-brain and blood-CSF barriers.

The steady-state relationships between acid-base components in arterial blood versus cisternal CSF in humans are shown in Figure 1-1. In general, the bicarbonate concentration is similar in blood and CSF (about 24 mmol/liter). The arterial pH (about 7.40) is higher than that in CSF (about 7.32) because the PCO_2 is about 48 mm Hg in CSF versus about 40 mm Hg in arterial blood. The buffering capacity of CSF is substantially less than that in blood. Much of this difference is due to the fact that the CSF protein concentration (about 4×10^{-2} gm/dl) is minute compared to that in plasma (about 7 gm/dl). However, the pH of CSF remains remarkably constant despite this apparent inferior buffering capacity and despite substantial changes in arterial pH. In those conditions characterized by acute alterations in systemic PCO_2 (respiratory alkalosis and acidosis), there are acute alterations in pH and PCO_2 of CSF that are directionally similar to those in arterial blood [23,127]. However, the changes in CSF pH are initially less than those observed in arterial blood, and within 1 hour, efficient compensatory mechanisms have been initiated. In certain unique clinical situations, such as the treatment of uremic patients with hemodialysis, or therapy of patients with metabolic acidosis with sodium bicarbonate infusion, the pH of CSF may move in a direction that is opposite to that of blood (Fig. 1-2) [15,23,137].

TRACE METALS AND THE CENTRAL NERVOUS SYSTEM: POSSIBLE TOXIC EFFECTS

There are a number of trace metals that have been found to be elevated in brain of patients with various systemic diseases. These include nickel, zinc, aluminum, cadmium, tin, calcium, strontium, copper, iron, molybdenum, manganese, cobalt, lead, arsenic, boron, mercury, selenium, tellurium, thallium, and vanadium [11,21,83,151,164]. A number of these metals may actually have toxic effects upon the brain. The available evidence for such toxic effects varies substantially from metal to metal, but in

Fig. 1-2. Changes in arterial blood and cerebrospinal fluid (CSF) during rapid hemodialysis (HD) in uremic dogs. As the arterial pH rises (from 7.22 to 7.31) the pH in CSF falls (from 7.33 to 7.19). (From A. I. Arieff, et al. [15].)

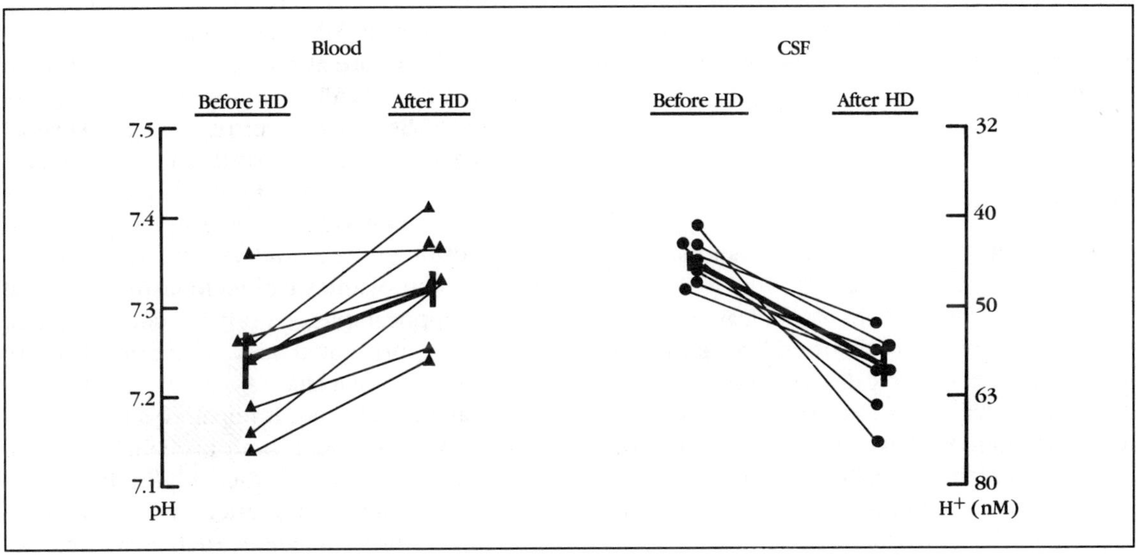

general, there has been either a known exposure followed by a clinical syndrome or the chemical isolation of a metal from central nervous tissue of a patient who has died from a clinical syndrome. Metals that have been so incriminated include tin, aluminum, calcium, manganese, silicon, and nickel in patients with renal failure [21,39,80,123,163], aluminum and tin in patients with renal failure and dialysis dementia [2–4,108], aluminum in patients with Alzheimer's disease [44,129,132], silicon in patients with Alzheimer's disease [35], aluminum in patients with amyotropic lateral sclerosis and parkinsonism dementia of Guam [130,132], aluminum in aging individuals [112], lead in individuals with encephalopathy [164] or mental retardation [121], and tin in patients with dementia and impaired vision [123,164]. Aluminum has received the most publicity, both in the scientific and lay press. Intraneuronal aluminum accumulation has been incriminated in the pathogenesis of several disorders of the central nervous system, including dialysis dementia, amyotropic lateral sclerosis, and parkinsonism dementia of Guam.

Mercury is toxic to various organ systems, particularly the kidneys. Mercury is used in combination with silver to form amalgam, which is used in dental fillings. The mercury has been shown to be released from dental amalgam fillings and to distribute itself in various tissues, including the brain [76]; neurotoxicity is possible but has not yet been shown to occur. Thus, much of the entire field of possible neurotoxicities of various trace metallic elements remains to be clarified.

ALZHEIMER'S DISEASE

There are both structural and metabolic abnormalities in the brain of patients with Alzheimer's disease, and the etiology is unclear. However, there is no shortage of theories. Because it is not clear that Alzheimer's disease is in fact a systemic disorder rather than a condition affecting only the brain, we have chosen not to include a chapter on Alzheimer's disease in this book. The disorder is of such importance, however, that it will briefly be covered here.

Alzheimer's disease is the leading cause of dementia in the United States, affecting about 4 percent of the population over age 65 and having a prevalence of about 20 percent among those over 80 years [96]. Among patients with established dementia, over 50 percent will probably have dementia of the Alzheimer's type [85,86,96,145]. Alzheimer's disease was probably the fourth leading cause of death in the United States in 1990 [85]. Although the diagnosis can be made with absolute certainty only by biopsy of the cerebral cortex, the clinical characteristics are distinctive enough that the diagnosis can be made with at least 80 percent accuracy [86].

The clinical manifestations of Alzheimer's disease have been well described in the medical literature. Briefly, there is an initial memory deficit that progresses, affecting both recent and remote memory. This is followed by a later confusional phase, with progressively more severe impairment of cognitive functioning [86,96,145]. Continuing deterioration of higher cortical functions, such as language, problem solving, and insight, is the rule. In the final stages, patients become aimless and often hallucinate, becoming restless, aphasic, and agitated. There are often associated abnormal neurologic reflexes, which are indicative of loss of higher neural inhibition.

Histologically, there is a loss of large neurons, particularly in the midfrontal and superior regions. In the cerebral cortex, there is a clumping of nerve cell fibers that forms neurofibrillary tangles. There are also degenerated nerve endings that form senile plaques. Paired helical filaments, a distinct type of pathologic neuronal fiber, are the principal constituents of the neurofibrillary tangles, and ubiquitin is a component of these filaments [120]. The plaques are of both the neuritic and amyloid variety. The distribution of such plaques can include the temporal lobes, hippocampus, entorhinal cortex, limbic structures, prefrontal area, anterior olfactory nucleus, and amygdala.

It may be that there is impaired axonal transport of neurofilament, both in Alzheimer's disease and in a number of other conditions characterized by dementia [66]. Such a defect could be due to a number of causes, such as trauma, genetic defects, toxins, nutrient deficiencies, slow virus infections, or deposition of trace metals, such as aluminum [60,66,96]. There are alterations in cytoskeletal proteins and there are also abnormal fibrous proteins, as well as granulovacuolar inclusions, of which tubulin is a major constituent. The tubulin may be abnormal due to effects of aluminum [105]. There are several abnormal fibrous proteins, such as vascular amyloid, neuritic plaque amyloid, and paired helical filaments. There may also be genetic defects in Alzheimer's disease. There is a tendency of the disorder to run in certain families, sometimes as an autosomal dominant. Patients with Down's syndrome who live past age 30 generally have neurofibrillary tangles and senile plaques in the brain that are similar to those observed in Alzheimer's disease. There is also mutation of a subsection of chromosome 21 in Alzheimer's disease, a defect that also occurs in Down's syndrome [49]. In particular, the mutation often appears to involve the proximal portion of the long arm of chromosome 21:21q11.2 21q22.2. Among the possible functional consequences of this mutation are a loss of natural cell barriers to aluminum [114]. As a result, aluminum may gain access to several brain sites, including the nuclear compartment of certain neurons. One important toxic action of aluminum in the brain may be an increase in the binding of histones to DNA, with reduced transcription. The reduced transcription may account for many metabolic abnormalities in cells, including regulation of phosphorylation, calcium homeostasis and neurotransmitter metabolism [114].

Neurochemical Abnormalities in Alzheimer's Disease

Perhaps as a consequence of some of the aforementioned abnormalities, there are a number of neurochemical disorders in the central nervous system of patients with Alzheimer's disease. Among the more important neurochemical findings in brain of Alzheimer's disease patients are decreased levels of certain enzymes in the temporal lobes. The most noteworthy enzyme deficiency observed to date probably is that of choline acetyltransferase [144], but deficiencies of gamma-aminobutyric acid (GABA), somatostatin, serotonin, and norepinephrine have also been reported [60, 128, 144]. The decreased brain levels of choline acetyltransferase are associated with impaired synthesis of acetylcholine in brain of patients with Alzheimer's disease [60]. It has been suggested that there may be decreased cerebral blood flow, along with impaired glucose and oxygen utilization, in brain of patients with Alzheimer's disease. The decreased glucose utilization may be related to impaired acetylcholine synthesis [60]. If this were important in the pathogenesis of Alzheimer's disease, there should be reduced ability of the brain to metabolize glucose. In fact, in vivo studies by positron emission tomography (PET) scanning of the brain of subjects with Alzheimer's disease demonstrate decreased glucose utilization in the temporoparietal cortex [64]. However, biopsies of cerebral cortex tissue from patients with Alzheimer's disease can as readily metabolize glucose to carbon dioxide as can a control population [150]. Thus, the reduced glucose utilization observed by PET scanning may actually reflect decreased cerebral energy requirements. The issue is still unresolved.

Among the more potentially important chemical findings in brain of patients with Alzheimer's disease is an increased level of aluminum in the cerebral cortex [44, 112, 130]. This finding has not been observed by all investigators [165]. It initially appeared that the aluminum was localized only to the nuclear regions of neurofibrillary tangles [130] in patients with Alzheimer's disease. More recent investigations reveal that, in fact, aluminum accumulates in at least a number of different sites [114]. Despite a tremendous amount of research on the role of aluminum in the pathogenesis of Alzheimer's disease, it is still unclear whether aluminum is important in the causation of Alzheimer's disease or is merely a paraphenomenon. However, recent data make it quite clear that continued extraordinarily large exposure to aluminum can lead to cognitive impairment [5, 140].

In general then, Alzheimer's disease may well be a form of metabolic encephalopathy, but the issue remains unresolved. Among the major issues in the causation of Alzheimer's disease is the role of the amyloid protein [109]. Some feel this is a "bystander" and of little or no importance in pathogenesis, while others believe that amyloid protein plays a major role in the pathogenesis of Alzheimer's disease. Recent data suggest that a fragment of the amyloid precursor may be neurotoxic [168]. Others believe that neurotoxic effects of aluminum may be important in the pathogenesis of Alzheimer's disease [44, 129, 130, 132]. Recent studies suggest a mechanism whereby aluminum may actually impair neurotransmitter synthesis in brain [4], and several possible mechanisms have been suggested for increased transport of aluminum into brain [54, 131]. The biochemical sequelae may lead to the cholinergic and glutamatergic dysfunction that is observed in Alzheimer's disease [125]. It must be emphasized that there is no established or even postulated relevance of Alzheimer's disease to dietary aluminum. The entire increase of aluminum in the brain of a patient with Alzheimer's disease is less than 4 mg, while the usual dietary intake of aluminum exceeds 100 mg/day [9]. Thus, the problem is not the availability of aluminum, but rather how it gets into the central nervous system.

OTHER METABOLIC ENCEPHALOPATHIES

Cerebral Hypoxia

Hypoxia and/or ischemia can eventually lead to cell death in the brain. However, when hypoxia/ischemia is of short duration (less than 1 hour) and the clinical situation that led to the insult is then removed, permanent brain damage often occurs nonetheless. The intervening stages that lead to eventual brain damage are discussed in Chapter 3, and it is clear that the later process is indeed a "metabolic encephalopathy"

Hypoxia can affect brain water and electrolyte composition. However, our understanding of the effects of hypoxia on brain water, electrolyte, and high-energy phosphate composition has been substantially altered in the past decade. The impression of many physicians is that hypoxia somehow leads to a decrease in high-energy phosphate concentration, with a loss of potassium and gain in sodium and chloride by cells, with resultant secondary influx of water resulting in cerebral edema [67, 90, 117, 122]. Many of these concepts result from observations now believed to be artifactual [122]. For example, a diagnosis of "brain edema" was often based on measurements of CSF pressure rather than actual brain water content. There are very few actual measurements of brain water content to document brain edema associated with hypoxia. Currently, brain water can be evaluated in vitro using such techniques as CT scanning or MRI [138].

Theoretically, in the strict biochemical sense, if severe hypoxia were present, there would be a decrease in high-energy phosphate compounds, such as adenosine triphosphate (ATP) and phosphocreatine. When this happens, it is suggested that there should be a failure of the mechanisms involved in active outward transport of sodium, such as the Na^+-K^+ ATPase system, with a resultant loss of potassium and gain in sodium by brain cells [117]. However such impressions are not supported by recent studies employing MRS to measure cerebral phosphate metabolites [28, 71].

Delayed Postanoxic Encephalopathy

A poorly understood but well reported subgroup of hypoxic brain damage is the entity of delayed postanoxic encephalopathy, or hypoxic-ischemic leukoencephalopathy. Delayed postanoxic encephalopathy has been known for over 60 years. The disorder can follow anoxia-hypoxia from any cause, but most cases are related to either carbon monoxide intoxication, strangulation, cardiopulmonary arrest, or various miscellaneous intoxications, with the vast majority of reported cases related to either carbon monoxide intoxication or cardiopulmonary arrest with resuscitation [35, 69, 70, 135]. Whatever the cause, patients are initially deeply comatose, often requiring artifical ventilation. Characteristically, they begin to regain consciousness within 1 to 3 days. As early as 2 days, or as late as several weeks, patients begin to relapse. The onset may be abrupt and heralded by disorientation, confusion, restlessness, apathy, or inappropriate behavior.

There may be cortical dysfunction, which may be multifocal in character, with dysphasias, agnosias, and apraxias. Motor control is impaired, with resultant rigidity or spasticity. Hypoxic-ischemic leukoencephalopathy is indeed a "metabolic encephalopathy," as the patients progress from an alert, lucid state to one of coma, paralysis, and dementia without a structural lesion of the brain. The exact pathologic-biochemical lesions whereby delayed hypoxic-ischemic leukoencephalopathy leads to permanent brain damage are not known. However, it is almost certainly secondary to a chain of events initiated by hypoxic-ischemic damage to the brain, leading to biochemical alterations in the brain that may eventually involve alterations of brain water and electrolytes. Often, cerebral demyelinating lesions develop in various parts of the brain, such as subcortical white matter, thalamus, pons, and basal ganglia. Such lesions are similar to those observed following other hypoxic states, such as cardiac arrest with survival or hyponatremic encephalopathy with respiratory arrest [8, 95].

Hypernatremia

There are a number of medical conditions that are commonly associated with hypernatremia, the etiologies of which are quite different in children and adults. In infants, gastroenteritis with diarrhea is the most common cause [43], while in elderly individuals, hypernatremia is often associated with elective surgery or infirmity, with a gradual excessive loss of free water [152]. Small children may also become hypernatremic after accidental administration of a high solute load, particularly accidental substitution of salt for sugar in preparation of formula [55] or improper dilution of concentrated formulas. Such situations are probably rare.

Generally, diabetes insipidus is associated with hypernatremia only under circumstances where the patient is unable to obtain water freely or when the lesion responsible for the diabetes insipidus also results in a decrease in thirst [106]. Severe hypernatremia has also been observed in patients inadvertently receiving intravenous hypertonic sodium chloride for therapeutic abortion [34] and may also occur in patients with metabolic acidosis who receive large quantities of intravenous sodium bicarbonate [110]. Another group of patients in whom there is a low index of suspicion for hypernatremia is the chronic alcholic with severe liver disease who presents with liver failure and hepatic encephalopathy. Such patients are often treated with oral lactulose as therapy for their hepatic encephalopathy. Hypernatremia as a result of osmotic diarrhea may complicate such therapy [89, 61]. The neurologic manifestations of hypernatremia are discussed in Chapter 5.

Phosphate Depletion

The clinical syndrome of phosphate depletion was orginally described in six patients who ingested magnesium–aluminum hydroxide gels for up to 130 days. The symptoms included weakness, bone pain, anorexia, and malaise and were rapidly reversed with phosphate repletion [103]. Similar clinical manifestations have been observed in patients with chronic renal failure receiving aluminum hydroxide and treated with hemodialysis [100].

A wide variety of clinical manifestations may accompany hypophosphatemia [92], and organ systems affected may include the neuromuscular, hematologic, hepatic, skeletal, muscular, pulmonary, cardiac, and central nervous systems. Most such patients also have multiple electrolyte and acid-base abnormalities involving, for example, sodium, magnesium, calcium, and potassium. The syndrome of phosphate depletion has been most commonly observed in alcoholic subjects and in those with chronic wasting medical conditions, such as malnutrition, hepatic cirrhosis, and renal insufficiency. The nervous system complications of phosphate depletion are discussed in Chapter 10.

Diabetic Comas

Coma as a complication of diabetes mellitus has been described for over 100 years [7]. Although most such patients have some depression of sensorium, such as impaired response to verbal or painful stimuli, many patients are alert and responsive and are therefore not "comatose."

Strictly speaking, diabetic "coma" implies depression of sensorium to at least a state of obtundation, which is defined as a state of dull indifference, where increased stimulation is required to evoke a response [33]. In clinical practice, most patients with hyperglycemia in excess of 450 mg/dl (25 mM) are said to have diabetic coma [10, 65]. If one excludes stroke, there are at least three syndromes of metabolic derangements associated with diabetes that can be classified as diabetic comas: These are diabetic ketoacidosis, nonketotic hyperosmolar coma with hyperglycemia (nonketotic coma), and hypoglycemia.

Hepatic Encephalopathy

Hepatic encephalopathy is a clinical syndrome characterized by abnormal mental status occurring in patients with severe hepatic insufficiency. It is a neuropsychiatric disorder associated with characteristic but nonspecific histologic lesions in the central nervous system [1, 94]. Cerebral edema is a common but not invariable finding in patients with acute fulminant hepatic failure [68, 161]. The clinical manifestations of hepatic coma are related at least in part both to the rapidity with which the hepatic failure develops and to the severity of liver failure. The causes are numerous and are reviewed in Chapter 9. With the advent of many new drugs that are hepatotoxic, a high consumption of alcohol in malnourished and homeless individuals, and an increased incidence of more virulent forms of hepatitis leading to liver failure, hepatic encephalopathy is a reasonably common disorder in most major metropolitan hospitals. Although the overall outlook for patients with hepatic encephalopathy is generally poor, the clinical manifestations of this disorder are often reversible. This is often achieved by such simple techniques as avoidance of alcohol (ethanol), a low-protein diet, and the appropriate use of lactulose and/or neomycin. Survival among patients with hepatic encephalopathy, although poor, is better than that for other forms of nontraumatic coma [98]. The neurologic manifestations of hepatic encephalopathy are discussed in Chapter 9.

Uremia

Technical improvements in dialytic therapy, better immunosuppression for renal transplantation, and improved medical management of end-stage renal disease have resulted in impressive modifications of both the duration and quality of life in patients with renal failure. However, patients who have renal failure continue to manifest a variety of neurologic disorders. Even after the institution of otherwise adequate maintenance dialysis therapy, patients may continue to manifest more subtle nervous system dysfunction, including impaired mentation, generalized weakness, and peripheral neuropathy. The central nervous system disorders of both untreated renal failure and that persisting despite dialysis are collectively referred to as uremic encephalopathy [62]. The dialytic treatment of end-stage renal disease has itself been associated with the emergence of two distinct disorders of the central nervous system: dialysis disequilibrium and dialysis dementia [9, 154]. The dialysis disequilibrium syndrome is a consequence of the initiation of dialysis therapy in some patients. Dialysis dementia is a progressive, generally fatal encephalopathy that can affect patients on chronic hemodialysis.

In addition to the neurologic diseases that are specifically related to uremia or dialysis, a number of other neurologic disorders occur with increased frequency in patients who have end-stage renal disease and are being treated with chronic hemodialysis. Subdural hematoma, electrolyte disorders, vitamin deficiencies, drug intoxications, hypertensive encephalopathy, and acute trace element intoxication are among the disorders that must be considered in any patient who has renal failure and presents with an altered mental status. The neurologic manifestations of renal insufficiency are discussed in Chapter 8.

REFERENCES

1. Adams, R. D., and Foley, J. M. The neurological disorders associated with liver disease. *Res. Publ. Assoc. Res. Nerv. Ment. Dis.* 32:198, 1953.

2. Alfrey, A. C., LeGrande, G. R., and Kaehny, W. D. The dialysis encephalopathy syndrome: Possible aluminum intoxication. *N. Engl. J. Med.* 294:184, 1976.
3. Alfrey, A. C., Mishell, J., Burks, S. R., et al. Syndrome of dyspraxia and multifocal seizures associated with chronic hemodialysis. *Trans. Am. Soc. Artif. Intern. Organs* 18:257, 1972.
4. Altmann, P., Al-Salihi, F., Butter, K., et al. Serum aluminum levels and erythrocyte dihydropteridine reductase activity in patients on hemodialysis. *N. Engl. J. Med.* 317:80, 1987.
5. Altmann, P., Dhanesha, U., Hamon, C., et al. Disturbance of cerebral function by aluminum in haemodialysis patients without overt signs of aluminum toxicity. *Lancet* 2:7, 1989.
6. Anderson, R. J. Asterixis as a manifestation of salicylate toxicity. *Ann. Intern. Med.* 95:188, 1981.
7. Arieff, A. I. Effects of Water, Acid Base, and Electrolyte Disorders on the Central Nervous System. In A. I. Arieff and R. A. DeFronzo (eds.), *Fluid, Electrolyte and Acid-Base Disorders.* New York: Churchill Livingstone, 1985. P. 969.
8. Arieff, A. I. Hyponatremia Associated with Permanent Brain Damage. In G. H. Stollerman, W. J. Harrington, J. T. LaMont, et al. (eds.), *Advances in Internal Medicine.* Chicago: Year Book, 1987. P. 325.
9. Arieff, A. I. Aluminum and the pathogenesis of dialysis dementia. *Environ. Geochem. Health* 12(1/2):89, 1990.
10. Arieff, A. I., and Carroll, H. J. Cerebral edema and depression of sensorium in nonketotic hyperosmolar coma. *Diabetes* 23(6):525, 1974.
11. Arieff, A. I., Cooper, J. D., Armstrong, D., et al. Dementia, renal failure and brain aluminium. *Ann. Intern. Med.* 90(5):741, 1979.
12. Arieff, A. I., and Graf, H. Pathophysiology of type A hypoxic lactic acidosis in dogs. *Am. J. Physiol.* 253(*Endocrinol. Metab.* 16):E271, 1987.
13. Arieff, A. I., and Guisado, R. Effects on the central nervous system of hypernatremic and hyponatremic states. *Kidney Int.* 10:104, 1976.
14. Arieff, A. I., Guisado, R., and Lazarowitz, V. C. Pathophysiology of Hyperosmolar States. In T. E. Andreoli, J. J. Grantham, and F. C. Rector, Jr. (eds.), *Disturbances in Body Fluid Osmolality.* Bethesda, MD: American Physiological Society, 1977. P. 227.
15. Arieff, A. I., Guisado, R., Massry, S. G., et al. Central nervous system pH in uremia and the effects of hemodialysis. *J. Clin. Invest.* 58:306, 1976.
16. Arieff, A. I., Kerian, A., Massary, S. G., et al. Intracellular pH of brain: Alterations in acute respiratory acidosis and alkalosis. *Am. J. Physiol.* 230(3):804, 1976.
17. Arieff, A. I., Kleeman, C. R., Kerian, A., et al. Cerebral edema in diabetic comas: II. Effects of hyperosmolality, hyperglycemia and insulin in diabetic rabbits. *J. Clin. Endocrinol. Metab.* 38(6):1057, 1974.
18. Arieff, A. I., Kleeman, C. R., Keushkerian, A., et al. Brain tissue osmolality: Method of determination and variations in hyper- and hypo-osmolar states. *J. Lab. Clin. Med.* 79(2):334, 1972.
19. Arieff, A. I., Kleeman, C. R., Keushkerian, A., et al. Studies on mechanisms of cerebral edema in diabetic comas: Effects of hyperglycemia and rapid lowering of plasma glucose in normal rabbits. *J. Clin. Invest.* 52(3):571, 1973.
20. Arieff, A. I., Llach, F., Massry, S. G., et al. Neurological manifestations and morbidity of hyponatremia: Correlation with brain water and electrolytes. *Medicine* (Baltimore) 55(2):121, 1976.
21. Arieff, A. I., and Massry, S. G. Calcium metabolism of brain in acute renal failure: Effects of uremia, hemodialysis, and parathyroid hormone. *J. Clin. Invest.* 53(2):387, 1974.
22. Arieff, A. I., and Massry, S. G. Dialysis Disequilibrium Syndrome. In S. G. Massry and A. L. Sellers (eds.), *Clinical Aspects of Uremia and Dialysis.* Springfield, IL: Thomas, 1976. P. 34.
23. Assal, J. P., Aoki, T. T., Manzano, F. M., et al. Metabolic effects of sodium bicarbonate in management of diabetic ketoacidosis. *Diabetes* 23:405, 1974.
24. Avison, M. J., Hetherington, H. P., and Shulman, R. G. Applications of NMR to studies of tissue metabolism. *Ann. Rev. Biophys. Biophys. Chem.* 15:377, 1986.
25. Ayus, J. C., Guntupalli, K., Guntupalli, J., et al. Effect of hyponatremia in hypoxic rats. *J. Am. Soc. Nephrol.* 1(4):317, 1990.
26. Bartko, D. Some Aspects of the Course of Acute Cerebral Hypoxia. In *Experimental Brain Hypoxia.* Baltimore, MD: University Park Press, 1971. P. 15
27. Baxter, C. F., Baldwin, R. A., Parsons, J. E., et al. Water homeostasis in CNS: Involvement of non-essential amino acids. *Proc. Am. Soc. Neurochem.* 19:80, 1988.
28. Behar, K. L., Den Hollander, J. A. D., Stromski, M. E., et al. High-resolution ^{1}H-nuclear magnetic resonance study of cerebral hypoxia in vivo. *Proc. Natl. Acad. Sci. U.S. A.* 80:4945, 1983.
29. Betz, A. L. Transport of ions across the blood-brain barrier. *Fed. Proc.* 45:2050, 1986.
30. Braakman, R., Avezaat, C. J. J., Maas, A. I. R., et al. Interobserver agreement in the assessment

of the motor response of the Glasgow "coma" scale. *Clin. Neurol. Neurosurg.* 80:100, 1977.
31. Bradbury, M. W. B. The structure and function of the blood-brain barrier. *Fed. Proc.* 43:186, 1984.
32. Brick, J. F., Gutrecht, J. A., and Ringel, R. A. Reflex epilepsy and nonketotic hyperglycemia in the elderly: A specific neuroendocrine syndrome. *Neurology* 39:394, 1989.
33. Brown H. W., and Plum, F. The neurologic basis of Cheyne-Stokes respiration. *Am. J. Med.* 30:849, 1961.
34. Cameron, J. M., and Dayan, A. D. Association of brain damage with therapeutic abortion induced by amniotic-fluid replacement: Report of two cases. *Br. Med. J.* 1:1010, 1966.
35. Candy, J. M., Klinowski, J., and Perry, R. H. Aluminosilicates and senile plaque formation in Alzheimer's disease. *Lancet* 1:354, 1986.
36. Caplan, L. R., and Scheiner, D. Dysconjugate gaze in hepatic coma. *Ann. Neurol.* 8:328, 1980.
37. Carroll, H. J., Gotterer, R., and Altshuler, B. Exchangeable sodium, body potassium, and body water in previously edematous cardiac patients: Evidence for osmotic inactivation of cation. *Circulation* 32:185, 1965.
38. Chan, P. H., and Fishman, R. A. Elevation of rat brain amino acids, ammonia and idiogenic osmoles induced by hyperosmolality. *Brain Res.* 161(2):293, 1979.
39. Cogan, M. G., Covey, C., Arieff, A. I., et al. Central nervous system manifestations of hyperparathyroidism. *Am. J. Med.* 65:963, 1978.
40. Conomy, J. P., and Swash, M. Reversible decerebrate and decorticate postures in hepatic coma. *N. Engl. J. Med.* 278:876, 1968.
41. Corbett, J. J., Jacobson, D. M., Thompson, H. S., et al. Downbeating nystagmus and other ocular motor defects caused by lithium toxicity. *Neurology* 39:481, 1989.
42. Cosgriff, T. M. Anisocoria in heroin withdrawal. *Arch. Neurol.* 29:200, 1973.
43. Covey, C. M., and Arieff, A. I. Disorders of Sodium and Water Metabolism and Their Effects on the Central Nervous System. In B. M. Brenner and J. H. Stein (eds.), *Sodium and Water Homeostasis: Contemporary Issues in Nephrology.* New York: Churchill Livingstone, 1978. P. 212.
44. Crapper, D. R., Krishnan, S. S., and Quittkat, S. Aluminum, neurofibrillary degeneration and Alzheimer's disease. *Brain* 99:67, 1976.
45. Davson, H. The Cerebrospinal Fluid. In H. Davson (ed.), *A Textbook of General Physiology* (4th ed.). Baltimore: Williams & Wilkins, 1970. P. 714.
46. Davson, H. The blood-brain barrier. *J. Physiol.* (Lond.) 255:1, 1976.
47. de Courten-Myers, G. M., Yamaguchi, S., Wagner, K. R., et al. Brain injury from marked hypoxia in cats. *Stroke* 16:1016, 1985.
48. Degos, J. D., Verroust, J., Bouchareine, A., et al. Asterixis in focal brain lesions. *Arch. Neurol.* 36:705, 1979.
49. Delabar, J. M., Goldgaber, D., Lamour, Y., et al. B amyloid gene duplication in Alzheimer's disease and karotypically normal Down syndrome. *Science* 235:1390, 1987.
50. Delaney, P., and Light, R. Gaze paresis in amitriptyline overdose. *Ann. Neurol.* 9:513, 1981.
51. Donat, J. R. Unilateral asterixis due to thalamic hemorrhage. *Neurology* (N. Y.) 30:83, 1980.
52. Douglas N. J. Control of ventilation during sleep. *Clin. Chest Med.* 6:563, 1985.
53. Duckrow, R. B., Beard, D. C., and Brennan, R. W. Regional cerebral blood flow decreases during hyperglycemia. *Ann. Neurol.* 17:267, 1985.
54. Farrar, G., Altmann, P., Welch, S., et al. Defective gallium-transferrin binding in Alzheimer disease and Down syndrome: Possible mechanism for accumulation of aluminum in brain. *Lancet* 335:747, 1990.
55. Finberg, L., and Harrison, H. E. Hypernatremia in infants: An evaluation of the clinical and biochemical findings accompanying this state. *Pediatrics* 16:1, 1955.
56. Finberg, L., Luttrell, C., and Redd, H. Pathogenesis of lesions in the nervous system in hypernatremic states: Experimental studies of gross anatomic changes and alterations of chemical composition of the tissues. *Pediatrics* 23:46, 1959.
57. Florkin, M., and Schoffeniels, E. Extra- and Intracellular Osmotic Regulations. In M. Florkin and E. Schoffeniels (eds.), *Molecular Approaches to Ecology.* New York: Academic, 1969. P. 112.
58. Florkin, M., and Schoffeniels, E. Isosmotic Intracellular Regulation. In M. Florkin and E. Schoffeniels (eds.), *Molecular Approaches to Ecology.* New York: Academic, 1969. P. 89.
59. Forster, R. P., and Goldstein, L. Intracellular osmoregulatory role of amino acids and urea in marine elasmobranchs. *Am. J. Physiol.* 230:925, 1976.
60. Francis, P.T., Palmer, A. M., Sims, N. R., et al. Neurochemical studies of early-onset Alzheimer's disease. *N. Engl. J. Med.* 313:7, 1985.
61. Fraser, C. L., and Arieff, A. I. Hepatic encephalopathy. *N. Engl. J. Med.* 313(14):865, 1985.
62. Fraser, C. L., and Arieff, A. I. Nervous system complications in uremia. *Ann. Intern. Med.* 109(2):143, 1988.
63. Fraser, C. L., and Arieff, A. I. Fatal central dia-

betes mellitus and insipidus resulting from untreated hyponatremia: A new syndrome. *Ann. Intern. Med.* 112(2):113, 1990.
64. Friedland, R. P., Budinger, T. F., Ganz, E., et al. Regional cerebral metabolic alterations in dementia of the Alzheimer type: Positron emission tomography with [18F] fluorodeoxyglucose. *J. Comput. Assist. Tomogr.* 7:590, 1983.
65. Fulop, M., Tannenbaum, H., and Dreyer, N. Ketotic hyperosmolar coma. *Lancet* 2:635, 1973.
66. Gajdusek, D. C. Hypothesis: Interference with axonal transport of neurofilament as a common pathogenetic mechanism in certain diseases of the central nervous system. *N. Engl. J. Med.* 312:714, 1985.
67. Garcia, J. H., Conger, K. A., Morawetz, R., et al. Postischemic Brain Edema: Quantitation and Evolution. In J. Cervós-Navarro and R. Ferszt (eds.), *Brain Edema: Pathology, Diagnosis, and Therapy. Advances in Neurology.* New York: Raven, 1980. P. 147.
68. Gazzard, B. G., Portmann, B., and Murray-Lyon, I. M. Causes of death in fulminant hepatic failure and relationship to quantitative histological assessment of parenchymal damage. *Q. J. Med.* 44:615, 1975.
69. Ginsberg, M. D. Delayed neurological deterioration following hypoxia. *Adv. Neurol.* 26:21, 1979.
70. Ginsberg, M. D., Hedley-Whyte, E. T., and Richardson, E. P., Jr. Hypoxic-ischemic leukoencephalopathy in man. *Arch. Neurol.* 33:5, 1976.
71. Gonzalez-Mendez, R., McNeill, A., Gregory, G. A., et al. Effects of hypoxic hypoxia on cerebral phosphate metabolites and pH in the anesthetized infant rabbit. *J. Cereb. Blood Flow Metab.* 5:512, 1985.
72. Granholm, L., and Siesjo, B. K. The effect of combined respiratory and nonrespiratory alkalosis on energy metabolites and acid-base parameters in the rat brain. *Acta Physiol. Scand.* 81:307, 1971.
73. Griggs, R. C., and Satran, R. Metabolic Encephalopathy. In R. N. Rosenberg (ed.), *Comprehensive Neurology.* New York: Raven, 1991. P. 525.
74. Grinstein, S., Cohen, S., Goetz, J. D., et al. Na^+/H^+ exchange in volume regulation and cytoplasmic pH homeostasis in lymphocytes. *Fed. Proc.* 44:2508, 1985.
75. Grinstein, S. A., Rothsteom, A., and Sarkadi, B., et al. Responses of lymphocytes to anisotonic media: Volume regulating behavior. *Am. J. Physiol.* 246(15):C204, 1984.
76. Hahn, L. J., Kloiber, R., Vimy, M. J., et al. Dental "silver" tooth fillings: A source of mercury exposure revealed by whole-body image scan and tissue analysis. *F.A.S.E.B. J.* 3:2641, 1989.
77. Hanly, P. J., Millar, T. W., Steljes, D. G., et al. The effect of oxygen on respiration and sleep in patients with congestive heart failure. *Ann. Intern. Med.* 111:777, 1989.
78. Hasan, D., Wijdicks, E. F. M., and Vermeulen, M. Hyponatremia is associated with cerebral ischemia in patients with aneurysmal subarachnoid hemorrhage. *Ann. Neurol.* 27:106, 1990.
79. Hawkins, R. Cerebral Energy Metabolism. In D. W. McCandless (ed.), *Cerebral Energy Metabolism and Metabolic Encephalopathy.* New York: Plenum, 1985. P. 3.
80. Hershey, C. O., Ricanati, E. S., Hershey. L. A., et al. Silicon as a potential uremic neurotoxin: Trace element analysis in patients with renal failure. *Neurology* 33:786, 1983.
81. Hitzig, B. M., Prichard, J. W., Kantor, H. L., et al. NMR spectroscopy as an investigavtive technique in physiology. *F.A.S.E.B. J.* 1:22, 1987.
82. Hornbein, T. F., Townes, B. D., Schoene, R. B., et al. The cost to the central nervous system of climbing to extremely high altitude. *N. Engl. J. Med.* 321(25):1714, 1989.
83. Indraprasit, S., Alexander, G.V., and Gonick, H. C. Tissue composition of major and trace elements in uremia and hypertension. *J. Chronic Dis.* 27:135, 1974.
84. Kalin, E. M., Tweed W. A., Lee, J., et al. Cerebrospinal fluid acid-base and electrolyte changes resulting from cerebral anoxia in man. *N. Engl. J. Med.* 292:1013, 1975.
85. Katzman, R. The prevalence of malignancy in Alzheimer's disease: A major killer. *Arch. Gen. Psychiatry* 40:140, 1976.
86. Katzman, R. Alzheimer's disease. *N. Engl. J. Med.* 314:964, 1986.
87. Katzman, R., and Pappius, H. M. Brain Ions. In R. Katzman and H. M. Pappius (eds.), *Brain Electrolytes and Fluid Metabolism.* Baltimore: Williams & Wilkins, 1973. P. 111.
88. Katzman, R., and Pappius, H. M. Fluid Compartments. In R. Katzman and H. M. Pappius (eds.), *Brain Electrolytes and Fluid Metabolism.* Baltimore: Williams & Wilkins, 1973. P. 33.
89. Kaupke, C., Sprague, T., and Gitnick, G. L. Hypernatremia after the administration of lactulose. *Ann. Intern. Med.* 86:745, 1977.
90. Klatzo, I. Neuropathological aspects of brain edema. *J. Neuropathol. Exper. Neurol.* 26:1, 1967.
91. Kleeman, C. R., Metabolic coma. *Kidney Int.* 36:1142, 1989.
92. Knochel, J. P. The pathophysiology and clinical characteristics of severe hypophosphatemia. *Arch. Intern. Med.* 137:203, 1977.
93. Kregenow, F.M. The response of duck erythrocytes to hypertonic media. *J. Gen. Physiol.* 58:396, 1971.
94. Krigman, M. R., and Bouldin, T. W. Acute He-

patic Encephalopathy. In S. S. Schochet (ed.), *Neuropathology. The Clinical Neurosciences,* Rosenberg, R. N. (series ed.). New York: Churchill Livingstone, 1983. P. 514.

95. Krigman, M. R., and Bouldin, T. W. Oxygen deficiency: Brain Hypoxia and Ischemia. In S. S. Schochet, Jr. (ed.), *Neuropathology. The Clinical Neurosciences,* Rosenberg, R. N. (series ed.). New York: Churchill Livingstone, 1983. P. 496.
96. Kwentus, J. A., Hart, R., Lingon, N., et al. Alzheimer's disease. *Am. J. Med.* 81:91, 1986.
97. Levin, E., Arieff, A. I., and Kleeman, C. R. Evidence of different compartments in the brain for extracellular markers. *Am. J. Physiol.* 221(5):1319, 1971.
98. Levy, D. E., Bates, D., Caronna, J. J., et al. Prognosis in nontraumatic coma. *Ann. Intern. Med.* 94(3):293, 1981.
99. Levy, D. E., Caronna, J. J., Singer, B. H., et al. Predicting outcome from hypoxic-ischemic coma. *J.A.M.A.* 253:1420, 1985.
100. Litchtman, M. A., Miller, D. R., and Freeman, R. B. Erythrocyte adenosine triphosphate depletion during hypophosphatemia in a uremic subject. *N. Engl. J. Med.* 280:240, 1969.
101. Lockwood, A. H. Acute and chronic hyperosmolality: Effects on cerebral amino acids and energy matabolism. *Arch. Neurol.* 32:62 1975.
102. Longo, D. L., and Witherspoon, J. M. Focal neurologic symptoms in hypercalcemia. *Neurology* 30:200, 1980.
103. Lotz, M., Zisman, E., and Bartter, F. C. Evidence for a phosphorus-depletion syndrome in man. *N. Engl. J. Med.* 278:409, 1968.
104. Maccario, M., Messis, C. P., Vastola, E. F. Focal seizures as a manifestation of hyperglycemia without ketosis. *Neurology* (Minneap.) 15:195, 1965.
105. MacDonald, T. L., Humphreys, W. G., and Martin, R. B. Promotion of tubulin assembly by aluminum ion in vitro. *Science* 236:813, 1987.
106. Maffly, R. H. Diabetes Insipidus: Diagnosis of Diabetes Insipidus. In T. E. Andreoli, J. J. Grantham, and F. C. Rector (eds.). *Disturbances in Body Fluid Osmolality.* Bethesda, MD: American Physiological Society, 1977. P. 289.
107. Mahoney, C. A., Arieff, A. I., Leach, W. J., et al. Central and peripheral nervous system effects of chronic renal failure. *Kidney Int.* 24(2):170, 1983.
108. Mahurkar, S. D., Dkar, S. K., Salta, R., et al. Dialysis dementia. *Lancet* 1:1412, 1973.
109. Marx, J. Alzheimer's pathology explored. *Science* 249:984, 1990.
110. Mattar, J. A., Weil, M. H., Shubin, H., et al. Cardiac arrest in the critically ill: II. Hyperosmolar states following cardiac arrest. *Am. J. Med.* 56:162, 1974.
111. Mayfrank, L., and Thoden, U. Downbeat nystagmus indicates cerebellar or brain-stem lesions in vitamin B_{12} deficiency. *J. Neurol.* 233:145, 1986.
112. McDermott, J. R., Smith, A. I., Iqbal, K., et al. Brain aluminum in aging and Alzheimer disease. *Neurology* 29:809, 1979.
113. McDowell, M. E., Wolf, A. V., and Steer, A. Osmotic volumes of distribution: Idiogenic changes in osmotic pressure associated with administration of hypertonic solutions. *Am. J. Physiol.* 180:545, 1955.
114. McLachlan, D. R. C., Lukiw, W. J., and Kruck, T. P. A. Aluminum, altered transcription, and the pathogenesis of Alzheimer's disease. *Environ. Geochem. Health* 12:103, 1990.
115. Melton, J. E., and Nattie, E. E. Brain and CSF water and ions during dilutional and isomotic hyponatremia in the rat. *Am. J. Physiol.* 244:R724, 1983.
116. Melton, J. E., Patlak, C. S., Pettigrew K. D., et al. Volume regulatory loss of Na, Cl, and K from rat brain during acute hyponatremia. *Am. J. Physiol.* 252(*Renal Fluid Electrolyte Physiol.* 21):F661, 1987.
117. Meyer, J. S., Gotoh, F., Ebihara, S., et al. Effects of anoxia on cerebral metabolism and electrolytes in man. *Neurology* 15:892, 1965.
118. Montgomery, P., and Pinner, C. A. Transient hypoglycemic hemiplegia. *Arch. Intern. Med.* 114:680, 1964.
119. Moonen, C. T. W., van Zijl, P. C. M., Frank, J. A., et al. Functional magnetic resonance imaging in medicine and physiology. *Science* 250:53, 1990.
120. Mori, H., Kondo, J., and Ihara, Y. Ubiquitin is a component of paired helical filaments in Alzheimer's disease. *Science* 235:1641, 1987.
121. Needleman, H. L., Gunnoe, C., Leviton, A., et al. Deficits in psychologic and classroom performance of children with elevated dentine lead levels. *N. Engl. J. Med.* 300:689, 1979.
122. Norris, J. W., and Pappius, H. M. Cerebral water and electrolytes: Effect of asphyxia, hypoxia, and hypercapnia. *Arch. Neurol.* 23:248, 1970.
123. Nunnelley, L. L., Smythe, W. R., Alfrey, A. C., et al. Uremic hyperstannum: Elevated tissue tin levels associated with uremia. *J. Lab. Clin. Med.* 91:72, 1978.
124. Oldendorf, W. H., and Davson, H. Brain extracellular space and the sink action of the CSF. *Arch. Neurol.* 17:196, 1967.
125. Palmer, A. M., and Gershon, S. Is the neuronal basis of Alzheimer's disease cholinergic or glutamatergic? *F.A.S.E.B. J.* 4:2745, 1990.

126. Parry, G. Osmotic adaption in fishes. *Biol. Rev.* 41:392, 1966.
127. Palvin, E. G., and Hornbein, T. F. Distribution of H^+ and HCO_3^- between CSF and blood during metabolic acidosis in dogs. *Am. J. Physiol.* 228:1134, 1975.
128. Pearce, B. R., Palmer, A. M., Bowen, D. M., et al. Neurotransmitter dysfunction and atrophy of the caudate nucleus in Alzheimer's disease. *Neurochem. Pathol.* 2:221, 1984.
129. Perl, D. P., and Brody, A. R. Alzheimer's disease: X-ray spectrometric evidence of aluminum accumulation in neurofibrillary tangle-bearing neurons. *Science* 208:297, 1980.
130. Perl, D. P., Gajdusek, D. C., Garruto, R. M., et al. Intraneuronal aluminum accumulation in amyotropic lateral sclerosis and parkinsonism dementia of Guam. *Science* 217:1053, 1982.
131. Perl, D. P., and Good, P. F. Uptake of aluminum into central nervous system along nasal-olfactory pathways. *Lancet* 329:1028, 1987.
132. Perl, D. P., and Good, P. F. Microprobe studies of aluminum accumulation in association with human central nervous system disease. *Environ. Geochem. Health* 12:97, 1990.
133. Plum, F., and Posner, J. The Pathological Physiological Physiology of Signs and Symptoms of Coma. In F. Plum and J. Posner (eds.), *The Diagnosis of Stupor and Coma.* Philadelphia: Davis, 1966. P. 25.
134. Plum, F., and Posner, J. B. *The Diagnosis of Stupor and Coma.* The Contemporary Neurology Series, edition 3. Philadelphia: Davis, 1980.
135. Plum, F., Posner, J. B., and Hain, R. F. Delayed neurological deterioration after anoxia. *Arch. Intern. Med.* 110:18, 1962.
136. Plum, F., and Price, R. W. Acid-base balance of cisternal and lumbar cerebrospinal fluid in hospital patients. *N. Engl. J. Med.* 289:1346, 1973.
137. Posner, J. B., and Plum, F. Spinal-fluid pH and neurologic symptoms in systemic acidosis. *N. Engl. J. Med.* 277:605, 1967.
138. Prichard, J. W., and Shulman, R. G. NMR spectroscopy of brain metabolism in vivo. *Ann. Rev. Neurosci.* 9:61, 1986.
139. Reuler, J. B., Girard, D. E., and Cooney, T. G. Wernicke's encephalopathy. *N. Engl. J. Med.* 312:1035, 1985.
140. Rifat, S. L., Eastwood, M. R., McLachlan, D. R. C., et al. Effect of exposure of miners to aluminum powder. *Lancet* 336:1162, 1990.
141. Risau, W. Differentiation of blood barrier endothelium. *N.I.P.S.* 4:151, 1989.
142. Roos, A. Intracellular pH and buffering power of rat brain. *Am. J. Physiol.* 221:176, 1971.
143. Ropper, A. H. Ocular dipping in anoxic coma. *Arch. Neurol.* 38:297, 1981.
144. Rossor, M. N., Iversen, L. L., Reynolds, G. P., et al. Neurochemical characteristics of early and late onset types of Alzheimer's disease. *Br. Med. J.* 288:961, 1984.
145. Schenk, N. K., Reisberg, B., and Ferris, S. H. An overview of current concepts of Alzheimer's disease. *Am. J. Psychiatry.* 139:165, 1982.
146. Schmidt-Nielsen, B. Comparative physiology of cellular ion and volume regulation. *J. Exp. Zool.* 194:207, 1975.
147. Seshia, S. S., Seshia, M. M. K. and Sachdeva, R. K. Coma in childhood. *Dev. Med. Child Neurol.* 19:614, 1977.
148. Simmons, M. A., Adcock, E. W., Bard, H., et al. Hypernatremia and intracranial hemorrhage in neonates. *N. Engl. J. Med.* 291:6, 1974.
149. Simon, R. P. Forced downard ocular deviation: Occurrence during oculovestibular testing in sedative drug-induced coma. *Arch. Neurol.* 35:456, 1978.
150. Sims, N. R., Bowen, D. M., Neary, D., et al. Metabolic processes in Alzheimer's disease: Adenine nucelotide content and production of $^{14}CO_2$ from [U-^{14}C]glucose in vitro in human neocortex *J. Neurochem.* 41:1329, 1983.
151. Smythe, W. R., Alfrey, A. C., Craswell, P. W., et al. Trace element abnormalities in chronic uremia. *Ann. Intern. Med.* 96:302, 1982.
152. Snyder, N. A., Feigal, D. W., and Arieff, A. I. Hypernatremia in elderly patients: A heterogeneous, morbid, and iatrogenic entity. *Ann. Intern. Med.* 107(3):309, 1987.
153. Tarsy, D., Lieberman, B., Chirico-Post, J., et al. Unilateral asterixis associated with a mesencephalic syndrome. *Arch. Neurol.* 34:446, 1977.
154. Teschan, P. E., and Arieff, A. I. Uremic and Dialysis Encephalopathies. In D. W. McCandless (ed.), *Cerebral Energy Metabolism and Metabolic Encephalopathy.* New York: Plenum, 1985. P. 263.
155. Thompson, H. S. Symposium: Pupil in clinical diagnosis. *Trans. Am. Acad. Ophthalmol. Otolaryngol.* 83:847, 1977.
156. Thurston, J. H., and Hauhart, R. E. Brain amino acids decrease in chronic hyponatremia and rapid correction causes brain dehydration: Possible clinical significance. *Life Sci.* 40(26):2539, 1987.
157. Thurston, J. H., Hauhart, R. E., and Schulz, D. W. Effect of chronic hypernatremic dehydration and rapid rehydration on brain carbohydrate, energy, and amino acid metabolism in weanling mice. *J. Neurochem.* 40:240, 1983.
158. Trauner, D. A., and Huttenlocher, P. R. Short chain fatty acid-induced central hyperventilation in rabbits. *Neurology* (Minneap.) 28:940, 1978.

159. Vesterhauge, S., and Peitersen, E. Effects of some drugs on the caloric induced nystagmus. *Adv. Otorhinolaryngol.* 25:173, 1979.
160. Walker, G. L., Williamson, P. M., Ravich, R. B., et al. Hypercalcaemia associated with cerebral vasospasm causing infarction. *J. Neurol. Neurosurg. Psychiatry* 43:464, 1980.
161. Ware, A. J., D'Agostino, A. N., and Combes, B. Cerebral edema: A major complication of massive hepatic necrosis. *Gastroenterology* 61(6):877, 1971.
162. Wasterlain, C. G., and Posner, J. B. Cerebral edema in water intoxication:I. Clinical and chemical observations. *Arch. Neurol.* 19:71, 1968.
163. Webster, J. D., Parker, T. F., Alfrey, A. C., et al. Acute nickel intoxication by dialysis. *Ann. Intern. Med.* 92:631, 1980.
164. Weiss, B. The behavioral toxicology of metals. *Fed. Proc.* 37:22, 1978.
165. Wisniewski, H. M., Moretz, R. C., Sturman, J. A., et al. Aluminum neurotoxicity in mammals. *Environ. Geochem. Health* 12:115, 1990.
166. Wolf, P. Periodic synchronous and sterotyped myoclonus with postanoxic coma. *J. Neurol.* 215:39, 1977.
167. Yancy, P. H., Clark, M. E., Hand, S. C., et al. Living with water stress: Evolution of osmolyte systems. *Science* 217:1214, 1982.
168. Yanker, B. A., Dawes, L. R., Fisher, S., et al. Neurotoxicity of a fragment of the amyloid precursor associated with Alzheimer's disease. *Science* 245:417, 1989.
169. Yarnell, P. R., and Caplan, L. R. Basilar artery narrowing and hyperparathyroidism: Illustrative case. *Stroke* 17:1022, 1986.

2 Prognosis of Metabolic Coma

David E. Levy

The brain depends on a stable internal environment for optimal function. To some extent, the other systems in the body serve the brain: They provide nutrients to the brain, remove products of metabolism from the brain, and protect the brain from external perturbations. Moreover, a blood-brain barrier, which is in fact multiple physical and chemical barriers, further protects the brain from variations in the blood-borne milieu. Whenever these external variables change to levels that cannot be controlled by the barrier or whenever the barrier itself is damaged, the brain fails to function properly; at the extreme, delirium, stupor, or unconsciousness ensues.

In general, restoration of the systemic metabolic imbalance also restores brain function. In some instances, however, brain damage and permanent disability result. The prognosis from metabolic coma is not therefore as straightforward as one might initially believe, since it depends both on the underlying condition and on the possibly permanent effect of the metabolic derangement on the brain.

This chapter deals with unconsciousness caused by metabolic disturbances and specifically with prognosis and factors influencing prognosis. In general, mechanisms of dysfunction or damage are discussed in other chapters. This chapter covers only those abnormalities that can be considered diffuse metabolic insults to the brain and not focal insults that may involve similar mechanisms, such as ischemic stroke, or nonmetabolic insults, such as trauma.

INTERFERENCE WITH THE SUPPLY OF BRAIN NUTRIENTS

The first group of metabolic disturbances to be considered are noteworthy not only because they cause brain dysfunction but also because they, more than abnormalities to be considered subsequently, can also permanently damage the brain. These disturbances interfere with the supply of oxygen or glucose to the brain.

Ischemia

The paradigm of a diffuse, ischemic brain insult is that caused by cardiac arrest. Neurologic damage after cardiac arrest is probably the most exhaustively studied of the metabolic disturbances to be considered in this chapter. Most reports have focused on clinical variables found to be associated with prognosis, but some have also concentrated on the electroencephalogram (EEG), on various evoked electrical responses, and even on positron emission tomographic (PET) studies of brain metabolism.

In general, the fate most potential patients wish to avoid [3] is that of irreversible unconsciousness (the vegetative state [33]). Karen Quinlan, Nancy Jobes, and other well-publicized cases of unconscious survival lasting many years have in part contributed to this general public awareness. The world's record for such survival is held by a Miami woman who died 37 years after initially losing consciousness. Several groups have reported on the long-term fate of vegetative patients. In Japan, a longitudinal study of 110 vegetative patients [28,29] (most secondary to trauma but some secondary to vascular disease) indicated that the mean survival was 38 months. Only 3 of 110 initially vegetative patients regained any communicative ability, and only one of these three regained any degree of independence in daily life; both of the others remained confined to wheelchairs, and one of these two spoke only rarely. Even this degree of "recovery" was not predicted on the basis of any earlier clinical observations. A clinical-pathologic study of 10 vegetative patients in the United States [16] indicated that a typical pathologic pattern of predominantly cortical neuronal loss was seen, even in patients who at times appeared to track movement with their eyes or had desultory nystagmus to icewater caloric stimulation.

Less well known are the consequences of retained consciousness but markedly impaired communication and self-help functions, the locked-in syndrome [49]. Haig and associates [27] recently followed 27 patients locked-in for at least 1 year and found that most (24) were still alive at the last evaluation, that a few gained additional communication skills, but that none achieved recovery of motor control sufficient "to move an extremity against gravity." In other words, all of them would be classified as severely disabled, depending on others for virtually all aspects of daily care. The longest survival in a locked-in state among these patients was over 12 years, showing as with vegetative patients the potential for prolonged survival with severe brain damage.

Clinical Variables

Coma caused by cardiac arrest carries a grave prognosis in all reported studies. In one [38], persistence of coma for at least 6 hours meant that only 10 percent of patients would survive at least 1 year, and only 13 percent at some point within that year would regain the ability to live independently. Another study [9] described 284 patients "successfully" resuscitated from cardiac arrest, 19 of whom were brain dead and 114 of whom were comatose. Grouping the brain dead and comatose patients together, only 15 (12%) were discharged from the hospital without a neurologic deficit, and another 10 (8%) were discharged with a persistent deficit. Discharge without a neurologic deficit was less likely the longer coma persisted, and the study concluded that "full recovery from coma of more than three days' duration [was] exceptional" [9]. Similar experiences have been reported from other centers [38]: Only 6 percent of 106 patients still comatose after 1 day regained independent function, and only 4 percent of 57 patients comatose after 3 days made a similar recovery.

Individual clinical signs can be used, however, to assist in making predictions about outcome in specific patients. Analysis of data in Figure 2-1 shows that verbal responses, eye opening, the pupillary light reflex, corneal reflex, spontaneous eye movements, oculocephalic responses, oculovestibular responses, and motor responses are all indicators of likely recovery [38]. For example, no patient lacking pupillary light reflexes at the initial evaluation ever regained the ability to live independently; only 3 of 52 even regained consciousness, and these 3 were left severely disabled. Similarly the absence of pupillary light reflexes or corneal reflexes after 1 day identified overlapping groups of patients, none of whom regained independence. After 3 days, the persistent absence of motor responses or even the presence of extensor (decerebrate) or flexor (decorticate) posturing was not associated with recovery to an independent existence. This observation contrasts with an earlier report [65] that any nonpurposeful movement even 1 hour after resuscitation was incompatible with nondisabled survival.

Oculovestibular (caloric) responses were specifically examined [45] in patients comatose from a variety of causes, including hypoxia-ischemia (mostly cardiac arrest) in 29; only 8 percent of patients with absent oculovestibular responses recovered fully or with minimal disability. On the other hand, neither age, sex, location at the time of coma onset, cause of coma, nor the presence of paroxysmal activity was associated in that study with recovery. Another group [57] similarly reported a lack of correlation between paroxysmal activity and survival, although there was a nonsignificant trend linking myoclonus to reduced chances of survival.

Multiple clinical signs are even more powerful in assessing the chances of recovery from coma caused by cardiac arrest. In one study [17], the absence of pupillary light reactions, oculocephalic reflexes, and purposeful motor responses to pain each reduced chances of recovery. Another group [56] noted that increased numbers of abnormal brain stem reflexes reduced chances for survival. Algorithms have been developed [38] in the form of decision trees that utilized multiple clinical signs to assign patients to relatively poor or good prognosis groups (Figs. 2-2 and 2-3). Thus, no patient in the poorest prognosis group at the initial evaluation ever regained independent function, and only one of the poor prognosis patients at 1 day regained independence in daily life. On the other hand, 41 percent of patients in the best prognosis group at the initial evaluation regained independent function, a level of recovery achieved by 63 percent of those in the best prognosis group at 1 day, 77 percent of those at 3 days, 72 percent of those at 1 week, and 81 percent of those at 2 weeks.

Another way of combining clinical variables is the Glasgow Coma Score [62], which has been considered [47] to be a predictor of recovery from out-of-hospital cardiac arrest; this score is the arithmetic sum of three subscores reflecting eye opening, verbal responses, and motor responses. Seventy-three patients had scores either at or below 4 at 2 days or at or below 8 at 6 days, and 71 of them were ultimately considered failures (either dying or being left vegetative). Sixty patients had scores either at or above 10 at 2 days or above 8 at 6 days, and 46 of them were ultimately considered successes (although some were left severely disabled).

Various laboratory variables have been reported to correlate with recovery from cardiac arrest, the most powerful being the admission blood glucose [41]. Among 224 patients with blood glucose values at admission for cardiac arrest, the mean value in patients who awakened was 249 mg/dl, whereas it was significantly higher at 332 mg/dl in patients who never awakened. Results of hematocrit and arterial blood gas determinations were not associated with recovery from coma caused by cardiac arrest.

Electrophysiologic Correlates with Outcome

Other groups have concentrated more heavily on electrophysiologic monitors of potential recovery. Hockaday and co-workers [30] found no survivors among 14 post-arrest patients with a flat or nearly flat EEG record and only 1 survivor among 11 with delta intermixed with isoelectric periods or an isoelectric recording. They also noted that all patients with a deteriorating EEG died. Jørgensen and Malchow-Møller [34] reported more fully on the temporal evolution of EEG changes, noting that failure of intermittent electrocortical activity to return within 200 minutes or of continuous electrocortical activity to return within 10.5 hours was incompatible with return of consciousness.

In recent years, several studies dealing with evoked responses have appeared. The major point made in initial studies of brain stem auditory evoked responses (BAERs) [58] was that

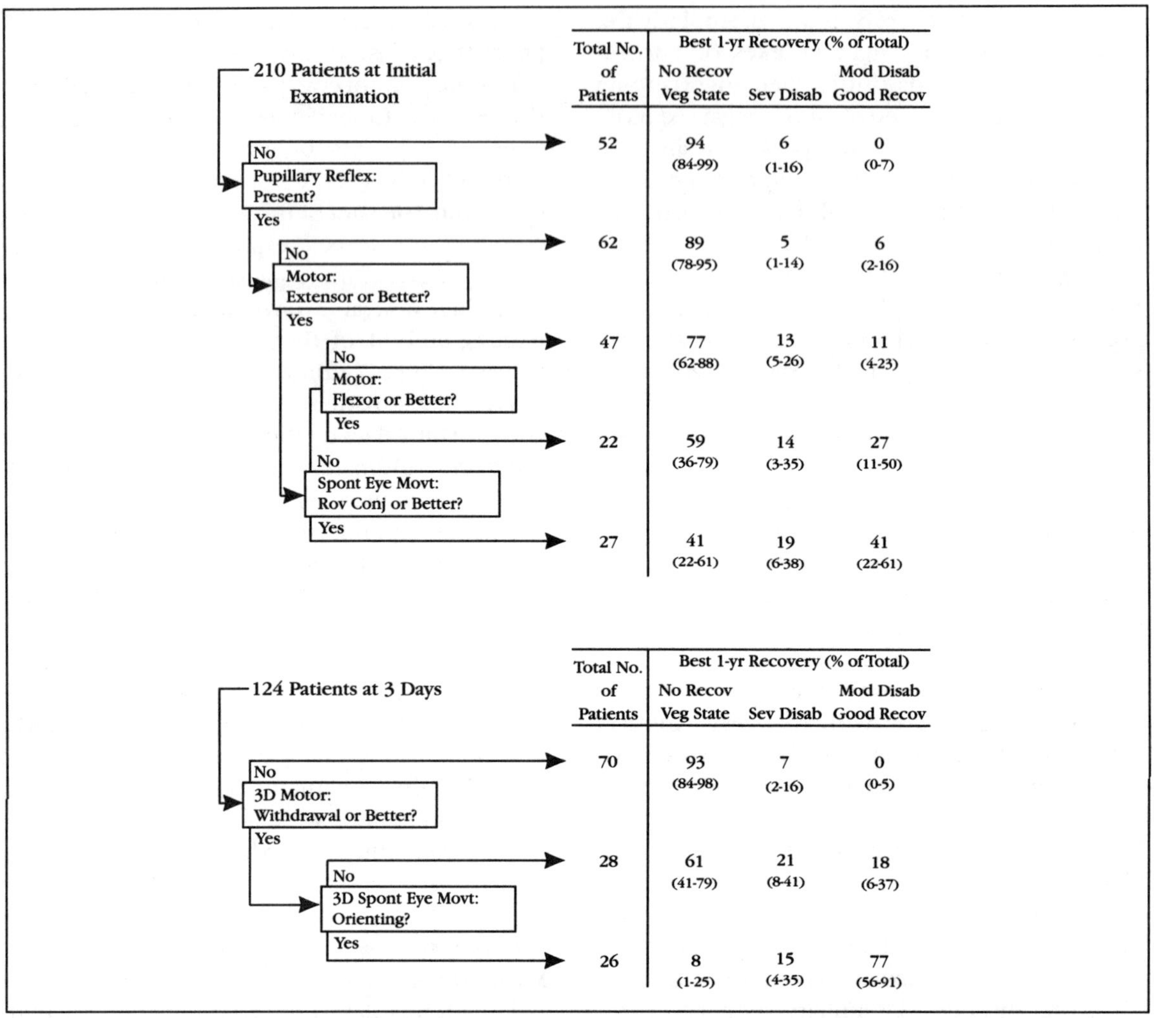

Fig. 2-1. Rules based on neurologic examination that classify patients in hypoxic-ischemic coma in accordance with their best functional state within first year. Figures in parentheses represent the 95% confidence intervals for percentages given immediately above. Abbreviations used in describing outcomes follow: recov indicates recovery; veg, vegetative; disab, disability; sev, severe; and mod, moderate. The following abbreviations are used in describing neurologic signs: spont eye movt indicates spontaneous eye movements; and rov conj, roving conjugate. Initial examination (*top left*) was obtained within 6 hours of onset of coma in 55% of patients and within 12 hours in 84%. Modifiers INIT, 1D, 3D, 1W, and 2W refer to initial, 0- to 1-day, 2- to 3-day, 4- to 7-day, and 8- to 14-day examinations, respectively. If no data are available, response to relevant question is considered to be "no." Where changes in clinical signs are utilized (*top right and bottom*), difference is between best response of previous time interval and best response of current interval. Physicians applying these rules must exercise caution when residual anesthetics or depressant drugs (including anticonvulsants) are present, should wait until the end of each time interval to make certain that the best clinical response has been observed, and should not use any rules that require responses that are unavailable for a specific patient. (Modified from D. E. Levy et al. [38].)

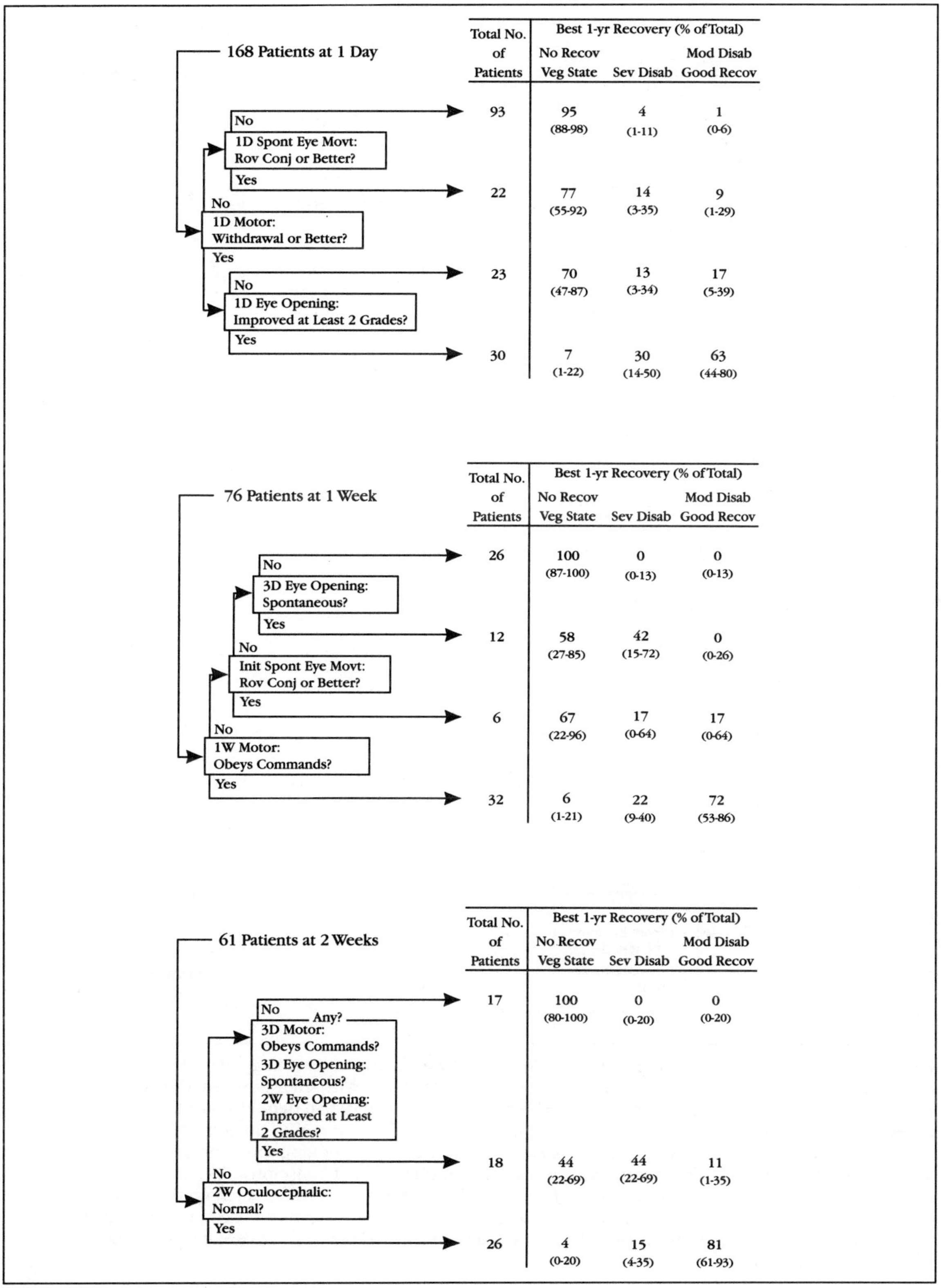

Fig. 2-1. (continued)

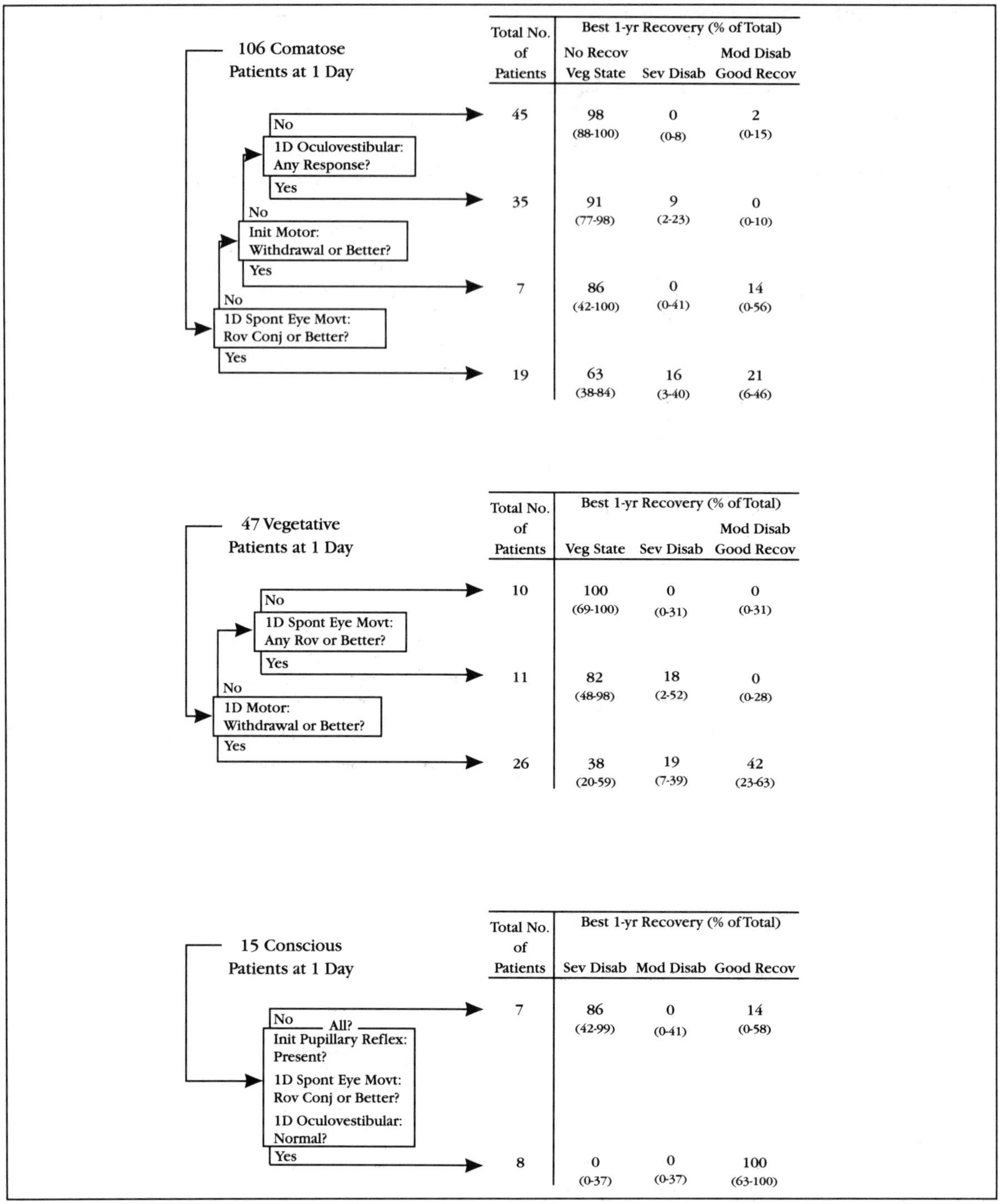

Fig. 2-2. Rules based on neurologic examination that classify patients surviving 1 day after hypoxic-ischemic coma with different levels of consciousness in accordance with their best functional state within first year. Abbreviations are as described for Figure 2-1. Operational definitions of levels of consciousness follow: coma (*top left*)—no eye opening regardless of stimulus, no comprehensible words, and commands not obeyed; vegetative state (*top right*)—eye opening spontaneously, to noise, or to pain, but no comprehensible words, and commands not obeyed; and consciousness (*bottom*)—comprehensible words or commands obeyed. These definitions, which were adopted on detailed examination of vegetative patients, were considered an improvement over those used at time study was begun and in previous publications because they distinguish coma from vegetative state. (From D. E. Levy et al. [38].)

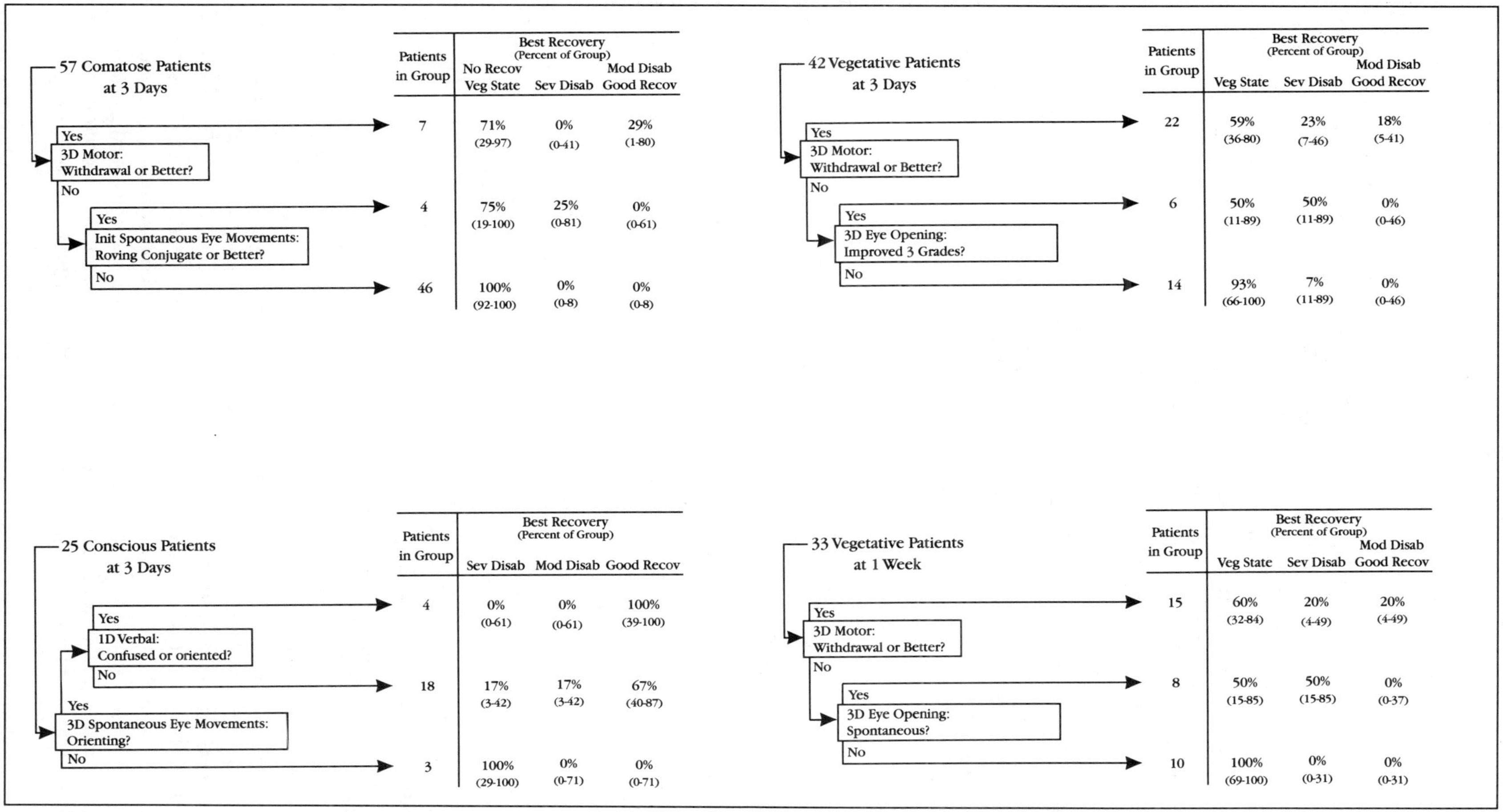

Fig. 2-3. These four prediction trees supplement those in Figure 2-2, providing breakdown by level of consciousness for patients surviving 3 days and for vegetative patients at 1 week. Other subgroups at 1 and 2 weeks are either too small or too homogeneous (with respect to outcome) for further analysis.

they were insensitive to depressant drugs and other metabolic causes of coma and might therefore be prognostically useful in coma caused by these conditions. Most studies attempting to relate evoked responses to prognosis from coma have concentrated on traumatic coma and are thus not germane to the present discussion. Rosenberg, Wogensen, and Starr [53], however, studied 25 patients in coma, of whom 13 had suffered hypoxia-ischemia. Although the evoked responses did not correlate with quality of survival, survival itself was related to simultaneous preservation of long- and middle-latency and brain stem evoked responses. The authors stress the importance of middle- and long-latency responses, noting only 1 survivor among the 8 patients with preserved brain stem evoked responses but neither of the other two evoked responses. By contrast, 6 of 9 patients with preservation of all three responses survived: Even for hypoxic-ischemic patients, there were no survivors among 5 patients with only brain stem responses but 3 survivors among 4 with preservation of all three. Kaga and associates [35] presented complementary data, showing for 54 comatose patients (7 hypoxic-ischemic) survival in 4 of 4 patients with all three responses but in only 10 of 17 patients with preserved brain stem responses alone.

Somatosensory evoked potentials (SSEPs) may more closely correlate with outcome from coma caused by cardiac arrest. Brunko and Zegers de Beyl [11] studied 50 adults in coma for at least 4 hours after cardiac arrest. Thirty of these patients lacked any cortical SSEPs, although most retained far-field, subcortical P14 potentials, and none of these 30 regained consciousness. By contrast, N20-P27 cortical SSEPs were seen in 10 patients and isolated N20 cortical SSEPs in another 10; 5 of these 20 patients regained consciousness, although one was left severely disabled. Ganes and Lundar [22] similarly performed EEG and SSEP determinations on 76 patients described as deeply comatose for various reasons, 16 of them because of cardiac arrest. The authors note that concern about head/neck movement because of trauma and concurrent medications interfered with the clinical examination in many of these patients. Thirty-seven had electrocerebral silence on the first EEG; none of these had SSEPs, and 33 of 33 patients who underwent cerebral angiography had full arrest of the cerebral circulation. Thirty-two patients had spontaneous EEG activity, and 12 of them had unilaterally or bilaterally maintained SSEPs. The only 2 patients in the entire group who survived were in the subgroup with some preservation of the SSEPs. Unfortunately, the quality of this survival is not indicated in the paper.

Metabolic Studies

The cerebral metabolic rate for glucose has recently been measured in seven vegetative patients [39], six of whom were unconscious as a result of diffuse hypoxia-ischemia, and in three locked-in patients. In the vegetative patients, the metabolic rate was depressed to approximately 40 percent of normal throughout all cortical gray structures (Fig. 2-4), a level seen only in very deep, surgical anesthesia and one also consistent with destruction of all neurons within the structures being measured. Although this investigation studied too few patients to be useful prognostically, the results suggest the extensive degree of brain destruction or dysfunction associated with chronic unconsciousness.

Hypoxia

Uncomplicated hypoxic insults to the brain are rare; usually the heart is also affected, and ischemia is thus added, resulting in a combined hypoxic-ischemic insult similar to that just described for cardiac arrest. Anesthesia misadventures, nitrogen inhalation, and carbon monoxide poisoning may sometimes, however, produce relatively pure hypoxic insults. The pathophysiology of underlying brain damage in this condition may differ in some respects from that of ischemia, representing primarily a leukoencephalopathy.

The more practical consideration of primarily hypoxic coma relates to the possible development of delayed postanoxic encephalopathy. In this condition, patients who initially appear to recover subsequently develop severe neurologic abnormalities, even leading to recurrent coma and death. The pathologic substrate is subcortical demyelination, consistent with the leu-

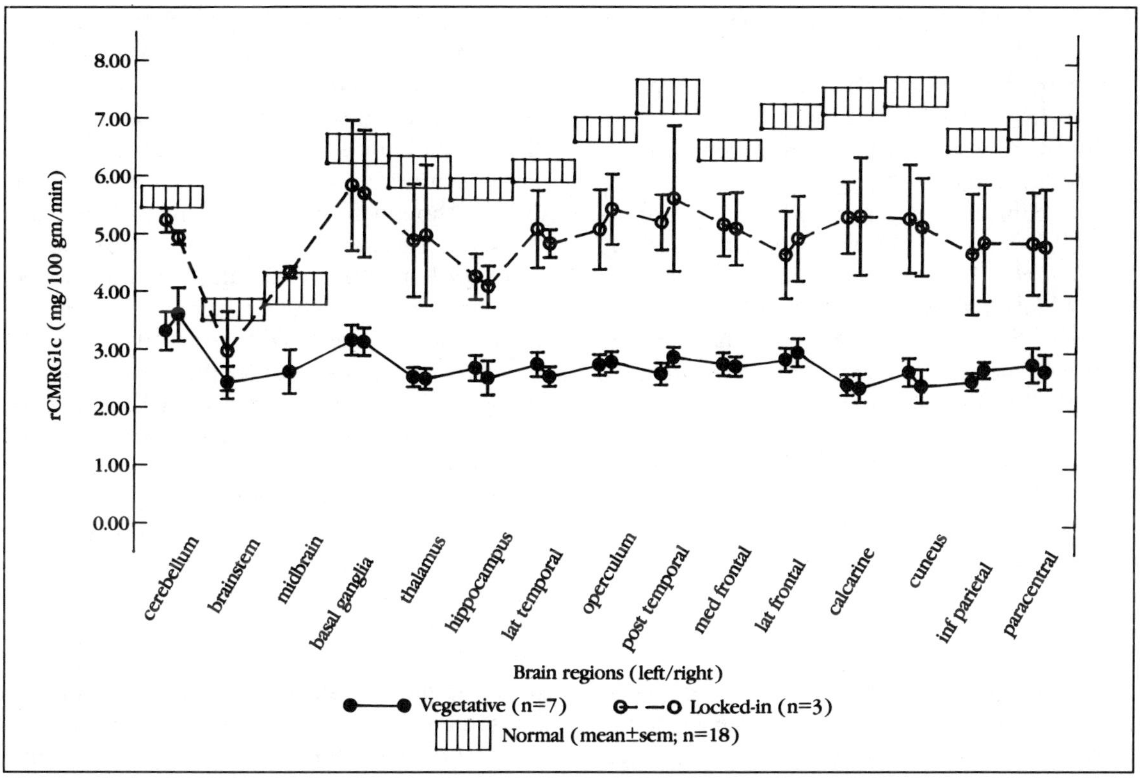

Fig. 2-4. Cerebral metabolic rate for glucose in vegetative and locked-in patients.

koencephalopathy produced experimentally with carbon monoxide [25]. An early clinical report [50] described patients exposed to carbon monoxide, pure anoxia, and anesthesia. Although initially comatose, the patients in this series typically regained consciousness within 1 day and then remained normal for a few days to several weeks. They then developed emotional and intellectual deterioration, followed by motor changes and, in some patients, recurrent coma leading to death. Subsequent reports have described this condition after other similar insults, but the frequency is not high. Other than recommending against overrapid mobilization of patients who appear initially to recover well from anoxic coma, no specific preventive or therapeutic measures have been advocated.

Carbon Monoxide Poisoning

Whether accidental or intentional, carbon monoxide poisoning is frequently fatal. Survivors can show extended periods of impaired consciousness, and other focal neurologic findings are present as well [23]. Smith and Brandon [55] obtained 3-year follow-up information on 46 patients after attempted suicide with carbon monoxide and another 28 accidentally exposed to the gas. Coma was relatively infrequent in both groups: 4 percent in the attempted suicide patients and 14 percent in the accidentally exposed. On the other hand, some impairment of consciousness was common: 80 percent of the attempted suicide group and 75 percent of the accidentally exposed. At 3 years, gross neuropsychiatric sequelae (irritability, aggressiveness, impulsiveness, violence, and memory loss) were found in approximately 10 percent of both groups of patients. The presence of these sequelae correlated with initial impairment of consciousness but not with reflex changes or with prolonged delirium. Despite the possibility of prolonged disability, anecdotal evidence [54] suggests that recovery from even prolonged unconsciousness caused by carbon monoxide poisoning might be better than from other types of serious hypoxic-ischemic injury.

Countries where coal is used extensively for indoor heating provide much of the recent, extensive clinical experience with carbon monoxide poisoning. Choi [15] reported a series of 549 inpatients with carbon monoxide poisoning in Korea, noting that 36 (6.6%) suffered delayed sequelae after a "clear" period ranging from 2 to 40 days (mean, 22 days). Symptoms included mental deterioration, urinary and/or fecal incontinence, gait disturbance, and, less frequently, motor and speech difficulties. Of the 36 patients with delayed sequelae, 27 (75%) recovered (5 with mild memory disturbances), but 6 (17%) exhibited no improvement.

Hypoglycemia

Just as oxygen deprivation can cause coma, so too can inadequate glucose delivery. Mechanisms of damage have recently been suggested, however, to differ from those operative in hypoxia-ischemia [8]. For example, in ischemia, cellular redox systems are reduced, whereas they are oxidized in hypoglycemia; in ischemia, brain acidosis is generally believed to develop, whereas alkalosis is more apparent in hypoglycemia. Energy levels do not fall as steeply in hypoglycemia as they do in hypoxia-ischemia: ATP levels are still over one-third normal when the EEG becomes isoelectric. Although the pathology of hypoglycemia was initially believed to be similar to that of hypoxia [10], more recent studies suggest that it too differs, at least topographically. In the rat, damage is related to cerebrospinal fluid (CSF) spaces [8], suggesting that a toxic substance in the CSF may be involved in the production of damage.

Clinical recognition of hypoglycemic coma is aided by its frequent occurrence in diabetics taking insulin and by the presence of prominent autonomic findings like sweating, pallor, and palpitations. Hypoglycemia can occur, however, in patients with liver disease and various systemic tumors. Seizures often herald the onset of hypoglycemic encephalopathy.

The precise correlation of clinical manifestations to blood glucose levels has been poorly established, but Pramming and colleagues [52] recently published a correlation of results on neuropsychological tests with blood sugars in diabetic patients given insulin under controlled circumstances and sham-treated diabetic controls. Although scores fell in many when the blood glucose was lowered from approximately 110 mg/dl to 50 mg/dl, there was a marked decline in all but 1 of 16 subjects when the glucose was further lowered to 30 mg/dl. No patient was unconscious at the lower level of hypoglycemia. In a subsequent investigation relating EEG to glucose, the same group [51] reported a decrease in alpha activity when the glucose fell to approximately 35 mg/dl. No patient showed any EEG changes at blood glucose levels above 55 mg/dl.

Although some well-publicized cases of prolonged unconsciousness resulting from hypoglycemia have appeared in the lay press, there are no large published series of these patients. Consequently, factors influencing prognosis cannot be cited. One would expect clinical and possibly also electrophysiologic predictors to be similar for hypoglycemic and hypoxic-ischemic coma, but that speculation cannot be sustantiated at this time.

OSMOLAR ABNORMALITIES

Changes in serum osmolality are relatively common, and they typically produce neurologic abnormalities. Most of these clinical alterations are nonspecific and mild (e.g., weakness, fatigue, nausea, and lethargy), but they can progress to marked stupor and coma as well. Associated neurologic complaints are often the first changes noticed by the patient, so that the clinician must be attuned to the possibility of an underlying osmolar abnormality. The most frequent osmolar abnormalities are hyperglycemia, either with or without ketosis, hypernatremia, and hyponatremia. Exogenous agents such as mannitol and glycerol can also produce hyperosmolality, but they will not be considered in this section. Although the following can be considered osmolar abnormalities, the pathophysiology of these conditions could involve other mechanisms.

Hyperglycemia

There are two forms of hyperglycemia, and both produce coma. They are diabetic ketoacidosis and nonketotic hyperosmolar hyperglycemia. Clinically the two forms can frequently be distinguished, since both seizures and focal neurologic abnormalities are more common in nonketotic hyperosmolar hyperglycemia than they are in diabetic ketoacidosis; moreover, diabetes is usually more apparent in the latter than in the former patients. As with most of the other conditions described in this chapter, correction of the underlying abnormality usually results in normalization of the neurologic state.

Diabetic Ketoacidosis

With inadequate endogenous and exogenous insulin, diabetic patients are unable to augment glucose entry from the extracellular to intracellular space, and the liver produces additional glucose as well. The result can be extreme hyperglycemia, with hyperosmolality and intracellular dehydration as secondary consequences. Inadequate insulin also results in increased lipolysis, and the resulting increased concentrations of free fatty acids are, in turn, metabolized to keto acids, which circulate in the blood and produce systemic acidosis.

The clinical manifestations are probably related to dehydration and acidosis and include nausea, vomiting, and labored, rapid respirations. Neurologically, patients become progressively stuporous and ultimately comatose. The precise mechanism of neurologic deterioration is, however, not known. Suggestions [26] have included neurologic depression caused by ketosis, vascular changes due to blood hyperviscosity, brain edema of unknown cause, and local biochemical abnormalities including impairment of phosphofructokinase and pyruvate oxidation and citrate accumulation. Fulop and co-workers [21] demonstrated in 70 patients a correlation of sensorium with calculated serum osmolality but not with acidosis or glucose level. As with many conditions, the cause may turn out to be multifactorial.

Coma may not always resolve as the hyperglycemic ketoacidosis is treated with insulin. Delays of hours to days have been noted, and some patients deteriorate clinically during insulin treatment. Although some have suggested that this might be caused by a lag in the correction of CSF glucose or by worsening brain acidosis, studies have failed to support this view, and the precise cause for delayed improvement is not established [26]. The long-term prognosis of coma caused by diabetic ketoacidosis is usually excellent, limited only by the underlying diabetic condition and, in some patients, associated intracranial vascular disease.

Nonketotic Hyperosmolar Hyperglycemia

Nonketotic hyperosmolar hyperglycemia develops more slowly than diabetic ketoacidosis and is often found in patients without overt diabetes. It is usually associated with even more extreme hyperglycemia than diabetic ketoacidosis, but ketosis and acidosis are not major components of the condition. Consequently, the clinical manifestations are related more directly to dehydration, and hypernatremia is often seen in conjunction with this dehydrated state.

Focal neurologic abnormalities, even including focal seizures, are common in nonketotic hyperosmolar hyperglycemia. The initial diagnosis in these patients is frequently that of stroke. It is tempting to speculate about a relationship of profound dehydration and secondarily impaired local blood flow, but pathologic confirmation is not available, and patients who recover typically lack any clinical evidence of a stroke [6].

In one series of 33 cases of coma caused by nonketotic hyperosmolar hyperglycemia [6], patients either died or fully recovered. Eleven patients died within 2 days of diagnosis; neither the blood glucose nor any other metabolic abnormality identified patients likely to die, but treatment with insulin was delayed longer in this group (33 hours) than in those who survived (12 hours). No surviving patient exhibited delayed neurologic deterioration that could not be explained by an intercurrent condition (e.g., infection). There were four additional patients in the series who did not develop coma. Interestingly, these patients differed in that their serum sodiums were not as high as in the comatose patients.

Hypernatremia

Neurologic manifestations are common in hypernatremia, often related to the speed with which the condition develops. Usually, the clinical change involves the sensorium, and deep stupor and coma are seen in patients with hypernatremia [61]. Most patients with acute coma caused by hypernatremia are young, and possibly as a result, the prognosis has been good. Among patients who die, venous occlusion, petechial hemorrhages, and vascular congestion are frequent [18]. In general, survivors (80% or more of all affected patients) recover fully, although some impairment of IQ has been noted among childhood survivors of hypernatremia [43, 44]. The actual level of hypernatremia has not been found to relate closely to recovery, but the degree of acute neurologic impairment does [43].

Hyponatremia

Hyponatremia is normally caused by either excessive sodium loss or water retention. The condition can develop either acutely or chronically; typically patients with acute hyponatremia are more symptomatic than patients whose illness develops more insidiously. Acute hyponatremia is usually caused either by iatrogenically administered fluids or by a syndrome of inappropriate antidiuretic hormone (ADH) secretion, sometimes related to surgery or to various drugs with antidiuretic effects [7]. The symptoms of acute hyponatremia include seizures, stupor, delirium, and even coma.

Restoration of normal serum sodium concentrations normally restores neurologic function. Patients who have died and had autopsies as a result of hyponatremic coma exhibited normal neuropathology [4]. In a more recent series, however, Arieff [5] reported on 15 previously healthy women who developed hyponatremia, seizures, and coma after initially awakening from uncomplicated surgery. Three died within 24 hours and at autopsy had evidence of herniation. After several days of coma and mechanical ventilation, 2 patients suspected of having herpes simplex encephalitis underwent open brain biopsies, which showed gray matter necrosis in the cerebral cortex.

In recent years, a fascinating condition, central pontine myelinolysis, has been linked to rapid correction of hyponatremia. Initially believed to occur in chronically debilitated patients [1], this demyelinating condition has now been shown both in animals [36] and humans [12] to be related to hyponatremia. Continuing research on the problem has shown that demyelination is more likely if serum sodium is increased by more than 12 mmol/liter/day than if a more cautious therapeutic approach is taken [60].

An additional delayed problem in patients recovering from hyponatremia was included in the series reported by Arieff [5]. Seven of the 15 patients initially in coma from hyponatremia awakened with treatment and were able to walk, eat, and talk, but after lucid intervals of at least 2 days, developed recurrent seizures and coma. One of these died (no autopsy), and the other 6 remained in a vegetative state after follow-up periods of at least 2 years. The author comments on the similarity of this course to cases of delayed postanoxic encephalopathy [50].

OTHER ABNORMALITIES OF THE BRAIN'S ENVIRONMENT

In general, these disturbances are not likely to lead to long-term brain damage. They can be considered similar to exogenous poisons such as barbiturates, where correction will restore normal brain function. In some instances, however, return of normal function is delayed, and in others, additional complications can develop.

Hypercalcemia

Calcium plays a central role in neurophysiology, and abnormalities of serum calcium are, not surprisingly, associated with clinical abnormalities. Although coma is sometimes correctly attributed to hypercalcemia, more commonly clinical depression, irritability, confusion, and fatigue develop. These symptoms can be accompanied by anorexia and headaches. Although hypercalcemia occurs with sarcoid and hyperthyroidism, its more common causes are hyperparathyroidism and cancer. The EEG is typically slow in hypercalcemic coma, and triphasic waves may be present.

What is particulary noteworthy with respect to prognosis is the poor correlation between recovery of normocalcemia and clinical and EEG normalization. One example is the report by Allen and colleagues [2] of 14 patients with hypercalcemia. Five of them underwent successful surgery for hyperparathyroidism, but despite rapid normalization of serum calcium in all 5 patients, the EEG frequency increased only after days or weeks, and clinical improvement was similarly slow.

Hepatic Failure

Hepatic coma is the most dramatic neurologic complication of liver disease, and milder forms of hepatic encephalopathy are relatively common in long-standing hepatic failure. In the staging system used for liver failure, hepatic coma is categorized as stage 4 (responds only to pain or no response at all). Like hypoxia-ischemia but unlike many of the other metabolic encephalopathies considered in this chapter, hepatic failure is associated with a characteristic neuropathologic change, an increase in the size and number of protoplasmic astrocytes, the Alzheimer type II astrocyte. The nuclei of these astrocytes are greatly enlarged and lobulated.

Although coma has been correlated with a number of specific biochemical metabolites in blood and CSF, including ammonia [20], glutamine [31], alpha-ketoglutaramate [63], and various neurotransmitter abnormalities such as elevated octopamine levels [19], the precise cause of neurologic dysfunction remains unclarified. Whether recovery from hepatic coma correlates with blood or CSF levels of any of these putative causative agents remains unestablished, but Steigmann and associates [59] reported that the ratio of aromatic and branched-chain amino acids in blood was related to the level of consciousness; they provided specific data showing that patients in hepatic coma had higher levels of glutamic acid and the aromatic amino acids methionine, phenylalanine, and tyrosine and lower levels of the branched-chain amino acids leucine and isoleucine than did noncomatose patients with liver disease.

The precise cause of hepatic encephalopathy is related to eventual outcome [24,48], with hepatitis A having the best prognosis for survival, hepatitis B an intermediate prognosis, and non-A, non-B hepatitis the worst. Mortality as high as 60 percent has been reported in some series of patients with acute hepatitis and coma. Halothane-induced liver failure and drug reactions were associated in one of these studies [48] with an even worse chance of recovery, whereas acetaminophen overdose had a better likelihood of survival than hepatitis A. One can thus speculate that ultimate recovery in liver parenchyma might determine improvement in brain function.

A recent hypothesis [46] has implicated an endogenous agonist for the benzodiazepine receptor in the pathogenesis of hepatic encephalopathy on the basis of elevated CSF levels of a substance that binds to benzodiazepine receptors and case reports of clinical improvement with administration of benzodiazepine receptor antagonists to patients with hepatic encephalopathy. Further investigation of this hypothesis might determine other factors associated with prognosis and, as suggested, offer directed treatment. At this point, however, despite claims for specific therapies, it is probably wisest to direct treatment to the general principles of support for the comatose patient and to the underlying hepatic dysfunction.

Prognosis from hepatic coma is also related to signs of neurologic dysfunction, as can be inferred from the study by Levy and co-workers [37]. Whereas only 12 percent of all patients in hypoxic-ischemic coma ultimately regained independent function, this proportion rose to 35 percent for hepatic coma. Presumably because it is not directly associated with pathologic damage, hepatic coma does not carry the same grave prognosis as hypoxic-ischemic coma.

Previously unpublished data from 51 patients in this series who were comatose at least 6 hours because of hepatic disease show correlations between clinical signs and ultimate recovery. Of 28 patients who exhibited a lack of motor responses or presence of posturing (extensor or flexor) at the initial examination, 8 (29%) ultimately regained independent function, whereas 16 (57%) died without awakening. By contrast, withdrawal from pain at the initial examination was associated with an eventual independent existence in 10 of 23 (43%) and with death without awakening in 9 (21%). No patient in hepatic encephalopathy who lacked either pupillary reactions to light or corneal reflexes at the initial (or subsequent) examination ever lived independently. Evaluation of spontaneous eye movements at the initial examination did not help: roving conjugate or orienting spontaneous eye movements at the initial examination were associated with an eventual independent existence in 10 of 30 (33%) and with death without awakening in 16 (53%), whereas absence of spontaneous eye movements or more primitive movements were associated with independent existence in 8 of 21 (38%) and failure to awaken prior to death in 9 (43%).

After 1 day, however, 16 of 32 (50%) of those with roving conjugate or orienting eye movements eventually regained independence, and 11 (34%) died without awakening, whereas of 13 patients with more primitive movements or with no spontaneous movements, only 2 (15%) recovered to an independent existence, and 9 (43%) died without first awakening. Motor responses were also more discriminating after 1 day, with independent existence noted by 2 of 2 (100%) who obeyed commands, 10 of 22 (46%) with withdrawal or localizing responses, and 8 of 28 (29%) with posturing or absent responses; by contrast, death without awakening occurred in 0 of 2 (0%) who obeyed commands, in 6 of 22 (27%) with withdrawal or localizing responses, and in 13 of 21 (62%) lacking any response or with posturing.

Although brain dysfunction associated with hepatic encephalopathy is reversible if hepatic abnormalities are corrected, long-term sequelae can develop, and these can create significant, permanent disability. The most prominent of these is acquired hepatocerebral degeneration [60], characterized by dementia, dysarthria, and ataxia. A tremor characterized by coarse, irregular, flexion-extension of the wrist and fingers is frequently seen, and less specific intention tremors and choreoathetosis can develop as well. Acquired hepatocerebral degeneration typically occurs in patients with prominent portal-systemic shunting.

The pathology of acquired hepatocerebral degeneration consists of spongy degeneration in the deep cortical layers and underlying white matter and, at times, pseudolaminar degeneration [64]. Giant Alzheimer type I astrocytes are sometimes seen. Unlike in Wilson's disease, Kayser-Fleischer rings are not found in this condition. Acquired hepatocerebral degeneration can lead to death within months, but in the original report [64], survival as long as 15 years was noted.

Renal Failure

Dialysis treatment of renal failure and increased use of renal transplantation have reduced the frequency of severe uremia with coma as an inevitable complication of end-stage renal disease. Patients may experience earlier, less severe central nervous system (CNS) symptoms of renal disease, including fatigue, impaired concentration, confusion, and seizures, but coma is now rare. The cause of coma, when more prevalent, was never entirely explained. The presence of high levels of urea alone did not explain the problem, and a variety of electrolyte abnormalities were proposed as explanations. The management of uremic coma is, like many of the conditions discussed in this chapter, that of the underlying condition, in this case dialysis.

It is important to recognize, however, that Wernicke's encephalopathy can complicate the picture in patients with renal failure, especially those undergoing dialysis. Initially noted in these patients in 1968 [42], Wernicke's encephalopathy has recently been reported in comatose patients on dialysis with renal failure [32]. The implication of these observations is that treatment with thiamine might reverse some of these neurologic complications, but this intervention has not been reported in any sizeable series to date.

Prognosis from coma associated with renal

failure was among the best of etiologically related causes of coma reported by Levy and coworkers [37]. Although renal failure composed only a small part of the group with miscellaneous causes of coma, 34 percent of these 58 patients eventually regained the ability to live an independent existence, and only 45 percent died without first awakening from coma. Here too, however, none of 8 patients lacking pupillary light reactions at admission ever regained consciousness, and the same was true for the small numbers of patients lacking oculovestibular responses (12) and motor responses (6). Other investigators have commented on various general factors relating to prognosis from renal failure with or without coma. Lohr and colleagues [40], for example, reported that failure to survive did not depend on age, gender, or indications for dialysis but did relate to hypotension, the need for assisted ventilation, congestive heart failure, sepsis, and gastrointestinal problems.

One distressing CNS complication of prolonged dialysis is an entity called dialysis encephalopathy [13], and when severe, this condition is also associated with coma. This is a progressive, sometimes fatal disorder, often beginning with dysarthria alone. In later stages, facial grimacing, chorea, asterixis, myoclonus, and generalized tremulousness develop, and later still, mental function deteriorates. Aluminum in the dialysate has been implicated in the pathogenesis [14], and resulting osteomalacia and abnormalities of parathyroid function have been described, although a relationship with hyperparathyroidism has been challenged [14]. Management directed to limiting aluminum exposure has reduced the incidence, and use of deferoxamine may be helpful in some patients.

CONCLUSION

Except for hypoxic-ischemic coma, specific predictors of outcome are lacking for most of the metabolic comas considered in this chapter. Although one might assume return to the premorbid state if the underlying disorder is successfully managed, evidence from many of these disorders suggests that a variety of disabling late sequelae do occur; these include demyelination following hyponatremia, acquired hepatocerebral degeneration following hepatic coma, dialysis dementia following uremic coma, and delayed postanoxic encephalopathy following carbon monoxide and hypoxic coma. The pathogenesis of most of these disorders is not currently known, one exception being demyelination with hyponatremia. A fruitful area for future investigation will be further clarification of those features predisposing to these sequelae in survivors of metabolic coma and measures designed to reduce their frequency. Additional studies designed to define variables with prognostic power in some of these conditions will be essential so that future treatment trials can be stratified appropriately.

REFERENCES

1. Adams, R. D., Victor, M., and Mancall, E. L. Central pontine myelinolysis. *Arch. Neurol.* 81:154, 1959.
2. Allen, E. M., Singer, F. R., and Melamed, D. Electroencephalographic abnormalities in hypercalcemia. *Neurology* 20:15, 1970.
3. American Medical Association. Most respondents favor ending life support. *Am. Med. News* 11/28:13, 1986.
4. Anderson, R. J., Chung, H.-M., Kluge, R., and Schrier, R. W. Hyponatremia: A prospective analysis of its epidemiology and the pathogenetic role of vasopressin. *Ann. Intern. Med.* 102:164, 1985.
5. Arieff, A. I. Hyponatremia, convulsions, respiratory arrest, and permanent brain damage after elective surgery in healthy women. *N. Engl. J. Med.* 314:1529, 1986.
6. Arieff, A. I., and Carroll, H. J. Nonketotic hyperosmolar coma with hyperglycemia: Clinical features, pathophysiology, renal function, acid-base balance, plasma-cerebrospinal fluid equilibria and the effects of therapy in 37 cases. *Medicine* 51:73, 1972.
7. Arieff, A. I., Llach, F., and Massry, S. G. Neurological manifestations and morbidity of hyponatremia: Correlation with brain water and electrolytes. *Medicine* 55:121, 1976.
8. Auer, R. N. Progress review: Hypoglycemic brain damage. *Stroke* 17:699, 1986.
9. Bell, J. A., and Hodgson, H. J. F. Coma after cardiac arrest. *Brain* 97:361, 1974.
10. Brierley, J. B., Brown, A. W., and Meldrum, B. S. The nature and time course of the neuronal alterations resulting from oligaemia and hypo-

glycaemia in the brain of macaca mulatta. *Brain Res.* 25:483, 1971.
11. Brunko, E., and Zegers de Beyl, D. Prognostic value of early cortical somatosensory evoked potentials after resuscitation from cardiac arrest. *Electroencephalogr. Clin. Neurophysiol.* 66:15, 1987.
12. Burcar, P. J., Norenberg, M. D., and Yarnell, P. R. Hyponatremia and central pontine myelinolysis. *Neurology* 27:223, 1977.
13. Burks, J. S., Alfrey, A. C., Huddlestone, J., et al. A fatal encephalopathy in chronic haemodialysis patients. *Lancet* 1:764, 1976.
14. Campistrus de Gencarelli, N., Cournot-Witmer, G., Zingraff, J., and Drüeke, T. The role of parathyroid function and parathyroidectomy in the outcome of aluminum-related dialysis encephalopathy. *Nephrol. Dial. Transplant.* 1:192, 1986.
15. Choi, J. S. Delayed neurologic sequelae in carbon monoxide intoxication. *Arch. Neurol.* 40:433, 1983.
16. Dougherty, J. H., Jr., Rawlinson, D. G., Levy, D. E., and Plum, F. Hypoxic-ischemic brain injury and the vegetative state: Clinical and neuropathologic correlation. *Neurology* 31:991, 1981.
17. Earnest, M. P., Breckinridge, J. C., Yarnell, P. R., and Oliva, P. B. Quality of survival after out-of-hospital cardiac arrest: Predictive value of early neurologic evaluation. *Neurology* 29:56, 1979.
18. Finberg, L., Kiley, J., and Luttrell, C. N. Mass accidental salt poisoning in infancy: A study of a hospital disaster. *J.A.M.A.* 184:187, 1963.
19. Fischer, J. E., and Baldessarini, R. J. False neurotransmitters and hepatic failure. *Lancet* 2:75, 1971.
20. Fischer, J. E., Rosen H. M., Ebeid, A. M., et al. The effect of normalization of plasma amino acids on hepatic encephalopathy in man. *Surgery* 80:77, 1976.
21. Fulop, M., Tannenbaum, H., and Dreyer, N. Ketotic hyperosmolar coma. *Lancet* 3:635, 1973.
22. Ganes, T., and Lundar, T. EEG and evoked potentials in comatose patients with severe brain damage. *Electroencephalogr. Clin. Neurophysiol.* 69:6, 1988.
23. Garland, H., and Pearce, J. Neurological complications of carbon monoxide poisoning. *Q. J. Med.* 36:445, 1967.
24. Gimson, A. E., White, Y. S., Eddleston, A. L., and Williams, R. Clinical and prognostic differences in fulminant hepatitis type A, B and non-A non-B. *Gut* 24:1194, 1983.
25. Ginsburg, M. D., Myers, R. E., and McDonagh, B. F. Experimental carbon monoxide encephalopathy in the primate: II. Clinical aspects, neuropathology, and physiologic correlation. *Arch. Neurol.* 30:209, 1974.
26. Guisado, R., and Arieff, A. I. Neurologic manifestations of diabetic comas: Correlation with biochemical alterations in the brain. *Metabolism* 24:665, 1975.
27. Haig, A. J., Katz, R. T., and Sahgal, V. Mortality and complications of the locked-in syndrome. *Arch. Phys. Med. Rehabil.* 68:24, 1987.
28. Higashi, K., Hatano, M., Abiko, S., et al. Five-year follow-up study of patients with persistent vegetative state. *J. Neurol. Neurosurg. Psychiatry* 44:552, 1981.
29. Higashi, K., Sakata, Y., Hatano, M., et al. Epidemiological studies on patients with a persistent vegetative state. *J. Neurol. Neurosurg. Psychiatry* 40:876, 1977.
30. Hockaday, J. M., Potts, F., Epstein, E., et al. Electroencephalographic changes in acute cerebral anoxia from cardiac or respiratory arrest. *Electroencephalogr. Clin. Neurophysiol.* 18:575, 1965.
31. Hourani, B. T., Hamlin, E. M., and Reynolds, T. B. Cerebrospinal fluid glutamine as a measure of hepatic encephalopathy. *Arch. Intern. Med.* 127:1033, 1971.
32. Jagadha, V., Deck, J. H. N., Halliday, W. C., and Smyth, H. A. Wernicke's encephalopathy in patients on peritoneal dialysis or hemodialysis. *Ann. Neurol.* 21:78, 1987.
33. Jennett, B., and Plum, F. Persistent vegetative state after brain damage: A syndrome in search of a name. *Lancet* 1:734, 1972.
34. Jørgensen, E. O., and Malchow-Møller, A. Natural history of global and critical brain ischaemia. Part III: Cerebral prognostic signs after cardiopulmonary resuscitation. Cerebral recovery course and rate during the first year after global and critical ischaemia monitored and predicted by EEG and neurological signs. *Resuscitation* 9:175, 1981.
35. Kaga, K., Nagai, T., Takamori, A., and Marsh, R. R. Auditory short, middle, and long latency responses in acutely comatose patients. *Laryngoscope* 95:321, 1985.
36. Kleinschmidt-DeMasters, B. K., and Norenberg, M. D. Rapid correction of hyponatremia causes demyelination: Relation to central pontine myelinolysis. *Science* 211:1068, 1981.
37. Levy, D. E., Bates, D., Caronna, J. J., et al. Prognosis in nontraumatic coma. *Ann. Intern. Med.* 94:293, 1981.
38. Levy, D. E., Caronna, J. J., Singer, B. H., et al. Predicting outcome from hypoxic-ischemic coma. *J.A.M.A.* 253:1420, 1985.
39. Levy, D. E., Sidtis, J. J., Rottenberg, D. A., et al. Differences in cerebral blood flow and glucose utilization in vegetative versus locked-in patients. *Ann. Neurol.* 22:673, 1987.
40. Lohr, J. W., McFarlane, M. J., and Grantham, J. J. A clinical index to predict survival in acute renal failure patients requiring dialysis. *Am. J. Kidney Dis.* 11:254, 1988.
41. Longstreth, W. T., Jr., Diehr, P., and Inui, T. S.

Prediction of awakening after out-of-hospital cardiac arrest. *N. Engl. J. Med.* 308:1378, 1983.
42. Lopez, R. I., and Collins, G. H. Wernicke's encephalopathy: A complication of chronic hemodialysis. *Arch. Neurol.* 18:248, 1968.
43. Macaulay, D., and Watson, M. Hypernatremia in infants as a cause of brain damage. *Arch. Dis. Child.* 42:485, 1967.
44. Morris-Jones, P. H., Houston, I. B., and Evans, R. C. Prognosis of the neurological complications of acute hypernatremia. *Lancet* 2:1385, 1967.
45. Mueller-Jensen, A., Neunzig, H.-P., and Emskötter, T. Outcome prediction in comatose patients: Significance of reflex eye movement analysis. *J. Neurol. Neurosurg. Psychiatry* 50:389, 1987.
46. Mullen, K. D., Martin, J. V., Mendelson, W. B., et al. Could an endogenous benzodiazepine ligand contribute to hepatic encephalopathy? *Lancet* 1:457, 1988.
47. Mullie, A., Verstringe, P., Buylaert, W., et al. Predictive value of Glasgow coma score for awakening after out-of-hospital cardiac arrest. *Lancet* 1:137, 1988.
48. O'Grady, J. G., Gimson, A. E., O'Brien, C. J., et al. Controlled trials of charcoal hemoperfusion and prognostic factors in fulminant hepatic failure. *Gastroenterology* 94:1186, 1988.
49. Plum, F., and Posner, J. B. *Diagnosis of Stupor and Coma.* Philadelphia: Davis, 1966. p. 197.
50. Plum, F., Posner, J. B., and Hain, R. F. Delayed neurological deterioration after anoxia. *Arch. Intern. Med.* 110:18, 1962.
51. Pramming, S., Thorsteinsson, B., Stigsby, B., and Binder, C. Glycaemic threshold for changes in electroencephalograms during hypoglycaemia in patients with insulin dependent diabetes. *Br. Med. J.* 296:665, 1988.
52. Pramming, S., Thorsteinsson, B., Theilgaard, A., et al. Cognitive function during hypoglycaemia in type I diabetes mellitus. *Br. Med. J.* 292:647, 1986.
53. Rosenberg, C., Wogensen, K., and Starr, A. Auditory brain-stem and middle- and long-latency evoked potentials in coma. *Arch. Neurol.* 41:835, 1984.
54. Shuttleworth, E. Recovery to social and economic independence from prolonged postanoxic vegetative state. *Neurology* 33:372, 1983.
55. Smith, J. S., and Brandon S. Morbidity from acute carbon monoxide poisoning at three-year follow-up. *Br. Med. J.* 1:318, 1973.
56. Snyder, B. D., Gumnit, R. J., Leppik, I. E., et al. Neurologic prognosis after cardiopulmonary arrest: IV. Brainstem reflexes. *Neurology* 31:1092, 1981.
57. Snyder, B. D., Hauser, W. A., Loewenson, R. B., et al. Neurologic prognosis after cardiopulmonary arrest: III. Seizure activity. *Neurology* 30:1292, 1980.
58. Starr, A., and Achor, L. J. Auditory brain stem responses in neurological disease. *Arch. Neurol.* 32:761, 1975.
59. Steigmann, F., Szanto, P. B., Poulos, A., et al. Significance of serum aminograms in diagnosis and prognosis of liver disease. *J. Clin. Gastroenterol.* 6:453, 1984.
60. Sterns, R. H., Riggs, J. E., and Schochet, S. S. Osmotic demyelination syndrome following correction of hyponatremia. *N. Engl. J. Med.* 314:1535, 1986.
61. Swanson, P. D. Neurological Manifestations of Hypernatremia. In P. J. Vinken and G. W. Bruyn (eds.), *Handbook of Clinical Neurology.* Amsterdam: North Holland, 1976. Pp. 443–461.
62. Teasdale, G., and Jennett, B. Assessment of coma and impaired consciousness: A practical scale. *Lancet* 2:81, 1974.
63. Vergera, F., Plum, F., and Duffy, T. E. α-Ketoglutaramate: Increased concentrations in the cerebrospinal fluid of patients in hepatic coma. *Science* 183:81, 1974.
64. Victor, M., Adams, R. D., and Cole, M. The acquired (non-Wilsonian) type of chronic hepatocerebral degeneration. *Medicine* 44:345, 1965.
65. Willoughby, J. O., and Leach, B. G. Relation of neurological findings after cardiac arrest to outcome. *Br. Med. J.* 3:437, 1974.

3 Hypoxia and the Central Nervous System

Robert C. Griggs and Allen I. Arieff

The average human brain weighs about 1.3 kg (1400 gm in adult males and 1240 gm in adult females) and thus represents only about 2 percent of body mass. Despite its modest mass, the brain receives about 20 percent of cardiac output, consumes about 65 percent of total glucose, and utilizes about 20 percent of the body's oxygen [20,69]. In addition, about 75 percent of total brain oxygen is used by cortical gray matter neurons, which constitute only about 20 percent of brain mass. The brain has enormous needs in terms of energy. About 85 percent of all glucose used by the brain is aerobically metabolized with oxygen, with about half of the energy produced utilized to maintain normal ionic gradients across brain cell membranes. The ionic gradients are needed to generate action potentials and conduct nerve impulses. If the brain does not obtain sufficient oxygen, glucose cannot be oxidized aerobically, with resultant decreased energy production by the brain. Anaerobic metabolism cannot supply enough energy for the brain to function. No measurable cerebral dysfunction occurs when cerebral oxygen utilization is maintained at a level of 50 percent of normal, which corresponds to an arterial PO_2 (PaO_2) of about 50 mm Hg. An acute lowering of PaO_2 below about 40 mm Hg results in measurable cerebral dysfunction, while PaO_2 below about 30 mm Hg (in unconditioned subjects) usually results in depression of sensorium. It is felt that chronic hypoxia, such as that experienced at high altitudes [135] is well tolerated, but this may not be true. A recent study of well-conditioned individuals at altitudes of up to 8848 meters demonstrated steady-state PO_2 of about 30 mm Hg at rest [77] and about 28 mm Hg with exercise. Such individuals were found to have developed persistent brain damage when subjected to a sophisticated battery of motor, intellectual, and psychological tests [77]. The PaO_2 level of about 27 mm Hg corresponds quite well to the minimum level in laboratory animals that is compatible with survival [13]. Despite a pronounced ability to survive at substantially reduced levels of PaO_2, brain survival is only possible for about 20 seconds in the total absence of oxygen [13]. Some understanding of how the body adapts to hypoxia can be obtained by the concept of the oxygen extraction reserve.

OXYGEN EXTRACTION RESERVE: BRAIN AND HEART

In the development of cerebral hypoxia, the oxygen extraction reserve is one of the major critical factors that determines the performance of the heart and lungs and the subsequent delivery of oxygen to the brain. Because of this, it is important to review the regulation of systemic oxygen delivery and utilization. Cerebral blood flow is a function of cardiac output, arterial blood pressure, and cerebral vascular resistance. In general, cerebral vascular resistance can respond to alterations in arterial blood pressure to provide a relatively constant cerebral blood flow. Impairment of autoregulation occurs with severe hypercapnia or hypoxia, both leading to increased cerebral blood flow. The heart usually plays a critical role in the development of hypoxia with resulting lactic acidosis [9]. Total body oxygen utilization can be substantially impaired without a measurable rise in arterial lactate [28], and measurements of arterial blood gases and lactate are often of no use in determining the acid-base and oxygenation status of the body [6,18,28]. It is now clear that arterial blood gases are at best a poor indication of the acid-base and tissue oxygenation status of the body and brain [2,6,14,28,64]. Measurements must be made of the arterial and mixed venous (pulmonary artery) gases, including oxygen content (which can be determined from the oxygen saturation and hemoglobin). As a practical matter, the central venous gases are similar enough to the mixed venous gases that they can be used when a pulmonary artery catheter cannot be placed in the patient [6]. Oxygen transport (or delivery) can be calculated using the product of the arterial oxygen content and blood flow (usually expressed as ml O_2/minute). It represents the quantity of oxygen available or delivered to the whole body or to individual organs or tissues and is maintained preferentially to the "vital organs" (heart and brain) during hypoxia by a number of adaptive mechanisms [25,26,34,78,121]. With mild hypoxemia (PaO_2 of 40–65 mm Hg), the oxygen content of arterial blood is relatively well preserved by virtue of the sigmoidal nature of the oxygen-hemoglobin binding curve [25,34]. Oxygen delivery declines only modestly (at most 20–30%), and the principal adaptation to this decline is a compensatory increase in tissue oxygen extraction.

The ability of tissues to increase oxygen extraction when oxygen delivery is inadequate is termed the oxygen extraction reserve or the oxygen utilization coefficient [25,67]. Since tissues are theoretically capable of extracting virtually all of the oxygen carried to them by hemoglobin in hypoxic states, the oxygen extraction reserve may be conveniently defined as the oxygen content of venous blood draining the tissue in question, which represents the amount of oxygen that is theoretically available but not extracted by that tissue. Under normal aerobic conditions, arterial blood is more than 95 percent saturated with oxygen, and the extraction reserve is quite large. Mixed venous blood is normally about 75 percent saturated with a corresponding oxygen content of 14 to 15 vol% [4,67]. Resting oxygen extraction is therefore only about 20 percent (95–75%) of that available, so that the reserve is about 75 percent, more than three times as large as the oxygen extracted. However, because resting oxygen requirements are higher per gram of tissue in the brain and heart than in any other organs, resting oxygen extraction is much higher in these tissues, about 60 to 65 percent [25]. Coronary sinus blood typically has an oxygen tension of 15 to 20 mm Hg with saturations in the 25 to 30 percent range. Consequently, the heart and brain have the smallest oxygen extraction reserve and can only increase resting oxygen extraction by a maximum of 50 percent of baseline

[73]. Thus, the body as a whole has an oxygen reserve that is over three times the normal resting oxygen extraction, and most organs can tolerate acutely PaO_2 of 40 mm Hg without difficulty. In the presence of hypoxemic stress however, the coronary oxygen reserve easily becomes exhausted, and circulatory adjustments become necessary in hypoxia to maintain adequate oxygen delivery to brain and myocardium [3,19]. Below a PaO_2 of about 40 mm Hg, there is a local vascular effect of hypoxia that causes direct vasodilation of both the coronary and cerebral circulations [42]. In the cerebral circulation, this effect may be partially mediated by increases in brain interstitial fluid potassium concentration [107]. Other vascular beds are minimally affected by the direct vascular effects of hypoxia. Sympathetic outflow to the coronary and cerebral vessels increases, augmenting vasodilation in these vascular beds and effectively redistributing blood flow from the "nonvital" to the "vital" organs [70]. Sympathetic outflow to the myocardium also increases, which increases the resting heart rate and contractile state of the myocardium. Stroke volume and cardiac output increase [15,70], and tissue oxygen delivery is improved by compensating the impaired arterial oxygen content with augmented blood flow. In the brain, cerebral circulation is "autoregulated" such that cerebral blood flow remains constant throughout a wide range of arterial blood pressure and cardiac output [20]. In general, cerebral vascular resistance can respond to alterations in arterial blood pressure as low as 30 to 50 mm Hg in laboratory animals and as low as 60 mm Hg or as high as 180 mm Hg in humans, by either vasoconstriction or vasodilatation, in order to provide a constant cerebral blood flow of 50 to 70 ml/100 gm/minute [93]. Major factors that can influence cerebral blood flow are the blood PO_2, PCO_2, and pH. In conditions characterized by hypocapnia or metabolic alkalosis, there is cerebral vasoconstriction, while both hypoxia and hypercapnia/metabolic acidosis result in cerebral vasodilatation. A breakdown of cerebral autoregulation occurs with severe hypercapnia or hypoxia, both leading to increased brain blood flow.

EFFECTS OF HYPOXIA ON THE BRAIN: CIRCULATORY ADJUSTMENTS

With profound hypoxia, therefore, circulatory adjustments become increasingly important to maintain adequate oxygen delivery to the heart and brain. Since blood flow must increase to compensate for any reduction of the oxygen content of arterial blood below the extraction reserve, myocardial mechanical function indeed becomes "vital" to outcome and survival, and thus brain and myocardial oxygen delivery must be defended at all costs. Unfortunately, there are untoward consequences of the circulatory adjustments that redistribute flow to vital organs. These sequelae can have a major impact on cerebral and myocardial function.

Vasoconstriction in the peripheral circulation [42] increases left ventricular afterload. Along with the heart rate and contractility increase, blood pressure rises. Consequently, myocardial oxygen requirements increase when oxygen delivery is compromised. To the extent that coronary blood flow can increase to augment myocardial oxygen delivery such that the increases in myocardial oxygen requirements are met, the enhanced contractile state of the myocardium will be maintained. There are also compensatory mechanisms whereby red blood cells are able to give up more of their bound oxygen despite decreasing PaO_2 [134]. Eventually, however, myocardial oxygen delivery will prove inadequate to meet oxygen requirements, and ischemia may develop [55]. With ischemia, the stroke volume and thereby systemic oxygen transport decrease. Perfusion pressure is reduced, particularly in the coronary vascular bed [73]. Increases in pulmonary venous pressure lead to interstitial edema, increasing the diffusion gradient for oxygen in the lungs and worsening pulmonary gas exchange. Secondarily, vasoconstriction of the splanchnic, renal, and skeletal muscular vascular beds reduces blood flow to these organs, reducing oxygen delivery and increasing anaerobic metabolism and hence lactate production [9,13]. In dogs with hypoxic lactic acidosis, the "whole body" oxygen use, which includes brain and heart, is normal to high, despite substantial decrements of oxygen use in carcass, gut, and liver [13]. Gluconeogenesis from lactate is also impaired in the liver and kidney, and thus lactate removal from the blood diminishes. Hydrogen ion also accumulates as a result of continued adenosine triphosphate (ATP) hydrolysis in the absence of adequate aerobic ATP formation and diminished gluconeogenesis from lactate [24,38,39,140]. The net result of the lactate and hydrogen ion accumulation is lactic acidosis.

Lactic acidosis is particularly detrimental to cerebral function. Unlike in other tissues, most of the lactate in brain is made within the brain [82], and its accumulation leads to a depression of intracellular pH (pHi) [75,82]. A consequence of the cerebral lactic acidosis is depression of respiration, which will further lower PaO_2 increase $PaCO_2$, and lower brain pHi [98]. Thus, a vicious cycle is initiated that, if not somehow interrupted, usually culminates in death.

EFFECTS OF HYPOXIA ON BRAIN COMPOSITION

Our understanding of the effects of hypoxia on brain water, electrolyte, and high-energy phosphate composition has undergone a substantial revision in the past decade. From a review of the literature prior to 1980, the impression is gained that hypoxia somehow leads to a decrease in high-energy phosphate concentration, with a loss of potassium and gain in sodium and chloride by cells, with resultant secondary influx of water resulting in cerebral edema [57,85,94,102]. Many of these concepts result from histopathologic findings now believed to be artifactual [85,102] or a diagnosis of "brain swelling" based on measurements of cerebrospinal fluid (CSF) pressure or mechanisms other than actual brain edema. There are very few actual measurements of brain water content to document brain edema associated with hypoxia. More recently, brain water can be evaluated in vitro using such techniques as computed tomography (CT) scanning or magnetic resonance imaging (MRI). Another problem has been the almost synonymous use of the terms *hypoxia* and *ischemia*. To understand the problems of brain edema and hypoxia, one must first differentiate hypoxia and ischemia.

Cerebral Hypoxia and Ischemia

Ischemia is a decrease or absence of blood flow to a tissue or organ. Ischemia will of course produce hypoxia, but if there is no blood flow (as in occlusion of an artery), the effects of an intact circulation cannot be evaluated. Hypoxia is a decrease in oxygen delivery to a tissue or organ, whatever the cause. The different types of brain tissue hypoxia-ischemia have been classified as follows [31]:

1. Ischemic hypoxia: There is complete cessation of blood flow to either the entire brain (global ischemia) or in the distribution of a single artery (regional ischemia).
2. Oligemic hypoxia: There is a global or regional reduction, but not an absence, of blood flow. This is often referred to as partial ischemia.
3. Anoxic hypoxia: The arterial oxygen tension is zero, due to a lack of transmission of oxygen into the bloodstream via the lungs for any reason.
4. Hypoxic hypoxia: The arterial oxygen is reduced to less than a critical level of about 40 mm Hg.
5. Anemic hypoxia: Oxygen delivery to tissues is reduced because of a reduced ability of the blood to carry oxygen or deliver it to the tissues.
6. Histotoxic hypoxia: There is poisoning of the enzymes involved in oxidative metabolism of the tissues.
7. Hypoglycemia: The blood glucose concentration is reduced below a certain critical level, usually 1.6 mM in women and 2.2 mM in men.

The above classifications have limited clinical application because many clinical circumstances dictate that more than one process is involved. For example, a reduction in blood flow to the brain (ischemic hypoxia, as in stroke) is often accompanied by hypoxic hypoxia (because of hypotension or lung disease). Partial ischemia due to hypotension frequently complicates anemic hypoxia (due to hemorrhage). However, the above classifications are generally useful if their limitations are appreciated.

Cerebral Biochemical Effects of Hypoxia

Theoretically, in the strict biochemical sense, if severe hypoxia were present, there would be a decrease in high-energy phosphate compounds, such as ATP and phosphocreatine. When this happens, it is suggested that there should be a failure of the mechanisms involved in active transport of sodium, with a resultant loss of potassium and gain in sodium by brain cells [94]. However, even older studies in laboratory animals suggest that this is usually not the case [27,102,132], and more recent studies employing magnetic resonance spectroscopy (MRS) to measure cerebral phosphate metabolites confirm these impressions [23,62]. With early (up to 3 hours) nonlethal hypoxia, there is actually only minimal brain edema. The edema is primarily present in astrocytes and is reversible [11,27,102,104,132]. Nonlethal levels of hypoxia (PaO_2 between 20 and 40 mm Hg) result in altered neuronal activity [107] and lead to an increase in cerebral extracellular potassium and glutamine concentrations, with a decrease of extracellular sodium [78,84]. Additionally, although brain concentrations of ATP and phosphocreatine are not appreciably altered by hypoxia (PaO_2 below 20 mm Hg) of short duration, lactate increases very quickly (after 15 minutes or more), as do brain total free fatty acids (FFA). Triacylglycerol-arachidonate and phosphatidylinositol are both decreased [79].

The cells that lose potassium are primarily astrocytes [104]. The potassium leaves the astrocytes via the astrocyte end-feet, and then enters brain capillaries. From the capillaries, it can freely diffuse into the CSF [99]. The increased extracellular potassium in the brain leads to cerebral arteriolar vasodilatation, with increased cerebral blood flow and resultant delivery of more oxygen to the brain [107].

Hypoxia and Cerebral Edema

There is apparently no substantial movement of sodium from blood into brain cells until there is irreversible cell damage that has been present for over 3 hours. Thus, global hypoxia that terminates in death within 3 hours will generally not be accompanied by cerebral edema. Regional brain death from anoxia-ischemia will eventually cause brain edema if the individual survives. This regional and localized swelling will raise intracranial and CSF pressure and give the appearance of generalized cerebral edema [72], as does any localized area of damaged brain [66]. This in fact makes perfect clinical sense. If hypoxia of short duration resulted in substantial global cerebral edema, all brains examined at autopsy would have to have cerebral edema. As a corollary, persons dying of cardiac arrest would not have cerebral edema, since they generally die within less than 3 hours. However, there is apparently some movement of potassium ion from intracellular space to extracellular space with modest hypoxia of short duration, and this process is reversible [78,94]. After hypoxia of more than 4 hours, such as occurs in asphyxia, there are more profound and irreversible changes. Following occlusion of the common carotid or internal carotid artery (in monkeys and gerbils) for greater than 4 hours, there are significant increases (7–20%) in the water content of cortex and subcortical white matter, and these are accompanied by corresponding increases of sodium content and decreases in potassium [27,63,132]. Thus, tissue death for an interval in excess of 3 hours, in the presence of an otherwise intact circulation, is probably necessary for substantial cerebral edema to occur.

Metabolic encephalopathies (hypoglycemia, hyponatremia, hepatic encephalopathy) may result in some degree of brain edema, and the presence of such edema along with hypoxia-ischemia often confounds so-called classic findings in the brain. The principal of "selective vulnerability" of the brain to ischemia generally dictates that certain parts of the brain are more vulnerable than others to ischemic damage [40]. The reasons for such selective vulnerability are not well known. The most vulnerable regions of the brain [32] are generally considered to be (1) layers 3, 5, and 6 of the cerebral cortex, (2) area h1 and areas h3, h4, and h5 of the hippocampus, (3) the central and basolateral portions of the amygdaloid nucleus, (4) Purkinje cells of the cerebellum, and (5) neurons of the caudate, putamen, globus pallidus, and thalamus. In adults with ischemia, the brain stem nuclei are usually not affected, and neurons of the spinal cord are least vulnerable to ischemia. However, the "classic" patterns noted above assume a relatively "pure" form of ischemia-hypoxia. There may be abnormalities in the distribution of cerebral blood flow (oligemic hypoxia) along with abnormalities in respiration (hypoxic hypoxia). There may also be systemic hypoglycemia, along with relative malfunction of enzymes involved in oxidative metabolism (histotoxic hypoxia) in addition to brain edema. In such instances, the classic patterns noted above would hardly be expected to occur. Such is the case in several of the metabolic encephalopathies, such as hypoglycemia, hyponatremia, hepatic encephalopathy, and phosphate depletion.

Biochemical Mediators of Ischemic Cerebral Damage

Recently, our knowledge of the possible mechanisms of selective vulnerability of the brain has expanded. It appears likely that excessive amounts of glutamate in brain extracellular fluid are at least a part of the pathogenesis for brain damage in ischemic states. Evidence for such a hypothesis has been accumulated from studies in laboratory animals. Ischemia causes an increase in glial production of glutamate, an effect mediated by peripheral chemoreceptors [74]. The release of glutamate into cerebral extracellular space leads to excitation of a subset of glutamate receptors, the *N*-methyl-D-aspartate (NMDA) receptor. Hypoxia increases excitation in neurons, particularly at the NMDA receptor. Excitation at this receptor then leads to an excessive influx of sodium ions and water [27]. Excitation, or increased synaptic activity, is an important factor in eventual cell death in hypoxic neurons [116]. Thus, the classic biochemical teachings where hypoxia-ischemia leads to a decrease of brain high-energy phosphate compounds, with a secondary influx of sodium, chloride, and water into brain (described above) are probably incorrect.

Incomplete injury may lead to the production of oxygen free radicals that have been demonstrated to injure cell membranes, mitochondria, and DNA [43]. In the setting of ischemic injury and low oxygen tension, arachidonic acid is converted to prostacyclin and leukotrienes. The enzymes involved in this conversion are cyclooxygenase and lipoxygenase. As a result of these conversions potentially injurious oxygen radicals are produced [35].

Another factor postulated to contribute to the hypoxic-ischemic injury is the phenomenon described by Ames, Wright, and Kowaela [5] termed no reflow. The mechanism underlying the restitution of usual blood flow after ischemia was attributed to capillary endothelial swelling. Swollen glial processes were considered to play a role in this failure of post-hypoxic recirculation. Others have studied this phenomenon of hypoperfusion after ischemia and observed that in the immediate postischemic period there is an initial hyperfusion [114]; however, with the passing of time a decline in blood flow occurs [46]. Electron-microscopic observations failed to confirm earlier studies of capillary changes [51]. The no reflow phenomenon was thought to be secondary to collections of red cell aggregates and heightened blood viscosity. Frank intravascular clotting was not observed [37]. Postischemic hypoperfusion can be favorably altered by filtration of blood before induction of hypoxic-ischemic injury [68], suggesting that a constituent of plasma may be involved in the vascular response to ischemia. A class of proteins termed heat shock proteins has been noted to increase in brain following hypoxic-ischemic injury [49]. The possibility has been raised that these proteins serve a protective role and their absence in areas prone to damage may contribute to selective vulnerability of that region to hypoxia (and other insults) [49].

Calcium Ions and Cell Death

A point is eventually reached where cerebral edema has occurred and cell viability is severely compromised. If the cellular damage continues, there follows an influx of calcium ions and a probable decrease in intracellular magnesium [130], which is at some point followed by permanent neuronal damage [44,112]. The actual event that leads to irreversible cell death in hypoxic brain is not entirely clear. A late event is the movement of calcium into hypoxic cells, and, in certain types of cell injury, calcium overload is the actual pathogenetic mechanism [36,44]. There are a number of theoretic reasons why calcium overload may be detrimental to cells. An increase in free cytosolic calcium can activate calcium-dependent phospholipases, resulting in the breakdown of cell membranes and production of substances that are toxic to cells, such as free fatty acids, lysozymes and phospholipids. Additionally, many important intracellular enzyme systems, such as ATPases, glycogen phosphorylase, and adenylate cyclase are regulated by calcium. Thus, a large increase of free cytosolic calcium can easily be conceived as upsetting the homeostasis between intracellular messengers, energy, and electrolytes. Elevations of free cytosolic calcium will increase Na^+-Ca^{+2} ATPase activity, resulting in an inhanced use of ATP, which is low in ischemic cells. Elevations in calcium can also lead to uncoupling of oxidative phosphorylation in mitochondria and deplete cells of chemical energy [36]. All of these findings, along with the fact that ischemic tissue contains large amounts of calcium, strongly suggest that ischemia leads to an uncontrolled increase in total cell calcium and cytosolic free calcium, which initiates a cascade of progressively deleterious events that terminate in cell death [36]. Additionally, magnesium is a necessary component of many intracellular enzyme systems [131]. Increased extracellular magnesium actually has a protective effect on hypoxic neurons [116]. Post-traumatic brain injury is associated with a decrease of intracellular magnesium [130], and alterations in cellular magnesium can have substantial effects on intracellular calcium current [136]. It is possible, but unproved, that the influx of calcium leads to a cellular exodus of magnesium following brain injury [40,48].

This biochemical pattern of cerebral injury is seen not only in ischemia, but also in traumatic brain injury [48]. There is thus evidence that both hypoxia and trauma can result in a "metabolic encephalopathy" after the initial insult has occurred. Therapy in experimental animals with competitive antagonists to NMDA receptors have been effective in preliminary studies, and such agents may have a role in the prevention of hypoxic or post-traumatic brain damage [48,83].

HYPOXIA ASSOCIATED WITH OTHER METABOLIC ENCEPHALOPATHIES

Cardiopulmonary Arrest

In the United States, an estimated 650,000 persons die each year from acute myocardial infarction. An estimated one million episodes of cardiac arrest occur each year in patients suffering from acute myocardial infarction. Thus, cardiopulmonary arrest is the most common cause of death in patients with coronary artery disease who suffer acute myocardial infarction. The high death rate from cardiopulmonary arrest underscores the generally dismal prognosis of this disorder. Several studies have recently documented these facts. Bedell and associates [22] found that among 294 patients who had coronary artery disease and suffered cardiopulmonary arrest, only 14 percent survived. The main negative factor determining survival was a resuscitation that took longer than 30 minutes [17]. In the most extensive study to date of the outcome of nontraumatic coma, Levy and coworkers [89] evaluated 500 comatose subjects. Of these, 210 patients had ischemic heart disease and had suffered cardiopulmonary arrest. Only 28 percent recovered from cardiac arrest, and of these, only 10 patients (5% of the total) were able to live independently and care for themselves. The prognosis is even worse if the patient is elderly. Murphy and colleagues [97] studied 503 patients who were over age 69 and suffered cardiopulmonary arrest. Overall, only 17 percent of these patients who had in-hospital cardiopulmonary arrest survived to discharge from the hospital, and when the arrest was unwitnessed, survival was only 4 percent. The limiting factor in all of these series was the presence of hypoxic brain damage that was global in nature. Thus, survival from global hypoxia complicating cardiopulmonary arrest is less than 30 percent overall and less than 20 percent in the elderly. However, at autopsy, the neurons in most such patients appear normal [40]. In addition, there is often a delayed progression of neurologic damage, which roughly corresponds to the histologic pattern of acute hypoxic injury. In another form of hypoxic hypoxia, carbon monoxide poisoning, a biphasic clinical course of delayed neurologic deterioration has been described [59]. This pattern also may occur after drowning, cardiopulmonary arrest with resuscitation, treated hyponatremia, and attempted strangulation. At autopsy, patients who had the clinical pattern of delayed neurologic deterioration frequently have white matter lesions of at least three different types [86]: (1) multiple small foci of white matter necrosis with demyelination, which are often found in subcortical white matter and optic tracts; (2) diffuse destruction of white matter, extending through deep white matter from frontal to occipital poles and corpus callosum; and (3) focal or confluent areas of primary demyelination, which are usually in deep hemispheric white matter and periventricular zones. Lesions of the first type correlate with a monophasic illness and death within 1 week; lesions of the second type correlate with a monophasic illness, coma, and death within 9 to 140 days; lesions of the third type correlate with a biphasic illness and often delayed neurologic deterioration, with a persistent vegetative state. Hyponatremia can also lead to delayed neurologic deterioration. Two patients who had hyponatremia, respiratory arrest, and a biphasic illness with delayed neurologic deterioration [7] remained in a coma and died after a mean of 2 years. At autopsy, both had white matter lesions corresponding to the third type of lesions described.

Hyponatremia, Hypoxia, and Delayed Postanoxic Encephalopathy

In the last 15 years, there have been a large number of studies of patients with hyponatremia who have developed cerebral demyelinating lesions [33,126,129]. Some of these investigators have suggested an association between hyponatremia or its therapy and central pontine myelinolysis (CPM), a rare neurologic disorder of uncertain etiology that is most often found in alcoholic malnourished individuals [1]. This disorder is discussed in detail in Chapter 14. However, more recent studies have suggested that the brain lesions associated with hyponatremia (hyponatremic encephalopathy) are in all probability due to a combination of hypoxic hypoxemia, herniation, and pressure necrosis [8,54]. Those associated with the therapy of hyponatremia occur in parallel with at least one of six different factors, which are discussed in detail in Chapter 4.

Cerebral demyelination occurring in hyponatremic subjects is usually secondary to a combination of anoxia-hypoxia and increased intracranial pressure (ischemic hypoxia) [138]. The clinical manifestations are sometimes delayed until after treatment has been completed, giving a false appearance of some relationship between cerebral demyelination and the therapy of hyponatremia. The laboratory of one of us has described the clinical course of seven patients who had severe symptomatic hyponatremia and developed permanent hypoxic brain damage (or death) following a series of two respiratory arrests separated by several days [7]. Although only recently recognized as being associated with hyponatremia, hypoxic brain damage appears to be an important factor in the neurologic disability observed in some hyponatremic subjects [7,54]. The syndrome of delayed postanoxic encephalopathy has been known at least since 1925 [59,60,109]. The disorder can follow anoxia-hypoxia from any cause, but most cases are related to either carbon monoxide intoxication, attempted strangulation, cardiopulmonary arrest, or various miscellaneous intoxications. The vast majority of reported cases are related to either carbon monoxide intoxication or cardiopulmonary arrest with resuscitation. The clinical characteristics of this condition have been well described [59]. Whatever the cause, patients are initially deeply comatose, often requiring mechanical ventilation. Characteristically, they begin to regain consciousness within 1 to 3 days. Initial improvement may be rapid enough that patients are discharged from the hospital within a week of the initial event. As early as several hours, or as late as several weeks (in exceptional cases, as late as 5–6 weeks), patients relapse. The onset may be abrupt and heralded by disorientation, confusion, restlessness, apathy, and irritability, often with agitation, mania, or other inappropriate behavior. There may be cortical dysfunction that is multifocal in character, with dysphasia, agnosia, or apraxia. Motor control is impaired, with associated rigidity.

There are no obvious features during the initial anoxic insult that serve to distinguish those patients destined to relapse from those who have uncomplicated recoveries. Many such patients are initially misdiagnosed and are felt to have primary cerebral pathology, such as subdural hematoma. In the hyponatremic patients, the diagnosis must be made on clinical grounds but appears to be the most likely cause of the relapsing encephalopathy, with either death or a persistent vegetative state as the usual outcome. An unfortunate clinical misinterpretation appears to have occurred in the clinical literature. Patients with symptomatic hyponatremia have been treated (usually with hypertonic NaCl) and appeared to improve [100,126,129]. Then, after several days, they deteriorated and often did not survive. At autopsy, these patients often had demyelinating lesions of the brain, usually subcortical white matter and basal ganglia, but sometimes including the pons [100,129]. Because of an occasional superficial anatomic similarity to central pontine myelinolyis, such patients were said to have such a lesion [127], even though the distribution of lesions invariably involved many other parts of the brain in addition to the pons. Hypoxia was usually not considered because the damaged areas of brain did not correspond to the principle of "selective vulnerability" [31]. However, it must be borne in mind that hyponatremia can lead to a 400 percent increase of intracranial pressure with a resultant decrease in cerebral blood flow of over 40 percent [115]. Increased intracranial pressure also leads to alterations in the brain's elastic response, further restricting cerebral blood flow [119]. The situation is further compounded by the fact that CPM is most common in subjects with cirrhosis, and such patients also have a high incidence of hyponatremia [106], hypotension [10], and respiratory alkalosis [53], which decreases tissue oxygen delivery at any given arterial PO_2. Thus, in patients with the combination of cirrhosis, hyponatremia, and neurologic deterioration, the cerebral demyelinating lesions found at autopsy were often diagnosed as related to the "therapy" of hyponatremia [100], even though many such patients had received no therapy at all [8,12,16,54]. In fact, the deterioration several days after therapy was virtually always associated with respiratory insufficiency, which had occurred before treatment [7,126], and the clinical picture and neuropathology were that of hypoxic encephalopathy, often with delayed postanoxic encephalopathy. It is now clear that such a sequence frequently occurs in the absence of therapy [7,18]. Similar pontine lesions are found in patients who have manifested increased intracranial pressure unrelated to hyponatremia [138], thus rendering any association with treatment of hyponatremia unlikely.

Focal Ischemia and Stroke

The incidence of stroke in the United States exceeds 250,000 cases per year. Strictly speaking, an ischemic stroke is an infarct of a portion of the brain, most often secondary to occlusion of a major or minor blood vessel. The sequelae of a particular stroke depend to a large extent on the location of the blood vessel, the extent of tissue damage, and the collateral circulation. These questions are beyond the scope of this chapter, and discussions can be found in textbooks of neurology. As a sequela of stroke, there is tissue death of a portion of the brain. Within the initial few hours after a stroke, and for a period of perhaps 1 to 3 days, there will be variable but progressive tissue edema and death in the area around the zone of infarction that is partially fed by the occluded vessel. Around the infarction is an ischemic penumbra, which has been proposed as an area of selective metabolic vulnerability, which represents a zone where electrical failure, but not ionic failure, is present [40]. In the area of selective metabolic vulnerability, cerebral blood flow has declined from the normal 40 to 60 ml/100 gm of brain to about 15 ml/100 gm of brain, and what viability remains is sustained by collateral flow [111]. As discussed, the stuctural integrity and metabolism of the neurons will probably fail if this state is present for more than 3 hours. Ultimately, the 30-day case fatality rate is about 20 percent for patients with nonhemorrhagic stroke. Of the survivors receiving rehabilitation, 50 percent will have persistent motor deficits, 20 to 30 percent will need assistance to move about, and 33 percent will require assistance for self care [45]. Current and anticipated concepts of stroke therapy might be directed at the prevention of delayed ischemic injury and clinical progression of stroke after the initial insult.

The probable presence of an ischemic penumbra provides the theoretic basis for virtually all therapy of stroke aimed at either improvement of cerebral blood flow (surgery, vasodilators, thrombolytic agents) or pharmacologic protection of neurons (calcium channel blocking agents, NMDA antagonists, anti–free radical agents, anion-exchange inhibitors). Such therapeutic interventions are attempts to reverse the effects of ischemia-hypoxia of this ischemic penumbra [16,48,83,120]. After the initial insult, most patients tend to worsen progressively after hospital admission for therapy of stroke. In the Pilot Data Bank of the NINCDS, 22 percent of stroke patients worsened after hospital admission. Such figures suggest that stroke may also be in effect a "metabolic encephalopathy." This description suggests that the initial insult leaves a zone of ischemic but potentially viable brain tissue that may be salvageable by pharmacologic means. The potentially viable tissue that does not survive is ultimately destroyed by secondary metabolic events occurring after the vessel occlusion. Attempts at limitation of stroke damage perhaps should be directed at the biochemical events described previously.

CLINICAL MANIFESTATIONS OF CEREBRAL HYPOXIC ISCHEMIA

The sequelae of cerebral hypoxic ischemia are most frequently the result of cardiac or respiratory failure. Diffuse signs are characteristic, but focal nervous system signs may occur if antecedent cerebrovascular disease was present.

In severe acute brain hypoxia, the patient does not respond to painful stimuli. Brain stem reflexes are absent: oculocephalic and caloric responses, corneal reflexes, and pupillary light reflexes. Motor responses such as defensive posturing and withdrawal are absent. Muscle stretch reflexes are depressed or absent. Recovery from this level of function is possible only if there is prompt restitution of brain perfusion and adequate oxygenation. Often only partial recovery occurs, depending on the duration of the coma and the failure of recovery of brain stem reflexes [21].

When recovery occurs, the clinical state changes beginning with the return of brain stem reflexes, followed by progressive restitution of more rostal functions. The critical time limits for recovery of respiratory function, pupillary light reflex responses, coughing, swallowing, ciliospinal reflex activity, and consciousness are measured in minutes [81]. Levy and associates [90] have set forth fundamental observations regarding reflexes, eye movements, motor responses, and responses to verbal commands that are of invaluable aid in helping predict the outcome after hypoxic-ischemic coma (see Chap. 2). For periods of up to 2 weeks important bedside observations have been recorded that are of additional prognostic value. Failure to improve after cardiopulmonary resuscitation depended most often on whether the blood pH was 7.2 or less at the end of the resuscitative effort [128]. Other factors that often contribute to mortality after resuscitation include pneumonia, electrolyte imbalance, and gastrointestinal bleeding [29].

Many survivors of brain hypoxic-ischemic injury regain consciousness but remain severely impaired. The term *vegetative state* has been proposed for this level of function by Jewett and Plum [80]. The vegetative state is defined as a persistent condition wherein eye opening may occur when the patient is challenged with verbal stimuli but no eye orienting occurs, no other verbal responses can be found, and limb movements are reflex and postural rather than voluntary. Both electroencephalographic and clinical observations show the occurrence of sleep cycles. The prognosis for survival and recovery of function from the vegetative state is unfortunately poor [71,88]. There nevertheless have been rare isolated instances of partial recovery of the ability to communicate and function [71].

THE CLINICAL EFFECTS OF CHRONIC HYPOXIA

Less dramatic but incapacitating deficits may occur as the result of chronic hypoxia. Some decline in cognition has been observed when oxygen tension falls below 50 mm Hg [113]. Patients hypoxic from chronic congestive heart failure and chronic obstructive pulmonary disease or restrictive lung disease may have fatigue, lethargy, early morning headache, tremor, asterixis, and myoclonus [52].

In patients with chronic obstructive pulmonary disease, mild alterations in cognition correlate with the degree of oxygen desaturation [65,110]. A decrease in the speed of test performance, impairment in abstract reasoning, and memory loss are frequent, and such patients are particularly vulnerable to further compromise in intellectual function by sedative drugs.

Chronic hypoxia occurs in the syndrome of sleep apnea, snoring, and excessive daytime sleepiness that is associated with abnormalities of the genioglossus muscle and velopharyngeal sphincter [133]. In such patients obesity [141] and hereditary factors [96] may modify the level of hypoxic ventilatory drive. Hypoventilation and hypoxia have been observed in quadriplegic patients as a result of weakness of thoracic musculature [61]. Chronic hypoxia also occurs in the setting of cirrhosis from abnormal pulmonary vasculature and shunting of blood [137]. There is also evidence that premature airway closure and trapping of air during ventilation are responsible for the arterial hypoxia observed in cirrhotic patients [56].

THERAPY

The fundamental therapy for the treatment of ischemic-hypoxic injury is to correct the cause. Many other therapies have been advocated for brain injury of hypoxic-ischemic origin. None has been found to restore function without neurologic deficit. It has been thought that osmotic diuretics might be successful in cases of brain swelling after hypoxic injury. Judicious administration of sodium bicarbonate in correcting the acidosis associated with cardiac arrest may improve the outcome, although this therapy in the newborn may result in hypernatremia [123] and has been noted to induce a hyperosmolar state [92]. It may also have a deleterious effect on cardiac function [17]. Vasodilating drugs including carbon dioxide, papaverine, and beta-adrenergic blockers have not been found to be of value in improving outcome.

It is recognized that at the time of ischemic-hypoxic injury there is often an associated loss of autoregulation of cerebral circulation such that further injury may be induced by hypotension [95]. Although hypertension may afford some protection in animals [50,118], its likelihood of causing brain hemorrhage has limited this type of treatment. Other modalities of therapy include corticosteroids, hypothermia, hemodilution, barbiturates, naloxone, calcium channel blockers, and prostacyclin. There is some evidence against the effectiveness of any and all of these treatments.

Dexamethasone has been used in animal models of ischemic brain edema with equivocal results [76,122]. The precise mechanism of steroid effect in preventing edema is unclear. In humans, these compounds do not improve neurologic recovery [47,102]. The side effects of corticosteroids in patients with stroke are often severe and include a worsening of diabetes mellitus and a susceptibility to infection and gastrointestinal hemorrhage [101, 105].

Hypothermia provides some protection against experimental cerebral ischemic injury, particularly when it has preceded the event [117]. This mode of therapy has been used after near-drowning [41]. In animals, hypothermia improved reperfusion following ischemic brain injury [103]. Profound hypothermia (21°C) prevents the usual neuropathologic changes observed in ischemic condition; however, prolonged hypothermia is not without potential injury [125]. Young and co-workers [139] observed in animals that progressive hypothermia was associated with maintenance of ATP levels. The combination of barbiturate with experimental hypothermia may be more effective than either modality alone [87]. Some type of multimodal treatment may be helpful in future therapy; however, hypothermia treatment for ischemic brain injury in humans has yet to be clearly established. Initial reports raised hopes for hemodilution treatment in acute brain infarction [58,91,124]. Subsequently, a regimen of venesection and administration of low-molecular-weight dextran in humans produced slight improvement in the first 3 months after an ischemic event [127]. The role of this type of treatment remains uncertain.

Calcium channel blockers have been proposed as a treatment for hypoxic-ischemic brain injury based on the hypothesis discussed above that calcium loading of cells leads to necrosis. A randomized study has shown that the calcium channel blocker lidoflazine is not beneficial in treatment [30]. The commentary on this report pointed out that devastating effect of cardiac arrest on heart muscle survival could result in such severe morbidity as to prohibit the detection of a beneficial effect of lidoflazine (or any treatment for that matter) on brain [108].

REFERENCES

1. Adams, R. D., Victor, M., and Mancall, E. L. Central pontine myelinolysis: A hitherto undescribed disease occurring in alcoholic and malnourished patients. *Arch. Neurol. Psychiatry* 81:154, 1959.
2. Adler, S., Simplaceanu, V., and Ho, C. Brain pH in acute isocapnic metabolic acidosis and hypoxia: A ^{31}P-nuclear magnetic resonance study. *Am. J. Physiol.* 258:F34, 1990.
3. Alella, A., Williams, F. L., Williams, C. B., and Katz L. N. Interrelation between cardiac oxygen consumption and coronary blood flow. *Am. J. Physiol.* 183:570, 1955.
4. Altman, P. L., and Dittmer, D. S. Blood Oxygen Dissociation Curves: Mammals. In *Biology Data Book.* Bethesda, MD: Federation of American Societies for Experimental Biology, 1974.
5. Ames, A., III, Wright, R. L., and Kowaela, M. P. Cerebral ischemia: II. The no-reflow phenomenon. *Am. J. Pathol.* 52:437, 1968.
6. Androgue, H. J., Rashad, N., Gorin, A. B., et al. Assessing acid-base status in circulatory failure: Differences between arterial and central venous blood. *N. Engl. J. Med.* 320:1312, 1989.
7. Arieff, A. I. Hyponatremia, convulsions, respiratory arrest, and permanent brain damage after elective surgery in healthy women. *N. Engl. J. Med.* 314:1529, 1986.
8. Arieff, A. I. Hyponatremia associated with permanent brain damage. *Adv. Intern. Med.* 32:325, 1987.
9. Arieff, A. I. Pathogenesis of lactic acidosis. *Diabetes Metab. Rev.* 5(8):637, 1989.
10. Arieff, A. I., and Chidsey, C. A. Renal function in cirrhosis and the effects of prostaglandin A1. *Am. J. Med.* 56:695, 1974.
11. Arieff, A. I., Doerner, T., Zelig, H., and Massry, S. G. Mechanisms of seizures and coma in hypoglycemia. *J. Clin. Invest.* 54:654, 1974.
12. Arieff, A. I., and Fraser, C. L. Detrimental consequences of untreated hyponatremia in children. *Kidney Int.* 31:190, 1987.
13. Arieff, A. I., and Graf, H. Pathophysiology of type A hypoxic lactic acidosis in dogs. *Am. J. Physiol.* 253:E271, 1987.
14. Arieff, A. I., Leach, W., Park, R., and Lazarowitz, V. C. Systemic effects of $NaHCO_3$ in experimental lactic acidosis in dogs. *Am. J. Physiol.* 242(*Renal Fluid Electrolyte Physiol.* 11):F586, 1982.
15. Arieff, A. I., Park, R., Leach, W. J., and Lazarowitz, V. C. Pathophysiology of experimental lactic acidosis in dogs. *Am. J. Physiol.* 239:F135, 1980.
16. Armstead, W. M., Mirro, R., Busija, D. W., and Leffler, C. W. Postischemic generation of superoxide anion by newborn pig brain. *Am. J. Physiol.* 255:H401, 1988.
17. Ayus, J. C., and Krothapalli, R. K. Effect of bicarbonate administration on cardiac function. *Am. J. Med.* 87:5, 1989.
18. Ayus, J. C., Krothapalli, R. K., and Arieff, A. I. Sexual difference in survival with severe symptomatic hyponatremia. *Kidney Int.* 33:181, 1988.
19. Baim, D. S., Rothman, M. T., and Harrison, D. C. Simultaneous measurement of coronary venous blood flow and oxygen saturation during transient alterations in myocardial oxygen supply and demand. *Am. J. Cardiol.* 49:743, 1982.
20. Bartko, D. Some Aspects of the Course of Acute Cerebral Hypoxia. In *Experimental Brain Hypoxia.* Baltimore, MD: Universtiy Park Press, 1971.
21. Bates, D., Caronna, J. J., Cartledge, E. F., et al. A prospective study of nontraumatic coma: Methods and results in 310 patients. *Ann. Neurol.* 2:211, 1977.
22. Bedell, S. E., Delbanco, T. L., Cook, E. F., and Epstein, F. H. Survival after cardiopulmonary

resuscitation in the hospital. *N. Engl. J. Med.* 309(10):569, 1983.
23. Behar, K. L., Den Hollander, J. A. D., Stromski, M. E., et al. High-resolution 1H-nuclear magnetic resonance study of cerebral hypoxia in vivo. *Proc. Natl. Acad. Sci. U.S.A.* 80:4945, 1983.
24. Berry, M. N., and Scheuer, J. Splanchnic lactic acid metabolism in hyperventilation, metabolic alkalosis and shock. *Metabolism* 16:537, 1967.
25. Bersin, R. M. Effects of Sodium Bicarbonate on Myocardial Metabolism and Circulatory Function During Hypoxia. In *Hypoxia, Metabolic Acidosis and the Circulation.* New York: Oxford University Press, 1990.
26. Bersin, R. M., Chatterjee, K., and Arieff, A. I. Metabolic and hemodynamic consequences of sodium bicarbonate administration in patients with heart disease. *Am. J. Med.* 87:7, 1989.
27. Betz, A. L., Ennis, S. R., and Schielke, G. P. Blood-brain barrier sodium transport limits development of brain edema during partial ischemia in gerbils. *Stroke* 20(9):1253, 1989.
28. Bihari, D., Smithies, M., Gimson, A., and Tinker, J. The effects of vasodilation with prostacylin on oxygen delivery and uptake in critically ill patients. *N. Engl. J. Med.* 317:397, 1987.
29. Bjork, R. J., Snyder, B., Campion, B. C., and Loewenson, R. B. Medical complications of cardiopulmonary arrest. *Arch. Intern. Med.* 142:500, 1982.
30. Brain Resuscitation Clinical Trial II Study Group. A randomized clinical study of a calcium-entry blocker (lidoflazine) in the treatment of comatose survivors of cardiac arrest. *N. Engl. J. Med.* 324:1125, 1991.
31. Brierley, J. B. Experimental hypoxic brain damage. *J. Clin. Invest.* 30(11):181, 1977.
32. Brierley, J. B., and Brown, A. W. The threshold and neuropathology of cerebral "anoxic-ischemic" cell change. *Arch. Neurol.* 29:367, 1973.
33. Burcar, P. J., Norenberg, M. D., and Yarnell, P. R. Hyponatremia and central pontine myelinolysis. *Neurology* 27:223, 1977.
34. Cain, S. M. Oxygen delivery and uptake in dogs during anemic and hypoxic hypoxia. *J. Appl. Physiol.* 42:228, 1977.
35. Chan, P. H., and Fishman, R. A. Transient function of superoxide radicals in polyunsaturated fatty acid induced brain swelling. *J. Neurochem.* 35:1004, 1978.
36. Cheung, J. Y., Bonventre, J. V., Malis, C. D., and Leaf, A. Calcium and ischemic injury. *N. Engl. J. Med.* 314(26):1670, 1986.
37. Chiang, J., Kowada, M., Ames, A., III and Wright R. L. Cerebral ischemia: III. Vascular changes. *Am. J. Pathol.* 52:455:1968.
38. Cohen, R. D., and Woods, F. Lactic acidosis revisited. *Diabetes* 32:181, 1983.
39. Cohen, R. D., and Woods, H. F. Type A Lactic Acidosis. In *Clinical and Biochemical Aspects of Lactic Acidosis.* Oxford: Blackwell, 1976.
40. Collins, R. C., Dobkin, B. H., and Choi, D. W. Selective vulnerability of the brain: New insights into the pathophysiology of stroke. *Ann. Intern. Med.* 110(12):992, 1989.
41. Conn, A. W., Edmonds, J. F., and Baker, G. A. Near-drowing in cold fresh water: Current treatment regimen. *Can. Anaesth. Soc. J.* 25:259, 1978.
42. Daugherty, R. M., Scott, J. B., Dabney, J. M., and Haddy, F. J. Local effects of O_2 on limb, renal and coronary vascular resistances. *Am. J. Physiol.* 213:1102, 1967.
43. DelMaestro, R. F., Thaw, H. H., Bjork, J., et al. Free radicals as mediators of tissue injury. *Acta Physiol. Scand. [Suppl.]* 492:43, 1980.
44. Dienel, G. A. Regional accumulation of calcium in postischemic rat brain. *J. Neurochem.* 43:913, 1984.
45. Dobkin, B. H. Neuromedical complications in stroke patients transferred for rehabilitation before and after diagnostic related groups. *J. Neurol. Rehab.* 1:3, 1987.
46. Drewes, L. R., Gilboe, D. D., and Betz, A. L. Metabolic alterations in brain during anoxic-anoxia and subsequent recovery. *Arch. Neurol.* 29:385, 1973.
47. Dyken, M., and White, P. T. Evaluation of cortisone in the treatment of cerebral infarction. *J.A.M.A.* 162:1531, 1956.
48. Faden, A. I., Demediuk, P., Panter, S. S, and Vink, R. The role of excitatory amino acids and NMDA receptors in traumatic brain injury. *Science* 244:798, 1989.
49. Ferriero, D. M., Soberano, H. Q., Simon, R. P., and Sharp, F. R. Hypoxia-ischemia induces heat shock protein-like (HSP72) immunoreactivity in neonatal rat brain. *Dev. Brain Res.* 53:145, 1990.
50. Fischer, E. G., and Ames, A. III. Studies on mechanism of impairment of cerebral circulation following ischemia: Effect of hemodilution and perfusion pressure. *Stroke* 3:538, 1972.
51. Fischer, E. G., Ames, A., III, Heddey-Whyte, E. T., and O'Gorman, S. Reassessment of cerebral capillary changes in acute global ischemia and other relationship to the "no reflow phenomenon". *Stroke* 8:36, 1977.
52. Flenly, D. C. Clinical hypoxia: Causes, consequences and correction. *Lancet* 1:542, 1978.
53. Fraser, C. F., and Arieff, A. I. Hepatic encephalopathy: Current concepts. *N. Engl. J. Med.* 313:865, 1985.
54. Fraser, C. F., and Arieff, A. I. Fatal central diabetes mellitus and insipidus resulting from un-

treated hyponatremia: A new syndrome. *Ann. Intern. Med.* 112(2):113, 1990.
55. Fulop, M., Horowitz, M., Aberman, A., and Jaffe, E. R. Lactic acidosis in pulmonary edema due to left ventricular failure. *Ann. Intern. Med.* 79:180, 1973.
56. Furukawa, T., Nobuyuki, H., Yasumoto, K., and Inokushi, K. Arterial hypoxemia in patients with hepatic cirrhosis. *Am. J. Med. Sci* 287:10, 1984.
57. Garcia, J. H., Conger, K. A., Morawetz, R., and Halsey J. H., Jr. Postischemic Brain Edema: Quantitation and Evolution. In *Brain Edema: Pathology, Diagnosis, and Therapy.* New York: Raven, 1980.
58. Gilroy, J., Barnhart, M. I., and Meyer, J. S. Treatment of acute stroke with dextran 40. *J.A.M.A.* 210:293, 1969.
59. Ginsberg, M. D. Delayed neurological deterioration following hypoxia. *Adv. Neurol.* 26:21, 1979.
60. Ginsberg, M. D., Hedley-Whyte, E. T., and Richardson, E. P., Jr. Hypoxic-ischemic leukoencephalopathy in man. *Arch. Neurol.* 33:5, 1976.
61. Goldman, A. L., and George, J. Postural hypoxemia in quadriplegic patients. *Neurology* 26:815, 1976.
62. Gonzalez-Mendez, R., McNeill, A., Gregory, G. A., et al. Effects of hypoxic hypoxia on cerebral phosphate metabolites and pH in the anesthetized infant rabbit. *J. Cereb. Blood Flow Metab.* 5:512, 1985.
63. Gotoh, O., Asano, T., Koide, T., and Takakura, K. Ischemic brain edema following occlusion of the middle cerebral artery in the rat: I. The time courses of the brain water, sodium and potassium contents and blood-brain barrier permeability to ^{125}I albumin. *Stroke* 16(1):101, 1985.
64. Graf, H., Leach, W., and Arieff, A. I. Evidence for a detrimental effect of bicarbonate therapy in hypoxic lactic acidosis. *Science* 227:754, 1985.
65. Grant, I, Heaton, R. K., McSweeny, A. J., et al. Neuropsychologic findings in hypoxic chronic obstructive pulmonary disease. *Arch. Intern. Med.* 142:1470, 1982.
66. Guisado, R., Arieff, A. I., and Massry, S. G. Effects of glycerol administration on experimental brain edema. *Neurology* 26(1):69, 1976.
67. Guyton, C. Transport of Oxygen in the Blood. In *Textbook of Medical Physiology.* Philadelphia: Saunders, 1986.
68. Hallenbeck, J. M. Prevention of post-ischemic impairment of microvascular perfusion. *Neurology* 27:3, 1977.
69. Hawkins, R. Cerebral Energy Metabolism. In *Cerebral Energy Metabolism and Metabolic Encephalopathy.* New York: Plenum, 1985.
70. Heistad, D. D., and Abboud, F. M. Circulatory adjustments to hypoxia. *Circulation* 61:463, 1980.
71. Higashi, K., Sakata, Y., Hatano, M., et al. Epidemiological studies on patients with a persistent vegetative state. *J. Neurol. Neurosurg. Psychiatry* 40:876, 1977.
72. Higuchi, T., Naruse, S., Horikawa, Y., et al. Pathophysiological investigation of experimental cerebral ischaemia using in vivo 31P-NMR spectroscopy and 1H-MRI. *Acta Neurochir. [Suppl.] (Wien)* 43:172, 1988.
73. Hoffman, J. I. E. and Buckberg, G. D. The myocardial supply: demand ratio—A critical review. *Am. J. Cardiol.* 41:327, 1977.
74. Hoop, B., Masjedi, M. R., Shih, V. E., and Kazemi, H. Brain glutamate metabolism during hypoxia and peripheral chemodenervation. *J. Appl. Physiol.* 69(1):147, 1990.
75. Hope, P. L., Cady E. B., Delpy, D. T., et al. Brain metabolism and intracellular pH during ischaemia: Effects of systemic glucose and bicarbonate administration studied by 31P and 1H nuclear magnetic resonance spectroscopy in vivo in the lamb. *J. Neurochem.* 50(5):1394, 1988.
76. Hoppe, W. E., Waltz, A. G., Jordan, M. M., and Jacobson, R. I. Effects of dexamethasone on distribution of water and pertechnetate in brains of cats after middle cerebral artery occlusion. *Stroke* 5:617, 1974.
77. Hornbein, T. F., Townes, B. D., Schoene, R. B., et al. The cost to the central nervous system of climbing to extremely high altitude. *N. Engl. J. Med.* 321(25):1714, 1989.
78. Hossmann, K. A., Sakaki, S., and Zimmerman, V. Cation activities in reversible ischemia of the cat brain. *Stroke* 8(1):77, 1977.
79. Ikeda, M., Busto, R., Yoshida, S., et al. Cerebral phosphoinositide, triacylglycerol and energy metabolism during severe hypoxia and recovery. *Brain Res.* 459(2):344, 1988.
80. Jewett, B., and Plum, F. Persistent vegetative state after brain damage: A syndrome in search of a name. *Lancet* 1:734, 1972.
81. Jorgensen, E. O., and Malchow-Moller, A. Cerebral prognostic sign during cardiopulmonary resuscitation. *Resuscitation* 6:217, 1978.
82. Kaasik, A. E., Nilsson, L., and Siesjo, B. K. The effect of asphyxia upon the lactate, pyruvate and bicarbonate concentrations of brain tissue and cisternal CSF, and upon the tissue concentrations of phosphocreatine and adenine nucleotides in anesthetized rats. *Acta Physiol. Scand.* 78:433, 1970.
83. Kimelberg, H. K., Rose, J. W., Barron, K. D., et al. Astrocytic swelling in traumatic-hypoxic brain injury: Beneficial effects of an inhibitor of anion exchange transport and glutamate uptake in glial cells. *Mol. Chem. Neuropathol.* 11(1):1, 1989.

84. Kirschner, H. S., Blank, W. F., Jr., and Myers, R. E. Brain extracellular potassium activity during hypoxia in the cat. *Neurology* 25(11):1001, 1975.
85. Klatzo, I. Neuropathological aspects of brain edema. *J. Neuropathol Exp. Neurol.* 26:1, 1967.
86. Krigman, M. R., and Bouldin, T. W. Intoxications and Deficiency Diseases. Oxygen Deficiency: Brain Hypoxia and Ischemia. In *Neuropathology.* New York: Churchill Livingstone, 1983.
87. Lafferty, J. J., Keykhah, M. M., Shapiro, H. M., et al. Cerebral hypometabolism obtained with deep pentobarbital anesthesia and hypothermia (30°C). *Anesthesiology* 49:159, 1978.
88. Levy, D. E., Knill-Jones, R. P., and Plum, F. The vegatative state and its prognosis following nontraumatic coma. *Ann. N.Y. Acad. Sci.* 315:293, 1978.
89. Levy, D. E., Bates, D., Caronna, J. J., et al. Prognosis in nontraumatic coma. *Ann. Intern. Med.* 94(3):292, 1981.
90. Levy, D. E., Caronna, J. J., Singer, B. H., et al. Predicting outcome from hypoxic-ischemic coma. *J.A.M.A.* 253:1420, 1985.
91. Mathews, W. B., Oxbury, J. M., Granger, K. M. R., and Greenhal, R. C. D. A blind controlled trial of dextran 40 in the treatment of ischemic stroke. *Brain* 99:193, 1976.
92. Mattar, J. A., Weil, M. H., Shubin, H., and Stein. L. Hyperosmolar state. *Am. J. Med.* 56:162, 1974.
93. Mchedlishvili, G., and Bevan, J. A. Cerebral arterial behavior providing constant cerebral blood flow, pressure and volume. *Arterial Behavior and Blood Circulation in the Brain.* New York: Plenum, 1986.
94. Meyer, J. S. Gotoh, F., Ebihara, S., and Tomita, M. Effects of anoxia on cerebral metabolism and electrolytes in man. *Neurology* 15:892, 1965.
95. Miller, J. R., and Myers, R. E. Neurologic effects of systemic circulatory arrest in the monkey. *Neurology* 20:715, 1970.
96. Moore, G. C., Zwillich, C. W., Battaglia, J. D., et al. Respiratory failure associated with familial depression of ventilatory response to hypoxia and hypercapnia. *N. Engl. J. Med.* 295:861, 1976.
97. Murphy, D. J., Murray, A. M., Robinson, B. E., and Campion, E. W. Outcomes of cardiopulmonary resuscitation in the elderly. *Ann. Intern. Med.* 111(3):199, 1989.
98. Neubauer, J. A., Simone, A., and Edelman, N. H. Role of brain lactic acidosis in hypoxic depression of respiration. *J. Appl. Physiol.* 65(3):1324, 1988.
99. Newman, E. A. High potassium conductance in astrocyte effect. *Science* 233:453, 1986.
100. Norenberg, M. D., Leslie, K. O., and Robertson, A. S. Association between rise in serum sodium and central pontine myelinolysis. *Ann. Neurol.* 11:128, 1982.
101. Norris, J. W. Steroid therapy in acute cerebral infarction. *Arch. Neurol.* 33:69, 1976.
102. Norris, J. W., and Pappius, H. M. Cerebral water and electrolytes: Effect of asphyxia, hypoxia, and hypercapnia. *Arch. Neurol.* 23:248, 1970.
103. Norwood, W. I., Norwood, C. R., and Casteneda, A. R. Cerebral anoxia: Effect of deep hypothermia and pH. *Surgery* 86:203, 1979.
104. Olson, J., Sankar, R., Holtzman, D., James, A., and Fleischhaker, D. Energy-dependent volume regulation in primary cultured cerebral astrocytes. *J. Cell. Physiol.* 128:209, 1986.
105. Ottonello, G. A., and Primavera, A. Gastrointestinal complication of high-dose corticosteroid therapy in acute cerebrovascular patients. *Stroke* 10:208, 1979.
106. Papadakis, M. A., Fraser, C. L., and Arieff, A. I. Hyponatremia in patients with cirrhosis *Q. J. Med.,* 76:675, 1990.
107. Paulson, O. B., and Newman, E. A. Does the release of potassium from astrocyte endfeet regulate cerebral blood flow? *Science* 237:896, 1987.
108. Plum, F. Vulnerability of the brain and heart after cardiac arrest. *N. Engl. J. Med.* 324:1278, 1991.
109. Plum, F., Posner, J. B., and Hain, R. F. Delayed neurological deterioration after anoxia. *Arch. Intern. Med.* 110:18, 1962.
110. Prigatano, G. P., Parsons, O., Wright, E., et al. Neuropsychologic test performance in mildly hypoxemic patients with chronic obstructive pulmonary disease. *J. Consult. Clin. Psychol.* 51:108, 1983.
111. Pulsinelli, W. A., Brierley, J. B., and Plum, F. Temporal profile of neuronal damage in a model of transient forebrain ischemia. *Ann. Neurol.* 11:491, 1982.
112. Rappaport, Z. H., Young, W., and Flamm, E. S. Regional brain calcium changes in the rat middle cerebral artery occlusion model of ischemia. *Stroke* 18:760, 1987.
113. Refsum, H. E. Relationship between state of consciousness and arterial hypoxaemia and hypercapnia in patients with pulmonary insufficiency breathing air. *Clin. Sci.* 25:361, 1963.
114. Rehncrona, S., Abdul-Raman, A., and Seisjo, B. K. Local cerebral blood flow in the post ischemic period. *Acta Neurol. Scand.* 72:294, 1979.
115. Rosomoff, H. L., and Zugibe, F. T. Distribution of intracranial contents in experimental edema. *Arch. Neurol.* 9:36, 1963.
116. Rothman, S. M. Synaptic activity mediates death of hypoxic neurons. *Science* 220:536, 1983.

117. Rueler, J. B. Hypothermia: Pathophysiology, clinical settings and management. *Ann. Intern. Med.* 89:519, 1978.
118. Safar, P., Stezosko, S. W., and Nemoto, E. M. Amelioration of brain damage after 12 minutes cardiac arrest in dogs. *Arch. Neurol.* 33:91, 1976.
119. Schettini, A., and Walsh, E. K. Brain tissue elastic behavior and experimental brain compression. *Am. J. Physiol.* 255:R799, 1988.
120. Scriabine, A., and van der Kerckhoff, W. Pharmacology of nimodipine: A review. *Ann. N. Y. Acad. Sci.* 522:698, 1988.
121. Shepherd, A. P., Granger, H. J., Smith, E. E., and Guyton, A. C. Local control of tissue oxygen delivery and its contribution to the regulation of cardiac output. *Am. J. Physiol.* 225:747, 1973.
122. Siegel, B. A., Studer, R. K., and Potchen, E. J. Steroid therapy of brain edema. *Arch. Neurol.* 27:209, 1972.
123. Simmons, M. A., Adcock, E. W., Bard, H., and Battaglia, F. C. Hypernatremia and intracranial hemorrhage in neonates. *N. Engl. J. Med.* 291:6, 1974.
124. Spudis, E. V., de al Torre, E., and Pikula, L. Management of completed stroke with dextran 40: A community hospital failure. *Stroke* 4:895, 1973.
125. Steen, P. A., Soule, E. H., and Michenfelder, J. D. Detrimental effect of prolonged hypothermia in cats with and without regional cerebral ischemia. *Stroke* 10:522, 1979.
126. Sterns, R. H., Riggs, J. E., and Schochet, S. S. Osmotic demyelination syndrome following correction of hyponatremia. *N. Engl. J. Med.* 314:1535, 1986.
127. Strand, T., Asplume, K., Eriksson, S., et al. A randomized controlled trail of hemodilution therapy in acute ischemic stroke. *Stroke* 15:980, 1984.
128. Sulaga-Pechtel, K., Goldberg, E., Strickson, P., et al. Cardiopulmonary resuscitation in a hospitalized population: Prospective study of factors associated with outcome. *Resuscitation* 12:77, 1984.
129. Tomlinson, B. E., Pierides, A. M., and Bradley, W. G. Central pontine myelinolysis: Two cases with associated electrolyte disturbance. *Q. J. Med.* 179:373, 1976.
130. Vink, R., McIntosh, T. K., Demediuk, P., et al. Decline in intracellular free Mg^{2+} is associated with irreversible tissue injury after brain trauma. *J. Biol. Chem.* 263(2):757, 1988.
131. Wacker, W. E. C., and Parisi, A. F. Magnesium metabolism. *N. Engl. J. Med.* 278:658, 1968.
132. Wantanabe, O., West, C. R., and Bremer, A. Experimental regional cerebral ischemia in the middle cerebral artery territory in primates: Part 2. Effects on brain water and electrolytes in the early phase of MCA stroke. *Stroke* 8(1):71, 1977.
133. Weitzman, E., Pollack, C., Borowiecki, B., et al. The Hypersomnia-Sleep Apnea Syndrome: Site and Mechanism of Upper Airway Obstruction. In C. Guilleminault and C. Dement (eds.), *Sleep Apnea Syndromes.* New York: Liss, 1978. P. 235.
134. Wells, R. M. G. The control of hemoglobin-oxygen binding in vertebrate animals. *News in Physiological Sciences* 4:242, 1989.
135. West, J. B. Acid-Base Status and Blood Lactate at Extreme Altitude. In *Hypoxia, Metabolic Acidosis and the Circulation.* New York: Oxford University Press, 1990.
136. White, R. E., and Hartzell, H. C. Effects of intracellular free magnesium on calcium current in isolated cardiac myocytes. *Science* 239:778, 1988.
137. Wolfe, J. D., Tashkin, D. P., and Holly, F. E. Hypoxemia of cirrhosis detection of abnormal small pulmonary vascular channels by a quantative radionuclide method. *Am. J. Med.* 63:746, 1977.
138. Wolman, L. Ischaemic lesions in the brain-stem associated with raised intracranial pressure. *Brain* 76:364, 1953.
139. Young, R. S. K., Olenginski, T. P., Yagel, S. K., and Towfighi, J. The effect of graded hypothermia in hypoxic-ischemic brain damage: A neuropathologic study in the neonatal rat. *Stroke* 14:929, 1983.
140. Zilva, J. F. The origin of the acidosis in hyperlactataemia. *Ann. Clin. Biochem.* 15:40, 1978.
141. Zwillich, C. W., Sutton, F. D., Pierson, J. D., et al. Decreased hypoxic ventilatory drive in the obesity-hypoventilation syndrome. *Am. J. Med.* 59:343, 1975.

4 Central Nervous System Manifestations of Hyponatremia

John Kucharczyk, Cosmo Lyle Fraser, and Allen I. Arieff

Hyponatremia is the most common electrolyte abnormality encountered in a general hospital population, with an incidence of about 1.0 percent. It is often seen in association with many different systemic disease states and represents a major public health problem with regard to morbidity and mortality. Hyponatremia is almost always the result of dilution, but the disorder may be either acute or chronic, and total body water may be high, low, or normal. In general, the causes of hyponatremia fall into nine major groups, depending on the patient's volume status, as well as the underlying causes [10].

In an overview, the major cause of hyponatremic encephalopathy is an osmotic imbalance between extracellular fluid and brain cells, leading to net movement of water into the brain with resultant cerebral edema. In most cases, the condition will be resolved, but if hyponatremia persists, the brain swelling will exert pressure upon the rigid skull. This can lead to pressure necrosis, and if the brain expands by more than about 5 percent of its volume [87], there will be possible cerebral herniation [80,81]. Whereas such a sequence doubtless plays a role in the pathogenesis of hyponatremic encephalopathy, it has recently become obvious that there are other major contributing factors. Studies have demonstrated that several steroid and peptide hormones can cause water movement in the central nervous system in the absence of a low serum sodium [167,174]. These include gonadal sex hormones, such as progesterone, estrogen, and testosterone, and vasoactive neuropeptides, such as vasopressin, atrial natriuretic peptide, and angiotensin [82,83]. These hormones have long been known to have widespread and diverse effects on body fluid-electrolyte homeostasis [111], but their involvement in the pathogenesis of symptomatic hypo-

Supported by the Research Service of the Veterans Affairs Medical Center, San Francisco, California.

natremia and hyponatremic encephalopathy has only recently come under investigation.

When hyponatremia occurs, the brain has only two basic responses: adaptation by a loss of osmotically active solute (primarily Na^+ and K^+) or gain in water. It is apparent that the latter can lead to brain edema, cerebral damage, possible herniation, and in some cases death. Solute extrusion, on the other hand, can minimize or altogether prevent cerebral injury associated with hypo-osmolar states. The pathogenesis of hyponatremic encephalopathy thus appears to involve an imbalance between selective loss of solute versus gain of water. The major objective of this chapter is to examine the multiple interactive factors that influence ion and water homeostasis in the central nervous system during severe symptomatic hyponatremia.

BRAIN LESIONS IN PATIENTS WITH SYMPTOMATIC HYPONATREMIA

Brain Pathology in Symptomatic Hyponatremia

Very few neuropathologic studies in patients who died of hyponatremia have been reported [13]. In one of the first published cases, the brain of a postoperative patient who had absorbed (rectally) 9 liters of tap water (serum sodium less than 110 mM) was studied 1 hour after death [96]. There was obliteration of the subarachnoid space, flattening of the cerebral gyri, obliteration of the sulci, and uniform swelling of the brain, and the ventricles were reduced in size. Microscopically, there was increased vacuolization and swelling of supportive (glial) structures, with cellular swelling confined to white matter. In more recent studies, brain edema with uncal and tonsillar herniation has been found in patients with symptomatic hyponatremia [80]. The primary lesion, however, is diffuse cerebral demyelination secondary to increased intracranial pressure and hypoxic brain damage. The hypoxic brain damage is caused by several factors, including a decrement in cerebral blood flow secondary to brain edema [176], as well as respiratory insufficiency or arrest caused by cerebral herniation leading to compression of the medullary respiratory centers [80]. The increased intracranial pressure can lead to ischemic lesions of the midbrain and pons [77,238], and these ischemic lesions are often mistakenly diagnosed as central pontine myelinolysis, even in the absence of pontine lesions {210,241].

Several investigators have studied the effects of acute water intoxication on brain in experimental animals. Considerably less swelling was found in the brain than in other tissues (liver, muscle). Edema was present in both gray and white matter of brain but was most pronounced in white matter. The blood-brain barrier was generally intact. Herniation is often the final event leading to death after acute water intoxication [12,14,17,18,22,80]. Hyponatremia may affect brain function and lead to permanent damage in a number of ways. The initial symptoms of symptomatic hyponatremia are probably due to brain swelling, with a secondary increase of intracranial pressure. The brain can expand by only about 5 percent of its volume because of the confines of the rigid skull [87]. Expansion by more than 5 percent leads to an enormous rise in intracranial pressure, resulting in a redistribution of intracranial contents, with loss of both blood and cerebrospinal fluid (CSF) from the brain [176]. With more prolonged hyponatremia, brain compensation leads to depletion of the intracellular content of Na^+, K^+, and perhaps amino acids, thereby limiting the increase in brain cell volume [16,134,177, 224]. The loss of brain Na^+ and K^+ may result in both inhibition in brain energy metabolism and interference with neurotransmitter (amino acid) release at the synaptic level. These changes may affect brain function and may in part be responsible for the encephalopathy of hyponatremia.

It has been suggested that symptomatic hyponatremia or its treatment with hypertonic NaCl may lead to central pontine myelinolysis (CPM), a rare neurologic disorder of uncertain etiology that was initially described in alcoholic malnourished subjects [130,135,147,225,241]. The lesion described in patients with CPM [1] involved the mediobasal pons and often extended from midbrain anteriorly to the nuclei of cranial nerves in the lower pons. Most medullary sheaths were destroyed within the area of the lesion. The destruction of myelin involved all tracts, but in contrast to the complete destruction of myelin, axis cylinders, nerve cells, and blood vessels were relatively well preserved [1].

In three large series of autopsied patients, the incidence of CPM has ranged from 0.17 to 0.28 percent, with a mean of about 23 cases per 10,000 autopsies [90,132,241]. Some patients with CPM may also have symmetric extrapontine demyelinating lesions [241], but these lesions may well be due to other disease processes. In earlier studies, CPM was generally diagnosed only by autopsy, but more recently radiologic criteria employing computed tomography (CT) or magnetic resonance imaging (MRI) of the brain have been utilized [138,218,225]. There have been considerable discussion and controversy about whether treatment of symptomatic hyponatremia with hypertonic NaCl may lead to central pontine myelinolysis. A recent study using autopsy, CT, and MRI data [19] found that most patients with symptomatic hyponatremia do not have CPM but are frequently misdiagnosed initially. However, in recent years the diagnosis of CPM has been ascribed to patients with pontine, extrapontine, and both pontine and extrapontine demyelinating lesions and even to patients with clinical manifestations similar to patients with CPM but lacking confirmation of central pontine demyelination by autopsy, CT, or MRI [147, 210]. To avoid such confusion, the term *cerebral demyelinating lesion* should be used to mean any cerebral demyelination that is confirmed by autopsy, MRI, or CT scanning, including both pontine and extrapontine myelinolysis. Patients with functional neurologic impairment without confirmed demyelinating lesions should not be considered to have either CPM or cerebral demyelinating lesions [21,80].

Because of the confines of the rigid skull, the brain is able to expand by only about 5 percent of its volume [87] before compression occurs [176]. When brain swelling exceeds about 5 percent of brain volume, herniation may occur, leading to a symptom complex that may include unequal pupils, fixed dilated pupils, hypoventilation, cardiovascular instability, impaired temperature regulation, urinary and/or fecal incontinence, and respiratory arrest [12,77,80,160]. Hypoxic brain damage will usually develop [238], and there may also be delayed postanoxic encephalopathy [12,161]. Increased intracranial pressure may lead to damage to other brain structures such as the pituitary gland, hypothalamus, or cranial nerves [80,160].

Permanent brain damage in such patients is virtually always associated with hypoxic injury, which is largely secondary to decreased tissue oxygenation after respiratory insufficiency or arrest [13,238]. The reported changes include anoxic lesions of the cerebellum, medulla, hypothalamus, pituitary, pons, and basal ganglia. Neurologic sequelae described in patients who have survived symptomatic hyponatremia are shown in Table 4-1.

Table 4-1. Neurologic sequelae of hyponatremia

Persistent vegetative state
Cortical blindness
Double vision
Dementia
Varying degrees of mental retardation
Varying degrees of motor impairment
Paralysis of arms and/or legs
Pituitary infarction with central diabetes mellitus and/or central diabetes insipidus
Quadriparesis
Deafness
Bulbar palsy
Dysarthria

Adaptation of the Brain to Hyponatremia: Effects on Brain Water, Electrolytes, and Structure

Adaptation of the brain to hyponatremia involves a redistribution of intracranial contents (Fig. 4-1). Initially, there is a loss of brain content of both blood and CSF so that brain water is increased much less than might otherwise occur [176]. The increase in intracranial pressure is also less than expected because when the brain expands, there are changes in its nonlinear elastic parameters. However, if intracranial pressure remains elevated, brain displacement and eventually herniation can occur [187].

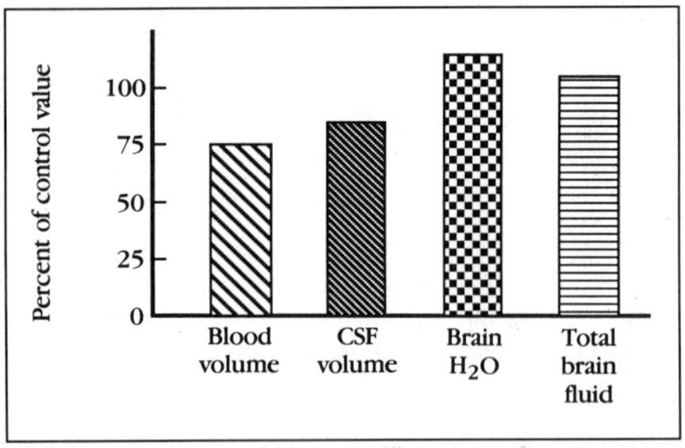

Fig. 4-1. The total intracranial fluid contents in hyponatremic brain as a percent of the control value. With hyponatremia, there is brain swelling with increased brain water, resulting in a decrease of both blood and CSF volume. The net result is that total brain fluid content is only minimally altered, but at the expense of a substantial decrease of cerebral blood flow. This leads to cerebral hypoxia. (Data from Rosomoff and Zugibe [176].)

Following the redistribution of intracranial contents, additional compensatory mechanisms can be activated (Fig. 4-2). Efflux of osmotically active cation (sodium and potassium plus cationic amino acids) [82,224] and gain of water can act to decrease brain intracellular osmolality and thereby minimize the increase in brain water. While both processes promote a reduction in brain intracellular osmolality, the balance between loss of solute versus gain of water effectively determines survival of the organism. For example, if plasma sodium in rabbits is lowered from 140 to 120 mEq/liter in 3 hours, there is 100 percent mortality, due principally to gain in brain water without loss of cation [18]. However, if the same change in plasma sodium occurs in rats and rabbits over 3 days, the brain loses cation (both Na^+ and K^+) and lowers its intracellular osmolality without a substantial

Fig. 4-2. Diagram showing adaptation of brain to hyponatremia. Following the diagram from the top left: (a) Infusion of hypontonic fluid leads to a fall in plasma osmolality from 285 to 225 mOsm/kg. (b) Because water freely moves across cell membranes and all compartments in the body must be in osmotic equilibrium, water moves into brain cells, resulting in a fall of brain osmolality from 285 to 225 mOsm/kg. The fall in brain osmolality can occur by either of two modalities, usually in combination: (c) a gain in water, resulting in brain swelling (*top right*); or (d) a loss of osmotically active solute, primarily Na and K, by various active transport mechanisms (*middle right*). The resolution of (c) versus (d) determines the extent of brain edema in response to hyponatremia.

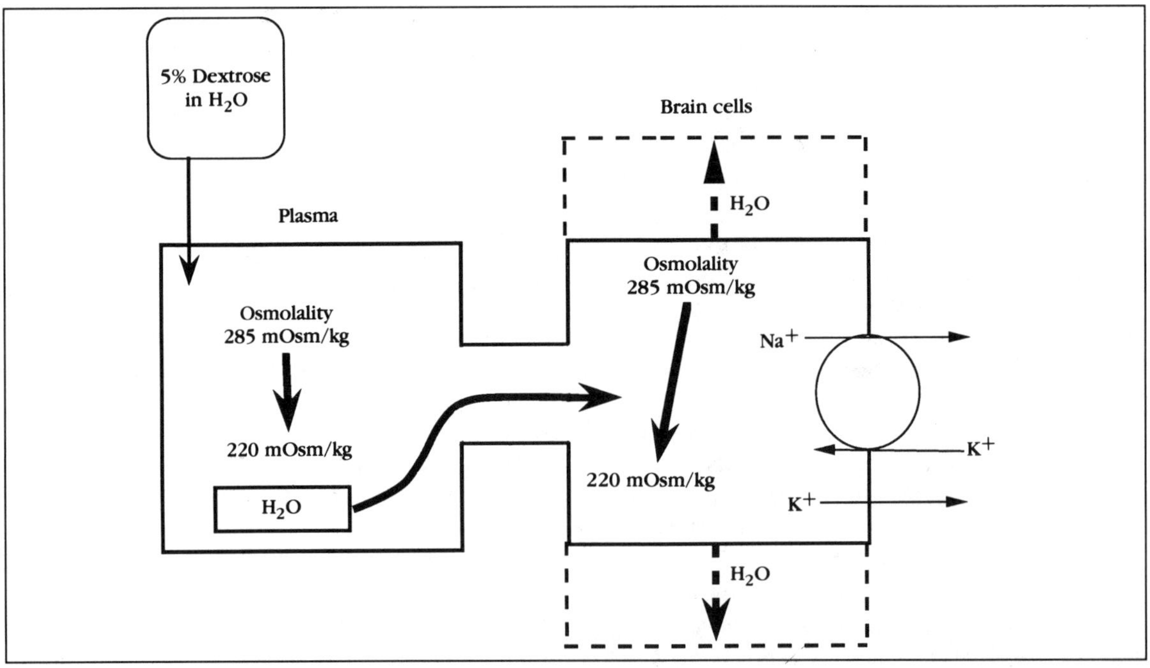

gain in water, with less than 30 percent mortality [18].

Although the mechanism of loss of cation from brain cells in hyponatremia is not totally understood, it probably has both active (related to a sodium-potassium pump) and passive (ouabain insensitive) components [82,83]. There are also doubtless specific sodium and potassium channels involved, as well as activation of the Na^+/H^+ antiporter system (7,145,150,184, 188]. In other cell types (lymphocytes, Ehrlich cells), there is a potassium conductive pathway that results in a loss of cell potassium when cells are placed in a hypo-osmotic medium [91,98]. In hypo-osmolar states, the passive component of potassium influx is also reduced [91], which would tend to increase loss of potassium from brain cells. When either the active component (probably Na^+-K^+ATPase mediated efflux) of sodium efflux, or the potassium conductive pathways are inhibited, sodium and potassium loss from the brain is impaired, leading to increase brain swelling with a higher morbidity [151].

Varying degrees of hyponatremia have been studied in several different animal species [11,16,18,47,121,134]. In general, the increase in brain water content seems to be greatest in animals with more symptomatic hyponatremia (1–4 hours). During more protracted hyponatremia, on the other hand, the increase in brain water content is lower than that predicted by the severity of hyponatremia and also lower than that seen in other tissues. Thus, the actual increase in brain water content in response to hyponatremia is determined both by the chronicity of hyponatremia and ability of the brain to extrude Na^+ and K^+ (Fig. 4-2). In animals made acutely hyponatremic (1–2 hours), brain water content is substantially elevated but the electrolyte content (mmol/kg dry weight) is only minimally decreased. By comparison, in chronic hyponatremia, there is a significant fall in brain content of Na^+, K^+, and Cl^-, which is proportional to the fall in serum sodium level, whereas water content is only minimally altered [18]. Moreover, in chronic hyponatremia the observed decrement in brain content of sodium and potassium results in a substantial decline in brain osmolality [18]. When similar degrees of hyponatremia are induced over a period of several days, brain osmolality falls progressively, eventually reaching levels similar to plasma. Recent evidence suggests that these compensatory mechanisms are more effective in males than in females [22,82,83].

As previously stated, in acutely water-intoxicated animals, the effects of hyponatremia on brain function are related to the early onset of cerebral edema, which occurred before the brain was able to undergo compensatory changes. Under these conditions, therapy in hyponatremic patients must be directed toward achieving an acute elevation in plasma osmolarity, which is necessary to decrease brain volume. An osmotic gradient of at least 25 mOsm/kg between plasma and brain appears to be necessary to promote an acute net loss or gain of water from the brain [17,208]. Thus, treatment of hyponatremia with water restriction or infusion of isotonic solutions (154 mM NaCl or Ringer's lactate) would not be expected to shrink acutely an already swollen brain.

Symptoms of Hyponatremia

The symptoms of hyponatremia are dependent on several factors, which include the age and sex of the patient as well as the etiology, magnitude, and acuteness of the condition. The symptoms of water intoxication are related to the age and sex of the individual, as well as the extent of the fall in serum Na^+ and the rapidity with which the serum Na^+ is lowered [81]. Neurologic manifestations of acute water intoxication may be observed when the plasma Na^+ is below 130 mM [80]. These include headache, nausea, and emesis in the vast majority of cases, as well as additional possible symptoms, which are shown in Table 4-2. More severe symptoms such as grand mal seizures, respiratory arrest, and coma occur in a substantial but undetermined number of patients. In general, symptoms are more severe and occur at a higher level of serum Na^+ in premenopausal women than in either men or postmenopausal women [22,81,209]. Symptomatic hyponatremia with plasma Na^+ below 120 mM is associated with mortality above 50 percent and substantial morbidity. However, when plasma Na^+ is lowered

Table 4-2. Symptoms of hyponatremia

Headache
Nausea
Emesis
Hallucinations (auditory and/or visual)
Urinary and/or fecal incontinence
Extrapyramidal-type reaction
Decorticate/decerebrate posturing
Fixed dilated pupils
Unilateral dilated pupil
Decreasing responsiveness
Lethargy
Weakness
Bradycardia
Hypoventilation
Respiratory depression
Respiratory arrest
Clonus
Seizure activity (focal or grand mal)

more slowly (several days to several weeks) to 120 mM or less in elderly subjects by a combination of salt depletion (often diuretic induced) and water ingestion, patients usually are less symptomatic. Male or postmenopausal female patients whose plasma sodium is above 120 mM are usually not symptomatic, and morbidity and mortality are minimal.

Patients with more protracted hyponatremia generally have less severe symptoms and a lower morbidity and mortality than patients with acute water intoxication. However, since chronic hyponatremia is more common in both men and elderly women, this may reflect the age, sex, and hormonal status of the patient rather than the degree or duration of the hyponatremia. Chronic hyponatremia is commonly observed in patients with any of several edematous states, such as congestive heart failure, nephrotic syndrome, renal insufficiency, or liver failure. In all these conditions, both total body water and Na^+ tend to be increased. It is also frequently seen in patients with the syndrome of inappropriate secretion of antidiuretic hormone (SIADH), which may be caused by tumors (which secrete ADH or similarly acting peptides), as well as a large variety of diseases of either the central nervous system, gastrointestinal system, or lungs. Among hospitalized patients, an SIADH-like syndrome is commonly seen in association with the administration of various drugs, including oral hypoglycemics, tricyclic antidepressant agents, certain anticancer agents, diuretics, clofibrate, and morphine-like analgesics. More protracted hyponatremia may also be seen in patients with salt-losing states, such as salt-losing renal disease, idiosyncratic reaction to diuretics, excessive sweating, Addison's disease, acquired immunodeficiency syndrome (AIDS), or gastrointestinal electrolyte loss. It has been reported in patients ingesting massive quantities of beer [59].

Chronic hyponatremia in children is less frequent, although acute water intoxication with seizures as well as SIADH syndromes have been described [51,52,228]. In unselected hyponatremic patients, the degree of hyponatremia does not always correlate with the severity of symptoms. Patients with serum Na^+ of 110 mM may be asymptomatic, while others whose Na^+ is as high as 128 mM may present in frank coma. The mental status of 65 consecutive hospitalized hyponatremic patients whose plasma sodium was 128 mM or less is plotted against plasma sodium in Figure 4-3. In general there is a good correlation, albeit with considerable overlap. Ubiquitously, however, when plasma sodium is below 120 mM, most patients are symptomatic with some depression of sensorium, and many have seizures. In this and other previous studies, age and sex were not taken into account.

HYPONATREMIA IN PATIENTS WITH LIVER DISEASE

Hyponatremia is a common disorder in patients with liver disease [15,32,153], and it is almost always associated with excessive retention of free water. Regardless of the volume status in such patients, the total body exchangeable cation (potassium + sodium) is "diluted" by relatively greater amounts of total body water [71]. Even in the setting of hypo-osmolality, ADH levels are not suppressed, which they normally would be. This may represent an effort to conserve "effective" intravascular volume [30,32,191,192,193], since physiologic regulations to maintain volume status generally super-

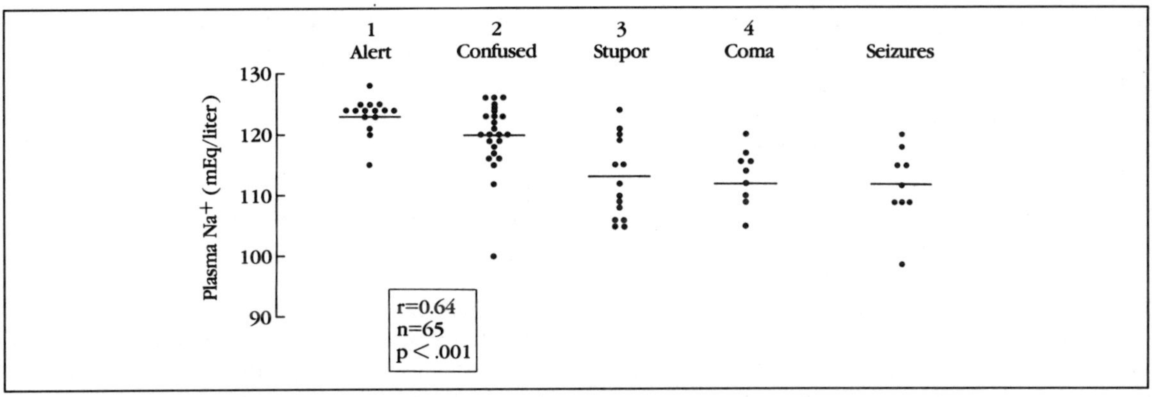

Fig. 4-3. The relationship between serum sodium (Na^+) and depression of sensorium in 65 consecutive patients with hyponatremia ($Na^+ \leq 128$ mEq/liter). (From Arieff, Llach, and Massry [18]. Copyright by Williams & Wilkins, 1976.)

cede the regulation of osmolality. In cirrhosis, a major mechanism for dilutional hyponatremia is the impaired ability of the kidneys to excrete free water [30]. Additionally, it is rare to lose any body fluid (such as urine, diarrhea, emesis) that is hypertonic with respect to the plasma sodium. Thus, hyponatremia can occur in patients with cirrhosis who are treated with either thiazide diuretics or large amounts of aldosterone-inhibiting agents, such as spironolactone. In patients with cirrhosis and hyponatremia, ADH levels are already elevated from nonosmotic stimuation, presumed to be secondary to decreased effective blood volume [30,31, 191,192].

Although the major cause of hyponatremia in liver disease is primarily dilutional, an etiologic component may be related to potassium deficiency. Edelman and associates [71] derived the following equation for the determination of serum sodium ($Na^+{}_s$):

$$(Na^+{}_s) = \frac{(K^+{}_e) + (Na^+{}_e)}{\text{TB } H_2O}$$

Serum sodium ($Na^+{}_s$) is thus a function of the total exchangeable sodium ($Na^+{}_e$), total exchangeable potassium ($K^+{}_e$), and total body (TB) water [32,71]. Reexamination of the original data demonstrates that in patients who had cirrhosis and ascites but were also hyponatremic, total body sodium and water were both within the normal range. However, total body potassium was significantly below control values. Thus, according to the above formula, the subjects are hyponatremic because of a deficiency of total body potassium stores and not because of an excess of total body water or low total body sodium. There are many possible reasons for the low body potassium. These include (1) loss of lean body mass (muscle) and replacement with fluid (ascites); (2) increased urinary potassium losses because of diuretic therapy or increased mineralocorticoid effect; (3) gastrointestinal losses of potassium (emesis and diarrhea) [153].

Despite the proposed theoretic relationship between hyponatremia and total exchangeable potassium, we are not aware of any clinical studies where potassium replacement has successfully corrected hyponatremia. On this basis, potassium replacement cannot be recommended as therapy for hyponatremia in patients with cirrhosis.

DIFFERENTIAL DIAGNOSIS OF HYPONATREMIC ENCEPHALOPATHY

In a patient who suddenly develops a symptom complex that can include opisthotonos, respiratory depression, impaired response to verbal or painful stimuli, bizarre behavior, incontinence of urine or feces, visual auditory hallucinations, lethargy, decorticate and decerebrate posturing, and seizure activity, the differential diagnosis is quite extensive. Patients with symptomatic hyponatremia may also develop respiratory arrest, fixed dilated pupils, and abnormal temperature regulation within 24 hours [81]. The respiratory arrest may be diagnosed as being related to the administration of morphine or meperidine (Demerol). However, in a generally healthy postoperative individual, although some respiratory depression may occur from a therapeutic dose of meperidine or morphine, respiratory arrest is extraordinarily rare. In patients with hyponatremia, there has been no response to the intravenous administration of naloxone hydrochloride (Narcan) [80]. Furthermore, following an overdose of morphine or meperidine, the pupils are constricted (pinpoint), while patients with hyponatremia and herniation often develop dilated pupils. The decorticate and decerebrate posturing is frequently diagnosed as a reaction to phenothiazine drugs (promazine [Sparine], promethazine hydrochloride [Phenergan], or prochlorperazine [Compazine]), which have been administered for nausea. These have been treated by discontinuing the agent and administrating diphenhydramine hydrochloride (Benadryl) or benztropine mesylate (Cogentin), again without any response. The sudden obtundation has occasionally been diagnosed as acute viral encephalitis, but this can generally be ruled out by examination of the CSF. However, the fixed dilated pupils are often thought to be indicative of brain death, and largely for this reason, many patients have received no therapy for their low serum sodium. However, in the presence of brain death, pupils are fixed and midpoint, not dilated [201]. The fixed dilated pupils are most likely caused by cerebral herniation, with pressure of the temporal lobe on the third cranial nerve or occlusion of the posterior cerebral artery near the third nerve. Many patients develop some combination of unilateral and then bilateral dilated pupils, absent pain response, apnea, and positive Babinski's sign. These signs and symptoms are frequently interpreted as being consistent with various drug reactions (see above) or acute intracranial events, such as subarachnoid bleeding episodes. Acute intracranial episodes can and should be ruled out by CT scan or MRI of the head. All of these events are consistent with acutely progressive brain herniation, and this can generally be diagnosed by modern imaging techniques (CT scan or MRI) [62,110].

DELAYED POSTANOXIC ENCEPHALOPATHY ASSOCIATED WITH HYPONATREMIA

An association between hyponatremia and CPM has been suggested by some investigators, but more recent studies have demonstrated that the brain lesions associated with hyponatremia (hyponatremic encephalopathy) are largely attributable to a combination of hypoxia, herniation, and pressure necrosis [14]. Demyelination is usually secondary to anoxia-hypoxia or increased intracranial pressure [238], and the clinical manifestations are sometimes delayed, giving a false appearance of some relationship to therapy. In a recent study, seven women developed a second episode of recurrent seizures and coma after correction of severe symptomatic hyponatremia [12]. In all cases, the second episode occurred while the serum sodium was above 128 mM. There have been a few additional cases described in hyponatremic patients that appear to be similar [240]. Four women had hyponatremia associated with acute polyneuropathy [162] and suffered cardiopulmonary arrest, and seven similar cases were reviewed. Among these 11 cases, the mean serum sodium (± SD) was 109 ± 8 mM. The clinical picture thus closely resembles the syndrome of delayed postanoxic encephalopathy that occurs after other causes of hypoxia-anoxia [88,89,161]. Figure 4-4 shows the clinical course of seven patients who had severe symptomatic hyponatremia and developed hypoxic brain damage following a respiratory arrest. Although only recently recognized as being associated with hyponatremia, hypoxic brain damage appears to be an important factor in the neurologic disability observed in some hyponatremic subjects [13]. The syndrome of delayed postanoxic encephalopathy has been known at least since 1925 [88,161]. This disorder can follow anoxia-hypoxia from any cause, but most reported cases were related to either carbon monoxide intoxication, attempted strangulation, cardio-

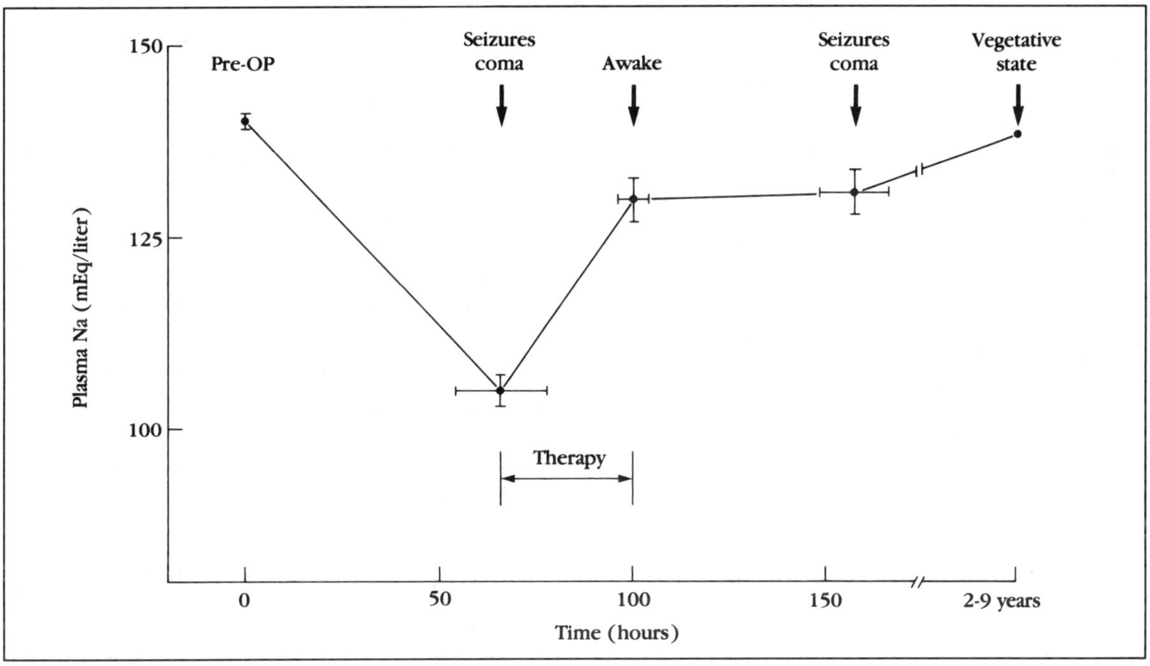

Fig. 4-4. The clinical course of seven women who developed symptomatic postoperative hyponatremia (serum sodium < 128 mM) but were treated and awoke. These seven patients again lapsed into coma, while their serum sodium was above 128 mM at all times. All had suffered a respiratory arrest prior to institution of therapy. The rate of correction of serum sodium was below 0.7 mmol/liter/hour in all cases. The patients suffered delayed postanoxic encephalopathy and did not recover. All either died or suffered permanent brain damage. (From Arieff [12].)

pulmonary arrest, or various miscellaneous intoxications. The clinical characteristics of this condition have been well described [88]. Whatever the cause, patients are initially deeply comatose, often requiring artificial ventilation. Characteristically, they begin to regain consciousness within 1 to 3 days. Initial improvement may be rapid enough that patients are discharged from the hospital within a week of the initial intoxication. As early as a day or as late as several weeks later, patients begin to relapse. The onset may be abrupt and heralded by disorientation, confusion, restlessness, apathy, and irritability, often with agitation, mania, or other inappropriate behavior. There may be cortical dysfunction that is multifocal in character, with dysphasias, agnosias, and apraxias. Motor control is impaired, with resultant rigidity or spasticity.

There are no obvious features during the intial anoxic insult that serve to distinguish those patients destined to relapse from those who have uncomplicated recoveries. Many such patients are initially misdiagnosed and are felt to have primary cerebral pathology, such as subdural hematoma. In hyponatremic patients, the diagnosis of postanoxic encephalopathy must be made on clinical grounds but appears to be the most likely cause of the recurrent seizures and coma, with death or a permanent neurologic disability a frequent outcome. A frequent clinical scenario has been reported among patients with symptomatic hyponatremia. These individuals have been treated (usually with hypertonic NaCl) and appeared to improve [147,210,225]. However, after several days, they deteriorated and often did not survive. At autopsy, these patients often had demyelinating lesions of the brain, sometimes including the pons [147,225]. Due to superficial anatomic similarity to CPM, such patients were diagnosed with CPM [210], even though the distribution of lesions invariably involved many other parts of the brain in an asymmetric manner [19].

The situation is further complicated by the fact that CPM is most commonly seen in subjects with cirrhosis, and such patients also have a high incidence of hyponatremia [152,153]. Thus, in patients with the combination of cirrhosis, hyponatremia, and neurologic deterioration, the cerebral demyelinating lesions found at autopsy were often mistakenly diagnosed as related to the "therapy" of hyponatremia [147], even in the absence of such therapy [13,21,135]. In fact, the deterioration several days after therapy was virtually always associated with a hypoxic event, usually respiratory embarrassment that occurred *before* treatment[12,13,210], and the clinical picture and neuropathology were that of hypoxic encephalopathy [109], often delayed postanoxic encephalopathy [12]. It is now clear that such a sequence frequently occurs in the *absence* of therapy [13,80,240]. Similar pontine lesions are found in patients who have manifested increased intracranial pressure unrelated to hyponatremia [77,238] or who had other disorders (burns, stroke, alcoholism, cirrhosis) but were never hyponatremic [33,132,138,181], thus rendering any association with hyponatremia or its treatment most unlikely.

POSSIBLE NEUROENDOCRINE CAUSES OF CENTRAL NERVOUS SYSTEM DAMAGE ASSOCIATED WITH HYPONATREMIA

Extracellular fluid movement in the central nervous system occurs principally at the blood-brain barrier (capillary endothelium) interfaces, blood-CSF barrier (capillary endothelium–choroid plexus), and CSF outflow system (dural sinus–arachnoid villi). Since the brain lacks a rigorous lymphatic drainage system and is encased within an unyielding skull, it is very susceptible to disruptions of normal fluid inflow-outflow dynamics. Growing evidence suggests that the regulation of the fluid-electrolyte environment of the brain is markedly influenced by a neuroendocrine system that affects the capillary endothelium, the choroid plexus, and the astroglia. Several of the barrier tissues at the interfaces of blood and brain or CSF and brain contain receptors or second messenger systems for endogenous neuropeptides that can affect water or ion movement. There is a growing awareness of the potent modulatory effects of sex hormones on these peptidergic mechanisms and the role of such interactions in diverse normal and pathologic states. There is also some recognition that a heterogeneous group of neurologic conditions are influenced by hormonal fluctuations associated with specific phases of the menstrual cycle, pregnancy, and use of steroid contraceptives [5,27,56,66,74,111,113,114,128,144, 157,189].

The results of our studies suggest that an interaction between endogenous vasoactive neuropeptides and gonadal steroid hormones may be an important factor in the female predeliction for hyponatremic encephalopathy [82]. This section will explore several possible neuroendocrine bases that could underlie the association between ovarian sex hormones and fluid-electrolyte balance in the central nervous system.

Sex Steroid Interactions with Central Nervous System Tissues

In mammalian species of both sexes, plasma sex hormones are derived directly from ovaries, testes, and adrenal glands and via enzyme-mediated conversions from prohormones in extraglandular tissues, such as adipose tissue and brain [142]. The unbound fraction of the circulating steroid hormone pool is highly lipophilic and exhibits rapid flux across the blood-brain barrier and neuronal cell membranes [81]. Sex steroids are now also known to influence rapid changes in neuronal functions via direct interactions with nerve cell membranes [213].

The concentrations of estrogen-binding neurons are highest in the forebrain and certain circumventricular organs [158,180]. Androgen and progestin target cells exhibit considerable anatomic overlap in the brain with the estrogen cell population [197]. A discrete subpopulation of periventricular astrocytes selectively binds estradiol and undergoes morphologic changes following estrogenic exposure [35]. These latter changes may be functionally significant insofar as the periventricular structures have repeatedly been implicated in the regulation of fluid-ion homeostasis [110,112,170,179,206,222, 223].

Gonadal sex steroids have long been known to exert important modulatory influences on fluid-electrolyte balance in peripheral tissues [69,117,120]. Estrogens operate via both renal and extrarenal mechanisms in producing their sodium- and water-retaining effects. In the rat, urine flow, urinary sodium concentration, and sodium excretion rate are lower at estrus than at diestrus, whereas urinary potassium concentration is higher [49]. Progesterone stimulates aldosterone hypersecretion by opposing the action of this mineralocorticoid on the distal tubule, with resulting natriuresis and reduced blood volume. Estrogens, on the other hand, seem to inhibit the natriuretic effect of progesterone and, in fact, appear to promote sodium absorption [166]. Data from several laboratories suggest that the sodium- and fluid-retaining action of estrogen is exerted via adrenal, pituitary, and cerebral hormonal mechanisms [81].

Sex steroids also directly influence a broad spectrum of central nervous system–mediated functions, including sexual differentiation of the brain, control of the hypothalamic-pituitary-gonadal secretions, temperature regulation and energy balance [189], and modulation of respiration [27]. Of particular interest is that sex steroids have been implicated as probable causative agents in a variety of disturbances of fluid-electrolyte balance and cerebro- and cardiovascular homeostasis. Relationships between endogenous sex hormones and stroke [54,66, 127,128] and migraine headache [74,144, 236] are well established. Fluctuations in circulating sex hormone levels may have direct adverse effects on the integrity of cerebral vessel walls, which could account for the high risk of hemorrhagic stroke in young women on oral contraceptives [157,189].

Some of the symptoms of migraine and premenstrual tension syndrome appear to be related to sex steroid–induced salt and water retention [74,144]. In many cases, migraine improves with gestation, and this occurs most frequently in patients whose headaches are linked to the menstrual cycle [74]. Estrogens may act directly on vascular smooth muscle [5], as well as modulate the activity of vasoactive substances at the neurovascular junction [236]. In women predisposed to mirgraine, premenstrual fluctuations in circulating estrogen levels may activate neurohypophyseal hormone release, leading to alterations in cerebrovascular tone [189]. Oxytocin, like vasopressin, is capable of inducing cerebral vasoconstriction [169], and the secretion of both peptides is influenced by circulating levels of estrogens [93,111,199]. External stimuli that can trigger estrogen release, such as strong emotional or sensory stimuli [189], may produce significant vascular changes in the brain via the release of posterior pituitary peptides [133,203]. Some data suggest that this effect is enhanced by sodium depletion and is virtually absent in the elderly [72]. As discussed later, this may be important in explaining the inappropriate release of antidiuretic hormone that occurs in adult premenopausal women during the postoperative recovery period.

A recent study found highly significant variations of synaptosomal Na^+-K^+ ATPase activity in the female rat hypothalamus and preoptic area during the estrous cycle and following ovariectomy and estrogen replacement therapy [173]. Estrogen treatment has also been shown to stimulate adenohypophyseal and uterine Na^+-K^+ ATPase levels of the cerebral cortex, preoptic area, and hypothalamus of male rats [92]. Orchidectomy, 4 weeks prior to sacrifice, decreased ATPase activity of the hypothalamus, whereas testosterone replacement caused a fourfold increase in Na^+-K^+ ATPase levels. These data indicate that gonadal sex steroids can have a strong influence on the major cation-transporting system in the brain.

Gonadal Steroid-Neuropeptide Interactions in Fluid Intake and Vasopressin Secretion

Body fluid homeostasis depends on the maintenance of a balance between fluid intake and water and electrolyte excretion. Fluctuations in fluid intake associated with the reproductive cycle are influenced by spontaneous variations in endogenous gonadal steroid hormones [55,76, 110,111,136,137,216,219,229,230]. In rats, the cyclic pattern of drinking can be abolished by bilateral ovariectomy [76] and restored by subsequent estradiol benzoate administration [216]. Chronic treatment with estradiol attenuates the response to a number of dipsogenic stimuli, including isoproterenol, epinephrine, serotonin, hypertonic saline, and components of the renin-angiotensin system [84,85,86,221]. However, estrogenic agents can also produce variable effects on fluid intake, including both increases and decreases, apparently related to the duration of steroid treatment [42].

Some reports suggest that gonadal steroids affect fluid-electrolyte balance by modulating both fluid intake and vasopressin secretion [24,159,171,205,217]. The marked fluctuations in drinking behavior observed during the estrous cycle of the female rat parallel the changes in plasma vasopressin and endogenous estradiol [111,199], peaking during early proestrus, falling in late proestrus, remaining low during estrus, and reaching a nadir at diestrus [199]. The decline in serum arginine vasopressin (AVP) during proestrus is accompanied by a trend toward a lower serum osmolality during the same stage [199]. Treatment with exogenous estrogenic agents, on the other hand, has less predictable influences on AVP levels. For example, in one study [42], administration of estradiol benzoate to ovariectomized rats for 14 weeks diminished urine concentrating ability during a 24-hour dehydration test, but exogenous AVP produced a normal renal concentrating response. This would suggest that estrogens can impair central AVP release. In another study, however, long-term administration of diethylstilbestrol, estrone, or progesterone and estradiol alone or in combination with progesterone to rats for 12 to 15 days had no effect on serum sodium, plasma osmolality, or plasma AVP [67]. Finally, treatment with estrogens for 1 to 2 weeks has also been reported to produce elevated serum vasopressin in rats [199] and in postmenopausal women [78].

Studies to determine whether there are interdependent alterations in plasma sodium, osmolality, or AVP during the female reproductive cycle have also yielded some conflicting results. During the human menstrual cycle, for example, Baylis [26] found a small but significant fall in mean plasma osmolality of the order of 2 mmol/kg during the luteal phase, but changes in serum sodium to account for the osmolality decrease were not statistically significant. Similar observations were made by Vokes and colleagues [229], who also noted no changes in serum sodium and plasma AVP concentrations but described a 5 mmol/kg fall in basal plasma osmolality in the luteal phase. Small but significant decrements in serum sodium and osmolality were found in postmenopasual women receiving an ester of ethinyl estradiol daily for 1 to 3 years [2]. However, there have also been reports of an absence of significant changes in serum sodium or plasma osmolality during the human menstrual cycle [57,79,163]. In still other studies, 3 to 10 days of estrogen treatment of men or postmenopausal women did not alter basal serum electrolytes [163], plasma osmolality [78], plasma AVP [164,237], or maximal urinary dilution after an oral water load [243]. The reasons for these apparently conflicting data are at present unclear, but they may be related to differences in the dose or duration of steroid administration. Alternatively, some other factor, possibly chorionic gonadotropin [172] or prolactin [106], may mediate the steroid influences on fluid-electrolyte balance.

Finally, it is interesting to note that a resetting of the osmotic threshold for vasopressin secretion as well as thirst occurs during gestation in the rat [164] and human [159], when a decrease in plasma osmolality of several milliosmoles is sustained until term. Similar "reset" phenomena leading to inappropriate vasopressin release have been observed in experimental metabolic alkalosis [156] and diabetes mellitus [154] in dogs and in various chronic disorders, such as hepatic cirrhosis and bronchogenic carcinoma [190], although patients with hyponatremia of hypothyroidism appear to have normal osmotic control of AVP release [97]. Angiotensin II may be secreted in response to hyponatremia in psychiatric patients [196]. This would result in increased fluid intake and vasopressin secretion, which aggravates the hyponatremia, resulting in further release of angiotensin. An accelerating vicious cycle is thereby established until medical intervention with sodium supplementation is instituted. A single case of severe water intoxication was recently treated successfully with angiotensin converting enzyme inhibitors [196]. Further research is needed to determine whether a reset of the osmotic threshold for vasopressin release might account for the inappropriately high levels of vasopressin observed in symptomatic hyponatremic patients with encephalopathy. In particular, since the renin-angiotensin system influences a variety of parameters that impact on fluid-electrolyte balance, its role in vasopressin hypersecretion merits close attention.

Brain Renin-Angiotensin System

Ovarian hormones may influence vasopressin secretion, blood pressure, and fluid intake by interacting with the cerebral renin-angiotensin system. A close correspondence has been found between brain regional angiotensinogen concentration, the state of hydration, and the levels of circulating estradiol [44]. Several of these areas of the brain, including the anterior hypothalamus, preoptic area, septum, and mesencephalic central gray matter contain neural pathways involved in fluid-electrolyte regulation [110,115]. Findlay, Fitzsimons, and Kucharczyk [76] found that fluid intake induced in adult female rats by intracranial injections of the dipsogenic hormone angiotensin II varied with the estrous cycle. Estrous cycle–related fluctuations in angiotensin-induced fluid intake were abolished by bilateral ovariectomy and were absent altogether in prepubertal female rats. It has since been shown that the estrogen attenuation of thirst stimulated by angiotensin injections is associated with decreased angiotensin binding in the preoptic area and anterior hypothalamus [103]. Pretreatment with prolactin increased fluid intake induced by angiotensin in female but not male rats [107]. Other studies have demonstrated that angiotensin-induced changes in blood pressure [103,214], anterior pituitary hormone [207], and vasopressin release may be modulated by estrogens at the level of the forebrain. It is also of potential importance that centrally injected angiotensin II has been shown to inhibit Na^+-K^+ ATPase pump activity and that this has been implicated in the development of some forms of hypertension [38].

Vasopressin

The possibility that gonadal steroids may affect brain fluid-electrolyte balance by interacting with vasopressin has only recently received some attention. In both males and females, hypovolemia and hyperosmolality are considered to be the most potent physiologic stimuli for vasopressin release [190]. As stated earlier, however, plasma vasopressin concentrations vary with the menstrual cycle in women, with the highest levels observed at midcycle, and estradiol administration increases plasma vasopressin in postmenopausal women. In laboratory animals, some investigators [199] have shown that plasma vasopressin levels in female rats were similar to or higher than those in males, depending on the phase of the estrous cycle, and that testosterone inhibited vasopressin release in females. Others [50] have found that treatment of castrated male rats with testosterone tended to increase plasma vasopressin, but estradiol, progesterone, and estradiol plus progesterone were without effect. Testosterone treatment of castrated male goats, on the other hand, did not influence vasopressin or oxytocin levels [220].

The importance of gonadal steroid influences on vasopressin secretion is likely related to the finding that vasopressin can significantly increase both brain capillary and ventricular ependymal cell water permeability [65,149,168, 175] and may be involved in the acute phase of cerebral vasospasm [39]. It is now generally accepted that the cerebral capillary endothelium represents the morphologic substrate of the blood-brain barrier. Specific transport mechanisms present there regulate the entry of fluid electrolytes, small molecules, and proteins, which determines the volume and composition of the brain interstitial fluid [34]. Increased intracranial pressure has been shown to cause vasopressin release into the CSF [204], and the addition of vasopressin to cisternal infusion fluids has been found to lower CSF pressure in rabbits [148]. Intracerebroventricular infusion of high doses of vasopressin into rats produced an increase in brain water content in the presence of water load [65]. Brain edema induced under these experimental conditions parallels the conditions (i.e., elevated vasopressin concurrent with plasma hypo-osmolality) observed in hyponatremic encephalopathy. Intraperitoneal administration of a vasopressin antagonist has been reported to decrease brain volume [68].

In the epithelial membranes of the kidney, vasopressin increases water permeability by the activation of cyclic adenosine monophosphate (AMP) [94], increasing the inward movement of sodium, which in turn activates a Na^+-K^+ ATPase on the basolateral surface to remove the excess sodium [186]. Clinical, morphologic, and experimental data indicate that injury to the central nervous system often produces increases in vasopressin, perhaps as a nonspecific effect of activation of the hypothalamic-neurohypophyseal system. For example, in one study, increases in intracranial pressure induced by injecting blood into the subarachnoid space of rats caused large increases in plasma vasopressin levels [200]. It has been suggested that the enhanced activity of the AVP neurosecretory cells in the supraoptic and paraventricular nuclei may have been stimulated by the effects of ischemic anoxia secondary to the decreased blood flow caused by the acute severe intracranial hypertension [118,131,243]. Although precise data concerning the effect of vasopressin on the cerebral microcirculation are not yet available, this peptide is known to influence CSF secretion by stimulating the choroid plexus [37,123,194]. The existence of vasopressin receptor sites in cerebral microvessels has recently been demonstrated in the pig brain by specific binding methods with [^{3}H] AVP as the ligand, which supports the hypothesis that the peptide plays a role in the control of the cerebral microcirculation [155]. It has also been found that circulating vasopressin, at concentrations similar to those observed during hemorrhage, selectively dilates large cerebral arteries and increases microvascular pressure without changes in cerebral blood flow [75]. Vasopressin-like peptides can cross the blood-brain barrier mainly by paracellular transport without significant carrier mediation [227]. Among its other varied effects in the central nervous system, vasopressin has been shown to influence arterial vasoconstriction [233], to reduce cerebral blood flow after intracarotid injection [124], and to reduce spinal cord blood flow after spinal subarachnoid injection [126]. These data point to a possible role for vasopressin in coordinating blood flow and cerebral permeability in accordance with local metabolic demand.

Vasopressin may also function as an endogenous analgesic [28]. The increases in blood pressure and arterial resistance induced by surgical stress in rats appear to be mediated by vasopressin and the renin-angiotensin system [133]. It is of some interest that recent studies have demonstrated a sex difference in endogenous opioid regulation of the vasopressin response to stress [215]. Naloxone significantly potentiated vasopressin secretion caused by immobilization but only in cyclic female and castrated male rats [43]. These data indicate that the neurochemical basis of the sex difference in vasopressin secretion may involve an opioid system that is modulated by circulating gonadal steroids. One possible neural level of interaction is the preoptic area, which projects to the sites of vasopressin biosynthesis in the supraoptic and paraventricular nuclei, and as well exhibits denser opioid binding sites in females compared with males [211].

Immunocytochemical studies have revealed the presence of extensive vasopressinergic projections from the suprachiasmatic nucleus to the limbic system and other brain areas. In the rat at least, from the twelfth postnatal day onward, males have a significantly higher density of vasopressin fibers in some areas of the forebrain than females [61]. However, the significance of this anatomic sex difference is currently unclear [36].

Vasopressin is synthesized in the brain and is carried in cortical cerebrospinal fluid from the hypothalamus to pituitary capillaries [75]. The hormone is secreted into the cerebrospinal fluid of the third ventricle. While in the cerebrospinal fluid, vasopressin binds directly to brain cells, where its cerebral effects are mediated by intracellular second messengers [174,175]. Vasopressin then migrates in the cerebrospinal fluid to the pituitary, from which the vasopressin is secreted into the bloodstream.

There are two major types of vasopressin receptors, which have been well described at this time: the V1 and V2 receptors. The V2 receptors are mostly located on the kidney. After binding to V2 receptors, vasopressin acts largely through activation of adenylate cyclase, elevating cyclic adenosine monophosphate (cyclic AMP) in the distal nephron. The vasopressin analogue desmopressin (DDAVP) also binds to V2 receptors, and thus has an action on the kidney that is similar to that of vasopressin. The V1 receptors are located in blood vessels, brain, and choroid plexus. Vasopressin binds to V1 receptors in brain and has intracellular actions that are mediated via any of several second messengers, which include cyclic guanosine monophosphate (cyclic GMP), nitric oxide, and inositol triphosphate. After vasopressin binds to V1 receptor sites on neurons and cerebral blood vessels, it has multiple cerebral effects. In rodents, vasopressin acts via cerebral V1 receptors, leading to water movement into brain in the absence of hyponatremia, a fall in brain intracellular pH, a significant decline in brain synthesis of adenosine triphosphate (ATP) [82], and decreased brain blood flow and production of cerebrospinal fluid [81]. When hyponatremia has been induced with either water alone or water plus DDAVP (which has no effect on the brain V1 receptor), the aforementioned cerebral effects of vasopressin are absent, demonstrating the probable importance of vasopressin in the pathogenesis of hyponatremic encephalopathy. These findings have implications for investigations into the pathophysiology of hyponatremic encephalopathy. Animal models that ultilize water plus DDAVP to induce hyponatremia have no relevance to human pathophysiology, as many of the cerebral effects of hyponatremia are secondary to effects of vasopressin on the brain [75,81,82,168].

Atriopeptins

Endogenous substances causing marked natriuresis have been demonstrated in the cardiac atria as well as mammalian brain. Immunoreactive atrial natriuretic polypeptide (ANP) is present in the hypothalamus, septum, and pons in rat [102,116,183,242] and human brain [146] and CSF [122]. Brain ANP may play a role in the central regulation of fluid and electrolyte balance, since central administration of this peptide causes significant suppression of vasopressin secretion and water intake [8,9,143,182]. Moreover, ANP receptors have been localized [99,165] and quantified [178] in circumventricular organs outside the blood-brain barrier, which are involved in the central control of blood pressure [119,234]. The close anatomic connections between the brain ANP system and the circumventricular structures suggest that ANP may participate in a coordinated peptidergic system regulating fluid volume and electrolyte balance [178].

ANP interactions with other peptidergic mechanisms are of considerable potential importance. ANP opposes the actions of vasopressin and angiotensin II by receptor-mediated actions in the kidney, adrenal gland, vasculature, and brain [40,165,182,232]. Several of the barrier tissues at the interfaces of blood and brain or CSF and brain, including circumventricular structures like the choroid plexus, subfornical organ, and organum vasculosum, contain receptors and second messenger systems for atriopeptins [206]. Atriopeptins can alter the rate of CSF production [29,129,206], which suggests that this endogenous peptide may participate in the physiologic regulation of water movement in the central nervous system by interacting with barrier tissues [206]. The presence of ANP binding sites in brain microvessels, ependyma, and ciliary bodies of the eye could be related to possible roles in the control of fluid production or ion fluxes across brain membranes [165,206]. This would correlate well with the established peripheral actions of ANP in stimulating both natriuresis and vasodilatation [40,185].

It appears that ANP may have opposite if not antagonistic actions to angiotensin and vasopressin in the regulation of central water and ion homeostasis [178]. In one study, AVP-positive vascular connections, investigated by immunoelectron-histochemistry, were found in close or direct contact with brain microvessels [64]. Central administration of vasopressin with or without an accompanying water load caused significant fluid accumulation. Brain edema induced by experimental subarachnoid hemorrhage had a significantly different time course in Wistar compared to vasopressin-deficient Brattleboro rats [64]. Central administration of rat ANF, on the other hand, prevented cerebral edema elicited by systemic hypo-osmolar fluid load and led to significant sodium loss from the central nervous system by altering capillary sodium permeability [64]. Considered together, these results indicate that brain barrier tissues, like the circumventricular organs, may play a role in water movement in the central nervous system and may be important target tissues for ANP and other peptides. The relevance of these findings to conditions of disordered water electrolyte homeostasis, such as cerebral edema or hyponatremic encephalopathy, is suggested by the finding that ANP binding sites in the rat choroid plexus are increased in hydrocephalis [226].

Another possible natriuretic factor in the central nervous system has potent Na^+-K^+ ATPase inhibiting activity [3,41], much like a cardiac glycoside, and reacts with the antidigoxin antibody [48]. Rat hypothalamus contains large quantities of an Na^+-K^+ ATPase inhibitor, which is normally stimulated by high sodium intake [3,139]. Recently, it was shown that ANP is capable of regulating the release from brain of an Na^+-K^+ ATPase inhibitor with similar chromatographic characteristics [48], which suggests that the two factors may be interrelated in the regulation of fluid-electrolyte balance. Activity of the Na^+-K^+ ATPase inhibitor was also detected in peripheral plasma, which changed in parallel with the hypothalamus [3]. Both natriuretic hormones are highly localized in the periaqueductal gray matter [198] just lateral to the dorsal raphe nucleus in the rat [183]. This is of interest because the periaqueductal gray matter is a major locus for the analgesic actions of morphine [239]. Opiates, especially morphine, have a powerful stimulatory action on the release of ANP-like immunoreactivity in the rat brain, although the mechanism has not yet been explained [100]. Thus it is also possible that the brain opioid peptides may also participate in the regulation of ANP secretion in the central nervous system of humans.

Prolactin

The effects of prolactin in the renal handling of water and salt were first examined 25 years ago [125]. More recent studies suggest that this classic "hormone of lactation" may influence cerebral water metabolism by centrally stimulating fluid intake. In human subjects acute administration of ovine prolactin has been reported to arouse thirst [101]. Ovine prolactin injected into rats is also dipsogenic [73], and it has been shown [105] that this increased drinking results from an exaggerated sensitivity of hyperprolactinemic rats to extracellular fluid deficits. Katovich and Simpkins [104] found that prolactin acts specifically on beta-adrenergic thirst mechanisms. This may account for the decreased drinking response to isoprenaline during estrus and proestrus [76], since serum prolactin levels are increased during these stages [6,202]. Isoprenaline-induced thirst is also attenuated in rats following estrogen treatment [221], which is known to increase serum prolactin levels significantly in this species [45]. Thus while a physiologic role for prolactin in fluid intake behavior during the estrous cycle has not been conclusively demonstrated, a variety of data suggest it may have primary dipsogenic activity. Although prolactin receptors have been identified in the brain [231], their direct relationship to cerebral water regulation has not been established. The significance of the recently demonstrated ANP inhibition [29] or angiotensin II stimulation [141] of prolactin secretion is also unclear at this time.

Hormones and Adaptation of Brain to Hyponatremia

There is increased morbidity and mortality from hyponatremia in females versus males [12, 14,22,240], and a major reason for this phenomenon appears to be a decreased ability of the female brain to defend itself against hyponatremia as compared to the male brain [81–83]. One of the primary mechanisms by which the brain can defend itself against hyponatremia is to extrude cations (sodium, potassium, amino acids) in order to lower its osmolality toward that of the plasma without a substantial gain of water

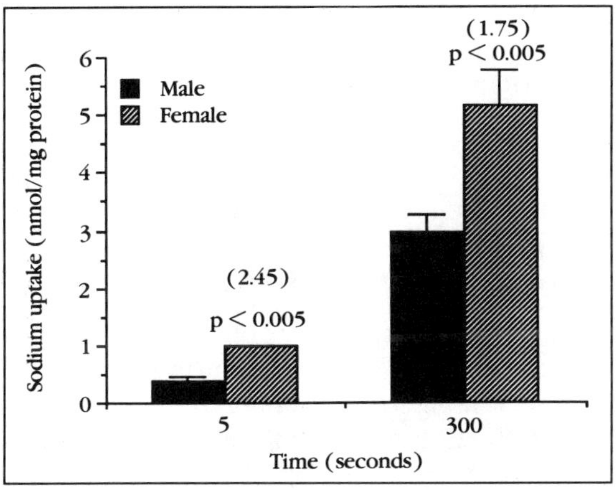

Fig. 4-5. The veratridine stimulated sodium uptake in synaptosomes from male versus female hyponatremic rat brain. The uptake is significantly greater in female rat brain after both 5 seconds and 300 seconds. The increased sodium uptake in female brain would theoretically lead to increased intracellular sodium and an increased tendency to brain edema associated with hyponatremia. (Data from Fraser et al. [82].)

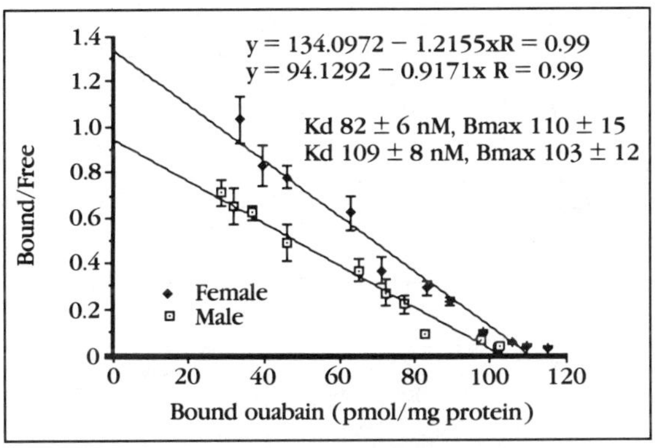

Fig. 4-6. Scatchard plot of ouabain binding in synaptosomes from male versus female hyponatremic rat brain. In males, Bmax = 103±12 pmol/mg of protein, and Kd = 109± 8 nM. In females, Bmax = 110± 15 pmol/mg of protein, and Kd = 82±6 nM. The lower Kd in females indicates that female brain has a greater affinity of its receptors for ouabain. (Bmax = maximum binding concentration; Kd = half maximal displacement concentration.) (From Fraser and Sarnacki [83].)

[16,18,134,177]. If this can be achieved, there will not be an osmolar gap from brain to plasma and less water will enter the brain, decreasing the magnitude of cerebral edema. However, if the brain is unable to lower cellular osmolality adequately by extrusion of cations, then the only other mechanism by which brain osmolality can be lowered is by an inward movement of plasma water into brain cells (see Fig. 4-2). If a sufficient amount of water enters the limited confines of the cranial vault, cerebral edema and herniation may follow [12,80]. There is preliminary evidence that suggests that the combination of estrogen and vasopressin may predispose to brain swelling. In laboratory animals, administration of vasopressin to normonatremic female rats resulted in brain edema, while the same treatment to male rats had essentially no effect [82]. Active extrusion of sodium from the brain to compensate for hyponatremia is probably accomplished at least in part through active transport by the Na^+-K^+ ATPase pump [83], and sex hormones can directly affect the function of this pump in intestine, liver, red blood cells, heart, and brain [81]. The Na^+-K^+ ATPase pump function in female rat brain synaptosomes has recently been shown to be significantly less effective than it is in male rats (Fig. 4-5). Among the reasons for this reduced pump activity in females is an increased affinity of the pump in female brain to bind ouabain and possibly ouabain-like substances (Fig. 4-6). This observation has substantial clinical implications, since there is now evidence that clearly shows that several female sex hormones have ouabain-like actions on the Na^+-K^+ ATPase pump in heart, brain, liver, and other tissues [81,92,117,120]. The binding of these hormones to the pump results in inhibition of pump function in a similar manner as observed with cardiac glycosides. Therefore, the increased affinity of the brain Na^+-K^+ ATPase pump of female rats for ouabain suggests that the female sex hormones may account for the observed decrease in pump function in this group [83]. In addition, the male sex hormone testosterone had no inhibitory effect on the pump, even at high concentrations [117]. As opposed to the inhibitory effects of the female sex hormones on the Na^+-K^+ ATPase pump, recent reports indicate that the male

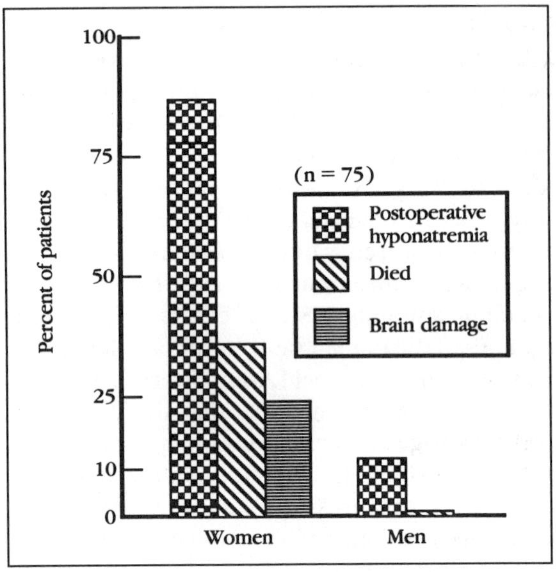

Fig. 4-7. The male versus female incidence of postoperative hyponatremia with brain damage. Included are those patients who developed symptomatic postoperative hyponatremia (serum sodium < 128 mM) in the absence of associated medical illness. Patients represent a comprehensive review of the literature as of Jan. 1, 1988. It can be seen that about 90% of all symptomatic postoperative hyponatremia occurs in women, while over 99% of associated morbidity and mortality occurs in women.

sex hormone testosterone stimulates Na^+-K^+ ATPase pump activity in the brain and other tissues [81,92].

Female Preponderance Among Patients Who Have Symptomatic Hyponatremia with Brain Damage

It is apparent from the previous discussion that there are multiple interactive hormonal mechanisms that regulate central nervous system water and electrolyte metabolism. From a clinical standpoint, it now appears likely that, although hyponatremic encephalopathy may occur in anyone, there is a clear predilection for women of reproductive age (13–50 years). Beginning in about 1950, there are several reports of symptomatic postoperative hyponatremia, often accompanied by coma and seizures, most of which appear in the older surgical literature [25,96, 195,244]. Despite the fact that serum sodium was below 120 mM and symptoms were present, neurologic morbidity and mortality were very infrequent. Since many of these patients were in generally good health and scheduled for elective surgical procedures, the ab-

Fig. 4-8. The clinical course of the syndrome of postoperative hyponatremia with brain damage described in Arieff [12]. Patients, generally young women, have a normal preoperative serum Na^+ and undergo surgery without incident. Following the surgery, they receive hypotonic fluid, and because the plasma vasopressin levels are always elevated after surgery, much of the administered fluid is retained. After a mean of about 2 days, the plasma Na^+ has fallen below 130 mM and patients manifest symptoms that usually include nausea, emesis, and headache but with only minimal impairment of sensorium. Then, over a period of about 20 minutes, the patients go from a state of alertness to seizures, respiratory arrest, and coma. The onset of seizure activity often coincides with brain herniation. (Data from Arieff [12], Ayus, Krothapalli, and Arieff [22], and Fraser and Arieff [80].)

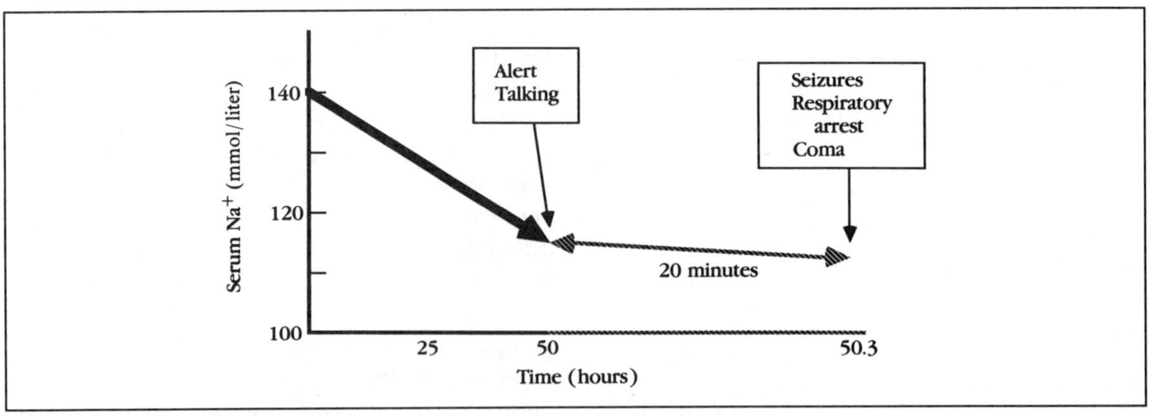

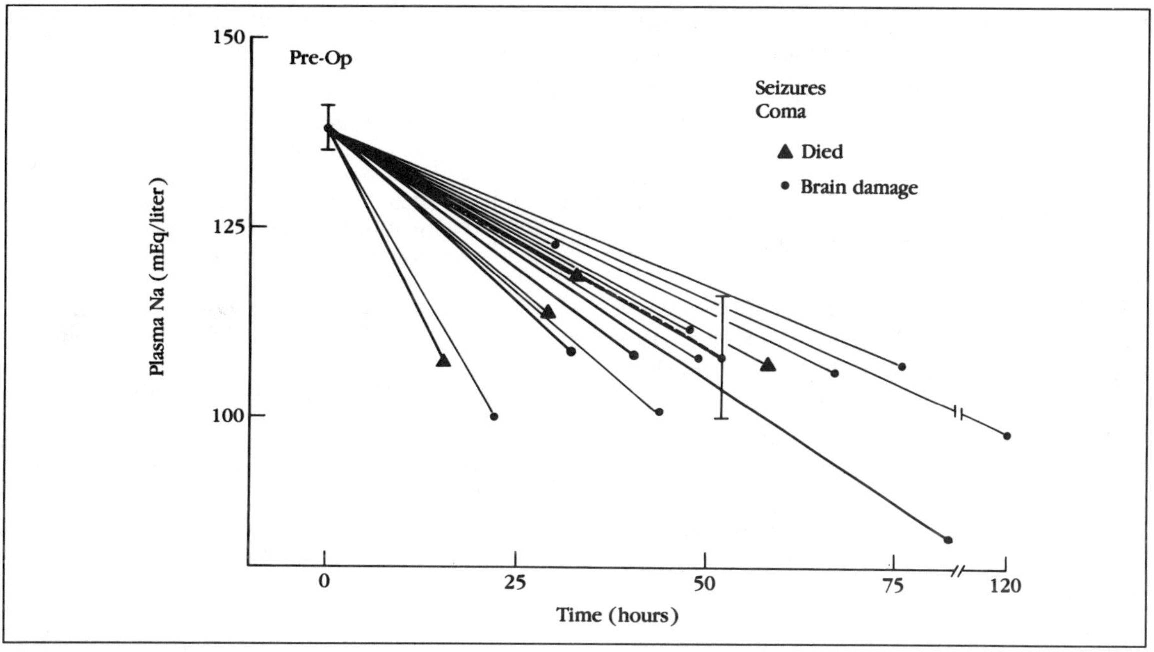

Fig. 4-9. The clinical course of 15 women who developed postoperative hyponatremia and died or suffered permanent brain damage. All 15 women had completely recovered from the effects of surgery and anesthesia and were awake and communicative when they developed seizures and coma. Seizures and coma were observed an average of 48 hours after surgery. (Data from Arieff [12].)

sence of serious associated medical illness was assumed to account for the low morbidity and mortality. However, recent studies clearly demonstrate that major determinants of brain damage in hyponatremia include the age and sex of the patient. In general, most patients with symptomatic hyponatremia (sodium below 120 mM) who did not suffer permanent neurologic damage were older women or men [25,209], while those who died or developed permanent brain injury have been younger women [12,22,240] (Fig. 4-7).

PRINCIPLES OF TREATMENT OF HYPONATREMIA

Any discussion of the therapy of hyponatremia must take into account both the underlying cause and the duration of the hyponatremia. Patients with low levels of plasma sodium who have volume expansion associated with hepatic cirrhosis, congestive heart failure, or nephrotic syndrome will probably not derive benefit from treatment with hypertonic NaCl. In such patients, there is probably a primary stimulus for renal retention of sodium and water, as well as elevated plasma ADH levels [191,192,212]. Patients with extrarenal losses of fluid (diarrhea, emesis, third space) resulting in dehydration may respond with elevations of plasma ADH. Subsequent ingestion of hypotonic fluid leads to water retention and hyponatremia. Such a sequence frequently occurs after surgery, and affected individuals may benefit from treatment with hypertonic NaCl. Increased vasopressin secretion activity may result from volume depletion secondary to blood loss, as well as any number of nonosmotic stimuli for vasopressin release, such as pain, fear anesthesia, emesis, nasogastric suction, prior diuretic administration, and decreased dietary sodium intake [113,190]. Therefore, when postsurgical patients are given predominantly hypotonic fluids, hyponatremia will occur frequently and may result in substantial morbidity and mortality (Figs. 4-8 and 4-9). Although such a sequence has received much attention recently [12,22,80,240], it has been known since at least 1935 [96] and frequently reported [18,25,60,195,244], although not with the understanding of pathogenesis currently available. Modification of this sequence by pretreatment with vasopressin antagonists may be appropriate in the near future [63,108]. Although women in their childbearing years are apparently far more susceptible to this syndrome than are males of any age, another group of patients who may develop acute symptomatic hyponatremia are those with SIADH who ingest or are given large quantities of water. These patients are often symptomatic from their hyponatremia, and therapy with hypertonic NaCl with or without a loop diuretic must be considered [12,25,244]. Patients who have SIADH on a chronic basis will often be relatively asymptomatic and are frequently male. Associated illnesses include cancer (lung, head, and neck) that is not operable and chronic pulmonary disease. Such patients can often be successfully managed with oral demeclocycline or lithium [140].

In patients with hormone deficiencies that may predispose to hyponatremia (hypothyroidism, adrenal insufficiency), treatment should be directed primarily at the underlying disorder. If the hyponatremia is symptomatic, NaCl should be administered along with the appropriate replacement hormone, since the plasma sodium is rarely below 125 mM, and therapy with hypertonic NaCl is rarely required. It is worth noting that hyponatremia is now frequently observed in patients with AIDS [53]. The hyponatremia in AIDS patients appears to be due to a combination of SIADH (from pulmonary or intracranial disease or various drugs), adrenal insufficiency, and loss of isotonic fluid (emesis or diarrhea) with replacement by water.

There are a vast number of pharmacologic agents that may interefere with the ability of the kidney to excrete a water load [140]. Included are large numbers of sedatives, hypnotics, analgesics, oral hypoglycemic agents, tranquilizers, antipsychotic agents, narcotics, and antineoplastic drugs. Hyponatremia associated with these agents may be acute, is often symptomatic, and may require treatment with hypertonic NaCl. Severe water intoxication may also occur in psychotic individuals even when they are not taking such drugs, and this is probably related to the fact that such individuals may have episodic

Table 4-3. Major risk factors that may lead to brain damage in patients with symptomatic hyponatremia

1. Delay in diagnosis and/or initiation of therapy resulting in respiratory depression or arrest, particularly when accompanied by seizure activity (definite hypoxic-anoxic episode)
2. Correction of hyponatremia to either normonatremic or hypernatremic levels within the initial 48 hours of therapy
3. Absolute change in serum sodium of greater than 25 mmol/liter within the initial 48 hours of therapy
4. Elevation of serum sodium to hypernatremic levels in patients with severe liver disease who may not have been hyponatremic
5. Symptomatic hyponatremia with serum sodium below 130 mmol/liter in women in their childbearing years (roughly ages 13–50 years)

Fig. 4-10. Prospective studies on the therapy of symptomatic hyponatremia in 88 patients. Prior to therapy, patients had a mean serum Na^+ of 108 mM, and none had suffered seizures or respiratory arrest. The serum Na^+ was increased from a mean of 108 to 127 mM in an average of 1 day, at an average rate of 1.7 mmol/liter/hour. The actual change in serum Na^+, the "delta," was 19 mmol over the initial 24 hours of therapy. No patient suffered brain damage as a result of therapy, and all survived. (Data from Ashouri [20], Ayus et al. [20, 21, 23], Cheng et al. [46], Decaux et al. [58], and Hartman et al. [95].)

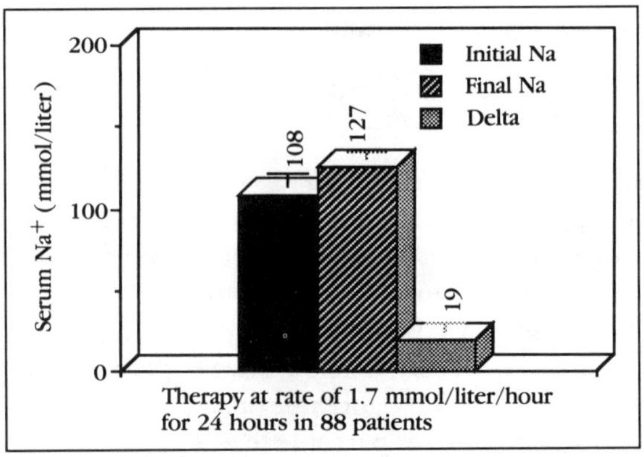

bursts of inappropriately elevated plasma vasopressin levels [196].

Clinical Outcome of Treatment

In devising general strategies for the treatment of symptomatic hyponatremia, certain principles seem pertinent [11]. First, it is likely that alcoholic/cachectic subjects represent a special case. If one reviews the literature for patients with symptomatic hyponatremia and serum sodium of either 120 mM or less or 106 mM or less who also had either chronic alcoholism, malnutrition, or cachexia, the mortality in the alcoholic/cachectic subjects was essentially double that in the other patients [11]. Thus, alcoholic/cachectic subjects with hyponatremia have an associated mortality that increases more with lower values of serum sodium than occurs with other individuals.

In general, many physicians do not employ hypertonic NaCl to treat symptomatic hyponatremia because of the presumed hazards of circulatory overload. This may be more of a theoretic hazard than a real one; few if any cases of circulatory overload complicating the treatment of hyponatremia have ever been reported. A major argument for "slow" correction of symptomatic hyponatremia is the possible development of cerebral demyelinating lesions [147,210]. At the present time, there are at least seven prospective studies involving over 100 patients who were treated with hypertonic NaCl where serum sodium was corrected at rates of 0.7 to 2.5 mmol/liter/hour (mean = 1.7 mmol/liter/hour) [20,21,23,46,58,95,240]. No patient had respiratory depression or arrest prior to therapy, and none of the other conditions shown in Table 4-3 were present. There was no neurologic deterioration or evidence of cerebral demyelinating lesions in any patient so treated (Fig. 4-10). Furthermore, a recent study clearly demonstrates that untreated symptomatic hyponatremia can result in virtually the same brain lesions that have been claimed in the past to be caused by "rapid" treatment [80]. Thus, based on a synopsis of all available prospective studies of therapy of symptomatic hyponatremic patients, the rate of correction of hyponatremia per se is not a factor in the development of brain lesions. As shown in Fig. 4-11, the rate of correction is the same, about 1 mmol/liter/hour, in patients with or without cerebral demyelinating lesions. However, the absolute change in serum sodium over the initial 24 hours of therapy appears to be a major factor in the possible development of cerebral demyelinating lesions (Fig. 4-12). An absolute change in serum sodium of more than 25 mmol in the initial 24 hours of therapy can lead to cerebral demyelinating lesions both in patients [21,210] and laboratory animals [81].

Hypoxic brain damage is often a major component of the neurologic disability observed in hyponatremic subjects. An hypoxic event such as respiratory insufficiency is a major factor militating against survival without permanent brain damage in patients with hyponatremia [12]. The combination of systemic hypoxemia and hyponatremia is far more deleterious than is either factor alone because hypoxia impairs the ability of the brain to adapt to hyponatremia, leading to a decrement of both cerebral blood flow and arterial oxygen content [19,176]. We have described more than 30 patients with symptomatic hyponatremia who had an arterial pO_2 below 40 mm Hg when the hyponatremia was diagnosed [19,22]. Such a degree of hypoxia without hyponatremia has been associated with substantial central nervous system morbidity or coma in healthy humans.

Hypoxic brain damage is a major component of the neurologic disability observed in some hyponatremic subjects [12,13,19,22]. Anoxia-hypoxia from any cause can be followed by the syndrome of delayed postanoxic encephalopathy, but most cases are related to carbon monoxide intoxication, strangulation, cardiopulmonary arrest, or various miscellaneous intoxications [88,89] with subsequent resuscitation. Patients are initially deeply comatose, usually requiring artificial ventilation. Characteristically, they begin to regain consciousness within several days but later relapse into coma from which recovery is infrequent. Recovery from coma followed by recurrent coma has often been observed in hyponatremic patients treated with hypertonic NaCl [12] and is similar to the sequence previously described in patients who have suffered hypoxic-anoxic episodes

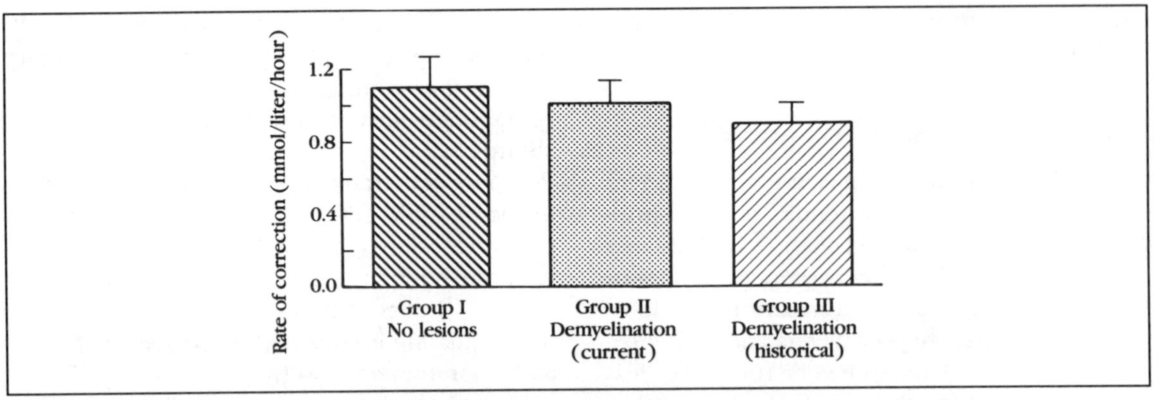

Fig. 4-11. The rate of correction of serum sodium among 33 patients with severe symptomatic hyponatremia (serum sodium < 128 mM) who recovered without neurologic sequelae or brain lesions (group I), among 12 patients with severe symptomatic hyponatremia who developed cerebral demyelinating brain lesions (group II), and among all patients in the literature as of January 1986 who had severe symptomatic hyponatremia (serum sodium < 120 mM) and developed cerebral demyelinating brain lesions (group III). It can be seen that the rate of correction of serum sodium is not different in all three groups. (Data from Ayus et al. [21].)

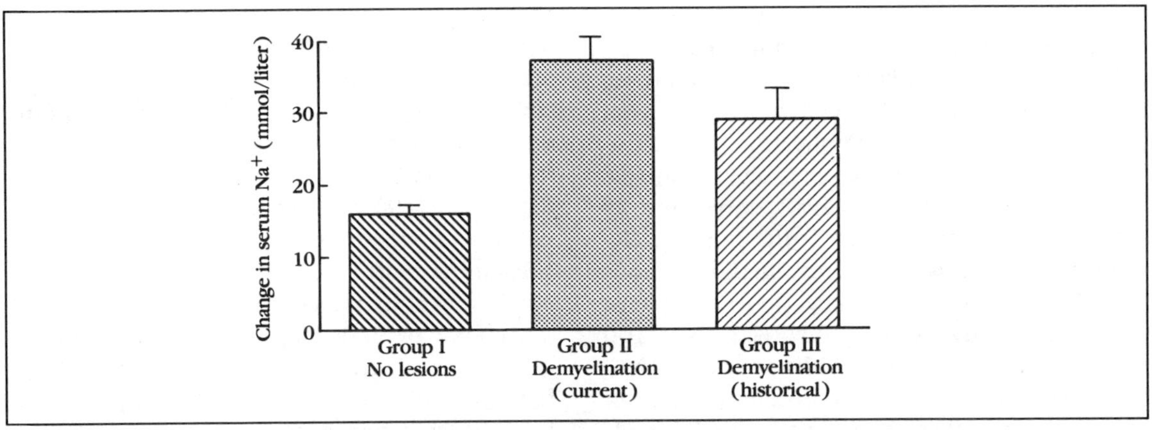

Fig. 4-12. The absolute change in serum sodium during the initial 48 hours of correction among 33 patients with severe symptomatic hyponatremia (serum sodium < 120 mM) who recovered without neurologic sequelae or brain lesions (group I), among 12 patients with severe symptomatic hyponatremia who developed cerebral demyelinating brain lesions (group II), and among all patients in the literature as of January 1986 who had severe symptomatic hyponatremia (serum sodium 128 mM) and developed cerebral demyelinating lesions (group III). It can be seen that the absolute change in serum sodium is significantly less between group I versus groups II and III. (Data from Ayus et al [21].)

from other causes [88]. In patients with hyponatremic encephalopathy, often the diagnosis is made on clinical grounds, but the radiology findings on CT or MRI are usually diffuse cerebral demyelinating lesions [19,21], which are similar to other clinical situations in which hypoxic encephalopathy occurs [109].

Therapy of Symptomatic Hyponatremia: Summary

In general, patients with symptomatic hyponatremia (serum sodium below 130 mM) should be treated with hypertonic (generally 514 mM) NaCl at a rate of infusion designed to raise

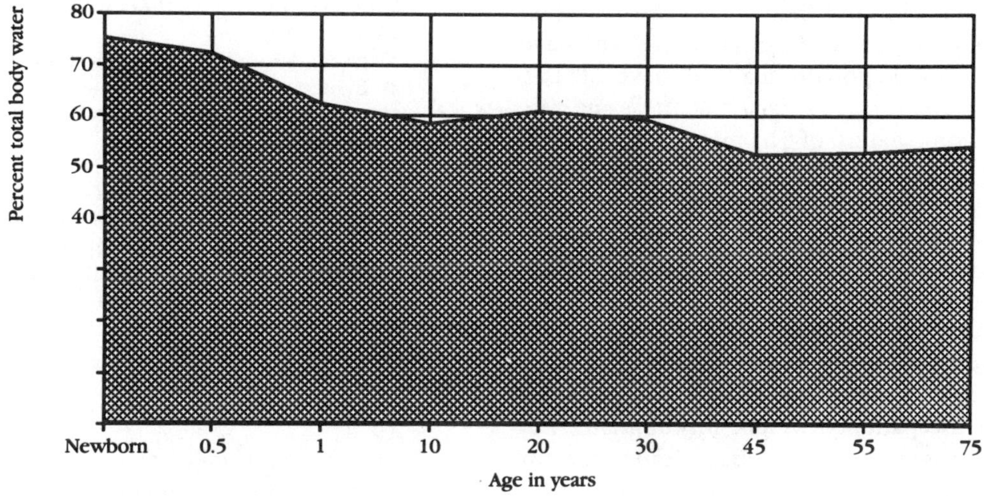

Fig. 4-13. The percent total body water in men as a function of age, weight, and sex. (Data from Altman and Dittmer [4], Edelman and Leibman [70], Park [155], and Weitzman and Kleeman [236].)

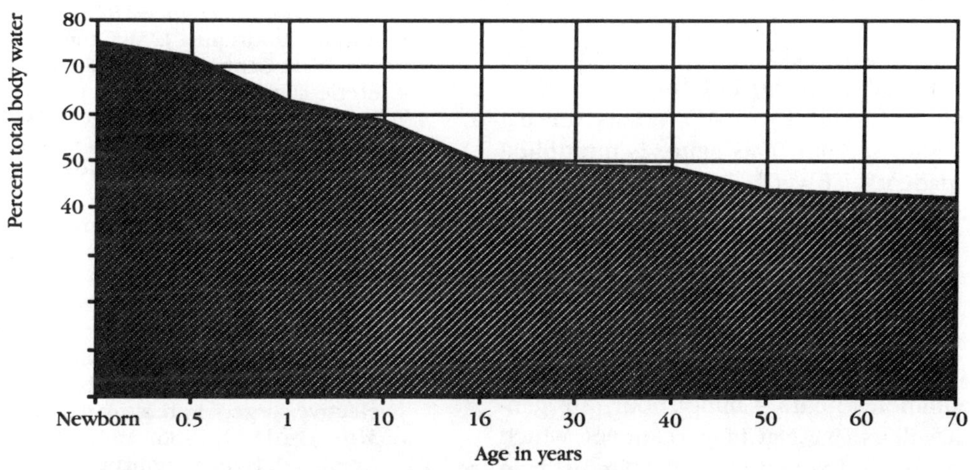

Fig. 4-14. The percent total body water in women as a function of age, weight, and sex. (Data from Altman and Dittmer [4], Edelman and Leibman [70], Park et al. [155], and Weitzman and Kleeman [236].)

plasma sodium at a rate of 1 to 2 mmol/liter/hour until the patient either becomes asymptomatic, the serum sodium is raised by 25 mmol/liter in the initial 48 hours of therapy, or a serum sodium of 125 to 135 mM is achieved. At this time hypertonic NaCl should be discontinued. This regimen may have to be modified in patients with severe hepatic, renal, or cardiac disease. Due to the possible dangers of cerebral demyelinating lesions, the serum sodium should never be increased to hypertonic levels; indeed, serum sodium should not be elevated acutely above 130 to 135 mM. Additionally, because cerebral demyelinating lesions have also been associated with abrupt acute changes in serum sodium (Fig. 4-12), the serum sodium probably should not be elevated by more than 25 mmol/liter during the initial 48 hours of therapy [21,132]. In patients who have symptomatic hyponatremia and have SIADH, plasma sodium can be raised at the same rate using a combination of 514 mM NaCl and intravenous furosemide [95]. The rate of correction of hyponatremia is not an important factor in the eventual outcome [21,240], but the absolute change in the initial 48 hours of therapy is (Figs. 4-10, 4-11, and 4-12).

Initially, one should determine the patient's estimated total body water (TBW). There is a traditional belief that this value is about 60 percent of the patient's weight in kilograms, but such an assumption is probably only true for young muscular males (Fig. 4-13). TBW varies based on age, sex, and weight, with infants having TBW of about 76 percent, and a low of about 36 percent occurring in elderly obese women [4,70,235]. In general, TBW is about 48 percent in hospitalized adults, but the best estimates can be obtained by extrapolation from Figures 4-13 and 4-14. The amount of sodium to be infused is then calculated as the goal of correction of serum sodium (about 130 mM), minus the patient's serum sodium. This figure is multiplied by the patient's TBW (in liters) to obtain the total mmoles to be infused. The number of hours of infusion is obtained by subtracting the patients serum sodium from 130, assuming a rate of correction of 1 mmol/liter/hour. To obtain the infusion rate, divide the number of millimoles to be infused by the number of hours, i.e., total millimoles/hours = mmol/hour. In general, one will use 3% NaCl for treatment, which is 514 mM NaCl. To obtain the rate of infusion in milliliters per hour (ml/hour), multiply millimoles per hour (mmol/hour) times 1000 and divide by 514.

REFERENCES

1. Adams, R. D., Victor, M., and Mancall, E. L. Central pontine myelinolysis: A hitherto undescribed disease occurring in alcholic and malnourished patients. *Arch. Neurol. Psychiatry* 81:154, 1959.
2. Aiken, J. J., Lindsay, R., and Hart, D. M. The redistribution of body sodium in women in long-term oestrogen therapy. *Clin. Sci. Mol. Med.* 47:179, 1984.
3. Alaghband-Zadeh, J., Fenton, S., Hancock, K., et al. Evidence that the hypothalamus may be a source of circulating Na-K-ATPase inhibitor. *J. Endocrinol.* 98:221, 1983.
4. Altman, P. L., and Dittmer, D. S. Total Body Water: Man. In *Biology Data Book* (2nd ed.). Bethesda, MD; Federation of American Societies for Experimental Biology, 1974. P. 1986.
5. Altura, B. Sex as a factor influencing the responsiveness of arterioles to catecholamines. *Eur. J. Pharmacol.* 20:261, 1972.
6. Amenomori, Y., Chen, C. H., and Meites, J. Serum prolactin levels in rats during different reproductive states. *Endocrinology* 86:506, 1970.
7. Amoroso, S., Schmid-Antomarchi, H. S., Fosset, M., et al. Glucose, sulfonylureas, and neurotransmitter release: Role of ATP-sensitive K^+ channels. *Science* 247:852, 1990.
8. Antunes-Rodriques, J., McCann, S. M., Rogers, L. C., et al. Atrial natriuretic factor inhibits dehydration- and angiotensin II-induced water intake in the conscious, unrestrained rat. *Proc. Natl. Acad. Sci. U.S.A.* 82:8720, 1986.
9. Antunes-Rodriques, J., McCann, S. M., and Samson, W. K. Central administration of atrial natriuretic factor inhibits saline preference in the rat. *Endocrinology* 118:1726, 1986.
10. Arieff, A. I. Central nervous system effects of disordered sodium metabolism. *Clin. Endocrinol. Metabol.* 13:269, 1984.
11. Arieff, A. I. Effects of Water, Electrolyte and Acid Base Disorders on the Central Nervous System. In A. I. Arieff and R. A. DeFronzo (eds.), *Fluid, Electrolyte and Acid-Base Disorders.* New York: Churchill Livingstone, 1985. P. 969.
12. Arieff, A. I. Hyponatremia, convulsions, respiratory arrest, and permanent brain damage after elective surgery in healthy women. *N. Engl. J. Med.* 314:1529, 1986.
13. Arieff, A. I. Hyponatremia associated with permanent brain damage. *Adv. Intern. Med.* 32:325, 1987.
14. Arieff, A. I. Osmotic failure: Physiology and strategies for treatment. *Hosp. Prac.* 23:173, 1988.
15. Arieff, A. I., and Chidsey, C. A. Renal function in cirrhosis and the effects of prostaglandin A_1. *Am. J. Med.* 56:695, 1974.
16. Arieff, A. I., and Guisado, R. Effects on the central nervous system of hypernatremic and hyponatremic states. *Kidney Int.* 10:104, 1976.
17. Arieff, A. I., Kleeman, C. R., Keushkerian, A., et al. Brain tissue osmolality: Method of determination and variations in hyper- and hypo-osmolar states. *J. Lab. Clin. Med.* 79:334, 1972.
18. Arieff, A. I., Llach, F., and Massry, S. G. Neuro-

logical manifestations and morbidity of hyponatremia: Correlation with brain water and electrolytes. *Medicine* (Baltimore) 55:121, 1976.
19. Arieff, A. I., Tien, R., Kucharczyk, W., et al. Hyponatremic brain damage: Is central pontine myelinolysis common? *Amer. J. Med.* 92 (in press), 1992.
20. Ashouri, O. S. Severe diuretic-induced hyponatremia in the elderly: A series of eight patients. *Arch. Intern. Med.* 146:1355, 1986.
21. Ayus, J. C., Krothapalli, R. K., and Arieff, A. I. Treatment of symptomatic hyponatremia and its relation to brain damage: A prospective study. *N. Engl. J. Med.* 317:1190, 1987.
22. Ayus, J. C., and Arieff, A. I. Effects of age and gender on outcome in patients with postoperative hyponatremia. *Ann. Intern. Med.* (in press), 1992.
23. Ayus, J. C., Olivero, J. J., and Frommer, J. P. Rapid correction of severe hyponatremia with intravenous hypertonic saline solution. *Am. J. Med.* 72:43, 1982.
24. Barron, W., Schreiber, J., and Lindheimer, M. D. Effect of ovarian sex steroids on osmoregulation and vasopressin secretion in the rat. *Am. J. Physiol.* 240:E352, 1986.
25. Bartholomew, L. G., and Scholz, D. A. Reversible postoperative neurological symptoms: Report of five cases secondary to water intoxication and sodium depletion. *N. Engl. J. Med.* 162:22, 1956.
26. Baylis, P. H. Vasopressin Secretion During the Menstrual Cycle: An Overview. In Allen W. Cowley, J.-F. Liard and D. A. Ausiello (eds.), *Vasopressin: Cellular and Integrative Functions.* New York: Raven, 1988.
27. Bayliss, D. A., Dean, J. B., Cidlowski, J. A., et al. The central facilitation of respiration by progesterone is estrogen-dependent. *Soc. Neurosci. Abstr.* 14:174, 1988.
28. Berkowitz, B. A., and Sherman, S. Characterization of vasopressin analgesia. *J. Pharmacol. Exp. Ther.* 220:329, 1982.
29. Bianchi, C., Gutkowska, J., Ballak, M., et al. Radioautographic localization of ^{125}I-atrial natriuretic factor binding sites in the brain. *Neuroendocrinology* 44:365, 1986.
30. Bichet, D., Szatalowicz, V., and Chaimovitz, C. Role of vasopressin in abnormal water secretion in cirrhotic patients. *Ann. Intern. Med.* 96:413, 1982.
31. Bichet, D. G., Van Putten, V. J., and Schrier, R. W. Potential role of increased sympathetic activity in impaired sodium and water excretion in cirrhosis. *N. Engl. J. Med.* 307:1552, 1982.
32. Birkenfeld, L. W., Leibman, J., O'Meara, M. P., et al. Total exchangeable sodium, total exchangeable potassium and total body water in edematous patients with cirrhosis of the liver and congestive heart failure. *J. Clin. Invest.* 37:687, 1958.
33. Boon, A. P., Carey, M. P., and Salmon, M. V. Central pontine myelinolysis not associated with rapid correction of hyponatremia. *Lancet* 2:458, 1988.
34. Bradbury, M. W. B. The structure and function of the blood-brain barrier. *Fed. Proc.* 43:186, 1984.
35. Brawer, J. R., Naftolin, F., and Mantin, J. Effects of a single injection of estradiol valerate on the hypothalamic arcuate nucleus and on reproductive function in the female rat. *Endocrinology* 103:501, 1978.
36. Brot, M. D., Miller, M. A., and Dorsa, D. M. Measurement of vasopressin receptors in the septum of male and female rats. *Soc. Neurosci. Abstr.* 14:145, 1988.
37. Brownfield, M. S., and Kozlowski, G. P. The hypothalamo-choroid tract:1. Immunohistochemical demonstration of neurophysin pathways to telencephalic choroid plexuses and cerebrospinal fluid. *Cell Tissue Res.* 178:111, 1977.
38. Buckley, J. P., Doursout, M. F., Liang, Y.-Y., et al. Centrally angiotensin II mechanisms and the sodium pump. *J. Hypertens.* 4(Suppl. 6):5465, 1986.
39. Cach, R., Durboraw, C., Smock, T., et al. Vasopressin mediation of microvascular spasm in the rat brain. *Soc. Neurol. Abstr.* 14:59, 1988.
40. Cantin, M. and Genest, J. The heart and the atrial natriuretic factor. *Endocrinol. Rev.* 6:107, 1985.
41. Carilli, C. T., Berne, M., Cantley, L. C., et al. Hypothalamic factor that inhibits (Na,K)ATPase from the extra-cellular surface: Mechanism of inhibition. *J. Biol. Chem.* 260:1027, 1985.
42. Carlberg, K. A., Fregley, M. J., and Fahey, M. Effects of chronic estrogen treatment on water exchange in rats. *Am. J. Physiol.* 247:E101, 1984.
43. Carter, D. A., et al. A sex difference in endogenous opioid regulation of the posterior pituitary response to stress in the cat. *J. Endocrinol.* 111:239, 1986.
44. Chen, F. M., Hawkins, R., and Printz, M. P. Evidence for a Functional Independent Brain-Angiotensin System: Correlation Between Regional Distribution of Brain Angiotensin Receptors, Brain Angiotensinogen and Drinking During the Estrous Cycle of Rats. In D. Ganten, M. P. Printz, M. I. Phillips, and B. A. Scholkens (eds.), *The Renin Angiotensin System in the Brain, Experimental Brain Research.* Berlin: Springer-Verlag, 1982. P. 157.
45. Chen, F. M., and Meites, J. Effect of estrogen and progesterone on serum and pituitary pro-

lactin levels in ovariectomized rats. *Endocrinology* :503, 1970.

46. Cheng, J. C., Zikos, D., Skopicki, H. A., et al. Correction of symptomatic hyponatremia. *Kidney Int.* 33:186, 1988.
47. Covey, C. M., and Arieff, A. I. Disorders of Sodium and Water Metabolism and Their Effects on the Central Nervous System. In B. M. Brenner and J. H. Stien (eds.), *Topics in Nephrology.* New York: Churchill Livingstone, 1978. P. 212.
48. Crabos, M., Ausiello, D. A., Haupert, G. T., Jr., et al. Atrial natriuretic peptide regulates release of Na^+-K^+-ATPase inhibitor from rat brain. *Am. J. Physiol.* 254 (*Renal Fluid Electrolyte Physiol.* 23):F912, 1988.
49. Crocker, A. D., and Hinsull, S. M. Renal electrolyte excretion during the oestrus cycle in the rat. *J. Endocrinol.* 55:XLII, 1972.
50. Crofton, J. J., Baer, P., Share, L., et al. Vasopressin release in male and female rats. *Endocrinology* 117:1195, 1985.
51. Crowley, D. M., Pabari, M., Sinton, T. J., et al. Pathogenesis of postoperative hyponatraemia following correction of scoliosis in children. *Aust. N.Z. J. Surg.* 58:485, 1988.
52. Crumpacker, R. W., and Kriel, R. L. Voluntary water intoxication in normal infants. *Neurology* 23:1251, 1973.
53. Cusaano, A. J., Thies, H. L., Siegal, F. P., et al. Hyponatremia in AIDS and ARC. *Kidney Int.* 35:215, 1988.
54. Dalen, J., and Hickler, R. Oral contraceptives and cardiovascular disease. *Am. Heart J.* 101:626, 1981.
55. Danielson, J., and Buggy, J. Depression of ad lib and angiotensin-induced sodium intake at oestrus. *Brain Res. Bull.* 5:501, 1980.
56. Davidson, J. M., Gilmore, E. A., Durr, J., et al. Altered osmotic thresholds for vasopressin secretion and thirst in human pregnancy. *Am. J. Physiol.* 246:F105, 1984.
57. Davison, J. M., Valloton, M. B., and Lindheimer, M. D. Plasma osmolality and urinary concentration and dilution during and after pregnancy: Evidence that lateral recumbency inhibits maximal urinary concentrating ability. *Br. J. Obstet. Gynecol.* 88:472, 1981.
58. Decaux, G., Unger, J., Brimioulle, S., et al. Hyponatremia in the syndrome of inappropriate secretion of antidiuretic hormone. *J.A.M.A.* 247:471, 1982.
59. Demanet, J. C., Bonnyns, M., Bleiberg, H., et al. Coma due to water intoxication in beer drinkers. *Lancet* 2:1115, 1971.
60. Deutsch, S., Goldberg, M., and Dripps, R. D. Postoperative hyponatremia with the inappropriate release of antidiuretic hormone. *Anesthesiology* 27:250, 1966.
61. DeVries, G. J., Buijs, R. M., and Swaab, D. F. L. Ontogeny of the vasopressinergic neurons of the suprachiasmatic nucleus and their extrahypothalamic projections in the rat brain: Presence of a sex difference in the lateral system. *Brain Res.* 218:67, 1981.
62. DeWitt, L. D., Buonanno, F. S., Kistler, J. P., et al. Central pontine myelinolysis: Demonstration by nuclear magnetic resonance. *Neurology* 34:570, 1984.
63. Dewolf, R., Jugus, M., Uyehara, C. F. T., et al. Correction of chronic hyponatremia by an alpha-2 adrenoceptor agonist. *Kidney Int.* 37:579, 1990.
64. Doczi, T., Joo, F., Szerdahelyi, P., et al. Neurohumoral regulation of brain water and electrolyte contents: Opposite action of central vasopressin and atrial natriuretic factor. *Proc. Second Int. Cong. Neurosci.,* August 1987. P. 412.
65. Doczi, T., Szerdahelgi, P., Gulya, K., et al. Brain water accumulation after the central administration of vasopressin. *Neurosurgery* 11:402, 1982.
66. Donaldson, J. *Neurology of Pregnancy.* Philadelphia: Saunders, 1978.
67. Durr, J. A., Stamoutsos, B., and Lindheimer, M. D. Osmoregulation during pregnancy in the rat. *J. Clin. Invest.* 68:3376, 1981.
68. Dytko, G., and Kinter, L. B. Prevention of Hyponatremia in Experimental Schwartz-Bartter Syndrome with the Vasopressin Antagonist SK & F 1010926. In H. F. Cserr (ed.), *The Neuronal Microenvironment.* New York: New York Academy of Sciences, 1986. P.369.
69. Dzau, V. J., Packer, M., Lilly, L. S., et al. Prostaglandins in severe congestive heart failure. Relation to activation of the renin-angiotensin system and hyponatremia. *N. Engl. J. Med.* 310(6):347, 1984.
70. Edelman, I. S., and Leibman, J. Anatomy of body water and electrolytes. *Am. J. Med.* 27:256, 1959.
71. Edelman, I. S., Leibman, J., O'Meara, M. P., et al. Interrelations between serum sodium concentration, serum osmolarity and total exchangeable sodium, total exchangeable potassium and total body water. *J. Clin. Invest.* 37:1236, 1958.
72. Engel, P. A., Rowe, J. W., Minaker, K. L., et al. Effect of exogenous vasopressin on vasopressin release. *Am. J. Physiol.* 246:E202, 1984.
73. Ensor, D. M., Edmondson, M. R., and Phillips, J. G. Prolactin and dehydration in rats. *J. Endocrinol.* 53:lix, 1972.
74. Epstein, M., Hockaday, J., and Hockaday, T. Migraine and reproductive hormones throughout the menstrual cycle. *Lancet* 1:543, 1975.
75. Faraci, F. M., Mayhan, W. G., Schmid, P. G., et al. Effects of arginine vasopressin on cerebral mi-

crovascular pressure. *Am. J. Physiol.* 25:H70, 1988.
76. Findlay, A. L. R., Fitzsimons, J. T., and Kucharczyk, J. Dependence of spontaneous and angiotensin-induced drinking in the rat upon the oestrous cycle and ovarian hormones. *J. Endocrinol.* 82:215, 1979.
77. Fisher, C. M. Acute brain herniation: A revised concept. *Semin. Neurol.* 4:417, 1984.
78. Forsling, M. L. Effect of ovarian steroids on vasopressin secretion. *J Endocrinol.* 95:147, 1982.
79. Forsling, M. L., Akerlund, M., and Stromberg, P. Variations in plasma concentrations of vasopressin during the menstrual cycle. *J. Endocrinol.* 89:263, 1981.
80. Fraser, C. L., and Arieff, A. I. Fatal central diabetes mellitus and insipidus resulting from untreated hyponatremia: A new syndrome. *Ann. Intern. Med.* 112(2):113, 1990.
81. Fraser, C. L., and Arieff, A. I. Water Metabolism and Its Disorders. In R. D. Cohen, K. G. M. M. Alberti, B. Lewis, and A. M. Denman (eds.), *The Metabolic and Molecular Basis of Acquired Disease.* London: Baillière Tindall, 1990.
82. Fraser, C. L., Kucharczyk, J., Arieff, A. I., et al. Sex differences result in increased morbidity from hyponatremia in female rats. *Am. J. Physiol.* 256 (*Regulatory Integrative Comp. Physiol.* 25):R880, 1989.
83. Fraser, C. L., and Sarnacki, P. Na^+-K^+ ATPase pump function in male rat brain synaptosomes is different from that of females. *Am. J. Physiol.* 257(20):E284, 1989.
84. Fregly, M. J. Attenuation of thirst in estrogen-treated rats. *Fed. Proc.* 37:2694, 1978.
85. Fregly, M. J. Effect of chronic treatment with estrogen on the dipsogen response of rats to angiotensin. *Pharmacol. Biochem. Behav.* 12: 131, 1980.
86. Fregly, M. J., and Thrasher, T. N. Attenuation of angiotensin-induced water intake in estrogen-treated rats. *Pharmacol. Biochem. Behav.* 9:509, 1978.
87. Garcia, J. H., Conger, K. A., Morawetz, R., et al. Postischemic Brain Edema: Quantitation and Evolution. In J. Cervós-Navarro and R. Ferszt (eds.), *Brain Edema: Pathology, Diagnosis, and Therapy. Advances in Neurology.* New York: Raven, 1980. P. 147.
88. Ginsberg, M. D. Delayed neurological deterioration following hypoxia. *Adv. Neurol.* 26:21, 1979.
89. Ginsberg, M. D., Hedley-Whyte, E. T., and Richardson, E. P., Jr. Hypoxic-ischemic leukoencephalopathy in man. *Arch. Neurol.* 33:5, 1976.
90. Goebel, H. H., and Zur, P. H.-B. Central pontine myelinolysis: A clinical and pathological study of 10 cases. *Brain* 95:495, 1972.
91. Grinstein, S. A., Rothsteom, A., and Sarkadi, B., et al. Responses of lymphocytes to anisotonic media: Volume regulating behavior. *Am. J. Physiol.* 246(15):C204, 1984.
92. Guerra, M., del Castillo, A. R., Battaner, E., et al. Androgens stimulate preoptic area Na^+, K^+-ATPase activity in male rats. *Neurosci. Lett.* 78:97, 1987.
93. Haigh, A., Kitchin, A., and Pickford, M. The effect of oxytocin on hand blood flow during the administration of estrogen and isoprenaline. *J. Physiol.* 169:161, 1963.
94. Handler, J. S., Strewler, G. J., and Orloff, J. Role of Protein Synthesis and Phosphoprotein Metabolism in Cellular Response to Vasopressin. In T. E. Andreoli, J. J. Grantham, and F. C. Rector, Jr. (eds.), *Disturbances in Body Fluid Osmolality.* Bethesda, MD: American Physiological Society, 1977. P. 85.
95. Hantman, D., Rossier, B., Zohlman, R., et al. Rapid correction of hyponatremia in the syndrome of inappropiate secretion of antidiuretic hormone: An alternative treatment to hypertonic saline. *Ann. Intern. Med.* 78:870, 1973.
96. Helwig, F. C., Schultz, C. B., and Curry, D. E. Water intoxication: Report of a fatal human case, with clinical, pathologic and experimental studies. *J.A.M.A.* 104:1569, 1935.
97. Hochberg, Z., and Benderly, A. Normal osmotic threshold for vasopressin release in the hyponatremia of hypothyroidism. *Hormone Res.* 17:128, 1983.
98. Hoffman, E. K. Role of separate K^+ and Cl^- channels and of Na^+/Cl^- co-transport in volume regulation in Ehrlich cells. *Fed. Proc.* 44:2513, 1985.
99. Holmes, H. R., Hurley, K. M., and Saper, C. B. Localization of atrial and brain natriuretic peptides in the rat brain. *Soc. Neurosci. Abstr.* 14:1988.
100. Horkey, K., Gutkowska, J., Garcia, R., et al. Effect of different anesthetics on immunoreactive atrial natriuretic factor concentrations in rat plasma. *Biochem. Biophys. Res. Commun.* 129:651, 1985.
101. Horrobin, D. F., Lloyd, I. J., Lipton, A., et al. Actions of prolactin on human renal function. *Lancet* 1:352, 1971.
102. Jacobowitz, D. M., Skofitsch, G., Keiser, H. R., et al. Evidence for the existence of atrial natriuretic factor-containing neurons in the rat brain. *Neuroendocrinology* 40:92, 1985.
103. Jonklaas, J., and Buggy, J. Angiotensin-estrogen interaction in female brain reduces drinking and pressor responses. *Am. J. Physiol.* 247:R167, 1984.
104. Katovich, M. J., and Simpkins, J. W. Effects of chronic hyperprolactinaemia on experimentally induced thirst in male rats. *J. Endocrinol.* 341:75, 1983.

105. Kaufman, S., and Mackay, B. J. Plasma prolactin levels and body fluid deficits in the rat: Causal interactions and control of water intake. *J. Physiol.* 336:73, 1983.
106. Kaufman, S., Mackay, B. J., and Scott, J. Z. Daily water and electrolyte balance in chronically hyperprolactinemic rats. *J. Endocrinol.* 321: 11, 1981.
107. Kaufman, S. F. A comparison of the dipsogenic responses of male and female rats to a variety of stimuli. *Can. J. Physiol. Pharmacol.* 58: 1180, 1980.
108. Kinter, L. B., Huffman, W. F., and Stassen, F. L. Antagonists of the antidiuretic activity of vasopressin. *Am. J. Physiol.* 254 (*Renal Fluid Electrolyte Physiol.* 23):F165, 1988.
109. Krigman, M. R., and Bouldin, T. W. Intoxications and Deficiency Diseases. Oxygen deficiency: Brain Hypoxia and Ischemia. In S. S. Schochet, Jr. (ed), *Neuropathology.* The Clinical Neurosciences, Rosenberg, R. N. (series ed.). New York: Churchill Livingstone, 1983. P. 496.
110. Kucharczyk, J. Localization of central nervous system structures mediating extracellular thirst in the female rat. *J. Endocrinol.* 98:183, 1984.
111. Kucharczyk, J. Neuroendocrine mechanisms mediating fluid intake during the estrous cycle. *Brain Res. Bull.* 12:175, 1984.
112. Kucharczyk, J., Assaf, S. Y., and Mogenson, G. J. Differential effects of brain lesions on thirst induced by administration of angiotensin II to the preoptic vegim, subfornical organ and anterior third ventricle. *Brain Res.* 198:327, 1976.
113. Kucharczyk, J., and Harding, R. K. Regulatory peptides and the onset of nausea and vomiting. *Can. J. Physiol. Pharmacol.* 1990.
114. Kucharczyk, J., Jamshaid, A., and Lemoine, J. Altered drinking responses in dogs with chronic metabolic alkalosis. *Peptides* 9:201, 1988.
115. Kucharczyk, J., Mogenson, G., and Rollin, C. Hypothalamic-Limbic Mechanisms in Body Fluid Homeostasis. In P. M. Gross (ed.), *Circumventricular Organs and Body Fluid Homeostasis.* West Palm Beach, FL: CRC, 1987. P. 105.
116. Kurihara, M., Saavedra, J. M., and Shigematsu, K. Localization and characterization of atrial natriuretic peptide binding sites in discrete areas of the rat brain and pituitary gland by quantitative autoradiography. *Brain Res.* 408:31, 1987.
117. LaBella, F. S., Bihler, I., and Kim, R.-S. Progesterone derivatives that bind to the digitalis receptor: Effects on ^{86}Rb uptake and contractility in the isolated guinea pig heart. *Can. J. Physiol. Pharmacol.* 62:1057, 1984.
118. Landolt, A. M., Yasargil, M. G., and Krayenbuhl, G. Disturbances of the serum electrolytes after surgery in intracranial arterial aneurysm. *J. Neurosurg.* 37:210, 1972.
119. Laragh, J. H., and Atlas, S. A. Atrial natriuretic hormone: A regulator of blood pressure and volume homeostasis. *Kidney Int.* 34(Suppl. 25):S64, 1988.
120. Lasker, N., Hoop, L., Grossman, S., et al. Race and sex differences in erythrocyte Na^+, K^+, and Na^+-K^+ adenosine triphosphatase. *J. Clin. Invest.* 75:1813, 1985.
121. Le Rudulier, D., Strom, A. R., Dandekar, A. M., et al. Molecular biology of osmoregulation. *Science* 224:1064, 1984.
122. Levin, E. R. Atrial natriuretic factor is detectable in human cerebrospinal fluid. *J. Clin. Endocrinol. Metab.* 66:1080, 1988.
123. Liszczak, T. M., Black, P. M., and Roley, L. Arginine vasopressin causes morphological changes suggestive of fluid transport in rat choroid plexus, opithelium. *Cell Tissue Res.* 246:379, 1986.
124. Lluch, S., Conde, M. V., Diegulz, G., et al. Evidence for the direct effect of vasopressin on human and goat cerebral arteries. *J. Pharmacol. Exp. Ther.* 228:749, 1984.
125. Lockett, M. F., and Neil, B. A comparative study of the direct renal actions of pituitary growth and lactogenic hormones. *J. Physiol.* 181:192, 1965.
126. Long, J. B., Martinez-Arizola, A., Johnson, S. H., et al. Arginine 8-vasopressin reduces spinal cord blood flow after spinal subarachnoid injection in rats. *J. Pharmacol. Exp. Ther.* 249:499, 1989.
127. Longstreth, W. T., Jr., Koepsell, T. D., and Yerby, M. S. Risk factors for subarachnoid hemorrhage. *Stroke* 16(3):377, 1985.
128. Longstreth, W. T., Jr., and Swanson, P. D. Oral contraceptives and stroke. *Stroke* 15(4):747, 1984.
129. Lynch, D. R., Braas, K. M., and Synder, S. H. Atrial natriuretic factors in rat kidney, adrenal gland and brain: Autoradiographic localization and fluid balance dependent changes. *Proc. Natl. Acad. Sci. U.S.A.* 83:3557, 1986.
130. Mahoney, C. A., and Arieff, A. I. Central and peripheral nervous system effects of chronic renal failure. *Kidney Int.* 24:170, 1983.
131. Matakas, F. M., Leipert, M., and Franke, J. Cerebral blood flow during increased subarachnoid pressure. *Acta Neurochir 45:19, 1971.*
132. McKee, A., Winkelman, M., and Banker, B. Central pontine myelinolysis in severely burned patients: Relationship to serum hyperosmolality. *Neurology* 38:1211, 1988.
133. McNeil, J. R., and Pang, C. C. Y. Effect of pentobarbital anesthesia and surgery on the control of arterial pressure and mesenteric resistance

in cats: Role of vasopressin and angiotensin. *Can J. Physiol. Pharmacol.* 60:363, 1982.

134. Melton, J. E., Patlak, C. S., Pettigrew, K. D., et al. Volume regulatory loss of Na, Cl, and K from rat brain during acute hyponatremia. *Am. J. Physiol.* 252 (*Renal Fluid Electrolyte Physiol.* 21):F661, 1987.

135. Messert, B., Orrison, W. W., Hawkins, M. J., et al. Central pontine myelinolysis: Considerations on etiology, diagnosis, and treatment. *Neurology* 29:147, 1979.

136. Michell, A. R. The influence of the oestrous cycle on electrolyte excretion in sheep. *Q. J. Exp. Physiol.* 64:77, 1979.

137. Michell, A. R. Sodium appetite and the oestrous cycle in sheep: Effects of oestrogen, progesterone and changes in food intake. *Q. J. Exp. Physiol.* 65:27, 1980.

138. Miller, G. M., Baker, H. L., Okazaki, H., et al. Central pontine myelinolysis and its imitators: MR findings. *Radiology* 168:795, 1988.

139. Morgan, K., Lewis, M. D., Spurlock, G., et al. Characterization and partial purification of the Na, K-ATPase inhibitor released from cultured rat hypothalamic cells. *J. Biol. Chem.* 260: 13595, 1985.

140. Moses, A. M., Blumenthal, S. A., and Streeten, D. H. P. Drugs and Water Metabolism. In A. I. Arieff and R. A. DeFronzo (eds.), *Fluid, Electrolyte and Acid-Base Disorders.* New York: Churchill Livingstone, 1985. P. 1145.

141. Myers, L. S., and Steele, M. K. Effect of angiotensin II (AII) and All) receptor blockers on prolactin (PRL) secretion. *Soc. Neurosci. Abstr.* 14:59, 1988.

142. Naftolin, F., Ryan, K., and Davies, I. The formation of estrogens by central neuroendocrine tissues. *Recent Prog. Horm. Res.* 31:295, 1975.

143. Nakamura, M., Katsuura, G., Nakao, K., et al. Antidipsogenic action of alpha-human atrial natriuretic polypeptide administered intracerebroventricularly in rats. *Neurosci. Lett.* 58:1, 1985.

144. Nattero, G. Menstrual Headache. In M. Critchley, A. Friedman, and S. Gorini (eds.), *Advances in Neurology.* New York: Raven, 1982.

145. Nilius, B. Gating properties and modulation of Na channels. *N.I.P.S.* 4:225, 1989.

146. Nimura, S., Mizuno, K., Ogawa, S., et al. Does atrial natriuretic peptide exist in human brain? *Igaku No Ayumi* 137:235, 1986.

147. Norenberg, M. D., Leslie, K. O., and Robertson, A. S. Association between rise in serum sodium and central pontine myelinolysis. *Ann. Neurol.* 11:128, 1982.

148. Noto, T., Nakajima, Y., Saji, Y., et al. Effect of vasopressin on intracranial pressure of rabbit. *Endocrinol. Jpn.* 25:591, 1978.

149. Noto, T., Nakajima, Y., Saji, Y., et al. Effects of vasopressin and cyclic AMP on water transport at arachnoid villi in cats. *Endocrinol. Jpn.* 26:239, 1979.

150. Okada, Y. and Hazama, A. Volume-regulatory ion channels in epithelial cells. *N.I.P.S.* 4:238, 1989.

151. Olson, J., Sankar, R., Holtzman, D., et al. Energy-dependent volume regulation in primary cultured cerebral astrocytes. *J. Cell. Physiol.* 128:209, 1986.

152. Papadakis, M. A., and Arieff, A. I. Unpredictability of clinical evaluation of renal function in cirrhosis. *Am. J. Med.* 82:945, 1987.

153. Papadakis, M. A., and Arieff, A. I. Hyponatremia and Hypernatremia in Patients with Liver Disease (3rd ed.). In M. Epstein (ed.), *The Kidney in Liver Disease.* Baltimore, MD: Williams & Wilkins, 1988, P. 73.

154. Paradis, H., Kucharczyk, J., Bichet, D., et al. Insulin-dependent mechanisms for the osmoregulation of thirst and vasopressin release in the diabetic dog. *Can. J. Physiol. Pharmacol.* 1990.

155. Park, R. A., Guisado, R., and Arieff, A. I. Nutrient Deficiencies in Man and Animals: Water. In *CRC Handbook of Nutrition and Food, Volume II, Section E: Nutritional Disorders.* West Palm Beach, FL: CRC, 1978. P. 363.

156. Peterson, L. N., Sztorc, D., Jamshaid, A., et al. Plasma AVP and renal concentrating defect in chloride depletion metabolic acidosis. *Am. J. Physiol.* 254:F15, 1988.

157. Petitti, D., and Wingred, J. Use of oral contraceptives, cigarette smoking, and risk of subarachnoid hemorrhage. *Lancet* 2:234, 1978.

158. Pfaff, D. W., Gerlack, J. L., and McEwen, B. S. Autoradiographic localization of hormone-concentrating cells in the brain of the female Rhesus monkey. *J. Comp. Neurol.* 170:279, 1976.

159. Phillips, P. A., Rolls, B. J., Ledingham, J. G. G., et al. Osmotic thirst and vasopressin release in humans: A double blind cross-over study. *Am. J. Physiol.* 248:R645, 1985.

160. Plum, F., and Posner, J. B. Supratentorial Lesions Causing Coma: Pathology and Pathological Physiology. In F. Plum and F. H. McDowell (eds.), *Diagnosis of Stupor and Coma.* Contemporary Neurology. Philadelphia: Davis, 1966. P. 48.

161. Plum, F., Posner, J. B., and Hain, R. F. Delayed neurological deterioration after anoxia. *Arch. Intern. Med.* 110:18, 1962.

162. Posner, J. B., Ertel, N. H., Kossmann, R. J., et al. Hyponatremia in acute polyneuropathy. *Arch. Neurol.* 17:530, 1967.

163. Preedy, J. R. K., and Aitken, E. H. J. The effect of estrogen, water and electrolyte metabolism. *J. Clin. Invest.* 35:423, 1956.

164. Punnonen, R., Viinamaki, O., and Multamaki, S.

Plasma vasopressin during normal menstrual cycle. *Hormone Res.* 17:90, 1983.
165. Quirion, R., Dalpe, M., and Dam, T.-V. Characterization and distribution of receptors for atrial natriuretic peptides in mammalian brain. *Proc. Natl. Acad. Sci. U.S.A.* 83:174, 1986.
166. Radev, A. I. Effect of the sequential use of estradiol and progesterone on the excretion of sodium and potassium and their level in kidney tissue. *Probl. Endokrinol.* 19:91, 1973.
167. Raichle, M. E. A central Neuroendocrine System Regulating Brain Volume. In J. Cervós-Navarro and R. Ferszt (eds.), *Advances in Neurology.* New York: Raven, 1980. P. 341.
168. Raichle, M. E., and Grubb, R. L. Regulation of brain water permeability by centrally-released vasopressin. *Brain Res.* 143:191, 1978.
169. Recht, L., Nilaver, G., and Abrams, G. Oxytocin innervation of cerebral blood vessels: A possible role in local vasoregulation. *Neurology* 32:110, 1982.
170. Robertson, A., Kucharczyk, J., and Mogenson, G. J. Drinking behavior following electrical stimulation of the subfornical organ in the rat. *Brain Res.* 274:197, 1983.
171. Robertson, G. I. Osmoregulation of Thirst and Vasopressin Secretion: Functional Properties and Their Relationship to Water Balance. In R. W. Schrier (ed.), *Vasopressin.* New York: Raven, 1985. P. 203.
172. Robertson, G. J. Physiology of ADH secretion. *Kidney Int.* 32 (Suppl. 21):S20, 1987.
173. Rodriquez del Castello, A., Battaner, E., Guerra, M., et al. Regional changes of brain Na^+, K^+-transporting adenosine triphosphate related to ovarian function. *Brain Res.* 416:113, 1987.
174. Rosenberg, G. A., et al. Effect of vasopressin on ependymal and capillary permeability to tritiated water in cat. *Am. J. Physiol.* 251:F485, 1986.
175. Rosenberg, G. A., Kyner, W. T., Estrada, E., et al. Effect of vasopressin on ependymal and capillary permeability to tritiated water in cat. *Ann. N.Y. Acad. Sci.* 481:383, 1986.
176. Rosomoff, H. L., and Zugibe, F. T. Distribution of intracranial contents in experimental edema. *Arch. Neurol.* 9:36, 1963.
177. Rymer, M. M., and Fishman, R. A. Protective adaption of brain to water intoxication. *Arch. Neurol.* 28:49, 1973.
178. Saavedra, J. M. Alterations in atrial natriuretic peptide receptors in rat brain nuclei during hypertension and dehydration. *Can. J. Physiol. Pharmacol.* 66:288, 1988.
179. Saikaley, A., Bichet, D., Kucharczyk, J., et al. Neuroendocrine factors mediating polydipsia induced by dietary electrolyte depletion. *Am. J. Physiol.* 251:R1071, 1986.
180. Sakuma, Y., and Akaishi, T. Cell size, projection path, and localization of estrogen-sensitive neurons in the rat ventromedial hypothalamus. *J. Neurophysiol.* 57:1148, 1987.
181. Salomon, A., Yeates, A. E., Burger, P. C., et al. Subcortical arteriosclerotic encephalopathy: Brain stem findings with MR imaging. *Radiology* 165:625, 1987.
182. Sampson, C. B. Atrial natriuretic factor inhibits dehydration and hemorrhage-induced vasopressin release. *Neuroendocrinology* 40:277, 1985.
183. Saper, C. B., Standaert, D. B., Currie, M. G., et al. Atriopeptin-immunoreactive neurons in the brain: Presence in cardiovascular regulating areas. *Science* 227:1047, 1985.
184. Sarkadi, B. R., Cheung, R., Mack, E., et al. Cation and anion transport pathways in volume regulatory response of human lymphocytes to hypoosmotic media. *Am. J. Physiol.* 248(*Cell Physiol.* 17):C480, 1985.
185. Sato, K., Murakami, K., Nishimura, K., et al. Possible involvement of sodium pump in the relaxation of rat aorta by α-human atrial natriuretic polypeptide. *Jpn. J. Physiol.* 38:187, 1988.
186. Schafer, J. A., and Andreoli, T. E. Action of Antidiuretic Hormone on Water and Nonelectrolyte Transport Processes in Mammalian Collecting Tubules. In T. E. Andreoli, J. J. Grantham, and F. C. Rector (eds.), *Disturbances in Body Fluid Osmolality.* Bethesda, MD: American Physiological Society, 1977. P. 57.
187. Schettini, A., and Walsh, E. K. Brain tissue elastic behavior and experimental brain compression. *Am. J. Physiol.* 255:R799, 1988.
188. Scheuer, T., Auld, V. J., Boyd, S., et al. Functional properties of rat brain sodium channels expressed in a somatic cell line. *Science* 247:854, 1990.
189. Schipper, H. M. Neurology of sex steroids and oral contraceptives. *Neurol. Clin.* 4:721, 1986.
190. Schrier, R. A., and Berl, T. Osmotic and nonosmotic control of vasopressin release. *Am. J. Physiol.* 236:F321, 1979.
191. Schrier, R. W. Pathogenesis of sodium and water retention in high-output and low-output cardiac failure, nephrotic syndrome, cirrhosis, and pregnancy: Part 1. *N. Engl. J. Med.* 319(16):1065, 1988.
192. Schrier, R. W. Pathogenesis of sodium and water retention in high-output and low-output cardiac failure, nephrotic syndrome, cirrhosis, and pregnancy: Part 2. *N. Engl. J. Med.* 319(17):1127, 1988.
193. Schrier, R. W., Caramelo, C., and Bichet, D. G. Vasopressin and Water Metabolism in Cirrhosis. In A. W. Crowley, J. F. Laird, and D. A. Ausiello (eds.), *Vasopressin: Cellular and Integrative Functions.* New York: Raven, 1988. P. 249.

194. Schultz, W. J., Brownfield, M. S., and Kozlowski, G. P. The hypothalamo-choroid tract: II. Ultrastructural response of the choroid plexus to vasopressin. *Cell Tissue Res.* 178:129, 1977.
195. Scott, J. C., Welch, J. S., and Berman, I. B. Water intoxication and sodium depletion in surgical patients. *Obstet. Gynecol.* 26:168, 1965.
196. Sebastian, C. S., and Bernardin, A. S. Role of angiotensin in the precipitation of severe self-induced water intoxication in a psychotic patient. *Soc. Neurosci. Abstr.* 14:41, 1988.
197. Sheridan, P. J. Autoradiographic localization of steroid receptors in the brain. *Clin. Neuropharmacol.* 7:281, 1984.
198. Skofitsch, G., Jacobowitz, D. M. Eskay, R. L., et al. Distribution of atrial natriuretic factor like immunoreactive neurons in the rat brain. *Neuroscience* 16:917, 1986.
199. Skowsky, V. R., Swan, L., and Smith, P. Effects of sex hormones on arginine vasopressin in intact and castracted male and female rats. *Endocrinology* 104:105, 1979.
200. Sladek, C. D., and Clough, R. W. Comparison of Vasopressin and Oxytocin Release from Hypothalamo-Neurohypophyseal Explants: Cholinergic and Osmotic Control. In A. W. Crowley, Jr., J.-F. Liard, and D. A. Ausiello (eds.), *Vasopressin: Cellular and Integrative Functions.* New York: Raven, 1988. P. 321.
201. Smith, M. C., and Bleck, T. P. Techniques for determining brain death. *J. Crit. Illness.* 4:67, 1988.
202. Smith, M. S., Freeman, M. E., and Neill, J. D. The control of progesterone secretion during the estrous cycle and early pseudopregnancy in the rat: Prolactin, gonadotropin and steroid levels associated with rescue of the corpus luteum of pseudopregnancy. *Endocrinology* 96:219, 1975.
203. Sorensen, P. S., Hammer, M., Gjerris, F., et al. Twenty-four-hour cerebrospinal fluid levels of vasopressin in hydrocephalic patients. *Regul. Pept.* 10:115, 1985.
204. Sorenson, P. S., et al. Cerebrospinal fluid vasopressin in benign intracranial hypertension. *Neurology* 32:1255, 1982.
205. Spruce, B. A., Baylis, P. H., Burd, J., et al. Variations in osmoregulation of arginine vasopressin during the human menstrual cycle. *Clin. Endocrinol.* 22:37, 1985.
206. Steardo, H., and Nathanson, J. A. Brain barrier tissues: End organs for atriopeptins. *Science* 235:470, 1987.
207. Steele, M. K., McCann, S. M., and Negro-Vilar, A. Modulation by dopamine and estradiol of the central effects of angiotension II on anterior pituitary hormone release. *Endocrinology* 33:722, 1982.
208. Stern, E. W., and Coxon, R. V. Osmolality of brain tissue and its relation to brain bulk. *Am. J. Physiol.* 204:1, 1964.
209. Sterns, R. H. Severe symptomatic hyponatremia: Treatment and outcome. A study of 64 cases. *Ann. Intern. Med.* 107:656, 1987.
210. Sterns, R. H., Riggs, J. E., and Schochet, S. S. Osmotic demyelination syndrome following correction of hyponatremia. *N. Engl. J. Med.* 314:1535, 1986.
211. Swanson, L. W., and Sawchenko, P. E. Hypothalamic integration: Organization of the paraventricular and supraoptic nuclei. *Ann. Rev. Neurosci.* 6:269, 1983.
212. Szatalowicz, V. L., Arnold, P. E., Chaimovitz, C., et al. Radiommunoassay of plasma arginine vasopressin in hyponatremic patients with congestive heart failure. *N. Engl. J. Med.* 305:263, 1981.
213. Szego, C. M., and Pietras, R. J. Membrane Recognition and Effector Sites in Steroid Hormone Action. In G. Litwack (ed.), *Biochemical Action of Hormones.* New York: Academic, 1981.
214. Takahashi, H., Iyoda, I., Okajima, H., et al. Vasopressor responses to centrally-administered steroid hormones are mediated via a renin-angiotensin system in the rat brain. *Clin. Exp. Hypertension* A6:2019, 1984.
215. Takahashi, L. K., Vanden Burgt, J. A., Barksdale, C. M., et al. Sex differences in behavioral and endocrinological responses to a controllable stressor applied repeatedly. *Soc. Neurosci. Abstr.* 14:209, 1988.
216. Tartellin, M. F., and Gorski, R. A. The effect of ovarian steroids on food and water intake and body weight in the female rat. *Acta Endocrinol.* 72:551, 1973.
217. Thompson, C. J., Bland, J., Burd, J., et al. The osmotic threshold for thirst and vasopressin release are similar in healthy man. *Clin. Sci.* 71:651, 1986.
218. Thompson, D. S., Hutton, J. T., Stears, J. C., et al. Computerized tomography in the diagnosis of central and extrapontine myelinolysis. *Arch. Neurol.* 38:243, 1981.
219. Thompson, J. S. An effect of estrogens on water intake. *Can. J. Biochem.* 33:10, 1955.
220. Thornton, S. N., Delaney, C. E., and Chapman, C. Plasma vasopressin and oxytocin levels in intact goats and in castrated goats given testosterone. *Acta Endocrinol. (Copenh.)* 117:260, 1988.
221. Thrasher, T. N., and Fregley, M. J. Responsiveness to various dipsogenic stimuli in rats treated chronically with norethynodel, ethinyl estradiol and both combined. *J. Pharmacol. Exp. Ther.* 201:84, 1976.
222. Thrasher, T. N., Keil, L. C., and Ramsay, D. J. Lesions of the organum vasculosum of the lamina terminalis (OVLT) attenuate osmotically

induced drinking and vasopressin secretion in the dog. *Endocrinology* 110:1837, 1982.
223. Thrasher, T. N., Simpson, J. B., and Ramsay, D. J. Lesions of the subfornical organ block angiotensin-induced drinking in the dog. *Neuroendocrinology* 35:68, 1982.
224. Thurston, J. H., and Hauhart, R. E. Brain amino acids decrease in chronic hyponatremia and rapid correction causes brain dehydration: Possible clinical significance. *Life Sci.* 40 (26):2539, 1987.
225. Tomlinson, B. E., Pierides, A. M., and Bradley, W. G. Central pontine myelinolysis: Two cases with associated electrolyte disturbance. *Q. J. Med.* 179:373, 1976.
226. Tsutsumi, K., Niwa, M., Himeno, A., et al. α-Atrial natriuretic peptide binding sites in the rat choroid plexus are increased in the presence of hydrocephalus. *Neurosci. Lett.* 87:93, 1988.
227. Van Bree, J. B., de Boer, A. G., Verhoef, J. C., et al. Transport of vasopressin fragments across the blood-brain barrier: In vitro studies using monolayer cultures of bovine brain endothelial cells. *J. Pharmacol. Exp. Ther.* 249(3):901, 1989.
228. Varavithya, W., and Hellerstein, S. Acute symptomatic hyponatremia. *J. Pediatr.* 71:269, 1967.
229. Vokes, T. J., Weiss, N. M., Schreiber, J., et al. Osmoregulation of thirst and vasopressin during normal menstrual cycle. *Am. J. Physiol.* 254:R641, 1988.
230. Wade, G. N. Sex hormones, regulatory behaviors and body weight. *Adv. Stud. Behav.* 6:201, 1976.
231. Walsh, R. J., Posner, B. I., Kopriva, B. M., et al. Prolactin binding sites in the rat brain. *Science* 201:1041, 1978.
232. Wang, M., Samson, W. K., Dudley, C. A., et al. Direct neuronal action of atrial natriuretic factor in the rat brain. *Neuroendocrinology* 44:49, 1986.
233. Webb, A. C., Ebenezer, I. S., and Burns, D. B. The effects of arginine-8 vasopressin on blood vessels supplying the cerebral cortex. *Reg. Pept.* 17:257, 1987.
234. Weidmann, P., Saxenhofer, H., Shaw, S. G., et al. Atrial natriuretic peptide in man. *J. Steroid Biochem.* 32:229, 1989.
235. Weitzman, R., and Kleeman, C. R. Water Metabolism and the Neurohypophyseal Hormones. In M. H. Maxwell and C. R. Kleeman (eds.), *Clinical Disorders of Fluid and Electrolyte Metabolism.* San Francisco: McGraw-Hill, 1980. P. 531.
236. Welch, K., Darnley, D., and Simkins, R. The role of estrogen in migraine: A review and hypothesis. *Cephalalgia* 4:227, 1984.
237. Williams, T. D. M., Edwards, A., Fairhall, K. M., et al. Influence of endogenous and exogenous oestrogens on posterior pituitary secretion in women. *Clin. Endocrinol.* 22:589, 1985.
238. Wolman, L. Ischaemic lesions in the brain-stem associated with raised intracranial pressure. *Brain* 76:364, 1953.
239. Wood, P. L. Multiple opiate receptors: Supports for unique mn, delta and kappa sites. *Neuropharmacology* 21:487, 1982.
240. Worthley, L. I. G., and Thomas, P. D. Treatment of hyponatremic seizures with intravenous 29.2% saline. *Br. Med. J.* 292:168, 1986.
241. Wright, D., Laureno, R., and Victor, M. Pontine and extrapontine myelinolysis. *Brain* 102:361, 1979.
242. Zamir, N., Skofitsch, G., Eskay, R. L., et al. Distribution of immunoreactive atrial natriuretic peptides in the central nervous system of the rat. *Brain Res.* 365:105, 1986.
243. Zerbe, R., and Robertson, G. Osmotic and Nonosmotic Regulation of Thirst and Vasopressin Secretion. In M. H. Maxwell, C. R. Kleeman, and R. G. Narins (eds.), *Clinical Disorders of Fluid and Electrolyte Metabolism.* New York: McGraw-Hill, 1987. P. 61.
244. Zimmermann, B., and Wangensteen, O. H. Observations on water intoxication in surgical patients. *Surgery* 31:654, 1952.

5 Neurologic Manifestations of Hypernatremia

Neal A. Snyder and Allen I. Arieff

The central nervous system is able to defend itself against certain systemic abnormalities, such as water and electrolyte disorders, by means of internal adjustments. Through such internal adjustments, the brain is able to maintain a normal cellular volume in the presence of such disorders as hypernatremia. Despite this ability, the central nervous system typically bears the brunt of end-organ damage caused by hypernatremic states: neurologic symptoms are the most prominent manifestations of hypernatremia. Conversely, central nervous system pathology can be a source for hypernatremia.

Hypernatremia occurs most commonly in people at the extremes of age, generally affecting the very old and the very young [6]. It is also among the most commonly encountered electrolyte abnormalities in hospital populations, with the reported incidence in adults ranging from 0.7 to 2.3 percent [11,75,138], or about one hospitalization per month per institution in adults [11] and an even higher incidence in children [10,37]. However, there remain a number of major unanswered questions concerning such issues as the actual potential danger of hypernatremia per se, as well as the appropriate types and rates of fluid replacement therapy. Central nervous system manifestations of hypernatremia have been well described [5], yet the clinical data on which these descriptions are based is largely derived from case series that are both small and heterogeneous. Additionally almost all of the patients have had severe concomitant diseases, making the precise attribution to hypernatremia of particular signs and symptoms difficult [5,75,138]. Most clinical studies focus on specific causes of hypernatremia, such as salt poisoning in children [48,55], enteral tube feedings [31,49,65,151], hypertonic sodium bicarbonate administration [102], or essential hypernatremia [27,40]. Therefore, few generalizations can be made concerning the clinical patterns of hypernatremic states. In many of these studies, the distinctions between damage associated with hypernatremia rather than subsequent iatrogenic damage from inappropriate fluid therapy is unclear, as is the distinction between brain damage specifically related to hypernatremia versus that of hyperosmolar states. There is also a paucity of experimental data, in either human subjects of laboratory animals, on the appropriate therapy for hypernatremia.

In this chapter we describe the normal water and solute composition of the central nervous system and review selected cellular and whole body mechanisms for the maintenance of sodium and water homeostasis, with special reference to the central nervous system. We then describe the clinical signs, symptoms, and anatomic manifestations of hypernatremia in both children and adults. The clinical situations that induce hypernatremic states as well as treatment, morbidity, and mortality are also discussed.

NORMAL BRAIN ELECTROLYTE CONTENT AND OSMOTICALLY ACTIVE SOLUTES

The major inorganic constituents of the cerebral cortex of various mammalian species (rat, cat, dog, human) in millimoles per kilogram wet weight are as follows: Na^+, 50 to 60 mmol/kg; K^+, 85 to 100 mmol/kg; Cl^-, 35 to 45 mmol/kg; Ca^{+2}, 1.0 to 2.8 mmol/kg; Mg^{+2}, 5 to 6 mmol/kg; bicarbonate, 10 to 12 mmol/kg [12,26,83,150]. The total brain inorganic cation concentration is approximately 170 mmol/kg (wet weight). The total brain inorganic and organic acid (such as lactate or glutamine) anion concentration is approximately 85 mmol/kg (wet weight) [150], with polyionic lipids and proteins composing the remainder. Since Cl^- is mostly extracellular, intracellular anions are organic and macromolecular [150]. The principal intracellular osmotically active cation is K^+, and a substantial portion of intracellular Na^+ is also probably osmotically active [73,83]. Although the amino acid content of brain in hypernatremia has been extensively studied, the actual osmotic activity of amino acids and other organic acids in the brain is uncertain [92,147,148].

Unlike plasma, cerebrospinal fluid (CSF) is essentially protein free and there is virtually no unmeasured anion. Therefore, $Na^+ + K^+ = Cl^- + HCO_3^-$. The Na^+ concentration of CSF generally parallels that of plasma water. This is in contrast to K^+, which has a relatively constant CSF concentration and generally does not vary with changes in plasma K^+ [25]. The CSF is identical with and a continuation of the extracellular fluid of the brain [28,39,84].

MECHANISMS OF ADAPTATION OF THE BRAIN TO HYPERNATREMIA

Cellular

Different species use different mechanisms to achieve intracellular volume regulation in the face of hyperosmotic challenges that tend to shrink cells (such as hypernatremia). In most tissues, these mechanisms often involve some combination or permutation of Na^+, K^+, and Cl^- influx (for example, in the duck, amphibian, dog, and human red blood cells) [13,56,89]. However, there is a substantial body of evidence suggesting that the brain undergoes osmotic adaptation in a manner distinctly different from that of other tissues. In both birds and mammals, muscle and nucleated red blood cells may adapt to hyperosmolar states such as hypernatremia by loss of water and gain in cation [13, 56, 89], while the brain adapts primarily by de novo generation of solute [13,18,104]. Thus, increases in plasma osmolality are accompanied by corresponding increments in brain tissue osmolality where the apparent net loss or gain of cellular water and commonly measured solute does not completely account for the change in brain osmole content (Figs. 5-1 and 5-2). This is particularly true when the hyperosmolar state has been present for more than several hours [10,13,56,104]. This undetermined solute has been called idiogenic osmoles [13,56,104]. In

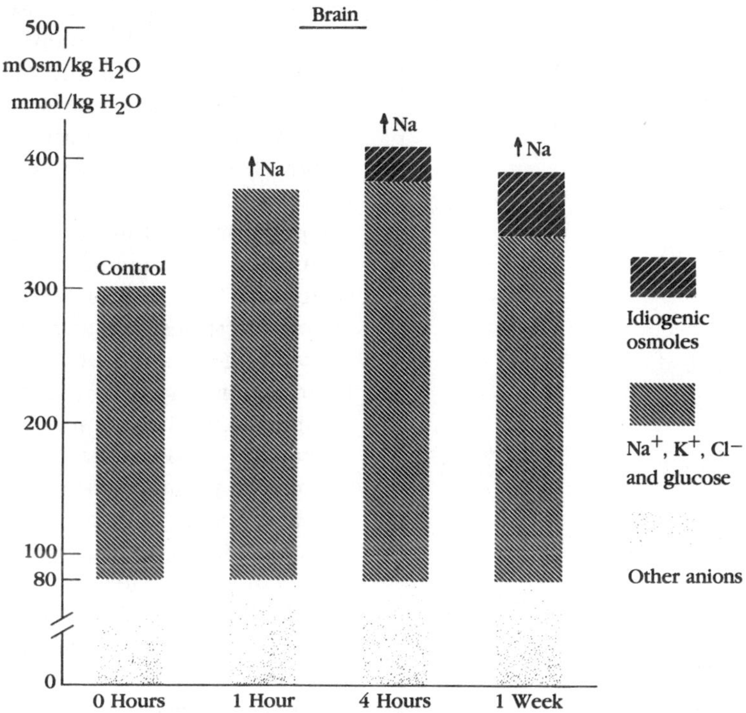

Fig. 5-1. The brain content of idiogenic osmoles in rabbits with hypernatremia for 1 hour to 1 week. Normally, all of the brain content of osmoles can be accounted for by known solutes. In hypernatremia, much of the brain osmole content after the initial 2 hours is found to consist of idiogenic osmoles. (From Arieff, Guisado, and Lazarowitz [11].)

animals with hypernatremia (mean serum Na^+ of 170–180 mM) for less than 3 hours' duration, there is a decrease in brain water and a rise in intracellular Na^+ and Cl^- concentration [10]. Potassium concentration increases minimally [25]. Virtually all of the increase in intracellular osmolality in these animals at 3 hours can be accounted for by the observed increases in measured brain electrolyte (Na^+, K^+, Cl^-) concentration. However, after sustained hypernatremia of several days' duration, brain water content is essentially normal [11]. In rabbits that have been hypernatremic (mean serum Na^+ of 173 mM) for 7 days, brain water content is normal, in spite of the fact that in these same animals there is still a marked loss of intracellular water in muscle tissue. Total brain Na^+ and Cl^- remain elevated in hypernatremic animals, but the increase in measured electrolytes (Na^+, K^+, Cl^-) is not sufficient to account for all of the measured increase in brain osmolality [10]. There is the appearance of unmeasured solute, which accounts for about 60 percent of the increase in brain intracellular osmolality in persistently (4–7 days) hypernatremic animals. These idiogenic osmoles begin to appear after several hours of hypernatremia and are not yet fully characterized. Rises in intracellular glutamine, alanine, inositol, aspartate, and glutamate have been observed in the brains of persistently hypernatremic animals and appear to contribute to the previously described rise in brain osmolality [11,92,96,147,148]. Similar studies have been reported in hypernatremic brain studies in vitro [32], and it has been observed that the brains of some vertebrates that live their lives in both saltwater and freshwater environments appear to have the ability to adapt to the changing osmotic environment by altering intracellular amino acid content [58,59]. These adaptive processes may have a limit. Four days of much more severe hypernatremia (serum Na^+ of

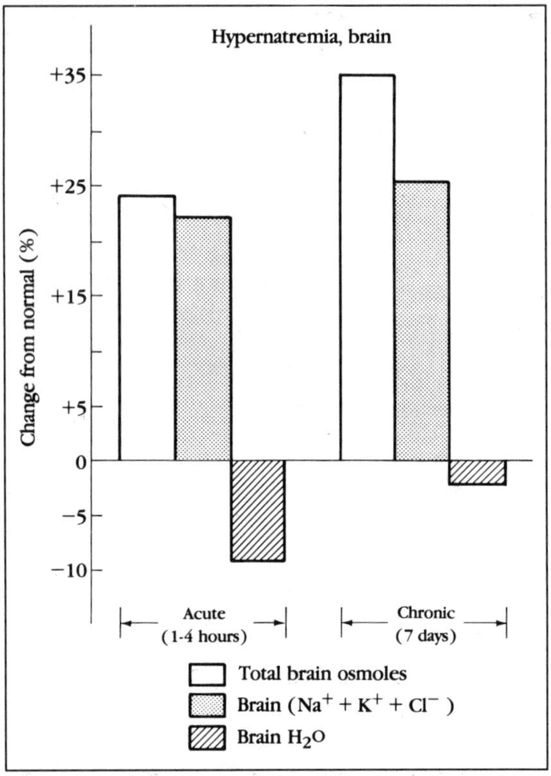

Fig. 5-2. The brain osmole content in laboratory animals with either acute (1–4 hours) or chronic (up to 1 week) hypernatremia. In acute hypernatremia, virtually all of the increase in brain osmole content is accomplished by a loss of water, with resultant increase in concentration of sodium, potassium, and cloride. In animals with chronic hypernatremia, brain water is almost normal, and much of the increase in brain osmole content is accomplished by the formation of idiogenic osmoles. (From Arieff and Guisado [10].)

164–208 mM) in very young mice resulted in persistently low brain water content [148].

Other, mostly hypothetic sources for this unidentified solute include the disassociation of intracellular protein-salt complexes, the action of hydrolytic enzymes in lysozymes activated by hyperosmolality, or some changes in intracellular metabolism leading to accumulation in brain of other low-molecular-weight substances [57,84]. Because this adaptive response of the brain is not immediate, overly rapid induction of hyperosmolality (e.g., hypernatremia) may be lethal [42,46,139]. It may also be that the time required for this adjustment in intracellular osmolality accounts for the fact that rapid correction of elevated serum Na^+ to normal (in rabbits, for example, with 140 mM glucose in water) has been shown to produce seizures [77]. Furthermore this adaptive response does not prevent symptoms in chronic hyperosmolar patients or experimental animals [10]. Either the process is not completely successful or the adaptive response has its own adverse sequelae.

By the generation of idiogenic osmoles, the brain is uniquely able to achieve osmotic equilibrium, minimize the loss of brain water, and defend cerebral cellular volume in the face of changes in plasma osmolality. It is likely that in the absence of this adaptive mechanism, the structural brain damage particularly associated with acute hypernatremic syndromes, including torn cerebral vessels and meninges and consequent hematoma (described below), would be far more prevalent than has been observed. The brain also generates idiogenic osmoles in cases of hyperglycemia, but in hyperglycemia these osmoles dissipate more quickly, probably explaining in part the clinical observation that one can safely correct hyperglycemia more quickly than hypernatremia [7,9,11].

In hyperglycemic subjects, such as those with nonketotic hyperglycemic states, the CSF osmolality remains in equilibrium with plasma osmolality, with continous reequilibration as changes occur in plasma osmolality [9]. Intracranial volume can often be altered by a change in the quantity of either blood or CSF without an actual change in brain volume [127], explaining in part perhaps why correction of dehydration with hypotonic solutions does not always cause a rise intracranial pressure [9].

Thirst

Intracellular volume and content are much more effectively regulated by alterations in water content than in salt content [116], that is, the initial response of dehydrated cells is to increase water content rather than to dump salt. Therefore, increasing water intake is a mechanism of primary importance in correcting or preventing hypernatremic dehydration and is, in fact, more important than regulation of renal water excretion. A major stimulus for thirst is an elevated plasma osmolality [38]. An increase in osmolality of only 1 to 2 percent is sufficient to stimulate thirst [124]. Both the thirst center and osmosensitive neurons are near the anterior hypothalamus. The level of plasma osmolality for thirst to occur is much higher than that which stimulates antidiuretic hormone (ADH) release (~280 versus 290 mOsm/kg)[123] and consequent renal water conservation. Thus, ADH can effectively conserve water without compelling increased drinking. ADH has also been found by some investigators to be dipsogenic [145], but the subject is beyond the scope of this chapter and is discussed elsewhere [62]. Sodium shares with other potent stimuli of thirst the characterisitc of limited entry into brain cells and, therefore, presumably limited entry into receptor cells [116]. The largest ADH response is elicited by sodium and its anions [124].

In dehydrated humans, drinking has been shown to abolish thirst rapidly and inhibit vasopressin secretion before any changes in blood volume or plasma osmolality occur, and the same is true of patients with hypernatremic states induced by hypertonic saline infusion [146]. This phenomenon may be related to the actual act of drinking water rather than its effect on plasma osmolality.

AGE-RELATED CHANGES IN SODIUM AND WATER HOMEOSTASIS

Hypernatremia is a frequent problem in older patients [75,128,128,158]. Thus, changes that may occur in the physiologic responses of the elderly to hypernatremia may be of particular interest in understanding the pathogenesis of hypernatremia in the elderly. When healthy elderly men are compared to younger controls, there are differences in the response to 24 hours of water deprivation [119]. In the older men, there are deficits in both the intensity and threshold of the thirst response to specific stimuli and the subsequent water intake that follows the thirst [156]. The ability to elaborate a concentrated urine during water deprivation also declines with advancing age [132]. This may be related to a relative increase in renal medullary blood flow [95], which washes out medullary tonicity; increases in solute load per nephron (because of nephron dropout), resulting in an obligate osmotic diuresis; or impairment of renal tubular responsiveness to osmolality-mediated vasopressin release [105]. Although there is an enhanced responsiveness to osmolality-mediated vasopressin release [74], there may be impaired responsiveness of vasopressin release to volume and pressure stimuli [130]. In addition, there is a high prevalence of bacteriuria in elderly patients [113], and such patients may exhibit impaired urine-concentrating ability [43]. Finally, there is both a decline in glomerular filtration rate [93,129] and an increased incidence of renal disease with advancing age [131], both of which may contribute to impaired ability to conserve water. There is a small but significant decrease in total body water in healthy people as they age, most of which can be accounted for by a decrease in the intravascular volume [141]; thus water losses of equal volumes in young and old patients may signify more severe dehydration in the more elderly [134].

CLINICAL MANIFESTATIONS OF HYPERNATREMIA

Pediatric Patients

Based on a review of the available literature, it appears that about 67 percent of children with hypernatremia have symptoms referable to the central nervous system. These include irritability, a high-pitched cry in infants, depression in sensorium ranging from lethargy to frank coma, occasional increases in muscle tone, and frank seizures [29,52,84]. In infants, chronic hypernatremia is usually caused by minor medical conditions, such as gastroenteritis, diarrhea, or fever [97,98]. There are several potential consequences of rapid correction of hypernatremia, including seizures [77]. Seizures are not commonly seen in chronic hypernatremia until therapy is initiated and may occur in up to 40 percent of cases [29,80,107]. The seizures that do occur in this group are usually generalized rather than focal and most often occur during the first 24 hours of therapy. Factors that may contribute to the development of seizures in these chronically hypernatremic children probably include the initial severity of the hypernatremia, the presence of significant azotemia, and acidosis [29,107,142]. Fever leading to febrile seizures may be a confounding co-morbid factor [80].

In pediatric subjects with acute hypernatremia, seizures are frequent and coma very common [54]. Unlike the situation in hypernatremia of a more gradual onset, seizures generally precede treatment. In a salt-poisoning episode that occured in Binghamton, New York, 14 infants in a hospital nursery were accidentally given formula containing 739 to 1170 mEq of NaCl per liter (salt was substituted for table sugar) [52]. Of the 14 infants, 11 had symptoms that included muscular twitching or frank convulsions, vomiting, or respiratory distress. The mean serum Na^+ in the 14 patients was 199 mM. These acutely hypernatremic infants displayed signs of avid thirst until they were quite ill. Other neurologic signs included hemiparesis and Babinski's sign. Two other children with hypernatremia after salt poisoning have been observed to have transient chorea [140]. Meningeal signs are usually not present, although the CSF will often have an elevated protein concentration without pleocytosis [83], which may on occasion reach levels greater than 1000 mg/dl [122] but almost always returns to normal in survivors [122]. Computed tomography of the brain of an infant with acute salt poisoning (serum Na^+ of 182 mEq/liter) and seizures revealed hypodense areas in the putamen which disappeared with restoration of normal serum sodium levels [72]. This is consistent with the extracellular edema and vascular changes described in the neuropathologic studies of salt poisoning (see below).

Adults

Hypernatremia in adults is most often a chronic process, usually occurring in the context of severe or catastrophic medical disease [37,86, 138,158]. Thus, it is difficult to know which signs and symptoms to attribute specifically to the presence of hypernatremia. It should be noted, however, that independent of the underlying disease, neurologic manifestations are nearly always present [37,86], supporting the notion that even in chronic hypernatremia in adults, hypernatremia is directly responsible for some of the morbidity experienced by these patients and that hypernatremia is not merely a biochemical marker for severe systemic disease.

Most of the signs and symptoms of hypernatremia are either nonspecific or inconsistent (in adults). The sensation of thirst, which is often intense, may not be verbalized because affected patients frequently have depression of sensorium. Furthermore, in older patients, physical signs that are commonly associated with dehydration, such as altered skin turgor and sunken eye sockets, may not be apparent because of the usual signs of aging. In addition, orthostatic changes in blood pressure may be present in from 10 to 30 percent of healthy elderly patients. Irritability, lethargy, stupor, or coma in varying degrees have been observed [46, 103,138]. In general, the higher the serum sodium, the greater the depression of state of consciousness [138], and greater depressions in the state of consciousness in hypernatremic patients correlate with increased mortality [138]. The incremental nature of the effects of hypernatremia on sensorium is less well understood, although progressive symptoms have occurred in experiments with animals with increasing hyperosmolality [5]. Additionally, progressive depression of sensorium with increasing osmolality has been observed in patients with other hyperosmotic states, such as nonketotic hyperglycemic coma [9] and diabetic ketoacidosis [64]. However, a number of patients with high plasma osmolality are alert, whereas those with lower levels of extracellular osmolality may be comatose [9,109,138]. Although distinguishing between the effects of hyperosmolality and hypernatremia is difficult, there may be some differences, particularly in the cardiovascular system [88]. Muscle irritability, hyperreflexia, and seizures have also been reported [46,84,140], but these occur rarely in chronic hypernatremia. No seizures were documented in one series of 162 hypernatremic patients [138]. Furthermore, it may be that seizures are related to therapy rather than to the hypernatremic state itself, as previously discussed. Muscle cramps are frequently seen in patients with dehydration and hypernatremia, particularly when the dehydration has occurred after exercise in hot climates [85].

A recently described but poorly understood consequence of hypernatremia may be a wasting cachectic state that is characterized by an actual negative nitrogen balance [15]. This clinical consequence appears to accelerate the mortality of hypernatremia in laboratory animals [15] and may contribute to the substantial mortality of hypernatremia observed in humans [52,55,138,158].

Animal Models

Hypernatremia produced in experimental animals (usually acute hypernatremia) represents "pure" hypernatremia in the sense that there is an absence of severe concomitant disease. In general, the animals manifest symptoms that appear to be similar to those described above. In rabbits infused intravenously with 1000 mM NaCl, severe central nervous system symptoms typically began to appear when plasma osmolality had reached 350 mOsm/kg. Initially the animals became alternately restless and lethargic and then went on to develop nystagmus and ataxia, followed by muscular twitching and trembling. Stupor then ensued. Many died of respiratory failure, in most cases at an "effective" plasma osmolality in excess of 400 mOsm/kg [42,139]. A similar picture has been observed in kittens made hypernatremic by intraperitoneal injection with hypertonic NaCl [56] and in animals with hyperosmolar states achieved by infusion of similar osmotic loads of sucrose or mannitol [139]. Recent studies in the hypernatremic rat demonstrate that hypernatremia is a hypercatabolic state, which leads to substantial nitrogen wasting [15]. The nitrogen wasting may be an important comorbid factor in the substantial mortality observed in hypernatremic patients.

Manifestations of Hypernatremia Outside the Central Nervous System

In infants with acute hypernatremia, the most commonly observed symptoms are emesis, fever (particularly beyond the neonatal stage [55]), and labored respirations [51,54,55]. Common laboratory abnormalities in these children with hypernatremia include hyperglycemia (most such children are nondiabetic), hyperkalemia, metabolic acidosis, and hypocalcemia [29,84,143]. Nausea and emesis are commonly associated with hypernatremia in children, particularly when the serum Na^+ exceeds 150 mEq/liter [46].

There are several endocrine abnormalities that are often associated with experimental hyperosmolar states such as hypernatremia [87]. These include impaired hepatic gluconeogenesis with peripheral insulin resistance, decreased muscular glucose utilization [126], and hypercatabolism [15]. Hypernatremic states are also associated with an increased risk of thrombosis. Although this is usually attributed to hyperviscosity and dehydration, at least one study suggests that a hypercoaguable state may be associated with experimental hypernatremia [71]. Severe cachexia has recently been described in laboratory animals.

Electroencephalographic Changes

In experimental animals, hyperosmolality results in a progressive slowing of background electroencephalogram (EEG) frequencies, but no spikes or paroxysmal discharges are seen [11,42,139]. These changes suggest alterations at different levels of the nervous system and probably include changes of spinal cord or peripheral nerve trunks function as well [42]. Other EEG abnormalities are observed at the time that symptoms of hyperosmolality become manifest. There is a generalized reduction in voltage, a disappearance of fast activity, and the appearance of bursts of 4 to 5 per second spindle-like activity. There is gradual progression to 1 to 3 per second high-voltage waves, with cessation of EEG activity at the time of respiratory arrest [139]. The EEG changes appear to be reversible with correction of plasma osmolality to normal [139].

In contrast to the findings in experimental animals, EEGs obtained in patients with hypernatremia have generally been normal. However, the EEGs of 10 to 52 hypernatremic children studied by Bruck, Abal, and Aceto [29] showed a decrease in amplitude similar to that observed in experimental animals, with generalized slowing of the background rhythm. All but two had returned to normal within 2 to 40 days after treatment. The two persistently abnormal EEGs showed typical seizure discharges.

Anatomic Changes in the Brain

In acute hypernatremia, as fluid from the intracellular space moves into the extracellular compartment to establish osmotic equilibrium, the cells initially lose volume [11]. In the brain, this loss of volume may put mechanical traction on delicate cerebral vessels to produce vascular damage [56]. Autopsies performed on children who died from acute salt poisoning have provided much of our information about the anatomic lesions produced in humans by acute hypernatremia [51]. In these children, there is evidence of widespread cerebrovascular damage. Capillaries and veins are markedly congested, with subcortical parenchymous hemorrhage and subarachnoid bleeding. Venous thromboses, sometimes leading to infarction, and occlusion of major venous sinuses have been observed. Although cerebral edema has been noted in some patients, it is more likely the result of overly rapid rehydration therapy rather than of hypernatremia per se.

The anatomic brain damage produced by acute hyperosmolality has also been studied in experimental animals. Shrunken, grossly dehydrated brains, engorged vessels, and petechial hemorrhages were observed in rabbits made hyperosmolar (mean plasma osmolality of 396 mOsm/kg) by the infusion of 1000 mM NaCl, with a 76 percent mortality [42,139]. Similarly, in the previously described study of kittens made hypernatremic by intraperitoneal injection of hypertonic saline or sodium bicarbonate, 85 percent of the animals had subdural hemorrhage with xanthochromia of the CSF, and 7 percent had subdural hematoma [56]. Central pontine myelinolysis, while typically associated with hyponatremia and its rapid correction [114], has been found in initially hyponatremic rats who were made acutely hypernatremic [14,76], although the gradual production of hypernatremia without preceding hyponatremia did not induce central pontine myelinolysis.

Similar findings of bleeding, petechial hemorrhages, and congested cerebral vessels have been observed in children dying of chronic hypernatremia [100], although to a lesser degree than in pediatric hypernatremia of more gradual onset. In chronically hypernatremic animals, dehydration and vascular congestion are present [147], although histologic changes are usually absent [11].

ETIOLOGIES OF HYPERNATREMIA

Numerous medical conditions are associated with or cause hypernatremia in adults (Table 5-1), whereas children typically have more circumscribed clinical scenarios producing hypernatremia. In fact, most clinical studies of hypernatremia have consisted of small, heterogeneous cause-specific case series, particularly in adults [138,158]. Since total body sodium content is the major determinant of extracellular fluid volume, causes of hypernatremia have usually been classified in terms of those that produce isolated decreases in total body water (pure water loss), those that produce decreases in total body effective solute accompanied by greater decreases in total body water (net hypotonic fluid loss), and those that produce gains in total body water accompanied by greater gains in solute (net hypernatremic gain) [3,20,112]. We have divided the medical conditions causing hypernatremia into adult and pediatric causes that usually bring about acute hypernatremia (within less than 24 hours) and those that cause hypernatremia to develop over longer periods of time, which better corresponds to the clinical patterns of the neurologic manifestations. These conditions are detailed in Table 5-1. Presented in more detail are the neurologic conditons that can produce hypernatremia.

Table 5-1. Hypernatremia in adults

Infirmity—inability to get water
Stroke
Dementia
Immobility
Delirium
Febrile illness
Nutritional supplementation
Tube feeding
Hyperalimentation
Increased oral NaCl intake
Diabetes mellitus
Diarrhea
Lack of adequate replacement of free water
Sorbitol with Kayexelate
Lactulose for therapy of hepatic encephalopathy
Intravenous administration of solute
Sodium
$NaHCO_3$
Cardiac arrest
Metabolic acidosis
Drug overdosage (to alkalinize urine)
NaCl
Mannitol
Radiologic contrast material
Gastrointestinal bleeding
Dialysis related
Hemodialysis
Peritoneal dialysis
Increased insensible water loss
Mechanical ventilation
Febrile illness
Increased ambient temperature
Diabetes insipidus
Central
Renal
Alcohol
Hypercalcemia
Postobstructive diuresis
Mineralocorticoid excess
Impaired thirst
Cerebral vascular disease
Cerebral tumors
Essential hypernatremia

Adult Hypernatremia

Acute hypernatremia in adults is usually the result of acute solute loading, particularly intravenous administration of hypertonic or isotonic sodium-containing solutions. Thus, it is almost always iatrogenic [3,81,138]. In one series of 12 patients receiving $NaHCO_3$ during cardiac arrest, the plasma osmolality rose to 377 ± 7 mOsm/kg, and none survived [102]. $NaHCO_3$ causing hypernatremia has also been reported during the treatment of metabolic acidosis [118,138] and alkalinization for drug overdosage [138]. This explains, in part, the diminished enthusiasm for the use of $NaHCO_3$ during advanced cardiopulmonary resuscitation [21,70]. The accidental introduction of hypertonic NaCl into the maternal circulation of patients undergoing therapeutic abortions has also been well documented [30,41]. Patients with burns often develop hypernatremia for a variety of reasons, many relating to increased water loss from the burn surface [105]. There is also some recent enthusiasm for the use of hypertonic lactated saline as part of the therapy of elderly patients with severe burns [24]. This regimen often leads to hypernatremia and may be a factor in the high mortality in such individuals. Fulminant hypernatremia has occurred with malfunction of hemodialysis proportioning systems as well as from improperly proportioned peritoneal dialysis solution [23,137,138]. Hot climate has caused an acute rise in serum Na^+ over a few hours [149]. Acute hypernatremia can occur in patients with heat stroke [90], in those who drown in seawater, and from massive ingestion of table salt [1,79].

Other causes of hypernatremia, usually associated with a more chronic process (and more typical of adult hypernatremia) include nasogastric enteral feeding [31,49,65,138], gastrointestinal bleeding [125,138], gastroenteritis, laxative abuse and oral administration of sorbitol [60,111,138,153], total parenteral nutrition [120,138,155], diabetes out of control and nonketotic hyperosmolar coma [138], acute renal failure, renal tubular damage, dehydration secondary to elevated ambient temperature, pituitary or renal diabetes insipidus, and hyperadrenocorticoid states (Fig. 5-3). Infirmities such as immobility as occurs in patients with strokes or in undiscovered patients with severe trauma who are unable to obtain water [117,138,158], delirium, and dementia are well described. Loop diuretics alone or in the context of concomitant intravenous salt loading [33,81,138] have also been reported to cause hypernatremia, particu-

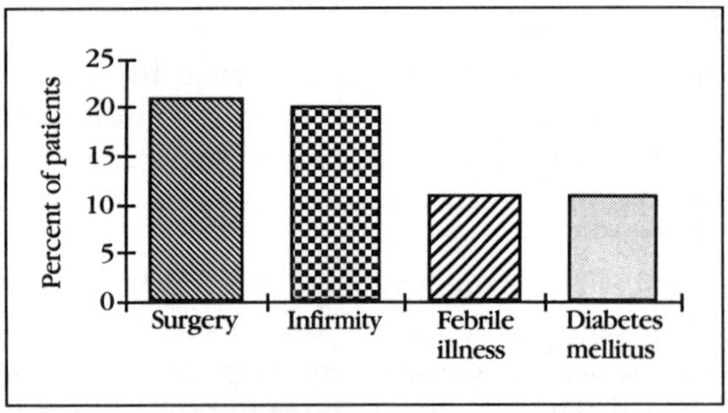

Fig. 5-3. The major causes of hypernatremia in a geriatric hospitalized population. About two-thirds of all cases are due to either surgery, infirmity, febrile illness, or diabetes mellitus. (Data from Snyder, Feigal, and Arieff [138].)

larly when the patients are dependent on the physician to ensure adequate water intake. The infusion of large amounts of isotonic sodium chloride (154 mM), particularly in older post-operative patients who may have had an impaired ability to concentrate the urine maximally, has also been described [138]. Even chicken soup [34,63], oral table salt ingestion [79], and meat tenderizer [157] have been implicated. A recently reported cause of acute hypernatremia is diabetes insipidus complicating untreated hyponatremia [61].

Geriatric Causes

A traditional, well-documented view of hypernatremia in elderly persons suggests that the condition usually occurs in those with infirmities [2,8,158], particularly in nursing home residents with dehydration. It is often alleged that the presence of hypernatremia suggests clinical neglect [75]. A recent report of a large series of hospitalized elderly patients with hypernatremia [138] is at variance with this view. In that current series, only a minority of patients developed hypernatremia because of infirmity; hypernatremia was most often both iatrogenic and multifactorial, with the majority of cases developing after admission to the hospital. Surgery (21%), febrile illness (20%), infirmity (11%), and diabetes mellitus (11%) were the four most common primary causal factors of hypernatremia in this series (Fig. 5-3). Both nutritional supplementation (often by nasogastric tube) and intravenous administration of sodium-containing solutions were commonly associated causal factors, particularly in post-operative patients. The probable interaction between age-associated changes in water metabolism (reviewed above) and previously described causes of hypernatremia such as administration of isotonic (154 mM) NaCl or loop diuretics was also documented.

Pediatric Causes

In infants, gastroenteritis with diarrhea is by far the most common cause of hypernatremia [52,121,128,136]. This is usually chronic hypernatremia, where the infant becomes gradually dehydrated over several days. These infants lose water in excess of sodium in their stool, leading to contraction of the extracellular fluid volume and subsequent hypernatremia. A second large group of children presenting with chronic hypernatremia are those with fever and tachypnea associated with infections [17,52]. There have also been reports of the disastrous substitution of sodium chloride for sugar in the preparation of infant formulas [48,55] presenting as acute hypernatremia (developing in less than 24 hours). The improper dilution of concentrated formula [36] and diets consisting exclusively of canned goods with high sodium concentrations (given to children with psychomotor retardation who could neither regulate their diets nor communicate thirst) have also been reported to lead to hypernatremia in small children [94]. Even breast-fed infants may be at risk for the development of hypernatremia as a consequence of inadequate intake of water, particularly if the sodium concentration of the breast milk is elevated [35]. Administration of large quantities of $NaHCO_3$ to newborn infants has been associated with acute hypernatremia and intracranial hemorrhage, with a mortality of 71 percent [135]. Chronic hypernatremia occurs very rarely in childhood and is usually associated with deficient osmoregulation of vasopressin secretion (see below). Other less common causes in children are described elsewhere [37].

Central Nervous System Causes of Hypernatremia

The central nervous system can influence the development of hypernatremia both by causing excessive losses of body water and by contributing to a failure of the individual to take in adequate amounts of water. Excessive water loss alone is usually not a sufficient explanation for the development of hypernatremia. Dehydration and hypernatremia are such a potent stimulus to thirst [123] that hypernatremia will develop only when there is either an abnormal impairment of thirst or the patient has limited access to water. This is true even in cases of diabetes insipidus with massive polyuria [20]. Patients with diabetes insipidus typically have normal serum Na^+ if conscious and able to obtain water. Hypernatremia will develop in such individuals only when the ability to obtain water is impaired, such as coma following head trauma [108].

Delirium and particularly dementia correspond to the well-described stereotype of hypernatremic dehydration in elderly patients. In a major review of hyperosmolar states [158], it was established that the hypernatremia in patients who were recovering from strokes was usually related to disabilities induced by their cerebrovascular disease (often cognitive impairments), in particular their inability to respond to thirst or to obtain water. Dehydration related to diabetes insipidus arising from their strokes was a rare cause of hypernatremia. In another study of elderly patients, a correlation was found between severity of mental impairment and degree of dehydration [133]. However, hypernatremia has also been reported in alert elderly persons with a history of stroke (not involving the pituitary gland or hypothalamus) who had hypodipsia without a clear explanation of the cause [106]. There have also been reports of hypernatremia in psychotic or demented patients who did not have identifiable central nervous system lesions. In these patients, the hypernatremia was most likely related to impaired intake of water [50,68,110]. Alert but demented patients with central nervous system disease such as diabetes insipidus are particularly vulnerable to dehydration and may require serial hospitalizations [138]. The hydration of cognitively impaired individuals requires careful attention. However, it should be emphasized that patients with these and other infirmities, which are often thought to cause most of the hypernatremia in older patients, may in fact represent only a small minority of such cases [138].

Central or neurogenic diabetes insipidus is caused by a deficiency of ADH release or by low levels of circulating arginine vasopressin in response to normal physiologic stimuli [62]. The clinical features include polyuria, excessive thirst (if the patient is conscious), polydipsia, and often enuresis in children. The onset is usually sudden. Adipsia or hypodipsia may result from impaired function of the hypothalamic thirst center because of extension of the same abnormality that caused the diabetes insipidus (see below), or dehydration may occur during periods of unconsciousness. When classified by pathophysiologic mechanism, there are four types of central diabetes insipidus [144]: (1) no releasable vasopressin present; (2) vasopressin released in response to hypovolemic stimuli, but not in response to osmotic stimuli; (3) higher set point for the osmoreceptors, that is, higher osmolalities are needed to produce release of ADH; and (4) ADH release begins at an appropriate osmolality but in subnormal amounts.

In a series of 104 patients with central diabetes insipidus of more than 6 months' duration [108], the most common pediatric causes were primary brain tumor (14 preoperative cases of which 50% had evidence of anterior pituitary insufficiency; 13 postoperative cases) and histiocytosis (4 cases). In fact, among children with histiocytosis, over 40 percent will probably eventually develop central diabetes insipidus [47]. Idiopathic central diabetes insipidus was the most common cause overall (28 cases, broad age range). In 50 percent of the cases of head trauma–related central diabetes insipidus (18 cases), there was severe accompanying permanent brain damage. Nonfunctioning pituitary tumors accounted for 5 cases, and metastatic tumors to the hypothalamus for 8. There were 7 cases of central diabetes insipidus following hypophysectomy for treatment of various endocrine and malignant diseases, and 5 cases developed following cerebral hypoperfusion. An important recently described cause of central diabetes insipidus is untreated hyponatremia [61]. Diabetes insipidus has been associated with cerebral hypoxia and cardiac arrest [19]. Additional sporadic causes of central diabetes insipidus either identified in this series or reviewed elsewhere include various infiltrative, vascular, or infectious processes involving the hypothalamus or pituitary gland [108].

In essential hypernatremia, the underlying diseases are usually the same as in diabetes insipidus, including surgical, infiltrative, granulomatous, or tumor [27,40,67,82,115,123,152]. In fact, essential hypernatremia might be understood as representing a special case of diabetes insipidus caused by the third pathophysiologic mechanism listed above: There is resetting of the "osmostat," so that body fluid tonicity is defended around a higher than usual value [4,27,40]. This disorder appears to manifest itself as impaired thirst sensation. It has been argued, however, that essential hypernatremia is probably not due to an elevation in the thirst threshold, but rather to a decrease in the sensitivity of the osmostats, usually limited to osmotic stimuli, since the arginine vasopressin (AVP) response to hypotension, nausea, and glucopenia ranges from normal to supernormal [124]. The syndrome has been described in fewer than 100 people [44]. Severe cases with nonfunctioning osmoreceptors have been described [124], and there are multiple reports with various congenital lesions in infants associated with other hypothalamic dysfunction such as temperature regulation and obesity. Essential hypernatremia is often accompanied by other anterior pituitary dysfunction [66]. Prescription of adequate water is the usual treatment. Other structural lesions in the central nervous system that may cause hypernatremia have been reviewed extensively elsewhere [10,37,138,158].

TREATMENT

It is often difficult to sort out the lethality of hypernatremia per se, as opposed to the lethality that may complicate its treatment. Overly rapid correction of hypernatremia by infusion of hypotonic solutions can cause seizures, cerebral edema, and death [11,30,41, 102,137]. There is little actual hard data to which the practicing physician may turn to determine the "correct" treatment. Replacement over 48 hours in both children and adults has been generally recommended [3,52,128]. In cases of very acute hypernatremia, it is likely that there are few idiogenic osmoles present so that more rapid correction is probably justified, particularly if neurologic signs or symptoms from the hypernatremia are manifest. There are several reports of fatal cases of cerebral edema and permanent brain damage with correction of more chronic hypernatremia within 24 hours [29,107,137]. Seizures with cerebral edema occurred in more than 50 percent of hypernatremic rabbits when plasma Na^+ was reduced from 185 to 142 mM in 4 hours [77]. In a similar study of treated chronically hypernatremic rabbits [78], brain water content was significantly greater in those animals with seizures compared to those without seizures, suggesting the importance of brain edema in the pathogenesis of seizure activity. The frequency of seizure activity was also directly proportional to the rate of administration of intravenous solutions utilized to correct hypernatremia. The use of fructose-containing solutions in rehydration therapy for hypernatremia has some intellectual appeal. However, the use of such solutions may cause serious metabolic complications, such as hyperlactemia, lactic acidosis, and circulatory shock due to decreased fructose tolerance [45]. Thus, there are some data that suggest which treatment regimens may be associated with adverse outcomes, but little actual data to suggest what is appropriate.

There have been several reviews of currently accepted regimens for children [37,52,53,128]. Oral fluid is sometimes preferable to intravenous administration in alert patients [3], presumably because the changes in serum osmolality would be less abrupt. However, poorly absorbed osmotic agents such as the unabsorbed carbohydrate in oral glucose-electrolyte solutions that have been used in the past in the treatment of diarrhea may actually intensify the hypernatremia by drawing free water into the intestines (via osmosis). The incremental loss of free water via diarrhea may have been partly responsible for the relatively high prevalence of hypernatremia in the 1950s [22,53]. In one study, infants who seized during treatment of chronic hypernatremia had their serum sodiums corrected at a rate of about 1 mmol/liter/hour, whereas in those who did not seize, the average fall in serum sodium was below 0.6 mmol/liter/hour [80]. Treatment of diarrhea in children with the World Health Organization rehydration packets (90 mmol of sodium per liter) may produce significantly more hypernatremia than would solutions of lower sodium concentrations (about 60 mmol/liter).

As mentioned above, rapid correction of hypernatremia that has developed acutely is probably relatively safe [8,16]. Current treatment recommendations for the chronic hypernatremia that is more typical of adults are as follows:

1. Support shock (if present) either with isotonic crystalloid or colloid; that is, address hypertonicity after the blood pressure has been stabilized.
2. Treat severe acidosis, but not if the pH is greater than about 7.15, since depression of cardiac function does not usually occur above this pH [69].
3. Estimate the fluid deficit [3,37] and replace over 48 hours (increase plasma osmolality by about 2 mOsm/liter/hour) with additional replacement for urinary and insensible losses. In cases of hypernatremia produced by solute and water excess, a loop diuretic may be of use to facilitate excretion of solute. In the face of already present neurologic consequences of hypernatremia, more rapid replacement may be justified.
4. Use hypotonic fluid, such as 280 mM glucose or 77 mM NaCl.
5. Monitor plasma electrolytes every 2 to 4 hours.
6. If possible, replacement fluid should be of a similar composition as that of the fluid lost (T tube, sweat, cecal fluid).
7. Specific therapies for hyperthermia and hyperventilation are often required.
8. Treat the underlying illness. This is especially important in cases where the hypernatremia is more of a paraphenomenon of severe systemic disease.

MORBIDITY AND MORTALITY

In adults, reported mortality rates range from 42 to greater than 70 percent [11,75,138]. Because the medical conditions associated with adult hypernatremia in themselves often carry a grave prognosis, and because most reported series of hypernatremic patients have been small and heterogeneous, it has been difficult to assess directly the morbidity and mortality attributable to hypernatremia [5,75,86,138,158] (Fig. 5-4). In 12 medically uncomplicated elderly patients with severe hypernatremia who were though to represent pure dehydration, only 2 died [138]. In the same study, hypernatremia accompanied by infection carried a particularly poor prognosis: a 63 percent mortality, as had been previously documented [101].

Coma associated with metabolic encephalopathy is said to be generally reversible with correction of the underlying abnormality [6]. In one series, metabolic coma (particulaly hepatic

Fig. 5-4. The mortality from hypernatremia in a geriatric hospitalized population, compared to a control population of similar age and illnesses in the same hospital over the same time interval. The mortality was increased sevenfold in patients whose serum sodium exceeded 149 mM. (Data from Snyder, Feigal, and Arieff [138].)

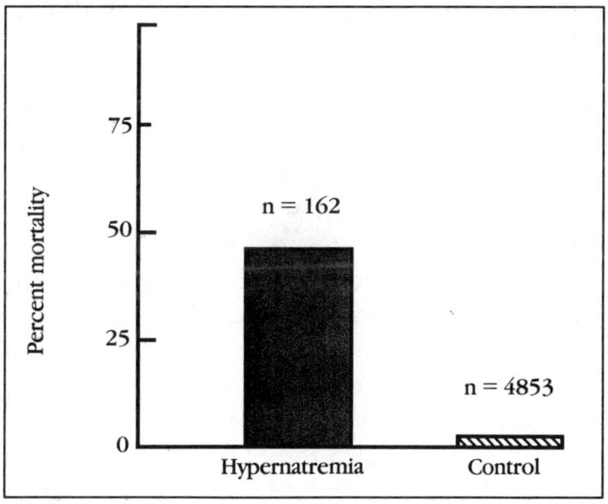

encephalopathy) had the best outcome of all causes of nontraumatic coma [91]. The applicability of this generalization to coma associated with hypernatremia is unproved. There are few data using neurologic status to predict the outcome of hypernatremia. In one series, hypernatremia-associated coma was associated with a poor outcome (11 out of 13 died) [138]. Estimates of the incidence of brain damage from hypernatremia are probably generally too low because many patients probably die before there is evidence of central nervous system damage. Estimates of morbidity as evidenced by brain damage may be too high if the follow-up period is not sufficiently long. This is particularly true in older patients, in whom delays in the recovery of cognitive function after resolution of metabolic derangements are common [131,138,154].

Mortality appears to be clearly related to the rate at which the hypernatremia develops. In one series [138], mortality was particularly high when the hypernatremia was produced acutely and iatrogenically in the hospital, when compared to patients with more gradual dehydration that had developed before hospitalization [138]. This was true despite higher serum sodium levels in the patients with more gradual dehydration. There is also a report of survival in an elderly patient with relatively uncomplicated gradual dehydration over several days with a serum sodium level of 202 mEq/liter [68]. A literature review of adult patients whose serum sodium levels were increased to at least 160 mM in less than 24 hours showed the mortality rate to be greater than 70 percent, whereas for patients with more gradual development of hypernatremia of this degree, the mortality rate was somewhat less (about 60%) [37] and marginally less (46%) with serum sodium levels measuring greater than 150 mM [75].

In fact, in two large series [101,138], the severity of hypernatremia did not predict mortality at all. It has been suggested that in patients with mild hypernatremia, recovery is the rule [158]. However, a mortality rate of 36 percent has been found for patients whose peak serum sodium levels measured only 149 mEq/liter [138]. In addition to the high mortality associated with adult hypernatremia, morbidity that is manifest as permanent brain damage with increased dependence on others for care is well documented [37,138].

One might conclude from the lack of correlation between the severity of adult hypernatremia and subsequent mortality and the apparent predictive power of particular disease states associated with the hypernatremia that hypernatremia is a paraphenomenon, being merely a marker of severe underlying systemic disease. In children, however, the confounding effects of co-morbid states are less prominent, since most cases of hypernatremia are associated with readily reversible underlying systemic illnesses. However, even in such hypernatremic children, there is still a high morbidity and mortality, caused primarily by neurologic damage that is a consequence of hypernatremia [17,29, 51,99,107]. This morbidity and mortality also varies with the rapidity with which the hypernatremic state is attained [6,138]. The mortality for children with acute hypernatremia (plasma Na^+ rising above 160mM in less than 24 hours) has ranged from 40 to 70 percent, with nearly two-thirds of the survivors having neurologic sequelae [37]. In those children who became hypernatremic over a period of several days (chronic), the mortality approximated 10 percent (range 7–29%) [37]. Among 100 patients with chronic hypernatremia [99], 8 sustained brain damage: 1 had tetraplegia, and 7 were either retarded, hyperkinetic, or clumsy. Among 32 chronically hypernatremic patients who were successfully treated and then followed up for 8 years, 1 was monoplegic, 2 had seizure disorders, and 8 had abnormal EEG findings [107]. In one study of seven children with dehydration and acute hypernatremia, all survived, but six of the seven had severe brain damage [54]. Overall, among 132 previously healthy children who developed hypernatremia, 6.8 percent suffered mental retardation and 25 percent had abnormal EEGs after the hypernatremia had been successfully treated [37].

Thus, it is highly probable that hypernatremia is by itself a potentially morbid condition. It should be noted that independent of the underlying disease, neurologic manifestations are nearly always present [37,86]. In addition to the morbidity and mortality in generally healthy children, accidental introduction of hypertonic sodium chloride (usually about 5 M) into the maternal circulation of mothers during therapeutic abortion also resulted in high percentage of morbid or mortal events [30,41]. Furthermore, as described, it has been shown in laboratory animals, children, and adults that acute hypernatremia secondary to infusion of either hypertonic sodium chloride or sodium bicarbonate can lead to abrupt shrinkage of the brain, with tearing of cerebral vessels and subarachnoid or subdural hemorrhage [42,56,79, 102,139].

The morbidity and mortality that can be attributed directly to hypernatremia of more gradual onset, however, are less easily distinguished from the effects of the associated diseases. As discussed, the defensive mechanisms of idiogenic osmole formation have time to come into play and the mortality is lower than that for more acute hypernatremia. This is true even when the serum sodium levels are much higher in the chronically hypernatremic patients. Furthermore, some patients with essential hypernatremia are asymptomatic despite moderate elevations in serum sodium levels for days to months [40].

REFERENCES

1. Addleman, M., Pollard, A., and Grossman, R. I. Survival after severe hypernatremia due to salt ingestion by an adult. *Am. J. Med.* 78:176, 1985.
2. Agate, J. Special Hazards of Illness in Later Life. In I. Rossman (ed.), *Clinical Geriatrics.* Philadelphia: Lippincott, 1986. Pp. 125–137.
3. Alvis, R., Geheb, M., and Cox, M. Hypo- and Hyperosmolar states: Diagnostic Approaches. In. A. I. Arieff and R. A. DeFronzo (eds.), *Fluid, Electrolyte, and Acid-Base Disorders.* New York: Churchill Livingstone, 1985. Pp. 200–207.
4. Arem, R., Rushford, F., Segal, J., et al. Selective osmoreceptor dysfunction presenting as intermittent hypernatremia following surgery for a pituitary chromophobe adenoma. *Am. J. Med.* 80:1217, 1986.
5. Arieff, A. I. Central nervous system manifestations of disordered sodium metabolism. *Clini. Endocrinol. Metab.* 13(2):269, 1984.
6. Arieff, A. I. Effects of Water, Acid-Base, and Electrolyte disorders on the Central Nervous System. In A. I. Arieff and R. A. DeFronzo (eds.), *Fluid Electrolyte, and Acid-Base Disorders.* New York: Churchill Livingstone, 1985. Pp. 969–1040.
7. Arieff, A. I. Cerebral edema complicating nonketotic hyperosmolar coma. *Miner. Electrolyte Metab.* 12:383, 1986.
8. Arieff, A. I. Osmoregulatory failure: Physiology and strategies for treatment. *Hosp. Prac.* 23:173, 1988.
9. Arieff, A. I., and Carroll, H. J. Cerebral edema and depresson of sensorium in nonketotic hyperosmolar coma. *Diabetes* 23(6):525, 1974.
10. Arieff, A. I., and Guisado, R. Effects on the central nervous system of hypernatremic and hyponatremic states. *Kidney Int.* 10:104, 1976.
11. Arieff, A. I., Guisado, R., and Lazarowitz, V. C. Pathophysiology of Hyperosmolar States. In T. E. Andreoli, J. J. Grantham, and F. C. Rector, Jr. (eds.), *Disturbances in Body Fluid Osmolality.* Bethesda: American Physiological Society, 1977. Pp. 227–250.
12. Arieff, A. I., Kerian, S. G., Massry, S. G., et al. Intracellular pH of brain: Alterations in acute respiratory acidosis and alkalosis. *Am. J. Physiol.* 230:804, 1976.
13. Arieff, A. I., and Kleeman, C. R. Studies on mechanisms of cerebral edema in diabetic comas: Effects of hyperglycemia and rapid lowering of plasma glucose in normal rabbits. *J. Clin. Invest.* 52:571, 1973.
14. Ayus, J. C., Krothapalli, R. K., Armstrong, D. L., and Norton, H. J. Symptomatic hyponatremia in rats: Effect of treatment on mortality and brain lesions. *Am. J. Physiol.* (*Renal Fluid Electrolyte Physiol.* 26) 257:F18–F22, 1989.
15. Ayus, J. C., Krothapalli, R., and Freigberg M. Role of hypercatabolism in mortality associated with chronic hypernatremia in rats. *Kidney Int.* 36:371, 1990.
16. Ayus, J. C., Krothapalli, R., Spark, J., and Freigberg, M. Severe hypernatremia in rats: Effect of treatment on brain function and histology. *Kidney Int.* 35:214, 1989.
17. Banister, A., Siddiqi, S., and Hatcer, G. W. Treatment of hypernatremic dehydration in infancy. *Arch. Dis. Child.* 50:179, 1975.
18. Baxter, C. F., Thurston, J. H., Arieff, A. I., and Bessman, S. P. Organic molecules involved in the osmotic regulation of nervous tissue. *Proc. Am. Soc. Neurochem.* 7:14, 1976.
19. Beasley, E. W., and Phillips, L. S. Polyuria and refractory hypernatremia after cardiopulmonary arrest. *Am. J. Med.* 82:347, 1987.
20. Berl, T., Anderson, R. J., McDonald K. M., and Schrier, R. W. Clinical disorders of water metabolism. *Kidney Int.* 10:117, 1976.
21. Bersin, R. M., Chatterjee, K., and Arieff, A. I. Detrimental effects of sodium bicarbonate in

patients with heart disease. *Am. J. Med.* 87:7, 1989.
22. Bhargava, S. K., and Sachdev, H. P. Complications of commercial rehydration packets. *Indian Pediatr.* 22(1):78, 1985.
23. Bluemle, L. W. Current status of chronic hemodialysis. *Am. J. Med.* 4:749, 1968.
24. Bowser-Wallace, B. H., Cone, J. B., and Caldwell, F. T. Hypertonic lactated saline resuscitation of severely burned patients over 60 years of age. *J. Trauma* 25(1):22, 1985.
25. Bradbury, M. W. B., and Kleeman, C. R. Stability of the potassium content of cerebrospinal fluid and brain. *Am. J. Physiol.* 213:519, 1967.
26. Bradbury, M. W. B., Kleeman, C. R., Bagdoyan, H., et al. The calcium and magnesium content of skeletal muscle, brain, and cerebrospinal fluid as determined by atomic absorption flame photometry. *J. Lab. Clin. Med.* 71:884, 1968.
27. Brezis, M., and Weiler-Ravell, D. Hypernatremia, hypodipsia and partial diabetes insipidus: A model for defective osmoregulation. *Am. J. Med. Sci.* 279(1):37, 1980.
28. Brightman, M. W., Shivers, R. R., and Prescott, L. Morphology of the Walls Around Fluid Compartments in Nervous Tissue. In H. F. Cserr, J. D. Fenstermacher, and V. Fencl (eds.), *Fluid Environment of the Brain.* New York: Academic, 1975.
29. Bruck, E., Abal, G., and Aceto, T. Pathogenesis and pathophysiology of hypertonic dehydration with diarrhea. *Am. J. Dis. Child.* 115:122, 1968.
30. Cameron, M. J., and Dayan, A. D. Association of brain damage with therapeutic abortion induced amniotic-fluid replacement: Report of two cases. *Br. Med. J.* 1:1010, 1966.
31. Cataldi-Betcher, E. L., Selter, M. H., Slocum, B. A., and Jones, K. W. Complications occurring during enteral nutrition support: A prospective study. *J. Parenter. Enteral Nutr.* 7(6):546, 1983.
32. Chan, P. H., and Fishman, R. A. Elevation of rat brain amino acids, ammonia and idiogenic osmoles induced by hyperosmolality. *Brain Res.* 161(2):293, 1979.
33. Chow, S., William, C., and Cole, E. Parathyroid storm: Rare manifestations of primary hyperparathyroidism. *Can. Med. Assoc. J.* 134:503, 1986.
34. Chu, E. Dangers of chicken soup (letter). *Pediatrics* 77(5):785, 1986.
35. Clarke, A. J., and Sibert, J. R. Hypernatremic dehydration and necrotizing enterocolitis. *Postgrad. Med. J. 61:65, 1985.*
36. Colle, E., Ayoub, E., and Raile, R. Hypertonic dehydration (hypernatremia) role of feedings high in solutes. *Pediatrics* 22:5, 1958.
37. Covey, C. M., and Arieff, A. I. Disorders of Sodium and Water Metabolism and Their Effects on the Central Nervous System. In B. M. Brenner and J. H. Stein (eds.), *Contemporary Issues in Nephrology.* New York: Churchill Livingstone, 1978. Vol. 1, pp. 212–241.
38. Cox, M., Gehab, M., and Singer I. Water Metabolism and the Regulation of Tonicity. In A. I. Arieff and R. A. DeFronzo (eds.), *Fluid, Electrolyte, and Acid-Base Disorders.* New York: Churchill Livingstone, 1985. Pp. 119–183.
39. Davson, H. The Extracellular Space of Brain and Cord. In H. Davson (ed.), *Physiology of the Cerebrospinal Fluid.* London: Churchill, 1968.
40. DeRubertis, F. R., Michelis, M. F., and Davis, B. B. "Essential" hypernatremia. *Arch. Intern. Med.* 134:889, 1974.
41. De Villota, E. D., Cavanilles, J. M., Stein, L., et al. Hyperosmolal crisis following infusion of hypertonic sodium chloride for purposes of therapeutic abortion. *Am. J. Med.* 55:116, 1973.
42. Dodge, P. R., Sotos, J. F., Gomstrop, I, et al. Neurophysiologic disturbances in hypertonic dehydration. *Trans Am. Neurol. Assoc.* 87:33, 1962.
43. Dontas, A. S., Papanayiotou, P., Marketos, S. G., and Papanicolau, N. T. The effect of bacteriuria on renal functional patterns in old age. *Clin. Sci.* 34:73, 1968.
44. Dow, S. W., Fettman, M. J., LeCouteur, R. A., and Allen, T. A. Hypodipsic hypernatremia and associated myopathy in a hydrocephalic cat with transient hypopituitarism. *J.A.M.A.* 191(2): 217, 1987.
45. Drumm, W., Kleinberger, G., Lenz, K., et al. Fructose-induced hyperlactemia in hyperosmolar syndromes. *Klin. Wochenschr.* 64:615, 1986.
46. Dubois, G. D., and Arieff, A. I. Clinical Manifestations of Electrolyte Disorders. In A. I. Arieff and R. A. DeFronzo (eds.), *Fluid, Electrolyte, and Acid-Base Disorders.* New York: Churchill Livingstone, 1087, 1985.
47. Dunger, D. B., Broadbent, V., Yeoman, E., et al. The frequency and natural history of diabetes insipidus in children with Langerhans-cell histiocytosis. *N. Engl. J. Med.* 321:1157, 1989.
48. Elton, N. W., Elton, W. J., and Nazareno, J. P. Pathology of acute salt poisoning in infants. *Am. J. Clin. Pathol.* 39:252, 1963.
49. Engel, F. L., and Jaeger, C. Dehydration with hypernatremia, hyperchloremia, and azotemia complicating nasogastric tube feeding. *Am. J. Med.* 17:196, 1954.
50. Farley, P. C., Kam-Yung, L., and Suba, S. Severe hypernatremia in a patient with psychiatric illness. *Arch. Intern. Med.* 146:1214, 1986.
51. Finberg, L. Pathogenesis of lesions in the nervous system in hypernatremic states: I. Clinical observations of infants. *Pediatrics* 23:40, 1959.
52. Finberg, L. Hypernatremic (hypertonic) dehy-

dration in infants. *N. Engl. J. Med.* 289:196, 1973.
53. Finberg, L. The role of oral electrolyte-glucose solutions in hydration for children: International and domestic aspects. *J. Pediatr.* 96:51, 1980.
54. Finberg, L., and Harrison, H. E. Hypernatremia in infants: An evaluation of the clinical and biochemical findings accompanying this state. *Pediatrics* 16:1, 1955.
55. Finberg, L., Kiley, J., and Luttrell, C. N. Mass accidental salt poisoning in infancy: A study of a hospital disaster. *J.A.M.A.* 184:187, 1963.
56. Finberg, L., Luttrell, C. N., and Redd H. Pathogenesis of lesions in the nervous system in hypernatremic states: Experimental studies of gross anatomic changes and alterations of chemical composition of the tissues. *Pediatrics* 23:46, 1959.
57. Fishman, R. A. Cell Volume, Pumps, and Neurologic Function: Brain's Adaptation to Osmotic Stress. In F. Plum (ed.), *Brain Dysfunction in Metabolic Disorders.* New York: Raven, 1974. Pp. 159–171.
58. Florkin, M., and Schoffeniels, T. Isosmotic Intracellular Regulation. In *Molecular Approaches to Ecology.* New York: Academic, 1969. Pp. 89–111.
59. Forster, R. P., and Goldstein, L. Intracellular osmoregulatory role of amino acids and urea in marine elasmobranchs. *Am. J. Physiol.* 230:925, 1976.
60. Fraser, C., and Arieff, A. I. Hepatic encephalopathy: Current concepts. *N. Engl. J. Med.* 313:865, 1985.
61. Fraser, C. L., and Arieff, A. I. Fatal central diabetes insipidus and mellitus resulting from untreated hyponatremia: A new syndrome. *Ann. Intern. Med.* 111: 1990.
62. Fraser, C. L., and Arieff, A. I. Water Metabolism and Its Disorders. In R. D. Cohen, K. G. M. M. Alberti, B. Lewis, and A. M. Denman (eds.), *The Molecular and Metabolic Basis of Acquired Disease.* London: Baillière Tindall, 1990.
63. Fujiwara, P., Berry M., Hauger, P., et al. Chicken-soup hypernatremia. *N. Engl. J. Med.* 313(18):1161, 1985.
64. Fulop, M., Tannenbaum, H., and Dreyer, N. Ketotic hyperosmolar coma. *Lancet* 2:635, 1973.
65. Gault, M. H., Dixon, M. E., Doyle, M., et al. Hypernatremia, azotemia, and dehydration due to high protein tube feeding. *Ann. Intern. Med.* 68(4):778, 1968.
66. Gill, G., Baylis, P., and Burn, J. A case of "essential" hypernatremia due to resetting of the osmostat. *Clin. Endocrinol.* 22:545, 1985.
67. Goldberg, M., Weinstein, G., Adesman, J., and Bleicher, S. J. Asymptomatic hypovolemic hypernatremia: A variant of essential hypernatremia. *Am. J. Med.* 43:804, 1967.
68. Goldszer, R. C., and Coodley, E. L. Survival with severe hypernatremia. *Arch. Intern. Med.* 139:936, 1979.
69. Graf, H., and Arieff, A. I. The use of sodium bicarbonate in the therapy of organic acidosis. *Intens. Care Med.* 12:1, 1986.
70. Graf, H., Leach, W., and Arieff, A. I. Evidence for a detrimental effect of bicarbonate therapy in hypoxic lactic acidosis. *Science* 227:754, 1985.
71. Grant, P. J., Tate, G. M., and Hughes, J. R. Does hypernatremia promote thrombosis? *Thromb. Res.* 40(3):393, 1985.
72. Habbick, B. F., Hill, A., and Tchang S. P. K. Computed tomography in an infant with salt poisoning: Relationship of hypodense areas in basal ganglia to serum sodium concentration. *Pediatrics* 74(6):1123, 1984.
73. Hanig, R. C., and Aprison, M. H. Determination of calcium, copper, iron, magnesium, manganese, potassium, zinc and chloride in several brain areas. *Anal. Biochem.* 21:169, 1967.
74. Helderman, J. H., Vestal, R. E., Rowe, J. W., et al. The response of arginine vasopressin to intravenous ethanol and hypertonic saline in man: The impact of age. *J. Gerontol.* 33:39, 1978.
75. Himmelstein, D. U., Jones, A. A., and Woolhandler, S. Hypernatremic dehydration in nursing home patients: An indicator of neglect. *J. Am. Geriatr. Soc.* 31:466, 1983.
76. Hirose, G., Kawada, J., Kitagawa, Y., et al. Changes of auditory brainstem responses in electrolyte-induced myelinolysis in rats: Role of hyponatremia and hypernatremia. *J. Neurol. Sci.* 69:59, 1985.
77. Hogan, G., Dodge, P. R., Gill, S. R., et al. Pathogenesis of seizures occurring during restoration of plasma tonicity to normal in animals previously chronically hypernatremic. *Pediatrics* 43:54, 1969.
78. Hogan, G. R., Pickering, L. K., Dodge, P. R., et al. Incidence of seizures that follow rehydration of hypernatremic rabbits with intravenous glucose or fructose solutions. *Exp. Neurol.* 87:249, 1985.
79. Johnston, J. G., and Robertson, W. O. Fatal ingestion of table salt by an adult. *West J. Med.* 125:141, 1977.
80. Kahn, A., Brachet, E., and Blum, D. Controlled fall in natremia and risk of seizures in hypertonic dehydration. *Intens. Care Med.* 5:27, 1979.
81. Kalter, S., and Reeves, W. B. Hypernatremia in cancer patients receiving normal saline, furosemide, and "salt-poor" albumin. *Texas Med.* 81:45, 1985.
82. Kampmeier, R. H., Gray, B., and Jordan, M. Hypernatremia, hypothermia, and disease of the pituitary gland in a schizophrenic patients. *South. Med. J.* 67(10):1155, 1974.
83. Katzman, R., and Pappius, H. M. Brain Ions. In

R. Katzman and H. M. Pappius (eds.), *Brain Electrolytes and Fluid Metabolism.* Baltimore: Williams & Wilkins, 1973. P. 111.

84. Katzman, R., and Pappius, H. M. Hypernatremia and Hyperosmolarity. In R. Katzman and H. M. Pappius (eds.), *Brain Electrolytes and Fluid Metabolism.* Baltimore: Williams & Wilkins, 1973. P. 278.

85. Knochel, J. P. Neuromuscular manifestations of electrolyte disorders. *Am. J. Med.* 72:521, 1982.

86. Knowles, H. C. Hypernatremia. *Metabolism* 5:508, 1956.

87. Komjati, M., Waldhausel, W., Kastner, G., and Barusch-Marrain, P. Effect of hyperosmolality on glucose uptake and ketogenesis in isolated rat hepatocytes. *Diabetes* 30(Suppl.):35 A, 1981.

88. Kozeny, G. A., Murdock, D. K., Euler, D. E., et al. In vivo effects of acute changes in osmolality and sodium concentration on mycardial contractility. *Am Heart J.* 109(2):290, 1984.

89. Kregenow, F. M. The response of duck erythrocytes to hypertonic media. *J. Gen. Physiol.* 58:396, 1971.

90. Levine, J. A. Heatstroke in the aged. *Am. J. Med.* 47:25, 1977.

91. Levy, D. E., Bates, D., Caronna, J. J., et al. Prognosis in nontraumatic coma. *Ann. Intern. Med.* 94:293, 1981.

92. Lien, Y. H. H., Shapiro, J. I., and Chan, L. Effects of hypernatremia on organic brain osmoles. *J. Clin. Invest.* (in press).

93. Lindeman, R. D., Tobin, J., and Shock, N. W. Longitudinal studies on the rate of decline in renal function with age. *J. Am. Geriatr. Soc.* 33(5):278, 1985.

94. Listernick, R., and Sidransky E. Hypernatremic dehydration in children with severe psychomotor retardation. *Clin. Pediatr.* 24(8):440, 1985.

95. Ljungqvist, A., and Lagergren, C. Normal intrarenal arterial pattern in adult and aging human kidney. *J. Anat.* 96:285, 1962.

96. Lockwood, A. A. H. Acute and chronic hyperosmolality: Effects on cerebral amino acids and energy metabolism. *Arch. Neurol.* 32:62, 1975.

97. Luttrell, C. N., and Finberg, L. Hemorrhagic encephalopathy induced by hypernatremia: I. Clinical, laboratory and pathological observations. *Arch. Neurol. Psychiat.* 81:424, 1959.

98. Luttrell, C. N., and Finberg, L. Hemorrhagic encephalopathy induced by hypernatremia: II. Experimental observations on hyperosmolality in cats. *Arch. Neurol.* 1:153, 1959.

99. Macauley, D., and Watson, M. Hypernatremia as a cause of brain damage. *Arch. Dis. Child.* 42:485, 1967.

100. Maffly, R. H., and Leaf A. The potential of water in mammalian tissues. *J. Gen. Physiol.* 42:1257, 1959.

101. Mahowald, J. M., and Himmelstein, D. U. Hypernatremia in the elderly: Relation to infection and mortality. *J. Am. Geriatr. Soc.* 29(4):177, 1981.

102. Mattar, J. A., Weil, M. H., Shubin, H., and Stein, L. Cardiac arrest in the critically ill: II. Hyperosomolal states following cardiac arrest. *Am. J. Med.* 56:162, 1974.

103. McCance, R. A., and Young, W. F. The secretion of urine during dehydration and rehydration. *J. Physiol. (Lond.)* 102:415, 1944.

104. McDowell, M. E., Wolf, A. V., and Steer, A. Osmotic volumes of distribution: Idiogenic changes in osmotic pressure associated with administration of hypertonic solutions. *Am. J. Physiol.* 180:545, 1955.

105. McKee, A. C., Winkelman, M. D., and Banker, B. Q. Central pontine myelinolysis in severely burned patients. *Neurology* 38:1211, 1988.

106. Miller, P. D., Krebs, R. A., Neal, B. J., and McIntyre, D. O. Hypodipsia in geriatric patients. *Am. J. Med.* 73:354, 1982.

107. Morris-Jones, P. H., Houston, I. B., and Evans, R. C. Prognosis of the neurological complications of acute hypernatremia. *Lancet* 2:1385, 1967.

108. Moses, A. M., Blumenthal, S. A., and Streeten, D. H. P. Acid-Base and Electrolyte Disorders Associated with Endocrine Disease: Pituitary and Thyroid. In A. I. Arieff and R. A. DeFronzo (eds.), *Fluid, Electrolyte, and Acid-Base Disorders.* New York: Churchill Livingstone, 1985. Pp. 851–872.

109. Nabarro, J. D. N. Hyperosmolar Non-ketotic Coma. In B. S. Liebel and G. A. Wrenshall (eds.), *On the Nature and Treatment of Diabetes.* New York: Excerpta Medical Foundation, 1965. Pp. 551–562.

110. Nadler, I. M., and Harprasad, M. K. Psychogenic oligodipsia with hypernatremia in a psychotic patient. *Am. J. Psychiatry* 137:1269, 1980.

111. Nanji, A.A., and Lauener, R. W. Lactulose-induced hypernatremia. *Drug Intell. Clin. Pharm.* 18:70, 1984.

112. Narins, G., Jones, E. R., Stom, M. C., et al. Diagnostic strategies in disorders of fluid, electrolyte and acid-base homeostasis. *Am. J. Med.* 72:496, 1982.

113. Nordenstam, G. R., Brandberg, C. A., Oden, A. S., et al. Bacteriuria and mortality in an elderly population. *N. Engl. J. Med.* 314(18):1152, 1986.

114. Norenberg, M. D., Leslie, K. O., and Robertson, A. S. Association between rise in serum sodium and central pontine myelinolysis. *Ann. Neurol.* 11:128, 1982.

115. Nussey, S. S., Ang, V. T. Y., and Jenkins, J. S. Chronic hypernatraemia and hypothermia following subarachnoid haemorrhage. *Postgrad. Med. J.* 62:467, 1986.
116. Oh, M. S., and Carroll, H. J. Regulation of Extra- and Intracellular Fluid Composition and Content. In A. I. Arieff and R. A. DeFronzo (eds.), *Fluid, Electrolyte, and Acid-Base Disorders.* New York: Churchill Livingstone, 1985. Pp. 1–38.
117. Park, G. R., and Flanagan, J. P. Hypernatremic dehydration following a road traffic accident. *J. R. Soc. Med.* 78:771, 1985.
118. Park, R., and Arieff, A. L. Lactic Acidosis: Current Concepts. In D. S. Schade (ed.), *Clinics in Endocrinology and Metabolism.* Vol. 12, No. 2. Philadelphia: Saunders, 1983.
119. Phillips, P. A., Rolls, B. J., Ledingham, D. M., et al. Reduced thirst after water deprivation in healthy elderly men. *N. Engl. J. Med.* 311(12):753, 1984.
120. Prescott, R. W. G., and Stoddart, J. C. Unrecognized dehydration during parenteral nutrition. *Br. Med. J.* 280:847, 1979.
121. Rapoport, S. Hyperosmolarity and hyperelectrolytemia in pathological conditions of childhood. *Am. J. Dis. Child.* 74:682, 1947.
122. Roach, E. S., Angelo, J. N., and Boyle, R. J. Hypernatremia with choroid plexus hematomas and elevated CSF protein level. *South. Med J.* 76:1055, 1983.
123. Robertson, G. L., Aycenina, P., and Zerbe, J. Neurogenic disorders of osmoregulation. *Am. J. Med.* 72:339, 1982.
124. Robertson, G. L. Abnormalities of thirst regulation. *Kidney Int.* 25:460, 1984.
125. Rodes, J., Arroyo, V., Bordas, J. M., and Bruguera, M. Hypernatremia following gastrointestinal bleeding in cirrhosis and ascites. *Dig. Dis. Sci.* 20(2):127, 1975.
126. Rosenthal, N. R., and Barrett, E. J. An assessment of insulin action in hyperosmolar hyperglycemic nonketotic diabetic patients. *J. Clin. Endocrinol. Metabol.* 60:607, 1985.
127. Rosomoff, H. L., and Zugibe, F. T. Distribution of intracranial contents in experimental edema. *Arch. Neurol.* 9:26, 1963.
128. Ross, E. J., and Christie, S. B. M. Hypernatremia. *Medicine (Baltimore)* 48:441, 1969.
129. Rowe, J. W., Andres, R. A., Tobin, J., et al. The effect of age on creatinine clearance in man: A cross sectional and longitudinal study. *J. Gerontol.* 31:155, 1976.
130. Rowe, J. W., Minaker, K. L., Sparrow, D., and Robertson, G. L. Age-related failure of volume-mediated vasopressin release. *J. Clin. Endocrinol. Metab.* 54:661, 1982.
131. Rowe, J. W., and Resnick, N. M. Disorders of the Kidney and Urinary Tract. In R. Andres, E. C. Bierman, and W. R. Hazzard (eds.), *Principles of Geriatric Medicine.* New York: McGraw-Hill, 1985. P. 616.
132. Rowe, J. W., Shock, N. W., and DeFronzo, R. The influence of age on urine concentrating ability in man. *Nephron* 17:279, 1976.
133. Seymour, D. G., Henschke, P. J., Cape, R. D. T., and Campbell, A. J. Acute confusional states and dementia in the elderly: The role of dehydration/volume depletion, physical illness and age. *Age Ageing* 9:137, 1980.
134. Shannon, R. P., Minaker, K. L., and Rowe, J. W. Aging and water balance in humans. *Semin. Nephrol.* 4:346, 1984.
135. Simmons, M. A. Adcock, E. W., Bard, H., and Battaglia, F. C. Hypernatremia and intracranial hemorrhage in neonates. *N. Engl. J. Med.* 291:6, 1974.
136. Skinner, A. L., and Moll, F. C. hypernataremia accompanying infant diarrhea. *Am J. Dis. Child.* 92:562, 1956.
137. Smith, R. J., Block, M. R., Arieff, A. I., et al. Hypernatremic, hyperosmolar coma complicating chronic peritoneal dialysis. *Proc. Dial. Transplant Forum* 3:96, 1974.
138. Snyder, N. A., Feigal, D. W., and Arieff, A. I. Hypernatremia in elderly patients: A heterogeneous, morbid, and iatrogenic entity. *Ann. Intern. Med.* 107:309, 1987.
139. Sotos, J. F., Dodge, P. R., Meara, P., and Talbot, N. B. Studies in experimental hypertonicity: I. Pathogenesis of the clinical syndrome, biochemical abnormalities and cause of death. *Pediatrics* 26:925, 1960.
140. Sparacio, R. R., Anziska, H. S., and Schutta, H. S. Hypernatremia and chorea: A report of two cases. *Neurology (N.Y.)* 26:46, 1976.
141. Steen, B., Isaksson, B., and Svanborg, A. Body composition at 70 and 75 years of age: A longitudinal population study. *J. Clin. Exp. Gerontol.* 1:185, 1979.
142. Stephenson, J. B. P. Uraemia as a determinant of convulsions in acute infantile hypernatremia. *Arch. Dis. Child.* 46:676, 1971.
143. Stevenson, R. E., and Bowyer, F. P. Hyperglycemia with hyperosmolar dehydration in non diabetic infants. *J. Pediatr.* 77:818, 1970.
144. Streeten, D. H. P. Moses, A. M., and Miller, M. Disorders of the Neurohypophyses. In R. G. Petersdorf, R. D. Adams, E. Braunwald, et al. (eds.), *Harrison's Principles of Internal Medicine* (10th ed.). New York: McGraw-Hill, 1983. P. 604.
145. Szcepanska-Sandowska, E., Sobocinska, J., and Sadowski, B. Central dipsogenic effect of vasopressin. *Am. J. Physiol.* 242:R372, 1982.
146. Thompson, C. J., Burd, J. M., and Baylis, P. H. Acute suppression of plasma vasopressin and

thirst after drinking in hypernatremic humans. *Am. J. Physiol.* 252:1138, 1987.

147. Thurston, J. H., Hauhart, R. E., Jones E. M., and Ater, J. L. Effects of salt and water loading on carbohydrate and energy metabolism and levels of selected amino acids in the brain of young mice. *J. Neurochem.* 24:953, 1975.

148. Thurston, J. H., Hauhart, R. E., and Schulz, D. W. Effect of chronic hypernatremic rehydration on brain carbohydrate, energy and amino acid metabolism in weanling mice. *J. Neurochem.* 40:240, 1983.

149. Toor, M., Wertheimer, E., Massry, S., and Rosenfeld, J. B. Development and correction of hypernatremia during a two hour hike at 42°C at Sodom. *Hasefuah (Tel Aviv)* 57:244, 1959.

150. Tower, T. B. Inorganic Constituents. In A. Lajtha (ed.), *Handbook of Neurochemistry: I. Chemical Architecture of the Nervous System.* New York: Plenum, 1969. P. 1.

151. Vanlandingham, S., Simpson, S., Daniel, P., et al. Metabolic abnormalities in patients supported with enteral tube feeding. *J. Parenter. Enteral Nutr.* 5(8):322, 1981.

152. Verdin, E., Smitz, S., Thibaut, A., et al. Adipsic hypernatremia in a patient with pseudotumor cerebri and the primary empty sella syndrome. *J. Endocrinol. Invest.* 8:369, 1985.

153. Warren, S. E., Mitas, J. A., and Swerdlin, H. R., Hypernatremia in hepatic failure. *J.A.M.A.* 243:1257, 1980.

154. Webb, A. K., Phillips, M. J., and Hanson, G. C. Iatrogenic nondiabetic hyperosmolar states. *J. R. Soc. Med.* 72:578, 1979.

155. Wyrick, W. J., Jr., Rea, W. J., and McClelland, R. N. Rare complications with intravenous hyper-osmotic alimentation. *J.A.M.A.* 211: 1967, 1970.

156. Yamamoto, H., Harada, H., Fukuyama, J., et al. Impaired arginine-vasopressin secretion associated with hypoangiotensinemia in hypernatremic dehydrated elderly patients. *J.A.M.A.* 259:1039, 1988.

157. Zarling, E. J., and Moeller, D. D. Bezoar therapy: Complication using Adolph's Meat Tenderizer and alternatives from literature review. *Arch. Intern. Med.* 141:1669, 1981.

158. Zierler, K. L. Hyperosmolarity in adults: A critical review. *J. Chronic Dis.* 7(1):1, 1958.

6 Neurologic Manifestations of Diabetic Coma

Jaime Uribarri and Hugh J. Carroll

Alterations in central nervous system (CNS) function in diabetes mellitus include those events common in nondiabetics but more common in diabetes mellitus, such as strokes and transient ischemic attacks. Our concern here, however, will be with those alterations in CNS functions that arise out of loss of control of glucose metabolism. This chapter will provide a description of the pathophysiology of uncontrolled diabetes in general and a more detailed description of two specific entities: diabetic ketoacidosis (DKA) and hyperosmolar nonketotic coma (NKC).

DIABETIC KETOACIDOSIS

The root cause of the metabolic alterations of DKA is lack of adequate insulin effect. In a minority of cases, the patient has neglected to take his insulin, but more often the patient is resistant to insulin for a number of reasons: elaboration of counter-regulatory (anti-insulin) hormones; insulin antibodies; in rare instances, antibody to insulin receptors; and resistance of an unknown nature through postreceptor mechanisms. The failure of cellular uptake of glucose leads to hyperglycemia, which in turn leads to osmotic diuresis, a stressful state that causes release of epinephrine and cortisol (Fig. 6-1). Reduction in cellular glucose leads to release of glucagon from the pancreatic alpha cells and of growth hormone from the pituitary. These four counter-regulatory hormones have profound effects on carbohydrate, protein, and lipid metabolism.

Hyperglycemia

Input into the extracellular glucose pool is from three sources: dietary, which is quite variable since the patient may be starving or ingesting sweetened fruit juice; glycogenolysis; and gluconeogenesis. Insulin lack is the primary cause

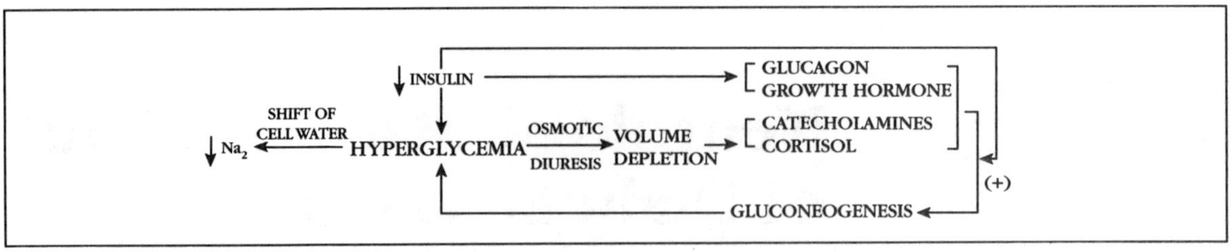

Fig. 6-1. Pathogenesis of hyperglycemia in diabetic ketoacidosis. The shift of cell water expands the extracellular fluid compartment and lowers serum sodium concentration. (From J. Uribarri et al., Water, electrolyte, and acid-base abnormality in diabetes mellitus. *Diabetic Nephropathy* 2:34, 1983.)

of glycogenolysis and gluconeogenesis, but the counter-regulatory hormones enhance these processes at various levels; for example, glucagon and epinephrine participate directly in the breakdown of hepatic glycogen to glucose. The entire glycogen depot of the liver supplies about 100 gm of glucose. Gluconeogenesis is accomplished by three mechanisms: the breakdown of tissue protein with conversion of the amino and carbon chains to glucose; lipolysis, which releases glycerol in quantities sufficient to supply a maximum of about 100 gm of glucose per day during the accelerated breakdown of triglycerides caused by insulin lack and the action of counter-regulatory hormones; and the conversion of glucose to lactate in many organs and particulary as a result of the breakdown of muscle glycogen. Gluconeogenesis occurs in both the liver and the kidney. Although accelerated hepatic output of glucose and diminished peripheral utilization provoke hyperglycemia, the efficiency of renal glucose clearance is such that maintenance of blood glucose at levels above 500 mg/dl requires sharp reduction of glomerular filtration rate [32,33]. The greater severity of volume depletion in nonketotic coma than in diabetic ketoacidosis is the explanation for the greater severity of hyperglycemia in NKC. Clearly then, hydration is one of the most important reasons for the decrease in blood glucose as decompensated diabetes mellitus is treated.

Effects of Hyperglycemia

The increase in osmolality of the extracellular space caused by hyperglycemia draws water from the intracellular compartment until equilibrium between the two compartments is achieved. Cellular dehydration alters significantly many cellular functions, particularly, as will be discussed later, brain function.

Water and Electrolyte Metabolism. As blood glucose increases, the filtered load of glucose soon exceeds the renal threshold, and glucose appears in the urine in increasing amounts. Glucose and other nonreabsorbable solutes, particularly sodium, force water to remain within the renal tubules, producing a progressive increase in urine flow; the quantity of water excreted is proportional to the rate of solute excretion. On the average, an adult with DKA has suffered a loss of about 4 liters of body fluid at the time of admission to the hospital. Although hyperglycemia causes an immediate rise in serum osmolality, it diminishes the release of antidiuretic hormone [62], presumably because glucose diffuses freely into the cerebral osmoreceptor cells, which are then bathed in a fluid whose sodium concentration has been reduced by the withdrawal of cell water from the rest of the body. In DKA, antidiuretic hormone (ADH) levels are elevated by volume depletion and possibly by insulin lack and other nonosmotic stimuli [59,61].

Since osmoreceptors for ADH release are similar to those related to the generation of thirst, a likely, but yet unproven, possibility is that thirst is also suppressed by hyperglycemia and that diabetic patients will develop polydypsia only after some degree of volume depletion is reached.

Sodium. Osmotic diuresis in patients with diabetic hyperglycemia leads to the loss of several hundred milliequivalents of sodium. The average serum sodium is 135 mEq/liter or slightly less, but the range is quite broad, as a result of several effects: The loss of body water in excess of sodium tends to raise the serum sodium, but osmotic withdrawal of cell water expands the extracellular fluid and lowers serum sodium. Each 100 mg/dl increase in glucose reduces serum sodium by about 1.5 mEq/liter. Serum sodium may be spuriously low because of the marked hyperlipidemia common in DKA; lipid displaces serum water and causes the delivery of reduced quantities of sodium into the flame photometer [44].

Potassium. Volume depletion causes a rise in serum aldosterone concentration. With the increased delivery of sodium to the distal nephron, aldosterone causes marked potassium loss in the urine. The delivery of poorly reabsorbable ketone anions to the distal nephron further increases kaliuresis. Kaliuresis is in a sense a fortunate event because potassium is rapidly entering the extracellular fluid (ECF) for a variety of reasons: (1) water drawn from cells to ECF by hyperglycemia carries some of the copious store of cell potassium with it—the phenomenon of "solvent drag"; (2) breakdown of glycogen releases potassium that is bound to the glycogen molecule; (3) buffering of acid by the cells releases cell potassium (administration of organic acids to dogs failed to raise serum potassium in some studies [50], but in others larger amounts of organic acid caused serum potassium to rise [56]); and (4) breakdown of tissue protein frees the potassium that serves as its counter ion. Serum potassium is usually normal or somewhat elevated in DKA, but with marked potassium depletion the serum potassium may be very low, even in the presence of marked acidosis [1,26,31].

Hyperglycemia and the Brain

The profound and potentially lethal alterations in brain volume and function in uncontrolled diabetes are not well understood, but extensive animal experimentation has provided some insight into the effects of the development and regression of hyperglycemia.

In diabetic rabbits, rapid elevation of plasma glucose to about 1100 mg/dl was associated with cerebral dehydration within 2 hours (Fig. 6-2) [8–10]. If the assumptions in that study concerning the distribution of cerebral chloride are correct, virtually the entire water loss was accounted for by shrinkage of cells; the brain extracellular volume was unchanged. With maintenance of hyperglycemia for 4 hours, brain water content returned to normal. The presumed sequence of events is as follows: Plasma hyperosmolality increases the permeability of the blood-brain barrier, and osmotic withdrawal of water reduces the brain extracellular volume and increases its salt concentration. The brain extracellular volume is rapidly restored by two mechanisms: (1) the accumulation in brain interstitium of glucose that osmotically shifts water from plasma across the blood-brain barrier and from the cerebrospinal fluid (CSF osmolality rises almost as rapidly as that of blood) (Fig. 6-3) and (2) osmotic with-

Fig. 6-2. The water content in brain (cerebral cortex) and skeletal muscle in normal rabbits and in those that had been rendered hyperglycemic for 2 hours or 4 hours, with plasma glucose maintained at about 60 mM (1080 mg/dl). After 2 hours of hyperglycemia, the water content of both brain (cerebral cortex) and skeletal muscle is significantly reduced. After 4 hours, brain water content is normal, while that in muscle remains low. (From Arieff, Kleeman, and Keushkerian [10].)

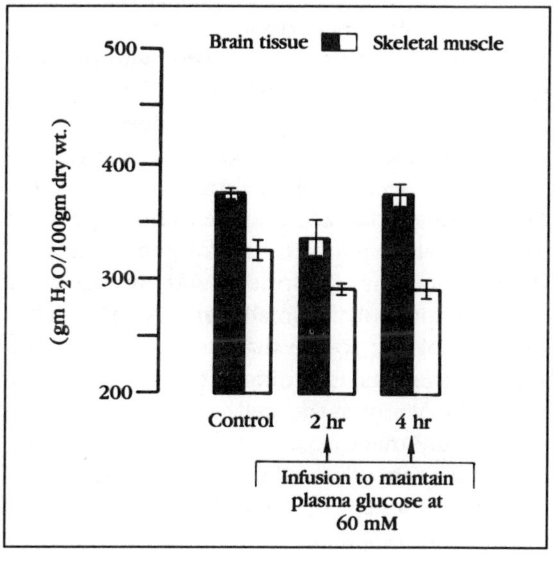

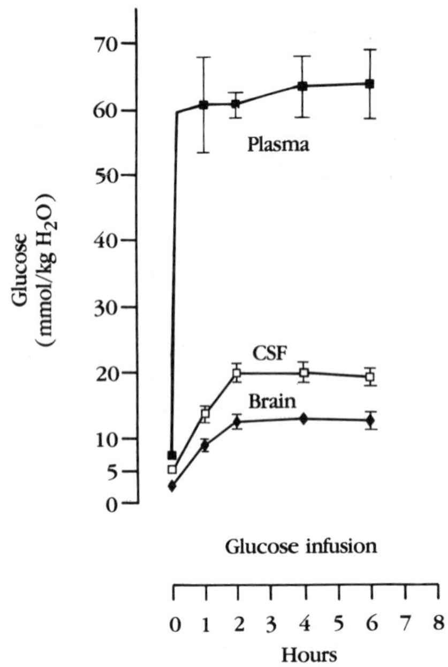

Fig. 6-3. The glucose levels in plasma, cerebrospinal fluid (CSF), and brain tissue in normal rabbits and in those that had been rendered hyperglycemic for 2 hours or 4 hours, with plasma glucose maintained at about 60 mM (1080 mg/dl). After 4 hours of hyperglycemia, the glucose in CSF is about 30 percent of that in plasma, while that in brain is about 20 percent of that in plasma. (Data from Guisado and Arieff [30].)

drawal of brain cell water caused by elevation in interstitial salt concentration.

Brain cell volume is restored within a few hours by the accumulation in the cells of osmotically active solute. Glucose does not contribute significantly to intracellular solute concentration because it is rapidly metabolized. Other solutes that accumulate in brain cells are only partially identified; the known solutes sodium, potassium, chloride, and amino acids account for only a small part. Nearly three-quarters of the solute that restored brain volume represents is "idiogenic osmoles," substances that enter the cell or change from an osmotically inactive state to an osmotically active state within the cell under the conditions of the experiment (Fig. 6-4). Regulation of brain volume in response to hyperglycemia most likely represents a specific homeostatic mechanism developed to avoid brain shrinkage with consequent alteration in brain function; generation of idiogenic osmoles is also observed with sustained hypernatremia but not when hyperosmolality is induced with mannitol (Fig. 6-5).

If the behavior of the brain of patients is analogous to that of the brain of diabetic rabbits, they should have normal brain volume on admission to the hospital, with some elevation in brain interstitial glucose and brain cell volume maintained largely by accumulation of some unidentified solute or by osmotic activation of some solute otherwise fixed and incapable of drawing water into the cell.

Ketogenesis and Acid-Base Metabolism

Although impaired peripheral utilization of keto acids may play some role, the major mechanism responsible for their accumulation in ketoacidosis is excessive production [23]. The production of keto acids requires two major metabolic steps: release of fatty acids by the adipose tissue and oxidation of these fatty acids to keto acids in the liver. Both steps are deranged in diabetic ketoacidosis (Fig. 6-6). Absence of insulin and increase in concentrations of catecholamines, growth hormone, glucagon, and glucocorticoids (lipolytic hormones) increase breakdown of tissue triglycerides. The released free fatty acids are carried to the liver, where they follow one of two courses: (1) they are reesterified with glycerol in the cytoplasm to form new triglycerides, which then bind to globulin to make very low density lipoproteins (VLDL), or (2) they enter the mitochondria and undergo beta oxidation to acetate. Normally this acetate can follow one of three routes: oxidation in the Krebs' cycle; conversion to fatty acids, which form VLDL; or conversion to keto acids. However, in the absence of insulin, acetate is predominantly converted to acetoacetic and beta-hydroxybutyric acids. The amount of fatty acid entering the hepatic mitochondria is determined by the activity of the enzyme carnitine palmitoyltransferase (CPT) located within the mitochondrial membrane. This enzyme is inhibited by increased cytoplasmic concentrations of

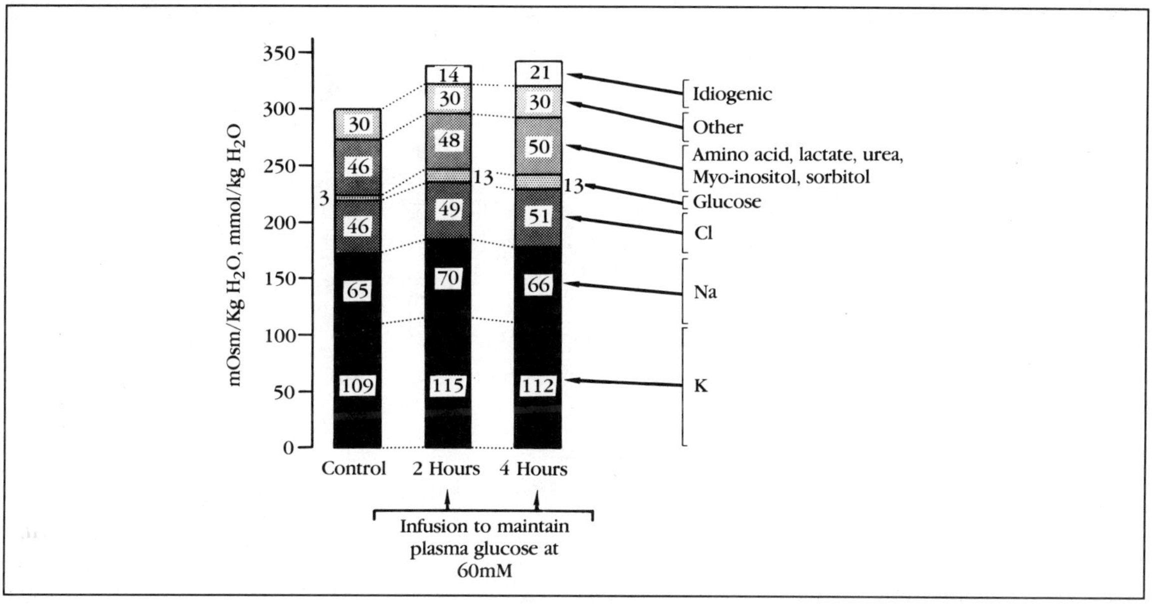

Fig. 6-4. Brain composition in normal rabbits and in those that had been rendered hyperglycemic for 2 hours or 4 hours, with plasma glucose maintained at about 60 mM (1080 mg/dl). After 4 hours of hyperglycemia, there is present in the brain 21 mOsm/kg of solute, which was not present in the control animal. This solute is none of the commonly measured solutes shown in the figure and is called idiogenic osmoles. (From Arieff, Kleeman, and Keushkerian [10]. By copyright permission of the American Society for Clinical Investigation.)

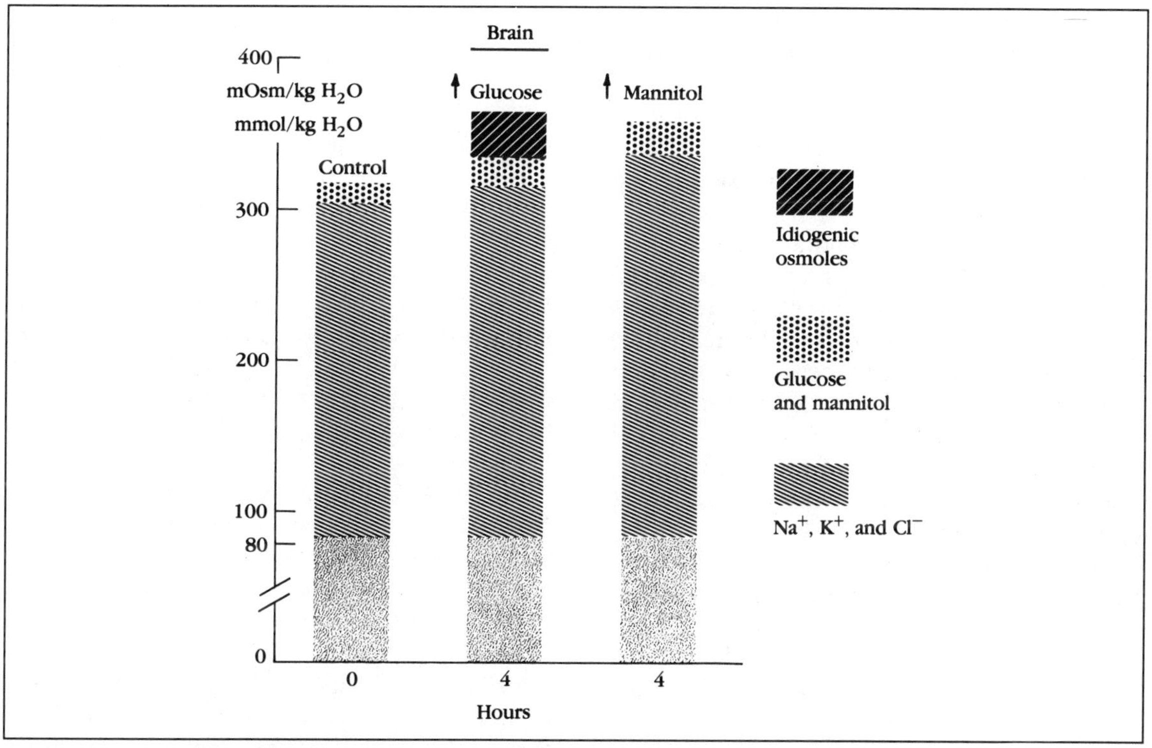

Fig. 6-5. The solute content in brain of rabbits rendered hyperosmolar by infusion of either glucose or mannitol for 4 hours. Idiogenic osmoles are present after 4 hours of hyperglycemia. Idiogenic osmoles are not present in brain after 4 hours of mannitol infusion. (From Arieff, Guisado, and Lazarowitz [8].)

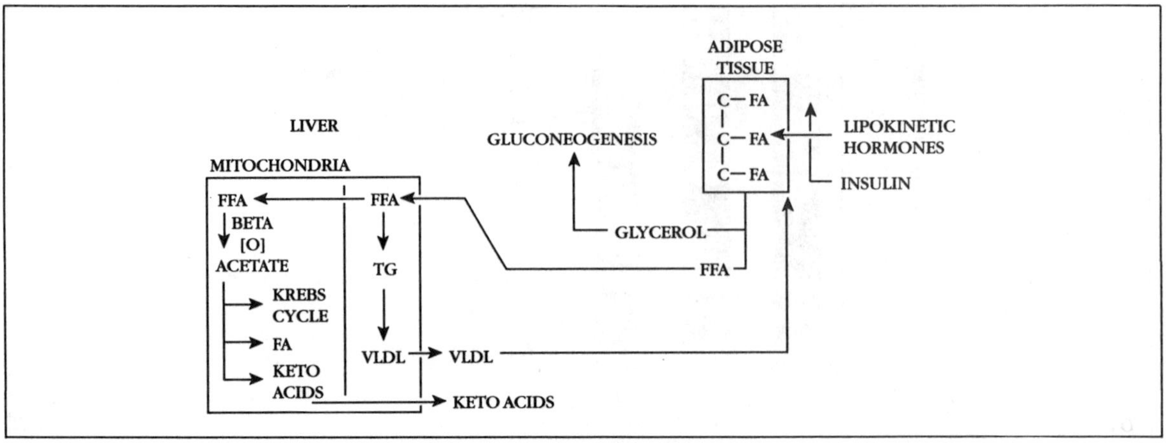

Fig. 6-6. Pathogenesis of ketosis. Increased lipokinetic hormones and lack of insulin allow mobilization of fat and transport of free fatty acids (FFA) to the liver. FFA form triglycerides (TG) in the liver and subsequently VLDL. FFA enter the mitochondria and undergo beta oxidation to acetate. The bulk of this acetate becomes keto acids (From J. Uribarri et al., Water, electrolyte, and acid-base abnormality in diabetes mellitus. *Diabetic Nephropathy* 2:34, 1983.)

malonyl coenzyme A (CoA), in turn regulated by glucagon. Glucagon inhibits malonyl CoA production by blocking both glycolysis and malonyl CoA carboxylase. Thus, during states of high glucagon activity, hepatic malonyl CoA levels are low, CPT activity is increased, and large amounts of free fatty acids are transferred into the mitochondria.

In patients whose mitochondria are in a poor state of oxidation, such as with hypotension or hypoxia, the reduced keto acid, beta-hydroxybutyric acid, may be formed to the near exclusion of the oxidized form, acetoacetic acid. This condition is called beta-hydroxybutyric acidosis [46]. Because the Acetest reaction measures acetoacetate and not beta-hydroxybutyrate in blood and urine, such a patient may not be recognized as having ketoacidosis.

The keto acids (HKA) are buffered by bicarbonate and by intracellular buffers in the following reactions:

$$\text{HKA} + \text{NaHCO}_3 = \text{NaKA} + \text{H}_2\text{CO}_3$$
$$\text{H}_2\text{CO}_3 \rightarrow \text{CO}_2 + \text{H}_2\text{O}$$

where NaKA = sodium ketoanion. The fall in serum bicarbonate leads rapidly to low blood pH and more slowly to low brain pH. This acidosis leads to compensatory hyperventilation:

$$\text{B}^+ \text{Buf}^- + \text{HKA} \rightarrow \text{HBuf} + \text{B}^+ \text{KA}$$

where B^+ = sodium or potassium and Buf^- = intracellular protein anion.

B^+ Buf^- is an intracellular protein or phosphate balanced by sodium or potassium. The potassium lost from cells in this reaction is excreted and replaced in the nephron by sodium, so that more NaKA accumulates in the body fluids. Some of the acetoacetic acid spontaneously decarboxylates into acetone, a volatile hydrocarbon appreciated by its fruity odor on the breath. A major part of the ketone anions is excreted in the urine.

The acidosis of diabetes is usually characterized by a high anion gap. Although in the average patient the fall in serum bicarbonate equals the rise in anion gap this equality is pure coincidence and does not hold for individual patients [2,3,27]. If the patient is not vomiting or receiving alkali, the serum bicarbonate is determined by only one factor: the quantity of bicarbonate titrated by acid. The anion gap, on the other hand, is determined by at least three factors: the quantity of keto acid produced, the quantity of ketone anion excreted, and the tendency for ketone anions to accumulate to a far greater extent in the extracellular fluid than in the cells. In well-hydrated patients with preserved renal function, large amounts of ketone may be excreted, leaving a smaller anion gap; the serum chloride will then be relatively elevated as electroneutrality is maintained. In more severely dehydrated patients, the anion gap tends to be higher and the serum chloride correspondingly lower.

The ketone salts are a major source of energy in the patients with DKA in whom glycolysis is slowed. The essential reaction is

$$NaKA + H_2CO_3 = HKA + NaHCO_3$$

If the HKA is acetoacetic acid, 2 mol of acetyl CoA will be oxidized with formation of adenosine triphosphate (ATP). Beta-hydroxybutyrate is oxidized to acetoacetate and oxidized through the reaction shown above with formation of HCO_3 and ATP. Note that every mole of ketone anion oxidized represents 1 mol of HCO_3 generated. In untreated patients, the formation of HKA exceeds its metabolism and body buffers are progressively utilized. With insulin therapy, conversion of KA^- to HCO_3 exceeds KA^- production, and acidosis is ameliorated. On admission to the hospital, the patients generally have a marked reduction in serum bicarbonate and a great deal of cellular buffer in the acid (HBuf) state.

Alterations in Mental Status

Some alteration in state of consciousness is often present in DKA, but it is less prominent than in patients with NKC. The pathophysiology of the altered mental state has not yet been elucidated, but several mechanisms have been postulated, principally the following: (1) metabolic acidosis, (2) ketosis, (3) hypotension, (4) cerebral hypoxia, (5) hyperosmolality, and (6) miscellaneous hematologic and biochemical alterations.

Acidosis was first examined in 1877 by Walther, who administered hydrochloric acid to rabbits and dogs and succeeded in producing a state resembling diabetic coma that could be completely relieved by administering alkali. However, subsequent clinical and experimental work has not supported this view. No other investigator has produced coma with hydrochloric acid, and acidosis in conditions such as uremia, renal tubular acidosis, and severe diarrhea is not associated with coma [51]. Furthermore, no correlation has been found between systemic pH and level of consciousness in patients with DKA. The argument could be made that the level of consciousness should be correlated with the brain intracellular pH rather than systemic pH, and while no experimental evidence exists of severely decreased brain pH in ketoacidosis, it is possible that extreme acidosis could lower brain pH to a level that could interfere with glucose metabolism and lead to subsequent depression of consciousness [11,53].

Schneider and Droller [54] produced a state resembling diabetic coma in rabbits by infusion of either acetoacetic acid or sodium acetoacetate but not with beta-hydroxybutyric acid, sodium beta-hydroxybutyrate, or hydrochloric acid. The possible pathogenetic role of acetoacetate was supported by the observation of Kety and associates [39] that cerebral utilization of oxygen declines with increasing plasma ketone levels. The main argument against this postulate is the lack of correlation between blood acetoacetate level and depth of coma in DKA. It is conceivable, however, that at an early stage of ketoacidosis, acetoacetate in high concentrations causes damage to the nervous system, which then recovers very slowly during metabolism and disappearance of acetoacetate.

Reduced cerebral perfusion due to dehydration or hypotension was an attractive hypothesis, but Kety and associates [39] found that cerebral blood flow is normal in comatose ketoacidotic patients. Nonetheless it seems possible that severely dehydrated and hypotensive patients may suffer sufficient reduction in cerebral perfusion to promote the development of coma.

Elevation in osmolality may lead to stupor and coma in the experimental animal, and a close correlation has been noted between osmolality of body fluids and level of consciousness in patients with NKC [7]. In the latter disorder, alteration in mental status was not a common finding in patients whose plasma osmolality was less than 350 mOsm/liter. However, Fulop and colleagues [25] found a close correlation between plasma osmolality and severity of alteration in mental status in 70 episodes of DKA when only 20 percent of patients had a plasma osmolality in excess of 350 mOsm/liter (Fig. 6-7). Several points are of importance in reconciling these two observations: (1) in NKC much of the rise in osmolality (mean, 30 mOsm/liter) was made up of urea, an ineffective osmole, while in DKA only 12 to 13 mOsm/liter are attributed to urea. (2) In DKA the rise in osmolality is likely to be extremely rapid, whereas the tendency in NKC is toward gradual accumulation of glucose with a sudden acceleration that rapidly raises osmolality. Hyperosmolality is a likely contributor to altered consciousness in DKA, particularly when the level is high and rapidly achieved.

Reduction in cerebral oxidative metabolism can produce stupor, coma, and death. In DKA the potential for cerebral hypoxia exists but it seems unlikely that this is a prominent mechanism. Erythrocyte 2,3-diphosphoglycerate (2,3-DPG) is low [38], but acidosis compensates for this deficiency and the hemoglobin-oxygen dissociation curve is normal. Blood viscosity is increased [52] but not to the point of limiting blood flow; in fact, cerebral blood flow is normal or even increased in DKA. Arterial oxygen tension often falls [28] in the treatment period, but before therapy it is usually normal. The consequences of reduced availability or utilization of oxygen by the brain should include reduction in adenine nucleotides, but in DKA they are normal [30].

Fig. 6-7. The relationship between depression of sensorium and plasma osmolality in 70 patients with diabetic ketoacidosis. There is some correlation, but with considerable overlap. (From Arieff and Carroll [7].)

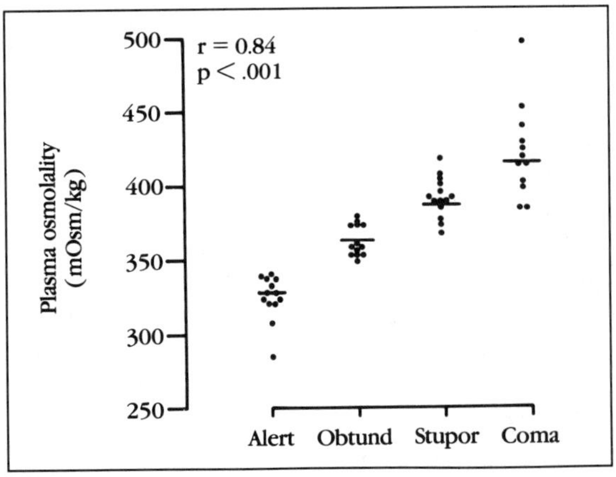

Timperley and co-workers [55] found evidence for intravascular coagulation that could have caused areas of ischemia by involvement of small vessels, but they considered this phenomenon at most a minor contributor to altered consciousness. Cerebral glucose metabolism may be impaired, such as through inhibition of phosphofructokinase activity caused by citrate, which accumulates in the brain in DKA. Pyruvate oxidation may also be impeded through inhibitory effects of excess acetyl CoA on pyruvate dehydrogenase. Other metabolic abnormalities have also been identified whose importance, like that of the biochemical abnormalities cited here, remains to be determined [30,53].

Clearly none of the factors discussed can, by itself, fully explain the depression of sensorium observed in patients with DKA, and it is likely that the pathogenesis of coma is multifactorial. Moreover, the severe associated illnesses frequently found in DKA may contribute to or in some instances completely account for the impaired state of consciousness. Whatever the mixture of causes of coma in DKA, decreased cerebral consumption of oxygen, the common denominator in all comatose conditions, is an important factor.

Clinical Presentation and Diagnosis of the Patient with DKA

The clinical diagnosis of DKA is usually straightforward, the clinical manifestations reflecting the major biochemical changes: hyperglycemia and glycosuria with ensuing volume depletion and metabolic acidosis with ketonemia and ketonuria. In some instances the major signs are those of the precipitating illness. The typical complaints are polyuria, thirst, weakness, malaise, and lethargy. Physical examination reveals signs of contracted interstitial and cellular volume: dry mucous membranes, poor skin turgor, loss of muscle bulk, and softness of the eyeballs. Low blood pressure, orthostatic hypotension, tachycardia, and diminished jugular volume and pressure indicate depleted vascular volume. Tachypnea with hyperventilation (Kussmaul's respiration) reflects compensation for metabolic acidosis; the odor of the breath indicates the presence of acetone. The skin may be warm and flushed in cases of moderate severity, but frank and severe hypothermia may be present in more severe disease. In such subjects resolution of DKA may be accompanied by hyperthermia; this poikilothermia reflects aberrant hypothalamic control. Acute abdominal pain is frequently present; its cause is unknown, but careful attention must be paid to the possibility of a serious intra-abdominal disorder. Hepatomegaly resulting from fatty infiltration may be present, especially after long periods of uncontrolled diabetes, and abnormalities of serum transaminases and amylase may futher complicate the evaluation of the abdomen. Gastroparesis with accumulation of large amounts of fluid in the stomach is fairly common in more seriously ill subjects and can be detected by the presence of a succussion splash; drainage of this fluid with a nasogastric tube may be necessary to prevent aspiration, especially since nausea and vomiting may complicate the picture. A frequent complaint is blurring of vision due to a lenticular refractive error induced by the accumulation of glucose and its metabolic products. Coma is far less common in DKA than in NKC, but some degree of drowsiness is almost universally present in DKA. Similarly focal neurologic signs and convulsions are common in NKC but are not part of the presentation of DKA.

Laboratory Abnormalities

The average blood glucose in one series was about 600 mg/dl with a range of 400 to 800 mg/dl. Some 15 percent of patients with DKA have blood glucose less than 300 mg/dl, but euglycemic (or even hypoglycemic) ketoacidosis suggests alcoholic ketosis. Since glucose levels in blood are closely dependent on renal function, a severely dehydrated diabetic may have ketoacidosis with blood glucose levels exceeding 2000 mg/dl; patients with what is essentially hyperosmolar nonketotic coma may have very mild ketonemia, while patients with DKA may have severe hyperosmolality.

Hematocrit, serum protein, and serum uric acid are characteristically elevated, reflecting volume depletion. Leucocytosis is also commonly seen and may be marked. Blood urea nitrogen (BUN) and serum creatinine are usually elevated because of volume contraction, although some patients may have intrinsic renal disease. Serum sodium is on the average lower than normal but with a wide range. Serum potassium may be normal, high, or low, but most patients present with normal or somewhat elevated serum potassium; severe hyperkalemia or hypokalemia may occur. Serum phosphorus and magnesium tend to be high despite depletion of both of these ions.

The hallmarks for the laboratory recognition of DKA are hyperglycemia, glycosuria, ketonemia, and ketonuria. Metabolic acidosis with an increased anion gap is the rule, but occasionally patients vomit so severely that alkalosis with a high anion gap is present.

Therapy

Treatment of DKA is directed at removal of the biochemical abnormalities described in the section on pathogenesis: insulin, to reverse hyperglycemia, ketonemia, and acidosis; water to reverse dehydration; sodium and potassium to replenish loss of these ions; and management of any concomitant illness. The need for phosphorus and magnesium is less clear.

Insulin stops the excessive gluconeogenesis, restores normal glucose metabolism, and causes rapid synthesis of glycogen; insulin also prevents lipid mobilization and thereby terminates the formation of keto acids. Low doses of regular insulin can be given by intravenous infusion (5–10 units/hour) or by intramuscular injection (10 units/hour), both approaches following an intravenous bolus of 10 units. Intramuscular administration probably should be avoided in hypotensive patients because of inadequate absorption of insulin from the injection site. The dosage of insulin infused can be halved when the blood glucose falls below 300 mg/dl; the end-point of urgent treatment is the disappearance of ketone anions [47].

Theoretically the ideal replacement solution should restore water in excess of salt and should consist of half-normal saline (77 mM NaCl). However, the concern that rapid administration of such a solution may provoke or worsen cerebral edema has led many authors to a compromise approach in which normal saline is given, alternating with half-normal saline. The rate of fluid administration varies with the perceived volume depletion, but a reasonable starting rate of fluid replacement is 500 to 1000 ml/hour. If the patient is hypotensive, normal saline should be given as quickly as possible; in many instances clinical need may call for replacement of plasma or blood as well. When the patient's blood glucose falls below 300 mg/dl (16.7 mM/liter), glucose-containing solutions should be started to avoid hypoglycemia.

Potassium replacement should begin promptly if the patient's urine output is normal and serum potassium is not elevated. A reasonable starting rate of infusion is 10 mEq of potassium per hour, which can then be modified according to subsequent serum potassium measurement. All of the potassium can be replaced as potassium chloride, but administration of half as potassium chloride and half as potassium phosphate will simultanously correct phosphate depletion. The beneficial effect of routine phosphate administration has not been clearly demonstrated [21], but theoretic advantages justify its use. Hypokalemic patients may require more than 10 mEq of potassium per hour; although the need seldom exceeds 20 mEq/hour, the physician must be prepared to administer potassium as rapidly as is necessary, for example, if a cardiac dysrhythmia complicates hypokalemia. When potassium is given at a rapid rate, the phosphate salt should not be given, since extreme hypocalcemia can result.

Bicarbonate is seldom given in DKA; effective conversion of ketone anions to bicarbonate with therapy and renal generation of bicarbonate obviate the need. Possible disadvantages of bicarbonate therapy include overshoot alkalosis, which shifts the hemoglobin-oxygen binding curve to limit tissue oxygen delivery, a particular hazard in patients with DKA who have low erythrocyte 2,3-DPG [38]. Selective accumulation of bicarbonate in the extracellular space leading to cerebral acidosis as hyperventilation wanes is a theoretic hazard without any documentation. Bicarbonate administration is reserved for the older diabetic with compromised myocardial reserve and arterial pH below 7.2, or the young diabetic with pH approaching 7.0. A dose of bicarbonate of about 150 mEq (2–3 ampules) is usually sufficient for an adult patient to overcome the severe phase of acidosis.

Course of Treated DKA and Subsequent Management

Blood glucose falls at an average rate of about 100 mg/dl/hour. Probably the most important determinant of the rate of decline in blood glucose is its rate of excretion in the urine.

Regression of Ketonemia and Amelioration of Acidosis

With cessation of keto acid production, the metabolic conversion of ketone salts into bicarbonate, abetted by insulin, and the continuing excretion of ketone anions lead to a fall in anion gap; generally within 8 hours of successful therapy serum ketones have disappeared and the anion gap has returned to normal. However, the rise in serum bicarbonate characteristically does not parallel the fall in anion gap; in one series [48] the average anion gap fell by 16.1 mEq/liter, while the serum bicarbonate rose by only 8.4 mEq/liter. This disparity may be explained by the following example. If a patient released 600 mEq of keto acid (HKA) into the circulation, he would buffer it with bicarbonate and cellular buffers and would create 600 mEq of NaKA. If he were anuric and excreted no bicarbonate precursor, the conversion of NaKA to $NaHCO_3$ with the administration of insulin would provide him with 600 mEq of alkali and his cellular buffers could be promptly titrated back to their normal state as serum bicarbonate rose to the level present before DKA developed. However, because patients with DKA regularly excrete large amounts of ketone anions in the urine, they arrive at the hospital with a quantity of potential buffer in the body that is considerably less than the amount needed to restore the body buffers (and serum bicarbonate) to normal. Hence, the disappearance of the abnormal anion gap is not accompanied by an immediate return to normal serum bicarbonate.

The concentration of organic anions in the extracellular space on admission is close to the deficit in extracellular bicarbonate because, as was previously noted, organic anions tend to accumulate in the extracellular space. Hence, although the patient has sufficient bicarbonate precursor in the extracellular space to restore extracellular bicarbonate to normal, the bulk of the bicarbonate formed from that NaKA is utilized by the cells to back-titrate cellular buffers, that is, the space of distribution of buffer deficit is greater than the space of distribution of potential buffers (organic anions) in the patient with DKA. The difference between the falling anion gap and the rising bicarbonate concentration is made up by an increase in serum chloride. Hence the patient with DKA very often passes through a phase of what appears to be classic hyperchloremic acidosis on his way to a cure. The serum chloride rises for two reasons: (1) return of buffer to the cell is accompanied by an osmotic shift of water from the extracellular compartment to the cells, which raises the extracellular chloride concentration directly; and (2) large amounts of NaCl are being administered. The explanation for hyperchloremic acidosis given here has been questioned [2,3], but a reexamination of the data in that study [49] shows them actually to be in keeping with the interpretation offered here. The failure of bicarbonate to rise promptly to normal does not mean that severe acidosis persists; hyperventilation continues and preserves an acceptable blood pH because brain bicarbonate does not rise as rapidly as serum bicarbonate and hence brain pH remains lower for a period of 24 to 36 hours. During these 24 to 36 hours the kidney excretes the excess chloride and replaces it with bicarbonate.

Brain Edema in DKA

Patients recovering from ketoacidosis, even those with few symptoms on admission, may manifest lethargy, drowsiness, and headache. Concurrently, and perhaps in a causal relationship, brain swelling appears as indicated by several lines of evidence: rising CSF pressure as demonstrated by Clements and associates [14] and echoencephalographic changes characteristic of edema found by Fein and colleagues [19]. A study using brain computed tomography (CT) scans in a pediatric population [41] showed that brain swelling was virtually a universal phenomenon during the treatment of DKA. In a rare case, usually that of a child or young adult, rapid deterioration of mental status, severe headache, abnormal respiratory pattern, and cranial nerve dysfunction such as pupillary dilatation indicates herniation of the brain with almost inevitable death [15,17,22,60]. The mechanism of edema formation, the role of treatment in causing herniation, and therapeutic measures to be taken in the face of herniation warrant exploration in some depth.

Several hypotheses have been offered to explain the development of brain edema during the treatment for DKA: (1) osmotic disequilibrium between blood and brain, (2) changes in oxygen delivery, (3) decreased plasma oncotic pressure as the result of volume loading with crystalloid, and (4) CNS acidosis.

Osmotic Disequilibrium

Due to Declining Blood Glucose. The hypothesis that an osmotic gradient is generated because blood glucose falls more rapidly than brain glucose during correction of hyperglycemia stems from animal experiments [13] and a few clinical observations [20,45]. Clements and associates [13] noted that dogs whose blood glucose was rapidly decreased from 400 to 600 mg/dl with isotonic saline infusion showed a consistent pathologic increase in their intracranial pressure, and their necropsy revealed brain edema; this effect, according to the authors, could not be attributed to fluid overload. Brains from these animals contained increased concentrations of glucose, sorbitol, and fructose, which were initially thought to explain a shift of water into the neurons. However, since the concentrations of fructose and sorbitol in the CSF were less than 1 mmol/liter and since the largest difference between plasma and CSF glucose concentrations was only 5.5 mOsm/

liter, these data, while they do not rule out an osmotic gradient between the brain and the plasma, do not support a role for glucose or its metabolites. This postulate of an osmotic gradient created by persistence of glucose in interstitium of the brain is theoretically unsound. The brain normally metabolizes glucose at a rate of about 150 gm/day (104 mg/minute), and in hyperglycemia the CNS glucose concentration is always less than 50 percent of that in plasma (see Fig. 6-3). If, for example, on admission the plasma glucose is 1600 mg/dl, the corresponding CNS glucose concentration would not exceed 800 mg/dl, and if total CNS fluid volume is 1.5 liters, the total brain glucose content would be 12 gm. Reduction in plasma glucose to 600 mg/dl over 4 hours would be accompanied by metabolism of 25 gm of glucose, and CNS glucose concentration would be much lower than that of plasma. Even if, in DKA, a considerable amount of brain energy were to be derived from metabolism of ketones, CNS glucose concentration would still fall at such a rate as to avoid osmotic disequilibrium with plasma. In previous analyses, the main route of disappearance for CNS glucose has been thought to be the relatively slow transfer to the circulation through the blood-brain barrier with no attention given to the rapid rate of glucose metabolism by the brain.

In the experiments of Arieff and co-workers [9] in which brain volume was maintained in the face of marked hyperglycemia, largely by the accumulation of "idiogenic osmoles," the response to rapid reduction in blood glucose depended on the method by which it was achieved. When blood glucose was quickly reduced from 60 mOsm/liter to a level greater than 14 mOsm/liter with insulin and hypotonic NaCl, the brain volume and solute content remained unchanged, that is, an osmotic gradient existed between brain and blood. This osmolar gradient is apparently due primarily to unidentified brain solute (the same osmolar gradient must exist between brain and CSF, since osmolality of CSF falls with that of plasma). When blood glucose was lowered to less than 14 mOsm/liter with insulin, the brain was apparently unable to maintain the osmolar gradient and edema rapidly developed; idiogenic osmoles increased in quantity, as did the content of sodium, potassium, and chloride. If, however, blood glucose was rapidly reduced by peritoneal dialysis, that is, without exogenous insulin, there was no accumulation of sodium, potassium, and chloride, idiogenic osmoles disappeared, and brain edema was much less severe than in the case of insulin administration. Some observers have interpreted these rather confounding results as suggesting that insulin somehow contributes to the persistence and even increase of idiogenic osmoles and accumulation of sodium, potassium, and chloride, as glucose rapidly declines. The application of this interpretation to clinical situations is, however, at odds with extensive experience in the management of NKC; even though the blood glucose and osmolality may fall at a very rapid rate, cerebral edema is exceedingly rare. For example, Arieff and Carroll [6] showed that a fall in plasma osmolality as fast as 7 mOsm/liter/hour during therapy for NKC was not associated with any signs of increased intracranial pressure either by clinical examination, measurement of CSF pressure, or necropsy findings. In contrast, patients being treated for DKA have developed brain edema at significantly lower rates of reduction of blood glucose: 27 mg/dl/hour and 70 mg/dl/hour in the two patients reported by Kanter, Gerson, and Bessman [38], compared with an average decline in blood glucose of 133 mg/dl/hour during the first 4.5 hours in the patients reported by Arieff and Carroll [6]. Accordingly, it seems unlikely that the combination of idiogenic osmoles, insulin, and rapidly falling glucose can alone account for cerebral edema in DKA.

Due to Hyponatremia, With Brain Herniation in Children. Duck and colleagues [16] described 40 children who suffered fatal brain herniation due to cerebral edema during treatment of DKA. All but 4 had received fluids at a rate equal to or greater than 4 liters/m^2/day, and their average serum sodium failed to rise as blood glucose fell from 600 to 334 mg/dl over a period of 7.4 hours. The persistence of initial hyponatremia was regarded as an index of excessive fluid retention, the latter ascribed to excessive fluid administration and also to a probable excessive secretion of ADH.

The authors raised the possibility that reduction in plasma osmolality may have worsened brain edema to the point of brain herniation.

This study is cited because the questions it raises are at the center of vigorous debate among pediatricians [16,34,36,42,43], although it is flawed on several counts: Several unwarranted assumptions are made; the statistics are far from compelling; and the decline in osmolality (calculated from the author's data) was only 2 mOsm/liter/hour (although this rate may not reflect the maximal rate of change in a given individual). The authors do not refer to alteration in oncotic pressure as such, but the inference might be drawn from their discussion that excessive decline in oncotic pressure, due to rapid administration of colloid-free fluid, might be an important fector. The role of lowered oncotic pressure in brain edema is tenuous at best and is dealt with in the section on oncotic pressure. Given all the caveats concerning the available data and their interpretation, it still seems warranted to suggest that the administration of copious amounts of hypotonic fluid to children, recommended in pediatric texts [36,43], be tempered somewhat [42]; herniation of the brain in DKA is extremely rare in adults, whatever the rate of fluid administration, but children could be predisposed to this devastating complication.

Decreased Oxygen Delivery

It has been postulated that rising blood pH in the presence of low levels of erythrocyte 2,3-DPG may so increase the affinity of hemoglobin for oxygen that oxygen delivery to the brain may decrease during the recovery phase of DKA. Hypoxemia, which is frequently observed in DKA, may be an additional factor. Hypoxia of the brain could in turn produce edema.

Decreased Plasma Oncotic Pressure

Fein and associates [19] studied 18 patients with DKA and found that plasma colloid osmotic pressure fell from 30.5 to 15.6 mm Hg during therapy of ketoacidosis and attributed these changes to a net fluid intake of 4544 ml of crystalloid solutions. Simultaneously, blood PO_2 fell from a mean of 113 to 80.4 mm Hg, with an increase in the alveolar-arterial gradient of 17.34 mm Hg; the latter phenomenon was attributed to pulmonary congestion. Serial echoencephalographic recordings in 9 of 11 patients in whom they were performed were highly suggestive of early cerebral edema, which the authors related to the decreased plasma oncotic pressure with some additive effect of hypoxemia. Under ordinary circumstances this thesis would be untenable on physiologic grounds; the blood-brain barrier is so tight that oncotic gradients do not promote fluid shifts [12,37,40]. However, it is possible that hyperosmolality of the blood or some other aspect of the altered biochemical environment in DKA may so increase the hydraulic conductivity of the blood-brain barrier as to permit a role for osmotic gradients in the transcapillary shift of water into the brain [35]. Studies such as this described by Fein and associates [19] have not been performed in patients with NKC, but although they receive much larger amounts of crystalloid solutions at a more rapid rate, and undoubtedly achieve at least the same fluid overload and decrease in oncotic pressure, the patients with NKC rarely develop brain edema [4,6].

CNS Acidosis

The suggestion has been offered that depression of consciousness may develop during therapy of DKA as the result of a worsening acidosis of the CSF and hence of the brain. According to this theory, as systemic pH rises with resolution of ketoacidosis, the stimulatory drive of peripheral chemoreceptors for the respiratory center diminishes and carbon dioxide retention begins. Since carbon dioxide equilibrates many times more rapidly across cell membranes than does bicarbonate, the increase in systemic PCO_2 is rapidly transmitted to the CSF while bicarbonate equilibration lags; thus CSF pH should fall while systemic pH rises. This low CSF pH might then adversely affect the tenuous central nervous system function. No substantiation of this proposal has appeared. More recently, Van Der Meulen and co-workers [57] have postulated that recovery from acidosis rather than cerebral acidosis itself explains the development of brain edema during therapy for DKA, through activation of the Na/H exchanger within the brain cells. This exchanger or antiport is a cell membrane transport mechanism that helps to regulate cell pH by pumping H^+ out of the cell in exchange for sodium. According to these authors, both the intracellular and the extracellular compartments in the brain are acidic before therapy, and the Na/H exchanger is inhibited. When therapy starts, the following three events facilitate cell swelling: (1) The extracellular proton concentration falls, eliminating its inhibitory influence on the transporter, and sodium moves into the cell in exchange for cytoplasmic H^+. This intracellular movement of sodium accompanied by increase in cell volume has been demonstrated experimentally [29]. (2) The simultaneous fall in extracellular osmolality due to other mechanisms would accentuate the effect of the newly accumulated intracellular osmoles. (3) Insulin therapy might activate even further the Na/H exchanger. This hypothesis is attractive but awaits experimental confirmation.

It seems likely that a combination of mechanisms related more to the biochemical abnormalities of DKA than of NKC is responsible for brain edema. While it is not possible to assign degrees of importance to various possible mechanisms, it would seem prudent to avoid volume overload, hyponatremia, and aggressive elevation of blood pH in the treatment of DKA, particularly in children. Brain edema almost invariably resolves with adequate therapy of DKA. In the patients with cerebral herniation, treatment (i.e., intravenous mannitol) is unlikely to be beneficial, but if it is to help it must be prompt.

HYPEROSMOLAR NONKETOTIC COMA

NKC is a clinical syndrome in which severe hyperglycemia is present without ketosis; the generally accepted definition of the "nonketotic state with hyperglycemia" is one in which the plasma Acetest reaction shows less than 2+ in a 1:1 dilution. The patient manifests depression of sensorium, marked dehydration, and often focal neurologic findings and seizures. In some cases, the syndrome is caused by interference with insulin secretion or action in combination with excessive carbohydrate intake. NKC occurs in nondiabetics and sometimes in insulin-dependent diabetics who have had previous episodes of DKA. Even with the increased awareness of the existence of this syndrome that has followed the development of a large literature on the subject, the diagnosis is commonly missed, although it can be readily made by bedside determination of blood glucose and ketone concentrations.

Distinction from DKA

In DKA mobilization of large amounts of free fatty acids from adipose tissue leads to production of ketoacids. Hyperventilation and evidence of altered mental status draw attention to the patient's illness, and the patient usually reaches the medical care facility without very severe dehydration. In NKC a more insidious onset and the absence of ketoacidosis remove the early signs of acute illness. In addition, patients with DKA are more likely to be younger and to be in an environment where illness is more readily noted. In NKC glycosuria and dehydration persist until the patient is grossly volume depleted and serum osmolality is markedly elevated. Cerebral hyperosmolality and reduced brain perfusion cause alterations in mental status from drowsiness to coma and a variety of other neurologic defects and abnormalities. Dehydration leads to marked diminution in glomerular filtration rate, and the inability to excrete glucose allows extremely severe hyperglycemia. The blood glucose may rise slowly until a fairly sudden deterioration of renal function allows the blood glucose to rise steeply. Commonly, there is a history of acute alteration in mental function after prolonged diuresis and polydipsia [6].

Predisposing Conditions

Patients who develop NKC are often bedridden and cared for by an aged spouse or a disinterested nursing home staff. Reduced access to fluid and diminished thirst in the face of ongoing polyuria lead to dehydration. When illness provokes the episode of decompensation, it is likely to be more severe than is the case with DKA. Nausea and vomiting are common. A variety of associated diseases may either precipitate the episode of NKC, hasten its development, or complicate the patient's recovery (Table 6-1). These disorders include pneumonia and other infectious processes, gastrointestinal bleeding, myocardial infarction, and uremia. A number of drugs known to interfere with insulin secretion or action commonly contribute to hyperglycemia, and include phenytoin, diuretics, glucocorticoids, chlorpromazine, and diazoxide. Cases have been described in which patients who have suffered an episode of DKA presented with NKC after initiation of therapy with propanolol, which inhibits the mobilization of free fatty acids. Patients may receive large amounts of carbohydrate in the form of sweetened fluids or through hypertonic peritoneal dialysis and hyperalimentation.

A syndrome of severe hyperglycemia with coma occurs in patients with head injury or recovering from neurosurgical procedures involving the hypothalamic-pituitary system or procedures interrupting the anterior blood supply to the brain [24]. The characteristic clinical pattern of these patients has consisted of central diabetes insipidus with large urine volumes, the latter replaced with glucose-containing solutions. Severe hyperglycemia leads to worsening polyuria and the need for increased administration of fluids containing glucose. The patients tolerate glucose poorly, probably because of stress, glucocorticoids given to limit brain edema, and phenytoin. Rapid losses of potassium in the urine may lead to inadequate or excessive potassium replacement; either may be lethal. The problem may be totally avoided by the prompt infusion of vasopressin as soon as the diagnosis of central diabetes insipidus is established. When vasopressin is given, close attention must be paid to serum sodium concentration; there is a tendency to overhydrate.

Table 6-1. Nonketotic coma: predisposing conditions

1. a. Serious illness
   b. Unobserved dehydration
   c. Fundamental metabolic change, permanent
   d. Increased carbohydrate intake, e.g., hemodialysis
   e. Inadequate insulin dosage
2. Combinations of transient reduction in carbohydrate tolerance with increased carbohydrate intake: e.g., burns, phenytoin, corticosteroids, parenteral hyperalimentation
3. Inhibition of fat mobilization in ketosis-susceptible subjects, e.g., propranol therapy
4. Other causes

Source: Data from one series of 37 cases. Arieff and Carroll [6].

Clinical Presentation in NKC

The most remarkable findings on physical examination are those associated with dehydration. Hypotension is common as well as dry mucous membranes, sunken eyeballs, and poor skin turgor. Abdominal distention and ileus may be present. Despite dehydration and hypotension, osmotic diuresis maintains the urine output. Patients present with a wide range of central nervous system manifestations, from mild mental clouding to severe coma. About half of the patients are comatose on admission. The severity of the mental status alterations correlates best with the degree of hyperosmolality. Most patients with a serum osmolality less than 350 mOsm/liter are alert [7].

Neurologic Manifestations in NKC

Depression of Sensorium

The correlation between serum osmolality and alteration in mental status is shown in Figure 6-7. The mechanism of coma is most likely cerebral dehydration similar to that which occurs in other hyperosmolar states. That autopsies performed in patients with NKC do not show evidence of cerebral dehydration suggests that volume regulation has been successful but does not eliminate the likelihood that brain dehydration initiated coma; once a particular brain dysfunction has been induced, a finite time may be required for its recovery.

Focal Neurologic Findings

Focal neurologic findings such as aphasia, hemiparesis, hyperreflexia, sensory defects, autonomic changes, and brain stem dysfunction can occur in NKC. In a large series of 33 episodes of NKC in 30 patients [6], the admitting diagnosis was acute stroke in 12 cases; 9 of these patients had Babinski's signs or evidence of hemiparesis. In none of these patients was the diagnosis of stroke ultimately verified. Other reports, however, suggest that acute stroke might have occurred. Remote cerebrovascular accident with persistent neurologic defect is a common explanation for the patient's inability to maintain hydration, and hence evidence of a remote stroke is fairly common. One might have expected a generalized rather than focal cerebral dysfunction produced by hyperosmotic dehydration, but most of the patients with the syndrome are elderly and likely to have areas in the brain where vascular supply is tenuous; these areas may be particularly sensitive to hyperosmotic dehydration. Faris and Poser [18] have shown that the simultaneous occurrence of locally compromised vascular supply and systemic metabolic abnormalities in the dog can lead to focal neurologic signs. Transient focal neurologic signs resulting from metabolic disturbances in patients with carotid stenosis have also been described.

Seizures

Generalized and focal seizures are common in patients with NKC but are distinctly unusual in patients with DKA. This observation has given rise to the concept that ketosis somehow prevents seizures, a concept supported by the apparent success of ketogenic diets in patients with certain types of seizures. However, it should be clear that many characteristics besides ketosis distinguish NKC from DKA.

An interesting hypothesis has been offered to explain the occurrence of seizures in DKA but not in NKC [30]. It is suggested that the brain of patients with NKC is depleted of gamma-aminobutyric acid (GABA) because Krebs' cycle activity is diminished; in DKA the brain content of GABA is normal because of the metabolism of large amounts of acetoacetate. GABA is an inhibitory substance found only in the central nervous system, and its depletion might give rise to seizures by causing neuronal hyperexcitability.

Laboratory Data

The admission laboratory data in one large series [6] of patients with NKC show the following: blood glucose 1166 mg/dl (range 650–2100 mg/dl), serum osmolality 384 mOsm/liter (range 351–452 mOsm/liter), and serum sodium 144 mEq/liter (range 118–162 mEq/liter). In cases outside of the series under discussion serum sodium in excess of 180 mEq/liter has been observed. Although balance studies have in general shown the loss of more than 250 mEq of sodium and nearly 200 mEq of potassium on the average, clinical observations of several patients with severe hypernatremia suggested that they had gained rather than lost sodium. Patients who ingest salt in liberal quantities during a phase of dehydration tend to retain salt because of volume depletion, despite ongoing osmotic diuresis. Serum potassium was 5.0 mEq/liter with a range from 2.7 to 8 mEq/liter. Although our own experience indicates that the average patient with NKC loses nearly 200 mEq of potassium, documentation exists for losses by individual patients of more than 700 mEq of potassium during an episode of NKC. The average hematocrit was 43 percent (range 14–49%); the low levels tended to be observed in patients with end-stage renal disease. Data comparing patients with DKA and NKC at the time of admission to the hospital are shown in Table 6-2. Analysis of body composition shows the following alterations: total body water reduced by 24.2 percent, extracellular fluid volume reduced by 25.3 percent, and intracellular volume reduced by 22.1 percent. The average water loss, 9.1 liters, was proportionately more than twice as great as the electrolyte loss; the appropriate repair solution would therefore be, in the absence of contraindications, a solution half-isotonic. A mild metabolic acidosis is a frequent finding in NKC; The anion gap is increased, and although it cannot be completely accounted for, it is attributable in significant measure to a combination of azotemia, increase in albumin concentration due to dehydration, and small amounts of ketone and lactate anions. Lactate accumulation is not significant unless the patient suffers from a disease

Table 6-2. Data for comparison of diabetic ketoacidosis (DKA) and hyperosmolar nonketotic coma (NKC)

	BUN (mg/dl)	*Blood glucose (mg/dl)*	*Plasma osmolality (mOsm/kg)*	*Water loss (liters)*	*Plasma ketones (Acetest)*	*Arterial pH*	*Mortality*
DKA	40	600	320	4–5	> 2+ (1:1)	<7.2*	5%
NKC	88	1200	388	8–9	< 2+ (1:1)	7.26	>50%

* Often less than 7.1.

that causes frank lactic acidosis; such disorders are no rare occurrence in elderly diabetics with severe infection. Although some of the patients with NKC have normal renal function, the majority have at least mild renal insufficiency and some have end-stage renal disease; the commonest renal syndrome is prerenal azotemia superimposed upon some degree of chronic renal insufficiency.

Biochemical Abnormalities in NKC

The reason for hyperglycemia in patients with NKC is straightforward: Inadequate insulin effect inhibits cellular uptake of glucose and permits increased gluconeogenesis. In all likelihood, the most significant reason for the failure of patients with NKC to develop ketosis is the failure to mobilize free fatty acids because of the presence of small amounts of insulin [5]; levels of insulin sufficient to prevent lipolysis may not be sufficient to inhibit gluconeogenesis or to permit normal glucose utilization. Several reports [58] have appeared showing high fatty acid levels in patients with NKC. In such patients it is likely that the levels of insulin in the portal venous blood are high enough to permit rapid conversion of free fatty acids into VLDL rather than allowing them to be shunted into the mitochondria where keto acid formation can take place. In some studies, the levels of lipokinetic hormones have been shown to be lower in NKC than in DKA, although glucagon levels are equally elevated in both conditions. In those patients who are ketosis prone but who present to the hospital with NKC, the usual story is that some small amount of insulin has been administered within 15 hours of the time of admission to the hospital, that is, a quantity of insulin sufficient to inhibit lipolysis but not sufficient to prevent hyperglycemia. It is not surprising that more insulin should be available in patients with NKC because these patients tend to be elderly type II diabetics in whom larger quantities of insulin are characteristically available; in DKA, insulin levels are either extremely low or completely absent at the time of admission to the hospital.

Treatment

Proper care of the patient with NKC requires recognition and management of any attendant illness; the majority of deaths in the syndrome are caused by the underlying medical problems rather than the metabolic abnormality.

Dealing with the metabolic abnormalities requires treatment of the following disorders: reduced organ perfusion as the consequence of dehydration; cerebral hyperosmolality; hyperglycemia with osmotic diuresis; and depletion of salt and potassium. Although considerable debate has attended the proper dosage of insulin in the treatment of NKC, our own experience leads us to apply the same rules of management for NKC as for DKA. A loading dose of 10 units of insulin intravenously is followed by an infusion of 5 to 10 units/hour. When blood glucose reaches 250 mg/dl, insulin infusion is stopped and insulin is subsequently given on the basis of need. It has been argued that half-normal saline cannot expand the extracellular fluid volume as rapidly as normal saline and in addition poses the hazard of contributing to the development of cerebral edema. The first point is easily answered by calculation of space of distribution of half-normal saline; approximately 70 percent of the fluid remains in the extracellular space. With regard to the second point, our experience and that of others indicates that cerebral edema is an extremely rare occurrence in patients with NKC, and most authors now favor the use of half-normal saline as the staple for volume replenishment. In those with unstable hemodynamics due to severe volume depletion, it may be appropriate to administer the first 1 or 2 liters rapidly as isotonic saline, and in some patients the use of volume expanders or blood may be necessary depending on the circumstance. In brief, half-normal saline has the advantage that it can rapidly expand extracellular fluid volume and at the same time lower the osmolality. Given the likelihood that extreme hyperosmolality is deleterious to cerebral function, it is to the patient's advantage that osmolality be reduced as rapidly as is consistent with the patient's well-being.

Osmotic Equilibrium Between Plasma and CSF During Treatment of NKC

Figure 6-8 shows data obtained by lumbar puncture in 21 patients on admission to the hospital [6]. The osmolality was identical in plasma and CSF. The glucose concentration in the CSF was about one-half the concentration in extracellular fluid, the difference in osmolality being made up by the higher concentration of sodium chloride in the CSF. The available information would suggest that the osmolality of the brain should be identical to that of plasma and CSF at this point. CSF pressure was normal on admission. The events that followed the administration of intravenous half-normal saline, during a period of several hours as the osmolality was declining to about 320 mOsm/liter and the glucose to about 250 mg/dl, are summarized as follows: (1) Plasma osmolality fell at an average rate of 8 mOsm/liter/hour, and CSF osmolality fell at approximately the same rate with a lag

Fig. 6-8. The solute equilibrium between plasma and cerebrospinal fluid (CSF) in 21 patients who had nonketotic hyperosmolar coma. The two compartments are in osmotic equilibrium, but the constituents are not. The concentrations of sodium and chloride are higher in CSF than in plasma, while the concentration of glucose is lower, which achieves osmotic equilibrium. Urea concentration is similar in plasma and CSF. (From Arieff and Carroll [7]. Copyright 1974, American Diabetes Association, Inc.)

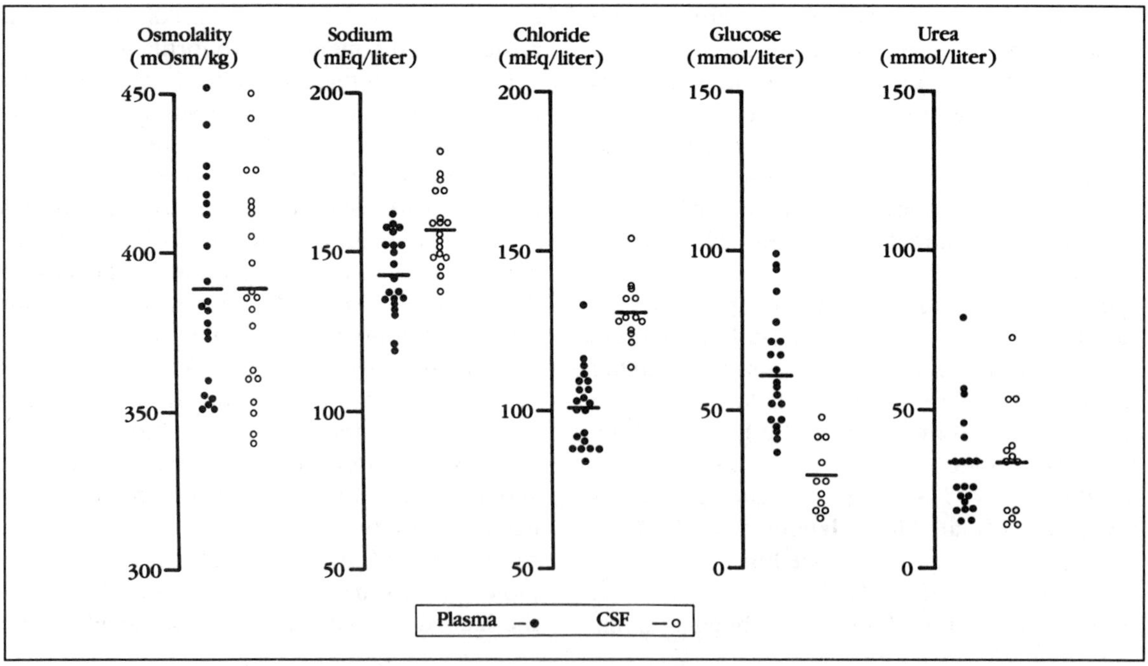

that averaged at any given point in time about 10 mOsm/liter; (2) blood glucose fell at a mean level of 133 mg/dl/hour for the first 6 hours; (3) the concentrations of all the solutes in CSF fell at about the same rate, suggesting that the major reason for the fall in osmolality in CSF was the entry of water into this compartment (Fig. 6-9); (4) despite the addition of water to CSF, serial lumbar punctures in eight patients showed no rise in CSF pressure; (5) no patient developed clinical evidence of cerebral edema, and autopsy in those patients who died showed no evidence of cerebral edema. This observation is in keeping with the previous evidence from CSF pressures that cerebral edema rarely occurs. Although a study has yet to be performed using CT scans, documented cases of cerebral edema in NKC are quite rare [4,6], in marked contrast to its ubiquity in DKA [30,41].

Conclusions

In summary, NKC occurs primarily in elderly type II diabetics, although it is occasionally observed in type I diabetics who have received inadequate quantities of insulin. The patients are severely dehydrated on admission to the hospital, and one must be cautious in using the serum sodium as an index of dehyration, since severe hypernatremia may be attributable in part to salt retention rather than water loss. Patients often have severe associated illness. Despite the loss of large quantities of salt, the extracellular fluid volume is depleted to about the same extent as the intracellular fluid volume because the glucose that accumulates in the extracellular space pulls water from the cells. The appropriate therapeutic approach is low-dose intravenous insulin and replenishment of salt, potassium, and water. Half-normal saline containing appropriate amounts of potassium is the ideal fluid; patients with unstable circulation may receive several liters of normal saline or plasma expanders before half-normal saline is begun. Experience shows that the osmolality of the extracellular fluid may be allowed to fall to about 320 mOsm/liter and the blood glucose to about 250 mg/dl without hazard; the cerebrospinal fluid pressure does not rise, there is no clinical evidence of cerebral edema, and autopsy findings suggest that cerebral edema is indeed quite rare in NKC. When the blood glucose is less than 300 mg/dl, the infusion of insulin may be terminated since by now the patient is secreting his own insulin; the solution may be changed to 5% dextrose containing whatever concentration of salt is required to allow the osmolality to fall to normal over the next 18 to 24 hours. Serum electrolytes, glucose, and osmolality should be checked every 2 hours. Subjects with severe hypernatremia may become even more hypernatremic as blood glucose falls; such patients should receive half-normal saline until the circulation is stable and then be treated with a program directed at lowering the serum sodium by about 0.7 mEq/liter/hour.

Fig. 6-9. A comparison of the relationship between osmolality and glucose concentration in plasma versus CSF in 8 patients who had nonketotic hyperosmolar coma and were being treated with insulin and intravenous hypotonic fluids (mainly 77 mM NaCl). The glucose falls at a much faster rate in plasma than in CSF, but there is no osmotic disequilibrium between the two compartments. (From Arieff and Carroll [7]. Copyright 1974, American Diabetes Association, Inc.)

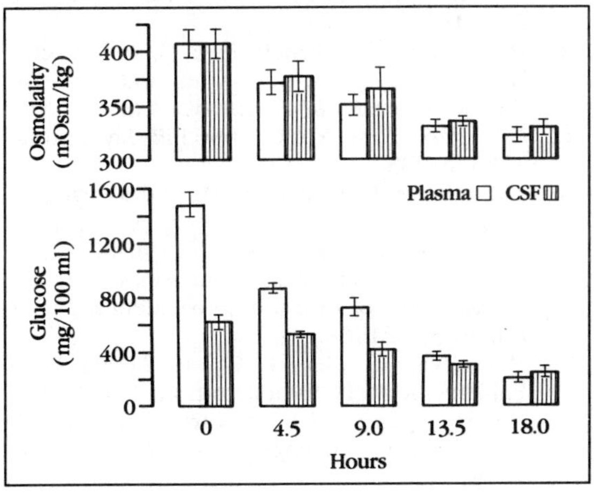

REFERENCES

1. Adrogue, H. J., and Madias, N. E. Changes in plasma potassium concentration during acute acid-base disturbances. *Am. J. Med.* 71:456, 1981.
2. Adrogue, H. J., et al. Plasma acid-base patterns in

diabetic ketoacidosis. *N. Engl. J. Med.* 307:1603, 1982.
3. Adrogue, H. J., et al. Diabetic ketoacidosis: Role of the kidney in the acid-base homeostasis reevaluated. *Kidney Int.* 25:591, 1984.
4. Arieff, A. I. Cerebral edema complicating nonketotic hyperosmolar coma. *Miner. Electrolyte Metab.* 12:383, 1986.
5. Arieff, A. I., and Carroll, H. J. Hyperosmolar nonketotic coma with hyperglycemia: Abnormalities of lipid and carbohydrate metabolism. *Metabolism* 20:529, 1971.
6. Arieff, A. I., and Carroll, H. J. Non-ketotic hyperosmolar coma with hyperglycemia. Clinical features, pathophysiology, renal function, acid-base balance, plasma-cerebrospinal fluid equilibria and the effects of therapy in 37 cases. *Medicine* 51:73, 1972.
7. Arieff, A. I., Carroll, H. J. Cerebral edema and depression of sensorium in non-ketotic hyperosmolar coma. *Diabetes* 23:525, 1974.
8. Arieff, A. I., Guisado, R., and Lazarowitz, V. C. Pathophysiology of Hyperosmolar States. In T. E. Andreoli, J. J. Grantham, F. C. Rector, Jr. (eds.), *Disturbances in Body Fluid Osmolality.* Bethesda, MD: American Physiological Society, 1977. P. 227.
9. Arieff, A. I., Kleeman, C. R., Kerian, A., et al. Cerebral edema in diabetic comas: II. Effects of hyperosmolality, hyperglycemia and insulin in diabetic rabbits. *J. Clin. Endocrinol. Metab.* 38(6):1057, 1974.
10. Arieff, A. I., Kleeman, C. R., Keushkerian, A., et al. Studies on mechanisms of cerebral edema in diabetic comas: Effects of hyperglycemia and rapid lowering of plasma glucose in normal rabbits. *J. Clin. Invest.* 52(3):571, 1973.
11. Beech, J. S., Williams, S. R., Cohen, R. D., et al. Gluconeogenesis and the protection of hepatic intracellular pH during diabetic ketoacidosis in rats. *Biochem. J.* 263:737, 1989.
12. Bradbury, M. W. B. The structure and function of the blood-brain barrier. *Fed. Proc.* 43:186, 1984.
13. Clements, R. S., Jr. et al. Acute cerebral edema during treatment of hyperglycemia. *Lancet* 2:384, 1968.
14. Clements, R. S., Jr., et al. Increased cerebrospinal-fluid pressure during treatment of diabetic ketosis. *Lancet* 2:671, 1971.
15. Dillon, E. S., et al. Cerebral lesions in uncomplicated fatal diabetic acidosis. *Am. J. Med. Sci.* 192:360, 1936.
16. Duck, S. C., and Wyatt, D. T. Factors associated with brain herniation in the treatment of diabetic ketoacidosis. *J. Pediatr.* 113:10, 1988.
17. Duck, S. C., et al. Cerebral edema complicating therapy for diabetic ketoacidosis. *Diabetes* 25:111, 1976.
18. Faris, A. A., and Poser, C. M. Experimental production of focal neurologic deficit by systemic hyponatremia. *Neurology* 14:206, 1964.
19. Fein, I. A., et al. Relation of colloid osmotic pressure to arterial hypoxemia and cerebral edema during crystalloid volume loading of patients with diabetic ketoacidosis. *Ann. Intern. Med.* 96:570, 1982.
20. Fernandez, J. P., et al. Cerebral edema from blood-brain glucose differences complicating peritoneal dialysis: Second membrane syndrome. *N. Y. State J. Med.* 68:677, 1968.
21. Fisher, J. N., and Kibatchi, A. E. A randomized study of phosphorus therapy in the treatment of diabetic ketoacidosis. *Clin. Endocrinol. Metab.* 57:177, 1983.
22. Fitzgerald, M. G., et al. Fatal diabetic ketosis. *Br. Med. J.* 1:247, 1961.
23. Foster, D. W., and McGarry, J. D. The metabolic derangements and treatment of diabetic ketoacidosis. *N. Engl. J. Med.* 309:159, 1983.
24. Freidenberg, G. R., et al. Hyperglycemic coma after suprasellar surgery. *N. Engl. J. Med.* 303:863, 1980.
25. Fulop, M., et al. Ketotic hyperosmolar coma. *Lancet* 2:635, 1973.
26. Fulop, M. Serum potassium in lactic acidosis and ketoacidosis. *N. Engl. J. Med.* 300:1087, 1979.
27. Gabow, P. A., Keahny, W. D., Fennessey, P. V., et al. Diagnostic importance of an increased anion gap. *N. Engl. J. Med.* 303:854, 1980.
28. Goldstein, D. A., et al. Transient hypoxemia in diabetic ketoacidosis. *Kidney Int.* 10:499, 1976.
29. Grinstein, S., et al. Amiloride-sensitive Na-H exchange in platelets and leucocytes: Detection by electronic cell sizing. *Am. J. Physiol.* 247:C293, 1984.
30. Guisado, R., and Arieff, A. I. Neurologic manifestation of diabetic comas: Correlation with biochemical alterations in the brain. *Metabolism* 24:665, 1975.
31. Halperin, M. L., Bear, R., Goldstein, M. B., et al. Interpretation of the serum potassium concentration in metabolic acidosis. *Clin. Invest. Med.* 2:55, 1979.
32. Halperin, M. L., Goldstein, M. B., Bear, R. A., et al. Diabetic Comas. In A. I. Arieff and R. A. DeFronzo (eds.), *Fluid, Electrolyte and Acid-Base Disorders.* New York: Churchill Livingstone, 1985. P. 933.
33. Halperin, M. L., Goldstein, M., and Richardson, R. Quantitative aspects of hyperglycemia in the diabetic. *Clin. Invest. Med.* 2:127, 1980.
34. Harris G. D., Fiordalisi, I., and Finberg, L. Safe management of diabetic ketoacidemia. *J. Pediatr.* 113:65, 1988.
35. Hasegawa, H., Allen, T. C., and Mehta, B. M. Enhancement of CNS penetration of methotrexate by hyperosmolar intracarotid mannitol in carcinomatous meningitis. *Neurology* 29:1280, 1979.

36. Jackson, R. L., and Guthrie, R. A. *The Child With Diabetes Mellitus,* Kalamazoo, MI: Upjohn, 1975.
37. Janzer, R. C., and Raff, M. C. Astrocytes induce blood-brain barrier properties in endothelial cells. *Nature* 325:253, 1987.
38. Kanter, Y., Gerson, J. R., and Bessman, A. N. 2,3-Diphosphoglycerate, nucleotide phosphate, and organic and inorganic phosphate levels during the early phases of diabetic ketoacidosis. *Diabetes* 26:429, 1977.
39. Kety S. S., et al. The blood flow and oxygen consumption of the human brain in diabetic ketoacidosis and coma. *J. Clin. Invest.* 27:500, 1948.
40. Kleeman, C. R. Metabolic coma. *Kidney Int.* 36:1142, 1989.
41. Krane, E. J., et al. Subclinical brain swelling in children during treatment of diabetic ketoacidosis. *N. Engl. J. Med.* 312:1147, 1985.
42. Krane, E. J. Cerebral edema in diabetic ketoacidosis. *J. Pediatr.* 114:166, 1989.
43. Krane, J. K. Diabetic ketoacidosis: Biochemistry, physiology, treatment and prevention. *Pediatr. Clin. North Am.* 34:935, 1987.
44. Ladenson, J. H., Apple, F. S., and Koch, D. D Misleading hyponatremia due to hyperlipidemia: A method dependent error. *Ann. Intern. Med.* 95:707, 1981.
45. Maccario, M., and Messis, C. P. Cerebral edema complicating treated nonketotic hyperglycemia. *Lancet* 2:352, 1969.
46. Marliss, E. B., Ohman, J. L., Aoki, T. T., et al. Altered redox state obscuring ketoacidosis in diabetic patients with lactic acidosis. *N. Engl. J. Med.* 283:978, 1970.
47. Narin, R. G., Kopyt, N. P., and Kleeman, C. R. Diabetic Acidosis and Coma: Insulin Administration. In M. H. Maxwell, C. R. Kleeman, and R. G. Narins (eds.), *Clinical Disorders of Fluid and Electrolyte Metabolism.* New York: McGraw-Hill, 1987. P. 657.
48. Oh, M. S., Banerjee, M. A., and Carroll, H. J. The mechanism of hyperchloremic acidosis during the recovery phase of diabetic ketoacidosis. *Diabetes* 30:310, 1981.
49. Oh, M. S., Uribarri, J. and Carroll, H. J. Mechanism of normochloremic and hyperchloremic acidosis in diabetic ketoacidosis. *Nephron* 54:1, 1990.
50. Perez, G. O., Oster, J. R., and Vaamonde, C. A. Serum potassium concentration in acidemic states. *Nephron* 27:233, 1981.
51. Posner, J. B., and Plum, F. Spinal-fluid pH and neurologic symptoms in systemic acidosis. *N. Engl. J. Med.* 277:605, 1967.
52. Reubi, F. C. Glomerular filtration rate, renal blood flow and blood viscosity during and after diabetic coma. *Circ. Res.* 1:410, 1953.
53. Ruderman, N. B., Ross, P. S., Berger, M., et al. Regulation of glucose and ketone-body metabolism in brain of anesthetized rats. *Biochem. J.* 138:1, 1974.
54. Schneider, R., and Droller, H. The relative importance of ketosis and acidosis in the production of diabetic coma. *Q. J. Exp. Physiol.* 28:3223, 1938.
55. Timperley, W. R., et al. Cerebral intravascular coagulation in diabetic acidosis. *Lancet* 1:952, 1974.
56. Uribarri, J., Oh, M. S., and Carroll, H. J. Hyperkalemia in diabetes mellitus. *J. Diabetic Compl.* 4:3, 1990.
57. van Der Meulen, J. A., et al. Possible mechanism for cerebral edema in diabetic ketoacidosis. *Lancet* 2:306, 1987.
58. Vinik, A., et al. Metabolic findings in hyperosmolar non-ketotic diabetic stupor. *Lancet* 2:797, 1970.
59. Vokes, T. P., Aycinena, P. R., and Robertson, G. L. Effect of insulin on osmoregulation of vasopressin. *Am. J. Physiol.* 252:E538, 1987.
60. Young, E., and Bradley, R. F. Cerebral edema with irreversible coma in severe diabetic ketoacidosis. *N. Engl. J. Med.* 276:665, 1967.
61. Zerbe, R. L., and Robertson, G. L. Plasma vasopressin in uncontrolled diabetes mellitus. *Diabetes* 28:503, 1979.
62. Zerbe, R. L., and Robertson, G. L. Osmoregulation of thirst and vasopressin secretin in man: The effect of various solutes. *Am. J. Physiol.* 244:E607, 1983.

7 Central Nervous System Manifestations of Hypoglycemia

L. Creed Pettigrew, Allen I. Arieff, and David W. McCandless

Hypoglycemia is a major complication of the therapy of diabetes mellitus, and also can complicate a number of other clinical conditions, such as sepsis, liver failure, renal failure, malnutrition, and the use of certain drugs [19,20,22,26]. Hypoglycemia is not merely a laboratory curiosity, but a major cause of morbidity and mortality in affected subjects. Virtually all of the morbidity associated with hypoglycemia is manifested in the central nervous system. However, despite extensive investigation for many years, the effects of hypoglycemia on central nervous system function are far from clear. To better understand how the clinical picture of hypoglycemia evolves, it is important to first review the metabolism of glucose by the brain.

This work was supported by Clinical Investigator Development Award NS01505 (L.C.P.) and the Veterans Administration.

CEREBRAL METABOLISM OF GLUCOSE

Glucose is the major fuel for metabolic function in normal adult brain [28,46]. Any interference with the regular supply of glucose may impair brain function. Other substrates such as ketone bodies (acetoacetate and beta-hydroxybutyrate) and lactate may serve as substrate under unusual circumstances, but the efficiency of their cerebral consumption remains speculative. The newborn brain may have a greater capacity to use these alternative substrates [31]. The rate of oxygen metabolism in brain is high compared to that of other organs, suggesting that cerebral extraction of glucose is not dependent on blood flow under most circumstances. Approximately 10 percent of blood glucose is extracted by normal resting brain; when flow drops, extraction tends to increase [36]. Transport of glucose into brain proceeds by facilitated diffusion, and the half maximal concentration (Km) for glucose transport ranges between 4 and 10 mM. Chronic hypoglycemia increases the transport of glucose across the blood-brain barrier [44]. The net levels of brain glucose are about 25 percent of those in blood, but under conditions of hyperglycemia, this ratio progressively decreases [5,6]. The net effect of insulin on glucose entry and metabolism in brain is unclear, but insulin alters the cerebral metabolic fate of glucose [4,6]. Insulin administration increases the blood-to-brain ratio of glucose in mice [50] and also increases incorporation of glycose into amino acids [6,65]. In vitro studies also show that rat spinal cord, cerebral cortex, and cerebellum take up glucose faster in the presence of insulin, although it has been suggested that the effect of insulin is on phosphorylation rather than uptake [15].

The oxidation of glucose (glucose + 6 O_2 + H_2O) has been shown to be the major route for generation of adenosine triphosphate (ATP) in the brain:

$$C_6H_{12}O_6 + 6\,O_2 + 38\,ADP + 38\,Pi \rightarrow 6\,CO_2 + 6\,H_2O + 38\,ATP$$

Where ADP = adenosine diphosphate and Pi = inorganic phosphate.

Other pathways such as the hexose monophosphate shunt are critical during early development but play limited roles in adult brain. Most glucose ends up going through aerobic pathways, with a small amount being metabolized through anerobic pathways generating lactate and pyruvate [35].

ETIOLOGY AND CLINICAL MANIFESTATIONS OF HYPOGLYCEMIA

Hypoglycemia is a common clinical disorder that is associated with a number of different medical conditions (Table 7-1). These include various problems with substrate availability, impaired gluconeogenesis, enzyme deficiencies, hormonal abnormalities, and increased substrate utilization. Hormone excesses that can lead to hypoglycemia, in addition to insulin, include insulin-related growth factor I [29] and insulin-related growth factor II [16]. Hormone deficiencies that can result in hypoglycemia include the counter-regulatory hormones epinephrine, glucagon, growth hormone, and cortisol. Of particular note is alcohol hypoglycemia [24], which can be refractory to therapy and is often fatal [7]. Hypoglycemia also complicates numerous medical and surgical conditions, many of which are shown in Table 7-1.

The clinical manifestations of hypoglycemia are primarily related to the central nervous system effects. These are shown in Table 7-2. It is noteworthy that seizures and coma are most commonly seen in those conditions characterized by an excess of insulin in blood, while lethargy is most common with hypoglycemia in the presence of a low plasma insulin [26,27,47]. A very common cause of hypoglycemia is the so-called reactive hypoglycemia, which probably represents a multitude of abnormalities [33]. The clinical signs and symptoms can be divided into two general catagories: adrenergic and neuroglucopenic [20] (Table 7-2).

The adrenergic symptoms are primarily due to hypoglycemia-induced release of the counter-regulatory hormone epinephrine and include symptoms such as cold perspiration, palpitations, anxiety, and tachycardia. It is particulary important to remember that such symptoms are due to stimulation of the sympathetic nervous system and are thus largely blocked by beta-blocking agents, such as propranolol. For this reason, agents such as propranolol should probably not be used in the treatment of hypertension in insulin-dependent diabetic subjects. Such drugs could largely eliminate the sympathetic overstimulation of hypoglycemia and thus impair the patient's awareness of the disorder. Thus, the propensity for brain damage could be substantially increased by propranolol.

The neuroglucopenic signs and symptoms include those due to the direct effects of decreased glucose on the central nervous system. Included are headache, weakness, confusion, and bizarre behavior. The most severe symptoms are those of seizures and coma, which can lead to permanent brain damage [20]. Even when the hypoglycemia has been successfully treated, there is substantial evidence that

Table 7-1. Derangements in mechanisms of glucose homeostasis leading to fasting hypoglycemia

Decreased Glucose Output

I. Decreased hepatic gluconeogenesis:
  A. Decrease in supply of substrate for gluconeogenesis:
    1. Decreased mobilization of certain amino acids from muscle
      (a) Hormonal excess—insulin, NSILA-s (nonpancreatic tumors), other polypeptides (nonpancreatic tumors)
      (b) Hormonal deficiency—cortisol, epinephrine
      (c) Idiopathic (ketotic hypoglycemia)
      (d) Depletion of muscle stores
    2. Increased uptake of amino acids by extrahepatic tissues
    3. Decrease in lactate & pyruvate originating from formed blood cells, renal medulla, nervous tissue, etc.:
      (a) Hormonal deficiency—growth hormone, cortisol, epinephrine
    4. Decreased mobilization of glycerol (& free fatty acids for energy requirements) from adipose tissue:
      (a) Hormonal excess—insulin, NSILA-s
      (b) Hormonal deficiency—glucagon, growth hormone, cortisol, ACTH, epinephrine
      (c) Depletion of adipose stores
  B. Decreased hepatic uptake of substrates:
      (a) Hormonal excess—insulin, NSILA-s
      (b) Hormonal deficiency—cortisol, growth hormone, epinephrine
  C. Deficiency in activity of rate-limiting hepatic enzymes (change in enzyme activation or synthesis—or both) involved in disposition of extracted substrate:
      (a) Hormonal excess—insulin, NSILA-s
      (b) Hormonal deficiency—glucagon, epinephrine, cortisol
      (c) Delay in maturation of enzyme synthesis (newborn of low birth weight)
      (d) Genetic enzyme deficiency (infancy & childhood)
  D. Decrease in substrate oxidation:
    1. Increase in $NADH_2$:NAD (alcohol)
    2. Decreased oxidation of long-chained fatty acids
  E. Extensive, diffuse hepatocellular damage
  F. Interference with hepatic blood flow

II. Decreased hepatic glycogenolysis:
  A. Deficiency in activity of hepatic enzyme:
      (a) Hormonal excess—insulin, NSILA-s
      (b) Hormonal deficiency—glucagon, epinephrine
  B. Genetic enzyme deficiency (infancy & childhood)
  C. Extensive, diffuse, hepatocellular damage

Increased Glucose Uptake

I. Liver:
  A. Hormonal excess—insulin, NSILA-s

II. Muscle:
  A. Hormonal excess—insulin, NSILA-s
  B. Hormonal deficiency—cortisol, growth hormone, epinephrine
  C. Exercise

III. Adipose tissue:
  A. Hormonal excess—insulin

IV. Conceptus

V. Tumor (extrapancreatic)

Increased Uptake of Amino Acids by Extrahepatic Tissues

I. Muscle:
  A. Excess—insulin, NSILA-s
  B. Deficiency—cortisol, epinephrine

II. Conceptus

III. Tumor (extrapancreatic)

Table 7-2. Clinical manifestations of hypoglycemia

Early manifestations
Quiet and withdrawn
Psychosis
Tachycardia
Ventricular premature beats
Hypothermia
Advanced manifestations
Involuntary twitching
Sensory aphasia
Apraxia
Emotional lability
Late manifestions
Unresponsiveness
Choreiform and athetoid movements
Tonic or clonic seizures
Adrenergic
Tremulousness
Anxiety
Hunger
Cold perspiration
Palpitations
Tachycardia
Neuroglucopenic
Headache
Weakness
Diplopia
Confusion
Amnesia
Bizarre behavior
Loss of motor skills
Seizures
Coma

permanent brain damage may occur. In the usual clinical setting, it is very difficult to estimate the exact duration of hypoglycemia in a given patient. It is not clear whether an episode of treated hypoglycemia leaves permanent residual effects. There have been several studies of long-term effects of hypoglycemia on the CNS [20]. Treated hypoglycemia has been shown to result in abnormalities of the Walton-Black test (suggesting general cerebral cortical damage) and an increased percentage of abnormalities of the electroencephalogram. Thus, it is more than likely that patients suffering repeated hypoglycemic episodes that are successfully treated often have subtle but persistent neurologic sequelae. Death is the ultimate complication of hypoglycemia, and if one surveys the literature, about 3 percent of deaths in younger insulin-dependent diabetic subjects are probably due to hypoglycemia [20].

Hypoglycemia remained unrecognized as a clinical syndrome until the discovery of insulin in 1921 [30]. The protean manifestations of symptomatic hypoglycemia were documented during the 1930s [71]. Plum and Posner [53] classified the neurologic symptoms of hypoglycemia into the four major categories of agitation, alteration of consciousness, seizures, and focal deficits. The series described by these authors is representative of most clinical reports in demonstrating that, of 56 hypoglycemic patients, 49 (88%) were diabetics taking insulin. The remaining 7 patients had tumors of the pancreas or were addicted to alcohol.

Two recent prospective studies of 262 admissions to Vanderbilt Medical Center and Harlem hospital made by 210 patients with symptomatic hypoglycemia has been reported [22,41]. Malouf and Brust [41] followed the classification scheme of Plum and Posner [53] by dividing the 125 admissions into 65 visits for alteration of consciousness such as coma, stupor, or obtundation (52%), 38 visits for agitation or bizarre affect (30.4%), 9 visits for generalized seizures (7.2%), and 3 admissions for hemiparesis of sudden onset (2.4%). The 3 patients with sudden hemiparesis demonstrated no other clinical signs of hypoglycemia and were thought initially to have cerebral infarction or hemorrhage. An additional 10 visits were prompted by dizziness or tremor (8%). All patients in the two studies had blood glucose levels ranging from 2 to 61 mg/dl. The blood glucose level could not be used to predict a specific clinical presentation. Diabetes, sepsis, renal insufficiency, malnutrition, liver disease, and alcohol abuse were the most common causes of hypoglycemia in these two series, accounting for 84 percent of the 262 episodes in the two studies [22,41]. The case fatality rate in the two series was 19 percent, although only one death could be attributed to hypoglycemic brain damage. Another 13 deaths resulted from associated or causative diseases such as sepsis, cancer, hepatic failure, and traumatic brain injury. The authors noted that a surprisingly low number of survivors retained focal neurologic deficits or cognitive impairment, although this observation may be related to lack of protracted follow-up supported with appropriate neuropsychological studies. Bale [11] found impaired cognitive skills in 100 insulin-dependent diabetics, whose poor performance was correlated with previous hypoglycemic episodes.

The intriguing phenomenon of hypoglycemic hemiplegia, as demonstrated by three of the patients in the survey by Malouf and Brust [41], returns to the question of selective vulnerability of neuronal populations. Cerebral blood flow remains normal or elevated during severe hypoglycemia, suggesting that alteration of neuronal function is not caused by vasospasm or obstruction of microcirculatory blood flow [3]. Focal neurologic deficits associated with hypoglycemia have been the subject of numerous case reports and clinical series [40,48,49,52,66]. Wallis and co-workers [66] described 16 patients who presented with unilateral hemiparesis, 10 of whom had blood glucose values less than 45 mg/dl and 6 of whom were being treated with an oral antihyperglycemic agent or insulin but were not tested for hypoglycemia. All 16 patients demonstrated resolution of hemiparesis with glucose treatment. One patient had two episodes of transient hemiparesis before she died of irreversible hypoglycemic encephalopathy. Postmortem examination revealed diffuse injury involving cortical neurons and Purkinje cells of the cerebellum but showed no evidence of focal infarction. Reproduction of symptoms following infusion of insulin was attempted in four patients but was successful in only one individual, who developed a transient right hemiparesis.

Another frequent cause of hypoglycemia is that of end-stage renal failure [26,27]. Such patients, although often developing blood glucose below 20 mg/dl [51], generally do not develop seizures, although they may lose consciousness [27,51]. It appears that the hypoglycemia of chronic renal failure is largely mediated by unavailability of substrate (amino acids) for gluconeogenesis [12,27]. The syndrome of hypoglycemia associated with chronic renal failure occurs most often in relatively cachectic individuals who do not consume adequate food for their metabolic needs [12]. Such individuals may become lethargic or even comatose, but seizure activity is rare.

What has been overlooked in the past is the substantial difference in the effects of hypoglycemia on the central nervous system between males and females. Merimee and Tyson [47] found that in premenopausal women subjected to a 3-day fast, blood glucose was significantly lower in the women, 48 ± 3 mg/dl, versus 66 ± 3 mg/dl in men ($p < .01$). The marked gender differences in glucose after a 3-day fast were accompanied by other biochemical changes. Women had significantly higher levels of glucagon and free fatty acids, while men had higher insulin levels. None of the individuals of either gender demonstrated central nervous system manifestations of their hypoglycemia [47], despite plasma glucose below 20 mg/dl in some women. Thus, as has recently been shown to occur in other types of clinical trials [10,57], there has been in the past a bias toward testing primarily men [32]. It is probable that women have a much lower threshold for central nervous system manifestations of hypoglycemia and can thus generally tolerate much lower levels of blood glucose than can men. It may be related to increased ability of women to mobilize free fatty acids, which can serve as fuel for the brain.

These findings all suggest that at least part of the effects of hypoglycemia on the central nervous system are due to effects of insulin rather than hypoglycemia per se. Subjects with blood glucose below 20 mg/dl may be asymptomatic [47] when insulin levels are low, while those with insulin-induced hypoglycemia often have seizures and coma [60]. However, another clinical manifestation of hypoglycemia, that of hypothermia, is apparently not due to an effect of insulin but to hypoglycemia per se [34]. Production of intracellular hypoglycemia by administration of 2-deoxy-D-glucose produced hypothermia in rats and human subjects, demonstrating that brain intracellular hypoglycemia was correlated with hypothermia independent of insulin [25].

An apparent exception to this appeared to be subjects with hypoglycemia related to large abdominal malignant tumors [38]. It was initially felt that such tumors produced hypoglycemia by actual metabolism of large amounts of glycose, independent of insulin. Many of these tumors in fact produce hypoglycemia by production of insulin-like growth factor II [16,61]. These peptides secreted by malignant tumors result in hypoglycemia with central nervous system effects in the absence of cachexia.

THERAPY OF HYPOGLYCEMIA

The principles of therapy of symptomatic hypoglycemia are those of elevation of plasma glucose and supportive maneuvers. There are now so many drugs that can cause hypoglycemia [19] that intravenous administration of 50% (2.8 M) glucose should probably be carried out in every unconsciousness patient. There is very little, if any possible harm to such a course of action, and the procedure may be lifesaving. One can draw a blood specimen for glucose analysis and then inject 50 ml of 2.8 M glucose without waiting for the laboratory value to become available. If the patient is indeed hypoglycemic, then 10% (0.56 M) glucose can be started and an infusion continued until the situation that led to the hypoglycemia has been controlled [60]. For a known diabetic who becomes mildly symptomatic but is alert, oral glucose-containing solutions, such as orange juice, may be adequate, as may injection of glucagon, if available [39]. If the patient does not regain consciousness within a few minutes, therapy with intravenous mannitol should be carried out. Steroids have been suggested to treat the cerebral edema that may be associated with hypoglycemia [39,60], but such therapy is unsupported by hard data. Steroids have been extremely useful in the treatment of other types of brain edema, particularly cerebral edema associated with neoplàsm of the brain [23,43]. The use of such agents in cerebral edema asociated with hypoglycemia is unproved, but such agents, particularly dexamethasone, have frequently been employed [39].

EXPERIMENTAL STUDIES

Experimental hypoglycemia in laboratory animals is most frequently induced by insulin administration. Doses vary between studies depending in part on the speed required for the induction of stupor and coma. The cerebral histologic events accompanying experimental hypoglycemia have been studied extensively. Two types of neuronal damage are seen in rat brain [2]. Early changes consist of cell shrinkage with nuclear condensation and scalloping of the cytoplasmic membrane. A second type of cell damage consists of swollen neurons containing vacuoles beneath the cytoplasmic membrane. Swollen neurons were seen in animals subjected to longer periods of hypoglycemia. These changes tend to revert to normal during a recovery phase. Only 2 percent of neurons appear abnormal after 4 hours of recovery. Neuronal damage does not occur if the electroencephalogram (EEG) does not show complete absence of cerebral activity [9]. Certain neuronal populations, including the superficial cortical layers, the dentate gyrus, and hippocampal pyramidal cells, appear to be selectively vulnerable to hypoglycemic injury [8,68,69].

"Selective vulnerability" of the brain is a principle describing the patterns of damage to the brain with hypoxia-ischemia. This principle generally dictates that certain parts of the brain are more vulnerable than others to ischemic damage [14] and probably is applicable to hypoglycemia as well [63]. The reasons for such selectivւ vulnerability of the brain are not well known. The most vulnerable regions of the brain are generally considered to be (1) layers 3, 5, and 6 of the cerebral cortex; (2) area h1 and areas h3, h4, and h5 of the hippocampus; (3) the central and basolateral portions of the amygdaloid nucleus; (4) Purkinje cells of the cerebellum; and (5) neurons of the caudate, putamen, globus pallidus, and thalamus [13]. In hypoglycemia, brain stem nuclei and neurons of the spinal cord are rarely affected.

EEG changes in hypoglycemic animals consist of a gradual slowing of activity as blood glucose levels reach 1 mM. Below 1 mM blood glucose results in an "isoelectric" EEG, signifying electrocerebral silence [37]. The overt behavior of chronically hypoglycemic mice and rats correlates with the blood glucose and EEG. Early stupor, characterized by impaired grooming and feeding, becomes obvious when blood glucose levels reach 1.5 to 2.0 mM.

The gradual slowing of EEG activity that accompanies a fall in blood glucose level to 1 mM in experimental animals has been confirmed in humans. Pramming and colleagues [54] performed serial EEGs on 13 insulin-dependent diabetics who were given intravenous insulin. Normal alpha rhythms became attenuated when the blood glucose level fell to 2 mM and were replaced with bisynchronous bursts of 2- to 4-Hz slow waves as it dropped to 1.3 mM. Alpha activity was restored promptly when glucose was infused to return the level to 2 mM.

Neurochemical studies of experimental hypoglycemia have focused on cerebral energy metabolism. ATP is the primary source of energy for cerebral function and is derived almost exclusively from glucose. Interestingly, results from several studies have shown that ATP depletion in hypoglycemic brain may not be responsible for the entire spectrum of metabolic impairment that characterizes this condition. Lewis and associates [37] measured high-energy phosphate metabolites in hypoglycemic rat brain at various EEG stages. Depletion of ATP and phosphocreatine occurred in the neocortex only when the EEG became isoelectric. The investigators concluded that energy failure was not responsible for the initial changes in EEG activity that preceded the isoelectric state. In another study in which recovery from hypoglycemia was examined, it was found that depleted ATP and phosphocreatine returned toward normal levels when the animals recovered [1].

Although parallels have been drawn between hypoglycemia and hypoxia, the effects of the two disorders on the brain are quite different. In hypoxia, there is an increase of brain lactate, a decline of brain intracellular pH (pHi) and an eventual decline in high-energy phosphate compounds (ATP, phosphocreatine) [17,55,56]. In hypoglycemia, there is generally not a detectable change in brain high-energy phosphate compounds until the EEG is isoelectric [21, 55,63]. Additionally, pHi is generally not affected by hypoglycemia, while inorganic phosphorus is increased in both conditions [55]. From the literature, the areas of the brain that suffer damage in hypoxia and ischemia are similar, but the pathology is quite different [62]. A number of studies in the older literature that have evaluated cerebral glucose metabolism have relied on the "freeze clamp" technique for evaluating brain metabolites [4,21]. Such measurements have been recently supplanted by more accurate techniques for evaluating brain high-energy phosphate compounds, such as magnetic resonance spectroscopy [56]. Some of the data in older studies may no longer be valid [55].

The large pieces of tissue used for neurochemical analysis must include a heterogenous population of cells. Since consciousness is mediated via the ascending reticular activating formation, study of this region without "contamination" by contiguous nonaffected tissue could yield more meaningful data. In one such project [45], young mice were made hypoglycemic with insulin. High-energy phosphates were measured in 100- to 500-ng samples of the ascending reticular activating system in the pontine region. Results obtained during early coma showed depletion of ATP to 30 percent of normal values and reduction of phosphocreatine to 55 percent of baseline. The levels of these high-energy phosphates returned to normal when the animals were in deep coma. These results suggest that there is a selective vulnerability in neurons of the reticular formation. The functional capacity of these cells and their synaptic connections with the cortex, as represented by the EEG activity, became impaired as they were depleted of ATP and phosphocreatine.

Although the preceding discussions have centered on cerebral energy metabolism in experimental hypoglycemia, other changes in compounds such as acetylcholine, cyclic nucleotides, and amino acids have been noted [63]. Several authors have presented work suggesting that increased amounts of the excitatory amino acid neurotransmitters glutamate and aspartate may be responsible for the pathologic changes observed with hypoglycemia [63,68,69]. The mechanisms appear to apply to hypoxic damage and probably apply to hypoglycemic damage as well. Excessive amounts of glutamate in brain extracellular fluid probably play a role in the pathogenesis of brain damage in hypoglycemia [63,68–70]. Severe and prolonged hypoglycemia causes a release of glutamate into cerebral extracellular space and may lead to excitation of a subset of glutamate receptors, the *N*-methyl-D-aspartate (NMDA) receptor. Excitation at this receptor then can lead to an excessive influx of sodium and water [62]. Continuous excitation, or increased synaptic activity, is an important factor in eventual cell death in hypoxic neurons [58] and may also be the case in hypoglycemia [68]. Competitive blockade of the NMDA receptor has been successful in preventing brain damage in metabolic encephalopathies that are unrelated to hypoglycemia, such as traumatic injury [18] and ischemia [64], and similar findings have been reported in experimental hypoglycemia as well [67]. Thus, brain damage from hypoglycemia, as is apparently the case in hypoxia and traumatic nervous system injury, may ultimately be mediated via continuous excitation, or increased synaptic activity, of specific neuronal receptors [42]. It appears that the classic biochemical teachings where hypoglycemia leads to a decrease of brain high-energy phosphate compounds, with a secondary influx of sodium, chloride, and water into brain, are probably not correct [21,62].

Auer [8] has shown that disruption of dendritic trees occurs with preservation of intermediate axons in brain subjected to experimental hypoglycemia, indicating that high tissue levels of a toxin similar to an excitatory amino acid may result in selective damage without causing infarction or necrosis associated with energy failure. The EEG silence associated with hypoglycemia is accompanied by marked increases in the extracellular concentrations of aspartate and glutamate [59]. Transection of glutamatergic fibers projecting from the cortex ameliorates damage to striatal neurons [70]. Wieloch [67] has shown that injection of a selective antagonist of the NMDA receptor for glutamate will limit cell necrosis in caudoputamen of rodent brain subjected to hypoglycemia.

REFERENCES

1. Agardh, C. D., Folbergrova, J., and Siesjo, B. K. Cerebral metabolic changes in profound insulin induced hypoglycemia, and the recovery period following glucose administration. *J. Neurochem.* 31:1135, 1978.
2. Agardh, C. D., Kalimo, H., Olsson, Y., et al. Hypoglycemic brain injury. *Acta Neuropathol.* 50:31, 1984.
3. Agardh, C. D., Rosen, I., and Ryding, E. Persistent vegetative state with high cerebral blood flow following profound hypoglycemia. *Ann. Neurol.* 14:482, 1983.
4. Arieff, A. I., Doerner, T., Zelig, H., et al. Mechanisms of seizures and coma in hypoglycemia. Evidence for a direct effect of insulin on electrolyte transport in brain. *J. Clin. Invest.* 54(3):654, 1974.
5. Arieff, A. I., Kleeman, C. R., Kerian, A., et al. Cerebral edema in diabetic comas: II. Effects of hyperosmolality, hyperglycemia and insulin in diabetic rabbits. *J. Clin. Endocrinol. Metab.* 38(6):1057, 1974.
6. Arieff, A. I., Kleeman, C. R., Keushkerian, A., et al. Studies on mechanisms of cerebral edema in diabetic comas: Effects of hyperglycemia and rapid lowering of plasma glucose in normal rabbits. *J. Clin. Invest.* 52(3):571, 1973.
7. Arky, R. A., Veverbrants, E., and Abramson, E. A. Irreversible hypoglycemia. *J.A.M.A.* 206:575, 1968.
8. Auer, R. N. Hypoglycemic brain damage. *Stroke* 17:699, 1986.
9. Auer, R. N., Olsson, Y., and Siesjo, B. K. Hypoglycemic brain injury in the rat. *Diabetes* 33:1090, 1984.
10. Ayus, J. C., and Arieff, A. I. Symptomatic hyponatremia: I. Making the diagnosis rapidly. *J. Crit. Illness* 5(8):846, 1990.
11. Bale, R. N. Brain damage in diabetes mellitus. *Br. J. Psychiatry* 122:337, 1973.
12. Block, M. B., and Rubenstein, A. H. Spontaneous hypoglycemia in diabetic patients with renal insufficiency. *J.A.M.A.* 213:1863, 1970.
13. Brierley, J. B., and Brown, A. W. The threshold and neuropathology of cerebral "anoxic-ischemic" cell change. *Arch. Neurol.* 29:367, 1973.
14. Collins, R. C., Dobkin, B. H., and Choi, D. W. Selective vulnerability of the brain: New insights into the pathophysiology of stroke. *Ann. Intern. Med.* 110(12):992, 1989.
15. Daniel, P. N., Love, E. R., and Pratt, O. E. Insulin and the way the brain handles glucose. *J. Neurochem.* 25:471, 1975.
16. Daughaday, W. H., Emanuelle, M. A., Brooks, M. H., et al. Synthesis and secretion of insulin-like growth factor II by a leiomyosarcoma with associated hypoglycemia. *N. Engl. J. Med.* 319:1434, 1988.
17. de Courten-Myers, G. M., Yamaguchi, S., Wagner, K. R., et al. Brain injury from marked hypoxia in cats. *Stroke* 16:1016, 1985.
18. Faden, A. I., Demediuk, P., Panter, S. S., et al. The role of excitatory amino acids and NMDA receptors in traumatic brain injury. *Science* 244:798, 1989.

19. Fajans, S. S., and Floyd, J. C., Jr. Fasting hypoglycemia in adults. *N. Engl. J. Med.* 294(14):766, 1976.
20. Feingold, K. R. Hypoglycemia: A pitfall of insulin therapy (Medical Staff Conference, University of California, San Francisco). *West. J. Med.* 139: 688, 1983.
21. Ferrendelli, J. A., and Chang, M. M. Brain metabolism during hypoglycemia. *Arch. Neurol.* 28: 173, 1973.
22. Fisher, K. F., Lees, J. A., and Newman, J. H. Hypoglycemia in hospitalized patients. *N. Engl. J. Med.* 315:1245, 1986.
23. Fishman, R. A. Brain edema. *N. Engl. J. Med.* 293:706, 1975.
24. Freinkel, N., Arky, R. A., Singer, D. L., et al. Alcohol hypoglycemia IV. *Diabetes* 14:350, 1965.
25. Freinkel, N., Metzger, B. E., Harris, E., et al. The hypothermia of hypoglycemia. *N. Engl. J. Med.* 287:841, 1972.
26. Frizzell, M., Larsen, P. R., and Field, J. B. Spontaneous hypoglycemia associated with chronic renal failure. *Diabetes* 22:493, 1973.
27. Garber, A. J., Bier, D. M., Cryer, P. E., et al. Hypoglycemia in compensated chronic renal insufficiency. *Diabetes* 23:982, 1974.
28. Gibbs, R. L., Lennox, W. G., Nims, L. F., et al. Arterial and cerebral venous blood: Arterial-venous differences in man. *J. Biol. Chem.* 144:325, 1942.
29. Guler, H. P., Zapf, J., and Froesch, E. R. Short-term metabolic effects of recombinant human insulin-related growth factor I in healthy adults. *N. Engl. J. Med.* 317:137, 1987.
30. Harris, S. Hyperinsulinism and dysinsulinism. *J.A.M.A.* 83:729, 1924.
31. Hawkins, R. A., Williamson, D. H., and Krebs, H. A. Ketone body utilization by adult and suckling rat brain in vivo. *Biochem. J.* 122:13, 1971.
32. Hilts, P. J. N.I.H. Starts Women's Health Office. *N.Y. Times,* Sept. 11, 1990, Science 3.
33. Hofeldt, F. D., Lufkin, E. G., Hagler, L., et al. Are abnormalities in insulin secretion responsible for reactive hypoglycemia? *Diabetes* 23:589, 1974.
34. Kedes, L. H., and Field, J. B. Hypothermia: A clue to hypoglycemia. *N. Engl. J. Med.* 271:785, 1964.
35. Kety, S. S. The General Metabolism of the Brain In Vivo. In D. Richter (ed.), *The Metabolism of the Nervous System.* London: Pergamon, 1957.
36. Laitha, A. L., Maker, H. S., and Clarke, D. D. Metabolism and Transport of Carbohydrates and Amino Acids. In G. J. Siegel, R. W. Albers, B. W. Agranoff, and R. Katzman (eds.), *Basic Neurochemistry.* Boston: Little Brown, 1981.
37. Lewis, L. D., Ljunggren, B., Ratcheson, R. A., et al. Cerebral energy state in insulin induced hypoglycemia related to blood glucose and EEG. *J. Neurochem.* 23:673, 1974.
38. Lyall, S. S., Marieb, N. J., Wise, J. K., et al. Hyperinsulinemic hypoglycemia associated with a neurofibrosarcoma. *Arch. Intern. Med.* 135:865, 1975.
39. MacCuish, A. C., Munro, J. F., and Duncan, L. J. P. Treatment of hypoglycaemic coma with glucagon, intravenous dextrose, and mannitol infusion in a hundred diabetics. *Lancet* 2:946, 1970.
40. MacDonald, J. T., and Brown, D. R. Acute hemiparesis in juvenile insulin-dependent diabetes mellitus (JIDDM). *Neurology* 29:893, 1979.
41. Malouf, R., and Brust, J. C. M. Hypoglycemia: Causes, neurological manifestations, and outcome. *Ann. Neurol.* 17:421, 1985.
42. Manev, H., Costa, E., Wroblewski, J. T., et al. Abusive stimulation of excitatory amino acid receptors: A strategy to limit neurotoxicity. *F.A.S.E.B. J.* 4:2789, 1990.
43. Marshall, L. F. Treatment of Brain Swelling and Brain Edema in Man. In J. Cervos-Navarro and R. Ferszt (eds.), *Advances in Neurology.* New York: Raven Press, 1980. P. 459.
44. McCall, A. L., Fixman, L. B., Fleming, N., et al. Chronic hypoglycemia increases brain glucose transport. *Am. J. Physiol.* 251:442, 1986.
45. McCandless, D. W. Insulin induced hypoglycemic coma and regional cerebral energy metabolism. *Brain Res.* 215:225, 1981.
46. McIlwain, H. (ed.), *Biochemistry and Central Nervous System.* Boston: Little Brown, 1966.
47. Merimee, T. J., and Tyson, J. E. Stabilization of plasma glucose during fasting. *N. Engl. J. Med.* 291:1275, 1974.
48. Meyer, J. F., and Portnoy, H. D. Localized cerebral hypoglycemia simulating stroke. *Neurology* 8:601, 1958.
49. Montgomery, B. M., Pinner, C. A., and Newberry, S. C. Transient hypoglycemic hemiplegia. *Arch. Intern. Med.* 114:680, 1964.
50. Nelson, S. R., Shulz, D. W., Passonneau, J. V., et al. Control of glycogen levels in brain. *J. Neurochem.* 15:1271, 1968.
51. Peitzman, S. J., and Agarwal, B. N. Spontaneous hypoglycemia in end-stage renal failure. *Nephron* 19:131, 1977.
52. Penman, W. A., and Johnson, J. K. Recurrent hemiplegia due to hypoglycemia. *Postgrad. Med. J.* 58:501, 1982.
53. Plum, F., and Posner, J. The Pathological Physiological Physiology of Signs and Symptoms of Coma. In F. Plum and J. Posner (eds.), *The Diagnosis of Stupor and Coma.* Philadelphia: Davis, 1966. P. 2.
54. Pramming, S., Thorsteinsson, B., Stigsby, B., et al. Glycaemic threshold for changes in electroencephalograms during hypoglycaemia in patients with insulin dependent diabetes. *Br. Med. J.* 296:665, 1988.
55. Prichard, J. W., Alger, J. R., Behar, K. L., et al.

Cerebral metabolic studies in vivo by ^{31}P NMR. *Proc. Natl. Acad. Sci. U.S.A.* 80:2748, 1983.
56. Prichard, J. W., and Shulman, R. G. NMR spectroscopy of brain metabolism in vivo. *Ann. Rev. Neurosci.* 9:61, 1986.
57. Purvis, A. Research for men only. *Time* 135:59, 1990.
58. Rothman, S. M. Synaptic activity mediates death of hypoxic neurons. *Science* 220:536, 1983.
59. Sandberg, M., Butcher, S. P., and Hagberg, H. Extracellular overflow of neuroactive amino acids during severe insulin-induced hypoglycemia: In vivo dialysis of the rat hippocampus. *J. Neurochem.* 47:178, 1986.
60. Seltzer, H. S. Drug-induced hypoglycemia. *Diabetes* 21:955, 1972.
61. Shapiro, E. T., Polonsky, K. S., Rubenstein, A. H. et al. Tumor hypoglycemia: Relationship to high molecular weight insulin-like growth factor II. *J. Clin. Invest.* 85:1672, 1990.
62. Siesjo, B. K. Oxygen deficiency and brain damage: Localization, evolution in time, and mechanisms of damage. *Clin. Toxicol.* 23:267, 1985.
63. Siesjo, B. K. Hypoglycemia, brain metabolism, and brain damage. *Diabetes Metab. Rev.* 4:113, 1988.
64. Simon, R. P., Swan, J. H., Griffiths, T., et al. Blockade of *N*-methyl-D-aspartate receptors may protect against ischemic damage in the brain. *Science* 226:850, 1984.
65. Stone, W. E., Tews, J. K., Whisler, K. E., et al. Incorporation of carbon from glucose into cerebral amino acids, proteins and lipids, and alterations during recovery from hypoglycemia. *J. Neurochem.* 19:321, 1972.
66. Wallis, W. E., Donaldson, I., Scott, R. S., et al. Hypoglycemia masquerading as cerebrovascular disease (hypoglycemic hemiplegia). *Ann. Neurol.* 18:510, 1985.
67. Wieloch, T. Hypoglycemia-induced neuronal damage prevented by an *N*-methyl-D-aspartate antagonist. *Science* 226:681, 1985.
68. Wieloch, T. Endogenous excitotoxins as possible mediators of ischemic and hypoglycemic brain damage. *Adv. Exp. Med. Biol.* 203:127, 1986.
69. Wieloch, T., Auer, R. N., Westerberg, E., et al. Hypoglycemic Brain Damage Is Mediated by Excitotoxins. In P. Roberts (ed.), *Excitatory Amino Acids.* New York: Macmillan, 1986. P. 127.
70. Wieloch, T., Engelsen, B., Westerberg, E., et al. Lesions of the glutamatergic cortico-striatal projections in the rat ameliorate hypoglycemic brain damage in the striatum. *Neurosci. Lett.* 58:25, 1985.
71. Wolf, A., Hare, C. C., and Riggs, H. W. Neurological manifestations in two patients with spontaneous hypoglycemia. *Bull. Neurol. Instit. N.Y.* 3:232, 1933.

8 Neurologic Manifestations of the Uremic State

Cosmo Lyle Fraser

Recent advances in the treatment of renal failure and its complications have resulted in marked improvement in both the duration and quality of life in these patients [50]. However, despite these therapeutic successes, patients with renal failure continue to manifest a number of neurologic disorders that have continued to be incapacitating. Patients with renal failure who are not yet on dialysis may develop symptoms such as mild sensorial clouding, tremor, asterixis, multifocal myoclonus, seizures, and even coma or death [50, 134]. Similarly, even after adequate maintenance dialysis therapy, they may continue to manifest nervous system dysfunctions such as impaired mentation, generalized weakness, and peripheral neuropathy. The central nervous system (CNS) disorders of both untreated renal failure and that persisting despite dialysis are referred to as uremic encephalopathy. Dialysis itself has also been associated with at least two distinct disorders of the CNS. These include dialysis disequilibrium syndrome and dialysis dementia, which occur in a small number of patients. Dialysis disequilibrium syndrome appears to be a consequence of the initiation of dialysis, while dialysis dementia is a progressive, generally fatal disorder that usually affects elderly patients on chronic hemodialysis, as well as children with chronic renal failure who have not been treated with dialysis [5, 18].

In patients with both advanced liver and renal diseases, it is often difficult to determine which of these conditions is responsible for the encephalopathy [49]. In fact, encephalopathy may be the result of both conditions. In such patients the blood urea nitrogen and serum creatinine do not always adequately reflect the degree of functional renal impairment [112]. Thus, many patients with cirrhosis, ascites, and normal blood urea nitrogen and creatinine may have a glomerular filtration rate that is below 30 ml/minute and may indeed have significant renal compromise [112]. Normally, protein and amino acids in the gastrointestinal tract are metabolized by bacteria and mucosal enzymes in the colon to form ammonia. Ammonia then enters the liver through the portal circulation, where it is converted to urea by the urea cycle [48, 49]. Most of the urea so produced is excreted in the urine, and the remainder enters the colon via hepatoenteric recirculation. However, in renal failure patients, the major route for the elimination of urea (i.e., the kidneys) is unavailable, so there is a rapid and sustained increase in blood urea nitrogen concentration. The elevated blood urea nitrogen level results in an increase in the amount of urea that enters the colon by recirculation. Thus, in uremic subjects, the additional urea in the gut is again acted upon by bacteria and mucosal enzymes, resulting in further ammonia production. This may then lead to increases of both plasma ammonia concentration and brain ammonia uptake in these subjects [40, 54].

UREMIC ENCEPHALOPATHY

Uremic encephalopathy is an organic brain syndrome that occurs with some frequency in patients with acute or chronic renal failure when glomerular filtration rate declines below 10 percent of normal [123]. As with other organic brain syndromes, patients display variable disorders of consciousness, psychomotor behavior, thinking, memory, speech, perception, and emotion [122]. They also frequently have features that suggest a functional psychiatric illness. Since these features may be different in different patients, other descriptions may be appropriately applied in specific clinical circumstances. These may include acute or chronic organic reaction, confusional state, clouding of consciousness, delirium, twilight state, coma, stupor, dementia, organic personality change, acute or chronic amnesic syndrome, and toxic psychosis.

The symptoms of uremia are usually quite variable in individual patients (Table 8-1) [134]. They may include sluggishness and easy fatigability; daytime drowsiness and insomnia with a tendency toward sleep inversion; itching; inability to focus or sustain attention or to perform mental (cognitive) tasks and manipulation; inability to manage ideas and abstractions; decreased flow and slurring of speech; anorexia, nausea, and vomiting (probably of central origin); restlessness; imprecise memory; diminished sexual interest and performance; volatile emotionality and withdrawal; feelings of coldness and hypothermia; myoclonus and "restless legs"; "burning feet"; asterixis; hiccoughs; paranoid thought content; disorientation and confusion with bizarre behavior; hallucinosis; muttering and mumbling; meningeal signs, amaurosis, nystagmus; vertigo and ataxia; transient pareses and aphasic episodes; torpor and preterminal coma and convulsions [50].

Certain salient characteristics of the symptoms of uremic encephalopathy are espe-

Table 8-1. Signs and symptoms of uremic encephalopathy

Mild (early)	*Moderate*	*Severe (late)*
Anorexia	Vomiting	Itching
Nausea	Sluggishness	Disorientation
Insomnia	Easy fatigability	Confusion
Restlessness	Drowsiness	Bizarre behavior
Decreased attention span	Sleep inversion	Slurring of speech
Inability to manage ideas	Volatile emotions	Hypothermia
Decreased sexual interest	Paranoia	Myoclonus
	Decreased cognitive function	Asterixis
	Inability to decipher abstractions	Convulsions
	Decreased sexual performance	Stupor
		Coma

cially noteworthy. They represent integrated behaviors in the whole organism. The severity and overall rates of progression of encephalopathy vary directly with the rate at which renal failure develops. Thus, uremic symptoms are generally more severe and progress more rapidly in patients with acute than in those with chronic renal failure. In slowly progressive chronic renal failure, the number and severity of symptoms also typically vary cyclically, with intervals of well-being in an otherwise inexorable downhill course. Patients' conditions are usually improved with maintenance dialysis and relieved entirely following restoration of renal function by successful renal transplantation [29].

DIFFERENTIAL DIAGNOSIS OF UREMIC ENCEPHALOPATHY

The diagnosis of uremic encephalopathy in most patients can be readily established by clinical history that is consistent with renal or urologic disease; by physical evidence such as hypertension, anemia, pruritus, or asterixis; and by laboratory findings of azotemia, acidosis, anemia, abnormal calcium, phosphate, and vitamin D metabolism, and hyperparathyroidism, with or without an active urinary sediment. However, since the presenting symptoms of uremia are nonspecific and are common among patients with many other encephalopathic states, the possibility of misdiagnosis certainly exists [50, 122].

The diagnosis of uremic encephalopathy may be further complicated by the fact that patients with renal failure are also subject to other intercurrent illnesses. Additionally, the treatments of these illnesses may induce symptoms that are due primarily to the side effects of drugs [134, 135]. Moreover, a drug or its metabolites with potential CNS toxicity that is normally excreted or significantly metabolized by the kidney may reach toxic levels at ordinary dose rates and produce symptoms of encephalopathy. Generally, in such patients, one or more dialyses may both restore normal body fluid composition and reduce drug levels, so that the question of whether the symptoms are due to uremia or to drug therapy remains moot while the patient recovers. Despite the possibilities that such multiple causes of encephalopathy might occur simultaneously, uremic encephalopathy may be successfully differentiated in most instances by means of the usual clinical methods (history, physical examination, and laboratory determinations) [50].

CENTRAL NERVOUS SYSTEM MANIFESTATIONS OF ACUTE RENAL FAILURE

Clinical Signs and Symptoms

The central nervous system manifestations of acute renal failure (ARF) have been studied in several large series of patients [38, 88, 137]. In these studies, mental state abnormalities have been noted as an early and sensitive index of neurologic disorder. The patient first developed lassitude and lethargy, which rapidly progressed to disorientation and confusion. Fixed attitudes, torpor, and other signs of toxic psychosis are also common, and if uremia is not treated and allowed to progress, coma will eventually supervene [50]. Though transient, cranial nerve signs are frequently common, as are nystagmus and mild facial asymmetries [50]. Visual fields, papilledema, and the optic fundi are usually normal in most patients. About half the patients have dysarthria and difficulty in protruding their tongue past the lips. Many have diffuse weakness and fasciculations of muscle groups. Marked variation of deep tendon reflexes in an asymmetric pattern is often noted in most patients. Very commonly, there is progression to hyperreflexia with unsustained clonus at the patella or ankle.

Electroencephalographic Changes of ARF

The electroencephalogram (EEG) in patients with ARF is usually abnormal within 48 hours of the onset of renal failure [38, 66, 71, 83, 88]. These abnormalities appear to be unaffected by dialysis for up to 3 weeks after treatment has been instituted (Fig. 8-1). In most instances, the percentage of EEG power less than 5 Hz and less

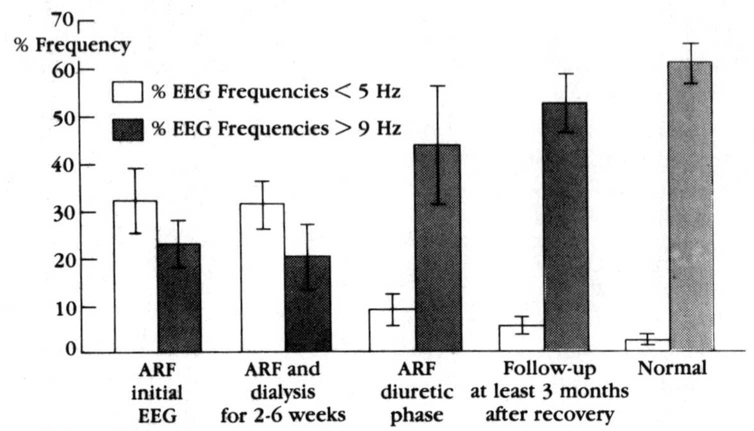

Fig. 8-1. Percentage of EEG frequencies below 5 Hz and above 9 Hz. Normal values are on the right. Patients with acute renal failure (ARF) have significant changes in both these frequencies above 9 Hz and those below 5 Hz. These changes are unaffected by dialysis but become normal with return of renal function. Data from 16 patients with ARF are illustrated. Data are mean ± SE. (From Cooper, Lazarowitz, Arieff [38].)

than 7 Hz (which are standard measurements of the percentage of EEG power devoted to abnormal [delta] slow wave activity) is more than 20 times the value observed in individuals without renal failure (Fig. 8-2)[38, 71]. The EEG is also abnormal with regard to the percentage of EEG frequencies above 9 Hz and those below 5 Hz. It may worsen both during and for several hours after hemodialysis and up to 6 months after the initiation of dialysis therapy [50]. Although EEG changes are not improved by dialysis, they will return to normal with recovery of renal function. These findings were also observed in experimental animals with renal failure [66].

CENTRAL NERVOUS SYSTEM MANIFESTATIONS OF CHRONIC RENAL FAILURE

Clinical Signs and Symptoms

The neurologic manifestations reported with chronic renal failure (CRF) are also quite numerous and have many similarities to those of ARF [50]. However, the symptoms tend to develop more slowly and may be more debilitating. Symptoms such as pruritus and bone and muscle pain are more commonly seen in CRF patients and are usually the result of secondary hyperparathyroidism [91, 134]. Additionally, patients with CRF tend to have less of a derangement in acid-base status for a given degree of renal impairment. This is due primarily to compensatory mechanisms by the chronically diseased kidney [90].

Electroencephalographic Changes of CRF

The EEG findings in patients with CRF are not as severe as those observed in patients with ARF. A good correlation exists between the percentage of EEG frequencies and power below 7 Hz and the decline of renal function as estimated by serum creatinine (Figs. 8-1 and 8-2) [137]. After the initiation of dialysis, there may be an initial period of clinical stabilization during which the EEG deteriorates (up to 6 months), but it tends to normalize thereafter [31, 83]. Since the EEG is not fully normalized with time, still more improvement is seen after renal transplantation

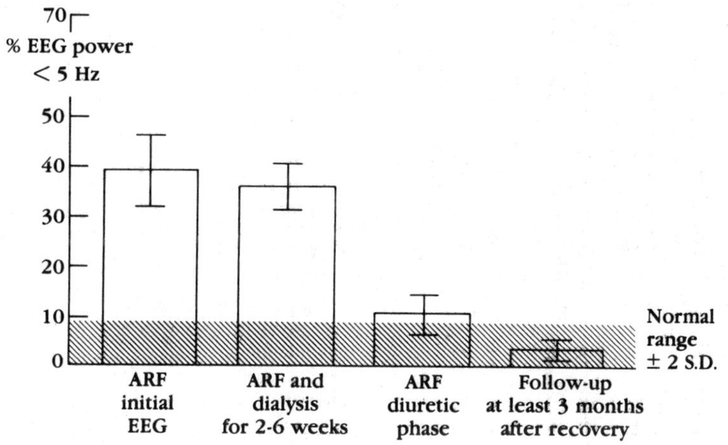

Fig. 8-2. Percent EEG power less than 5 Hz in 16 patients with acute renal failure (ARF). The normal range is shown in the cross-hatched area. In patients with ARF, there is a highly significant increase in the percent EEG power below 5 Hz, which is an indicator of the presence of abnormal slow waves. This is not affected by dialysis but becomes normal with return of renal function. (From Cooper, Lazarowitz, and Arieff [38].)

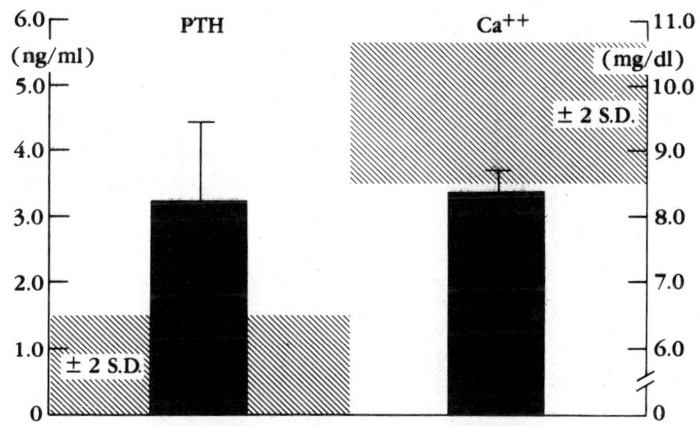

Fig. 8-3. Plasma levels of parathyroid hormone (PTH) and Ca^{+2} in patients with acute renal failure (ARF). PTH levels are more than twice the upper limit of normal ($p < .01$) and plasma Ca^{+2} is significantly less than normal ($p < .01$). The shaded areas show normal ranges for Ca^{+2} and PTH. (From Cooper, Lazarowitz, and Arieff [38].)

[71, 83]. The causes of the EEG abnormalities in uremic patients are probably multifactorial, but there is evidence that a major causative factor may be parathyroid hormone (PTH)[63, 66, 91, 130]. In experimental animals with acute or chronic renal failure, many of the EEG abnormalities are related to a direct effect of PTH on brain (Fig. 8-3). Studies in patients with either acute or chronic renal failure suggest a similar effect of PTH [36, 63, 66, 91].

Central nervous system dysfunction in uremia can also be quantitated by cognition-dependent performance measures. The cognitive functions known to be impaired in uremia include sustained attention, selective attention, speed of decision making, short-term memory, and mental manipulation of symbols [50]. The choice reaction time (CRT) test, which measures sustained attention as well as speed of decision making, is probably the most useful test to determine cognitive function on uremia.

BIOCHEMICAL CHANGES IN UREMIC BRAIN

Many studies have previously been carried out to determine the likely causes for the EEG abnormalities and the clinical symptoms that are found in patients with either acute or chronic renal failure. To this end, measurements of brain intracellular pH and the concentrations of Na^+, K^+, Cl^-, aluminum, Ca^{+2}, Mg^{+2} (Fig. 8-4), urea adenine nucleotides (creatine phosphate, adenosine triphosphate [ATP], adenosine diphosphate [ADP], adenosine monophosphate [AMP]), lactate, and Na^+-K^+-activated adenosine triphosphatase (ATPase) enzyme activity have all been determined [7]. In patients with ARF, the brain content of water, K^+, and Mg^{+2} is normal, while that of Na^+ is modestly decreased. Aluminum content is slightly elevated and cerebral cortex Ca^{+2} is almost twice the normal value (Fig. 8-5). Movement of Na^+ into the brain is decreased in uremia, while that of K^+ is increased. These changes have also been observed in dogs with ARF [1, 7, 50, 92, 93].

In brain of rats [116, 129, 140] with ARF, creatine phosphate, ATP, and glucose are said to be increased, but with a corresponding decrease in AMP, ADP, and lactate. It has been suggested that the uremic brain utilizes less ATP and thus does not produce ADP, AMP, and lactate at normal rates. The brain energy charge and the redox state are said to be normal [93, 140]. Its metabolic rate is decreased and is associated with a corresponding decrease in cerebral oxygen consumption. Brain glucose is elevated, however. In humans with renal failure, the pH of cerebrospinal fluid, liver, muscle, and brain is normal, despite a decreased blood pH [8] (Fig. 8-6). Patients with chronic renal insufficiency

Fig. 8-4. The postmortem calcium and magnesium contents in brain tissue from normal control subjects and from patients with chronic renal failure and secondary hyperparathyroidism are shown. Means ± SE are illustrated, with significance ($p < .05$, unpaired t test) denoted by an asterisk (*). A significant increase in cerebral cortical calcium, but not magnesium, is found in the brains of patients with secondary hyperparathyroidism. (From Cogan et al. [36].)

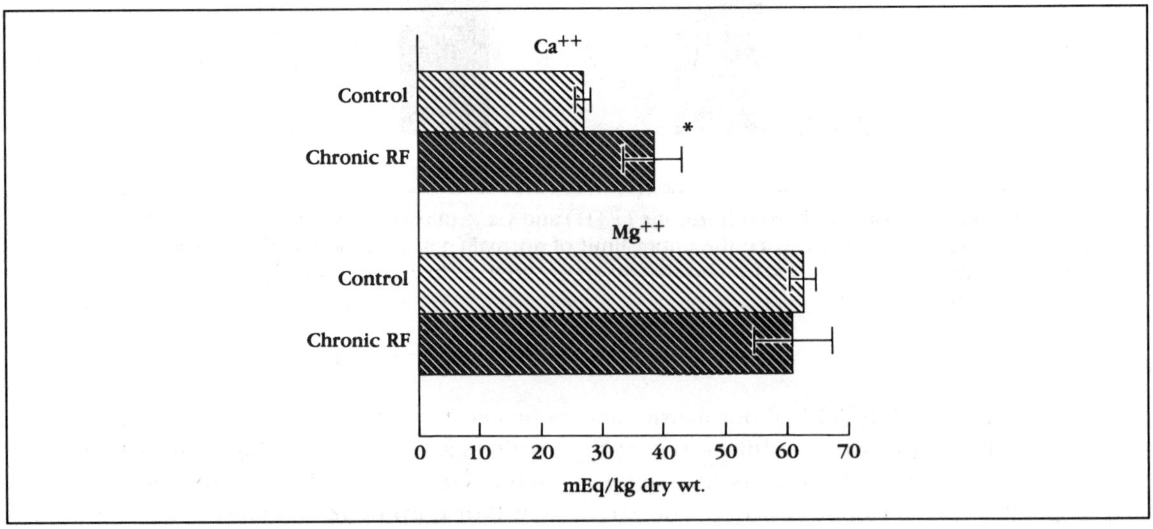

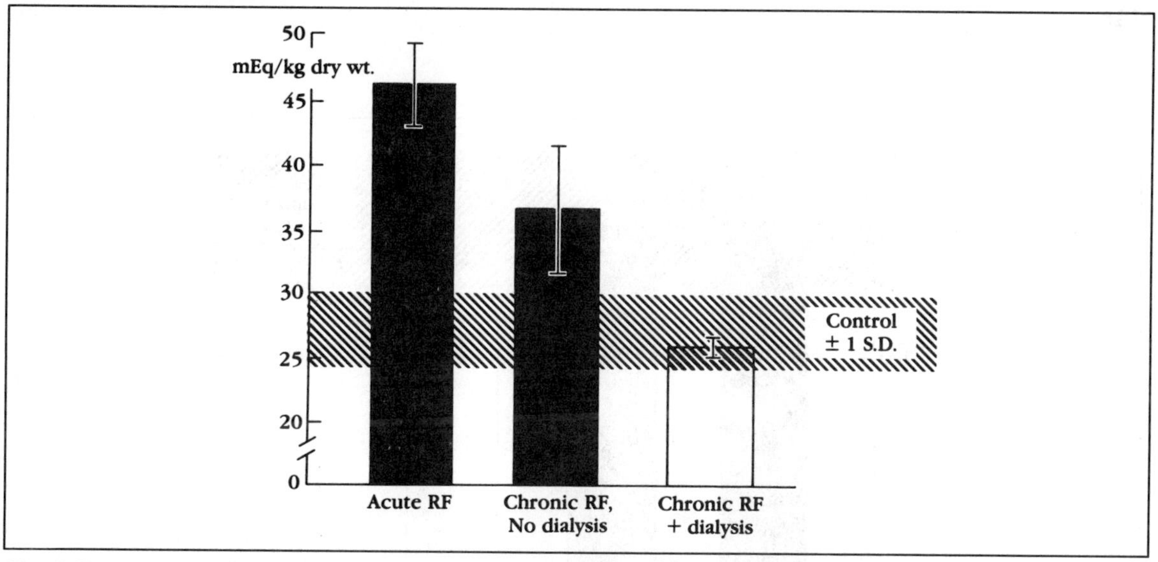

Fig. 8-5. The brain (cerebral cortex) content of calcium (Ca^{+2}) in patients who had acute renal failure, those with chronic renal failure treated with dialysis, or patients with end-stage chronic renal failure treated for at least 2 years with hemodialysis. Brain Ca^{+2} content is significantly greater than control values in patients who had acute renal failure ($p < .001$) or chronic renal failure not treated with dialysis ($p < .03$). However, in patients treated with dialysis, brain Ca^{+2} content is normal. RF = renal failure; data are means ± SE (From A. I. Arieff, Neurological Complications of Uremia. In B. M. Brenner and F. C. Rector, Jr. (eds.), *The Kidney.* Philadelphia: Saunders, 1986. Pp. 1731–1758.)

Fig. 8-6. The effects of 4 months of chronic renal failure (CRF) on the intracellular pH (pHi). In dogs with CRF, the arterial pH is significantly below control values. However, pHi is normal in brain white and gray matter, the liver, and skeletal muscle (*$p < .01$). (From Mahoney and Arieff [92].)

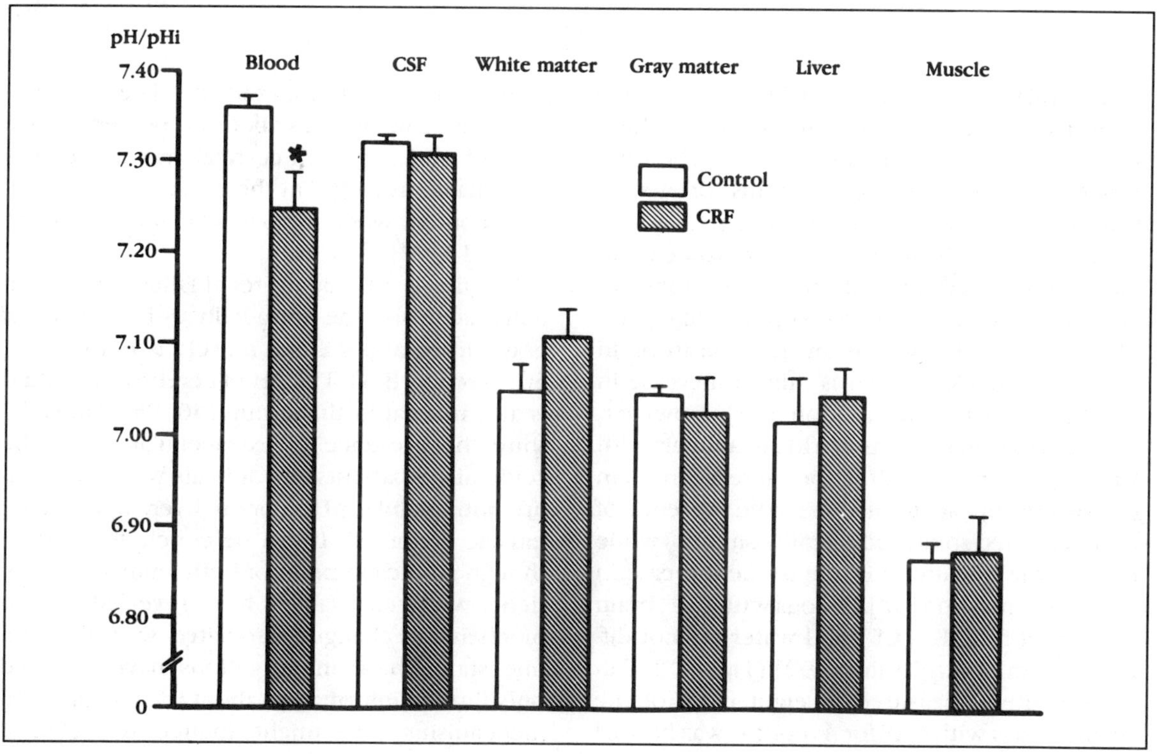

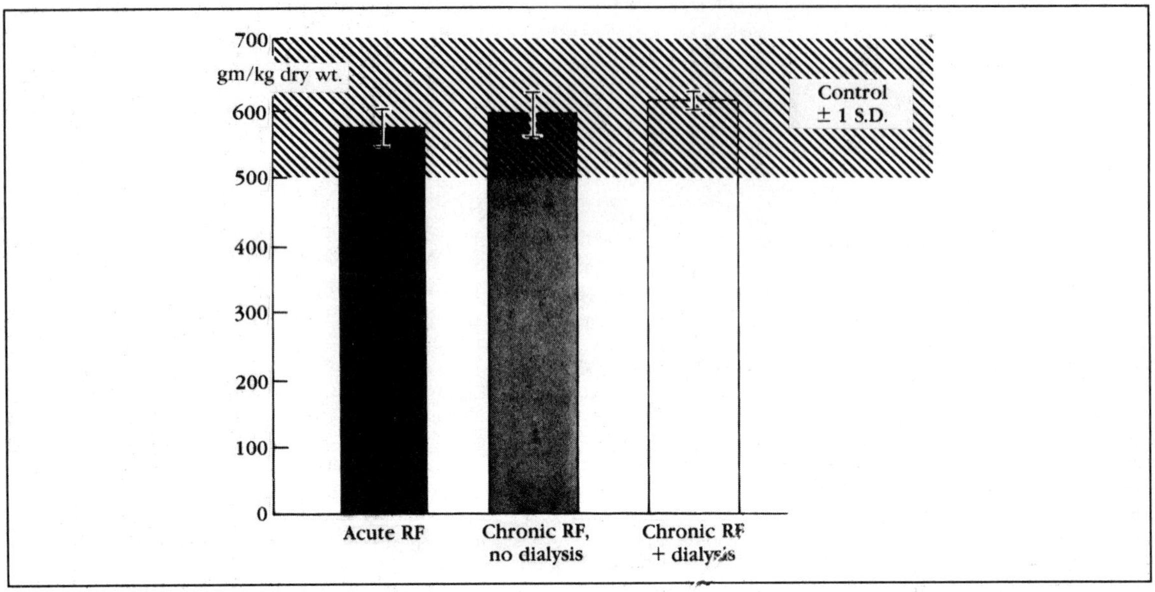

Fig. 8-7. The brain (cerebral cortex) water content in patients who had either acute renal failure (n = 10); chronic renal failure without dialytic therapy (GFR < 20 ml/minute, n = 6); or chronic renal failure treated with hemodialysis for at least 2 years (n = 6). RF = renal failure. The control value is the mean from nine patients who had no evidence of renal disease, stroke, parathyroid disease, or cancer. The water content was normal in cerebral cortex in all groups of patients with renal failure and was also normal in brain subcortical white matter. Tissue was obtained from autopsy specimens. (Data from Arieff et al. [10], Cogan et al. [36], Cooper, Lazarowitz, and Arieff [38], and A. I. Arieff, unpublished data, 1979.)

(glomerular filtration rate [GFR] below 20 ml/minute) have decreased brain uptake of glutamine and increased ammonia uptake. The relevance of these findings in terms of neurotransmitter regulation is unknown [42].

In animals with either acute or chronic renal failure, both urea concentration and osmolality are similar in brain, cerebrospinal fluid, and plasma [14, 92]. There is an increase in brain osmolality in ARF, which is due to increase in the brain urea concentration [14]. However, contrary to observations in ARF, in animals with CRF approximately half of the increase in brain osmolality appears to be due to the presence of undetermined solute (idiogenic osmoles) while most of the remainder is due to the increase in urea concentration [92]. In dogs with CRF, brain content of Na^+, K^+, Cl^-, and water are not different from control values [92] (Fig. 8-7). Calcium content measured in eight parts of the brain in dogs with CRF for 4 months was normal in the subcortical white matter, pons, medulla, cerebellum, thalamus, and caudate nucleus. However, calcium was about 60 percent above control values in both cortical gray matter and hypothalamus [92]. On the other hand, magnesium content was normal in all eight parts of the brain [13, 92].

In animals with acute renal failure and metabolic acidosis, the intracellular pH (pHi) of brain, liver, and skeletal muscle is normal [11, 50] (see Fig. 8-6). The pH of cerebrospinal fluid is also normal in this group [40, 75]. Thus, despite the presence of extracellular metabolic acidemia in patients and animals with renal failure, intracellular pH in brain, liver, and skeletal muscle is normal. It can be concluded that although studies in brain of both animals and patients with renal failure have revealed several biochemical changes associated with the uremic state, these investigations have revealed only limited information about the fundamental mechanisms that might induce the clinical symptoms of uremic encephalopathy.

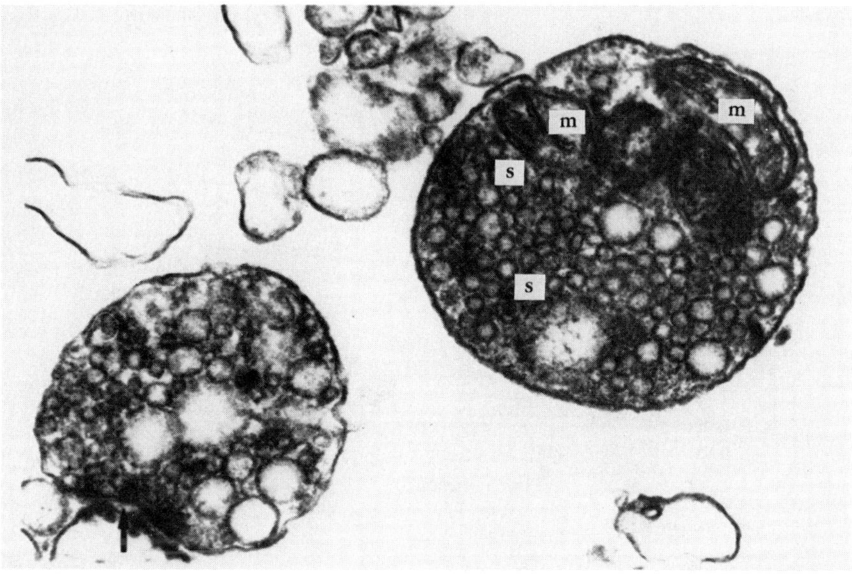

Fig. 8-8. Electron micrograph of synaptosomes from our preparation. Synaptosome at upper right contains numerous mitochondria (m) and many synaptic vesicles (s). ↑ shows synaptic cleft where communication is carried out between nerve cells (i.e., chemical or electrical transmission between presynaptic and postsynaptic terminals). Synaptic cleft is either a distinct separation (chemical injunction) or continuation on the cytoplasm of one cell to the other (electrical junction). Dark area adjacent to cleft represents accumulation of cellular constituents in the presynaptic (synaptic vesicles) and postsynaptic receptor area (ribosomes, endoplasmic reticulum). (From Fraser and Sarnacki [52].)

SUBCELLULAR EXCHANGES IN UREMIC BRAIN

Because of the difficulty of establishing a causal relationship between brain calcium, PTH, and symptoms of uremic encephalopathy, investigators have recently been studying the effects of uremia on the brain by studying subcellular fractions in brain. This subcellular analysis has been undertaken primarily with brain synaptosomes (Fig. 8-8) [48, 51–54]. Synaptosomes are vesicles derived from the presynaptic nerve terminal in brain [144, 145]. The reason for studying synaptosomal function in uremia was based on their anatomic location and the physiologic role they play in vivo, in the processing of information in the CNS [30, 33, 77].

When a neuron in the CNS is stimulated, an action potential is generated that travels the length of the axon to the nerve terminal. This results in an increase in the membrane permeability of the plasma membrane to calcium. This change reduces calcium influx from the extracellular space to the cytosol of the nerve terminal [48, 76, 77]. The mechanisms by which calcium enters cells include sodium channels, calcium channels, and the Na/Ca exchanger [48, 54]. As opposed to nonexcitable cells where the Na/Ca exchanger participates only in calcium efflux [23, 48, 54], in excitable cells such as neurons and myocardium, the exchanger participates in both calcium influx and efflux [23]. To maintain calcium balance, calcium that enters the cell from the extracellular space has to be pumped out after the physiologic response has been achieved. The outward movement of calcium is accomplished by both the Na/Ca exchanger and the Ca ATPase pump. These two mechanisms are the primary exporters of calcium from either excitable or nonexcitable cells [23, 117]. The relative importance of these transport systems in different tissues is quite variable, since a calcium channel that is specific for excitable tissues may not be as important or

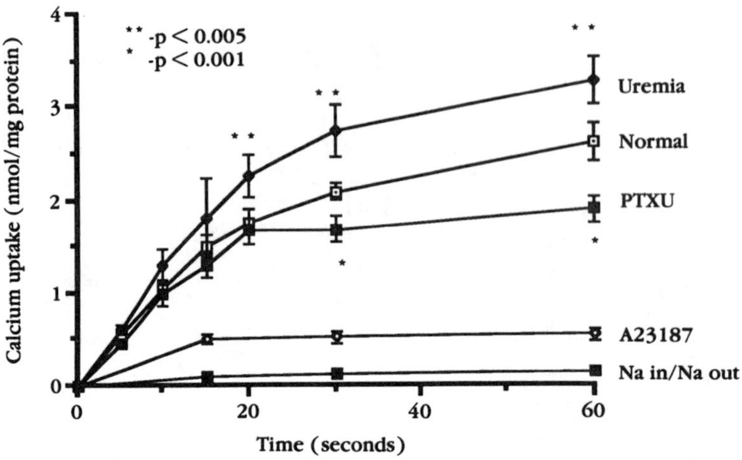

Fig. 8-9. Calcium uptake by sodium-calcium exchange mechanism in synaptosomes isolated from brains of normal, uremic, and uremic parathyroidectomized (PTX-U) rats. Uptake in uremia (**) is sigificantly greater ($p < .005$) than normal, as indicated. Uptake in PTX-U rats (*) is significantly less than in vesicles from uremic ($p < .001$) rats. Graph also shows effect of calcium ionophore A23187 and absence of a sodium gradient (Na in/Na out) on calcium uptake. Synaptosomes from three rats were pooled for each experiment, and eight experiments were performed. Data are means ± SE (From Fraser and Sarnacki [52].)

even exist in nonexcitable tissues [23]. For instance, the Ca ATPase of the liver is felt to be different from that of many other plasma membrane Ca ATPases [34]. However, regardless of the transporter that is utilized, the overall effect of these transporters is to maintain a calcium gradient of 10,000 : 1 (outside-inside cells). In the steady state, a net calcium flux of zero is maintained across the plasma membrane. The Na/Ca exchanger, which operates electrogenically (exchanging three Na^+ for one Ca^{+2}), is a high-capacity low-affinity system, while the Ca ATPase is a low-capacity high-affinity system that continuously pumps calcium out of cells. Thus, in cellular regulation of calcium, the Ca ATPase pump modulates subtle changes in cytosolic calcium, while the Na/Ca exchanger is important in regulating major changes in calcium fluxes [34].

The reason for the rapid entry of calcium into nerve terminals after the action potential increases the membrane permeability is quite complex. However, it appears that for neurotransmitter substances to be released within the synaptic junction, intracellular calcium must first be increased [48]. With the rise in cytosolic calcium, the neurotransmitter-containing vesicles (synaptic vesicles) aggregate at the affector surface of the presynaptic terminal and then liberate their content into the synaptic space [45, 144]. The transmitter substance bathes the receptor area of the receptor neuron, and the process is repeated until the appropriate information is successfully transferred. Since patients and animals with severe uremia displayed poor mentation and abnormal behavior, it was felt that either one or many of the processes responsible for information transfer within the CNS may be abnormal.

Utilizing synaptosomes. Fraser and associates [51–54] have shown that there are indeed many defects in synaptosomal function in the brains of uremic rats. Both the Na/Ca exchanger and the Ca ATPase pumps were shown to be abnormal

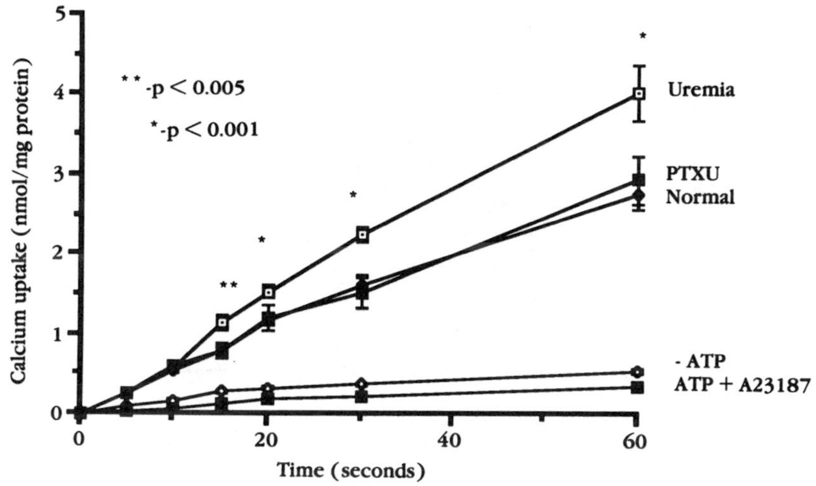

Fig. 8-10. Effect of parathyroidectomy on ATP-stimulated calcium uptake in plasma membrane vesicles from normal, uremic, and uremic parathyroidectomized (PTX-U) rat brain. *Significant ($p < .005$) increase in uptake in uremia as compared with vesicles from normal rats. Parathyroidectomy resulted in no increase in calcium uptake in uremia. In the absence of ATP and in the presence of calcium ionophore A23187, calcium uptake was eliminated. Values are means ± SE of eight experiments. (From Fraser and Sarnacki [52].)

in the brains of uremic rats [52, 55]. The presence of uremia resulted in an enhancement of calcium transport by both transport mechanisms (Figs. 8-9 and 8-10). These defects were shown to be primarily dependent on PTH, as PTH administered to nonuremic rats could also reproduce these abnormalities (Fig. 8-11)[54]. Further studies by this group have demonstrated that PTH action on calcium transport in these uremic synaptosomes were independent of cyclic AMP [51]. In this study it was shown that although PTH stimulates calcium transport in brain synaptosomes (Fig. 8-12), it was unable to stimulate cyclic AMP production in the synaptosomes (Table 8-2)[51, 55]. It has also recently been shown that the content of the neurotransmitter substance, norepinephrine, in synaptosomes may be altered in rats with CRF [132].

In other studies in synaptosomes, it was shown that the Na-K ATPase pump function was affected by uremia [53, 55]. The ouabain-sensitive component of both sodium and potassium transport was significantly decreased in the brains of uremic rats. In crude brain preparation, Na-K ATPase enzyme activity was found by other investigators to be either normal or decreased [104, 140]. Contrary to the detrimental effects that uremia has on ion transport in brain, water and urea transport do not appear to be affected by uremia [141].

There is a substantial body of work to indicate that neurotransmitter substance regulation may be altered in acute uremia. Since the mid-1960s, it has been shown that neurotransmitter substances such as norepinephrine, 5-hydroxytryptamine, acetylcholine, and dopamine are transported in the brain by sodium-dependent mechanisms [24–26, 28, 37, 39, 58, 73]. It has also been shown that the Na-K ATPase and potassium participate directly in the transport of the biogenic amines [27, 28, 37, 85, 113]. Ouabain, an inhibitor of the Na-K ATPase pump, is not only capable of inhibiting the pump, but it also inhibits neurotransmitter transport [21, 28, 138]. Inhibition of the pump results in inhibi-

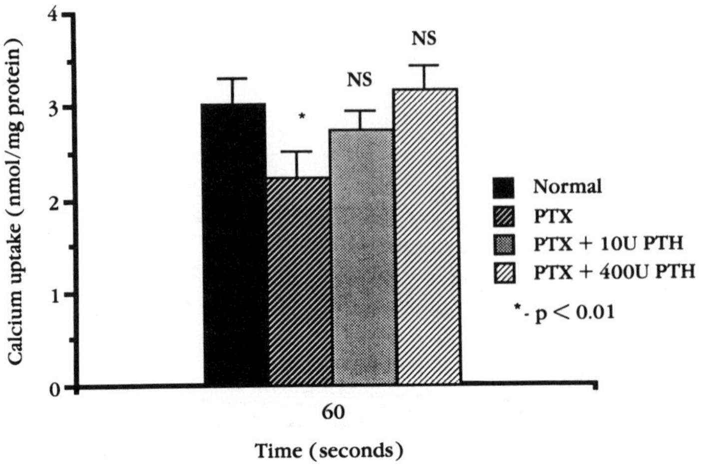

Fig. 8-11. Effect of parathyroid hormone (PTH) on the sodium-calcium exchange in synaptosomes from normal rats. When normal rats were parathyroidectomized, synaptosomal calcium uptake was significantly decreased ($p < .01$). With either 2.8 μg or (110 μg) 400 units of PTH, uptake was increased to values not significantly different from normal control. Values are means ± SE of six experiments. (From Fraser and Sarnacki [52].)

Fig. 8-12. This graph shows the effects of three different PTH molecules on calcium uptake in synaptosomes. Uptake in the presence of either 100 ng/ml of parathyroid extract or 10^{-7}M 1-34 bPTH significantly increased calcium uptake above control at 5 seconds ($p < .001$). 10^{-7}M 3-34 bPTH had no stimulatory effects on uptake. At 30 seconds, uptake of all three groups was not different from control. Data are expressed as mean ± SE of eight experiments. (From Fraser, Sarnacki, and Budayr [55]. Copyright permission of the American Society for Clinical Investigation.)

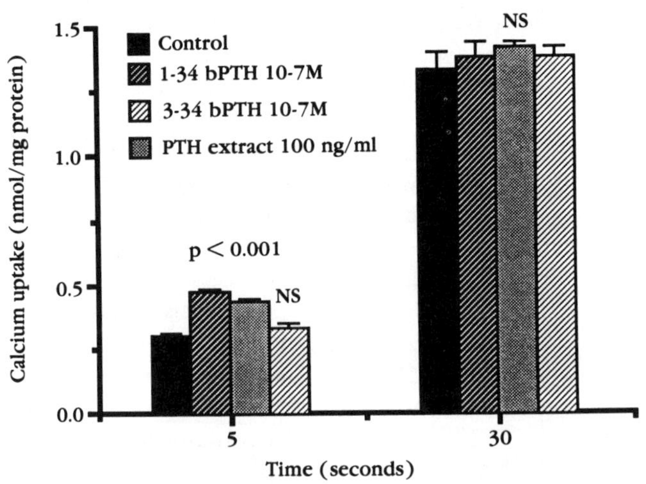

Table 8-2. Effects of PTH, forskolin, and sodium fluoride on adenylate cyclase activity in canine renal cortical plasma membrane versus synaptosomes

		Adenylate Cyclase Activity (pmol cyclic AMP/mg protein 30 minutes)	
Agents	*Concentration*	*CRCPM**	*Synaptosomes**
1-34 bPTH (ng/ml)	0	278 ± 11	911 ± 51
	30	763 ± 25 (2.7)	—
	300	1230 ± 36 (4.4)	953 ± 57
	100,000	1411 ± 40 (5.1)	922 ± 44
1-84 bPTH (ng/ml)	0	250 ± 15	1300 ± 98
	10	519 ± 22 (2.1)	1357 ± 34
	500	1036 ± 45 (4.1)	1290 ± 75
Forskolin (μM)	0	239 ± 34	911 ± 51
	0.1	3330 ± 145 (14)	7466 ± 420 (8.2)
NaF (μM)	0	239 ± 34	911 ± 51
	100	6669 ± 310 (28)	3562 ± 248 (4)

CRCPM = canine renal cortical plasma membrane.
* Five experiments. Data are expressed as mean ± SE.

tion of the neurotransmitter. In uremic rats, norepinephrine uptake, tyrosine hydroxylase activity, and catecholamines, such as dopamine, norepinephrine, and epinephrine concentrations, were found to be substantially decreased [3, 70]. Autopsy of brains of patients who have been on hemodialysis and died with renal failure showed a 40 percent decrease in gamma-aminobutyric acid content and a 25 to 35 percent decrease in acetylcholine transferase activity [116]. This decrease in transferase activity could result in decreased synthesis of acetylcholine. Our findings in brain synaptosomes, which showed decreased function of the Na-K ATPase pump and decreased transport of both sodium and potassium in acutely uremic rat brain, are consistent with these observations [53]. Taken in total, the evidence indicates that there are fundamental defects in the uremic brain that might explain many of the clinical manifestations of uremic encephalopathy.

BRAIN PATHOLOGY IN RENAL FAILURE

Results of pathologic studies from the brains of over 400 patients who died with CRF have shown that, in the past, subdural hemorrhages occurred in 1 to 3 percent of uremic patients [50]. Intracerebral hemorrhages were reported in about 6 percent of these patients, but the data may have been influenced by the fact that many patients were receiving oral anticoagulants at the time of death. Cerebral edema, once thought to be a common finding in uremic patients, is no longer felt to be present in the brains of either patients or laboratory animals with CRF [50]. Generalized but variable neuronal degeneration is often present but is inconsistent in location. Other findings reported in patients dying of uremia include necrosis of the granular layer of the cerebral cortex, small intracerebral hemorrhages, necrotic foci, and focal glial proliferation. In general, changes in brain of patients who died with CRF are probably nonspecific and are related more to some concomitant underlying disease state.

PATHOPHYSIOLOGY OF UREMIC ENCEPHALOPATHY

Although there are a multitude of factors that contribute to uremic encephalopathy, many investigators have shown no correlation between encephalopathy and any of the commonly measured indicators of renal failure. In recent years, there has been considerable discussion about the possible role of PTH as a uremic toxin. There is presently a substantial amount of evidence to suggest that PTH can produce toxic effects on the CNS in both in vivo and in vitro models, in humans and in laboratory animals [36, 38, 54, 62, 66].

Role of Parathyroid Hormone as a Possible CNS Uremic Toxin

Patient Studies

PTH is known to produce CNS effects in humans with normal renal function, and neuropsychiatric symptoms are reported to be among the most frequent manifestations of primary hyperparathyroidism [69]. Patients with primary hyperparathyroidism also have EEG changes that are similar to those observed in patients with ARF [36]. The common denominator appears to be the elevated plasma levels of parathyroid hormone. In patients with ARF, the EEG is abnormal within 18 hours of the onset of renal failure and is generally not affected by dialysis for periods of up to 8 weeks [38]. In patients with either primary or secondary hyperparathyroidism, parathyroidectomy results in an improvement in both the abnormalities of the EEG and psychological testing, suggesting a direct effect of PTH on the CNS [38, 62]. It has also been shown that dialysis therapy results in the return of brain (cerebral cortex) calcium toward normal in both patients and laboratory animals with renal failure and is associated with improvement of the EEG [13, 66]. In uremic patients, both the EEG changes and psychological abnormalities are improved by either parathyroidectomy or by medical suppression of PTH [36]. The mechanism by which PTH might disturb CNS function is not well known. The increased calcium content in such diverse tissues as skin, cornea, blood vessels, brain, and heart in patients with hyperparathyroidism suggests that PTH may facilitate the entry of Ca^{+2} and lead to cell death. Thus, PTH and/or a high brain calcium content is probably responsible for some of the clinical manifestations of the encephalopathy of renal failure.

Animal Studies

Dogs with acute or chronic renal failure show an increase in brain gray matter calcium and in EEG pattern that are similar to those seen in humans with renal failure [13]. In dogs, both the EEG and brain calcium abnormalities can be prevented by parathyroidectomy [66]. Conversely, these abnormalities can be reproduced by administration of PTH to normal animals. The abnormalities are not induced by elevation of the (calcium × phosphate) product or by hypercalcemia produced by vitamin D intoxication. In rats with ARF and encephalopathy, calcium transport in brain synaptosomes was found to be abnormal [54]. This abnormality was prevented by parathyroidectomy and could be duplicated by the administration of PTH [52, 54]. The mechanism by which PTH influences calcium transport in brain appears to be independent of cyclic AMP (see Table 8-2)[51].

The finding of increased calcium content in the brain of both dogs and patients with either acute or chronic renal disease and secondary hyperparathyroidism is consistent with the conception that part of the CNS dysfunction and EEG abnormalities found in acute or chronic renal failure may be due to PTH-mediated increase in brain calcium. Since calcium is essential for the function of a large number of intracellular enzyme systems [123], and an increase in brain calcium content could disrupt cerebral function, it appears that the elevated PTH associated with renal failure may have a detrimental effect on the CNS through a calcium-mediated mechanism.

Role of Aluminum as Possible CNS Uremic Toxin

Recent observations have shown that aluminum content in brain of patients with CRF (creatinine clearance less than 20 ml/minute) who had been taking aluminum hydroxide for at least 5 years before death was lower [2] but not significantly different from that of patients with dialysis dementia [10, 91]. Studies from several laboratories have shown that although mean brain aluminum is consistently higher in patients with dialysis dementia as compared with dialyzed uremic patients without dementia, there is considerable overlap between the groups [81, 102, 103]. Furthermore, aluminum is also elevated in cerebral cortex of patients with ARF, as well as in subcortical white matter of patients with acute or chronic renal failure. Thus, it would appear that the presence of increased quantities of aluminum in brain might occur as a consequence of the uremic state.

Aluminum is absorbed after oral administration of aluminum-containing antacids, and the rentention of aluminum after oral administration of aluminum salts is greater in patients with renal failure than in normal subjects [74, 75]. The typical daily dietary aluminum intake in the United States is 10 to 100 mg [33]. This 1-day quantity of dietary aluminum is more than enough to account for the entire increase in brain aluminum that is observed in patients with dialysis dementia. Among 22 such patients, the mean brain aluminum content was 22 mg/kg dry weight. The normal human male brain weighs about 1500 gm and is about 80 percent water, or 300 gm dry weight. Thus, the total increase in aluminum content for the whole brain is less than 7 mg in patients with dialysis dementia [50]. Therefore, the entire increase of brain aluminum in such patients can theoretically be accounted for by dietary aluminum alone. However, aluminum stores may also result from aluminum contamination from other sources, such as aluminum in dialysate water, dialysis system aluminum pipes, or aluminum leaked from anodes. Thus, the problem is not where the aluminum comes from, but rather how it gets into the brain. In both dialysis encephalopathy and Alzheimer's disease, abnormalities of the blood-brain barrier are probably important in the entry of aluminum into the brain. Thus, aluminum might be expected to be elevated in brain of patients with diseases that are associated with blood-brain barrier abnormalities. These include metastatic cancer and hepatic encephalopathy [50]. In fact, cerebral cortex aluminum is increased in patients with renal failure, hepatic coma, metastatic cancer, senile dementia, and Alzheimer's disease. Recent evidence also suggests that brain aluminum content may also increase as a function of the aging process (Fig. 8-13) [10, 102, 103].

In both rats and dogs receiving oral aluminum salts, there is a significant increment in brain aluminum content [10, 20, 100, 101]. However, it was also observed that the administration of PTH to rats receiving aluminum salts resulted in an additional increment of brain aluminum con-

Fig. 8-13. Brain content of various elements in patients with dialysis dementia. The content of bromine (Br) and rubidium (Rb) are below normal, while those of iron (Fe), calcium (Ca), copper (Cu), manganese (Mn), strontium (Sr), aluminum (Al), and tin (Sn) are above normal values. For each trace element, the bar represents the ratio of the value in patients with dialysis dementia to the value in normal individuals. (From Fraser and Arieff [50].)

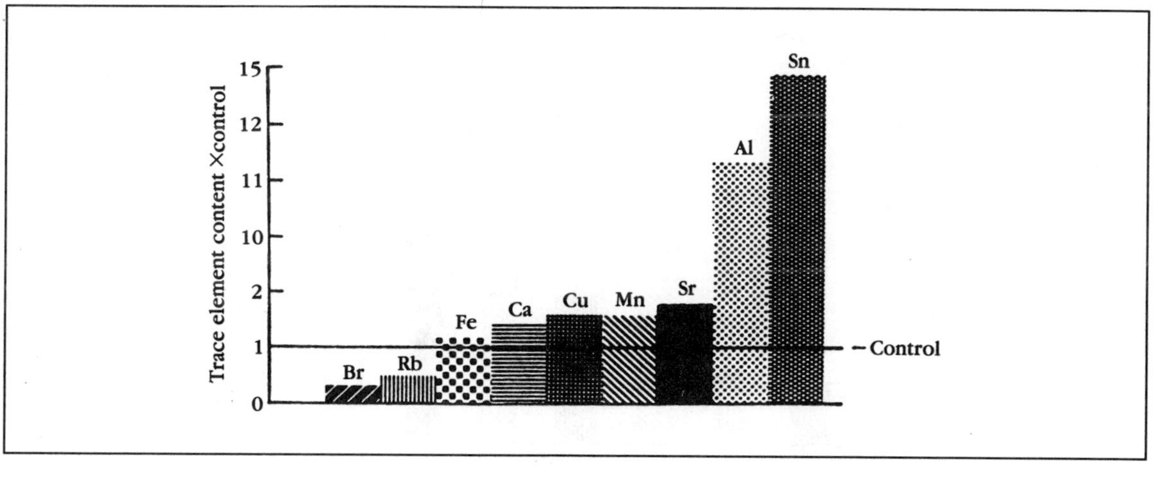

tent. Thus in laboratory animals, either a chronic increase in oral aluminum ingestion or PTH excess can lead to increased cerebral cortex aluminum, even in the absence of renal failure. Epidemiologic evidence also suggests that high levels of aluminum in water may be due to the use of aluminum salts in water purification systems. It has been suggested that the once high frequency of dementia at Cook County Hospital, Chicago, Illinois, may have been related to higher than normal levels of aluminum in water [44, 94]. However, an "epidemic" of dialysis dementia was reported from Nashville, Tennessee, at a time when dialysate water aluminum levels were virtually undetectable [19, 43]. In an earlier study from the University of British Columbia, Vancouver, B.C., Canada, dialysis dementia was reported to be one of the major causes of death. Just about 150 km away at Washington University School of Medicine in Seattle, Washington, there were fewer than two cases a year of dialysis dementia [7]. Presently, there is a decrease in the number of cases of dialysis dementia, which appears to parallel the removal of aluminum with deionizers from the water source. However, it may be that the deionizers may also be removing additional contaminants besides aluminum (Fig. 8-14). Thus, although there is a relationship between high aluminum in dialysate and the increased incidence of dialysis dementia, other factors may also play an important role as well.

There are other forms of encephalopathy that may be related to increased aluminum levels in brain. These include amyotropic lateral sclerosis, parkinsonism-dementia of Guam, and Alzheimer's disease [32, 40, 56, 84, 100, 101, 115]. Recent evidence suggests that some patients with dialysis encephalopathy have senile plaques and neurofibrillary tangles in their brains that are similar to those observed in patients with Alzheimer's disease [32, 84]. In Alzheimer's disease, the plaques and neurofibrillary tangles contain aluminum [40, 41, 115]. While the exact localization in the brain cells of the aluminum in patients with dialysis encephalopathy is unknown, it may be that aluminum in the presence of an abnormal blood-brain barrier produces toxic effects on the CNS. If this is the case, it may be that aluminum may be involved in the pathogenesis of several different forms of dementias, and dialysis encephalopathy is only one such disorder.

A possible mechanism of aluminum toxicity

Fig. 8-14. Brain aluminum content in patients who are more than 70 years old or have Alzheimer's disease, hepatic coma, metastatic cancer (not metastatic to brain), acute renal failure (ARF), chronic renal failure (CRF), or dialysis dementia. For each clinical condition, the bar represents the ratio of the aluminum content in patients to the value in normal persons. (From Fraser and Arieff [50].)

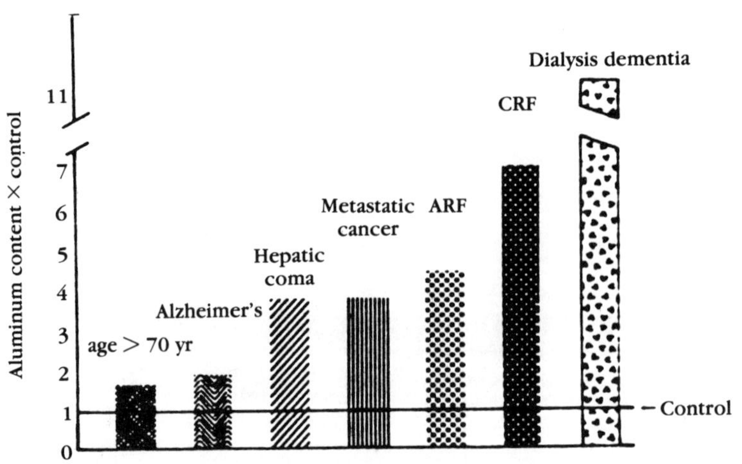

on the CNS can be inferred from the following. Tetrahydrobiopterin, a protein that is required for the synthesis of several different neurotransmitter substances in the brain, is reduced in dialysis patients [5]. The enzyme dihydropteridine reductase, which is necessary to maintain normal brain concentration of tetrahydrobiopterin, is also reduced in patients with renal failure. In dialysis patients with mean plasma aluminum levels greater than 13 times the control value, red blood cell activity of dihydropteridine reductase was reduced and was inversely related to plasma aluminum level [5]. The erythrocyte dihydropteridine reductase activity was shown to increase after plasma aluminum was removed by deferoxamine. Although these enzymes were not studied in brain tissue, they may have important ramifications for the future.

COMPLICATIONS OF THE THERAPY OF RENAL FAILURE

Dialysis Disequilibrium Syndrome

In patients with CRF, there are several central nervous system disorders that may occur after the patients are already on dialysis. Dialysis disequilibrium syndrome (DDS) is one such disorder. It is described as a clinical syndrome that occurs at the onset of hemodialysis in patients with renal failure. The syndrome has been described since the early 1960s [78–81] and is felt to include symptoms such as headache, nausea, emesis, blurring of vision, muscular twitching, disorientation, hypertension, hypotension, tremors, and seizures [7, 65, 125]. The EEG may be abnormal [125], but this has been disputed [71, 83, 137]. More recently, the syndrome of DDS was described in patients with milder symptoms, such as muscle cramps, anorexia, restlessness, and dizziness [65, 111, 125]. Although DDS has been reported among all age groups, it is more common among elderly patients and children [7]. The syndrome is most often associated with rapid hemodialysis of patients with ARF [7], but it also has been reported following maintenance hemodialysis of patients with CRF [125]. There has been much debate about the pathogenesis of DDS, and this is summarized elsewhere [7, 50]. Mild forms of DDS may be manifested by no more than restlessness and severe headache, which may occur during or soon after hemodialysis. This is commonly followed by nausea and vomiting, often accompanied by blood pressure elevation. These symptoms may be accompanied by disorientation and tremors. Seizures and cardiac arrhythmias have been reported but are uncommon. The symptoms are usually self-limited, but recovery may take several days. In some instances the seizures may lead to coma. It appears that the modern methods of dialysis have altered the clinical picture of DDS. Most reports of seizures, coma, and death were reported prior to 1970. It is also unclear whether any patient ever actually died from DDS or from other associated neurologic complications of dialysis, such as acute stroke, subdural hematoma, subarachnoid hemorrhage, or hyponatremia. Recently, the diagnosis of DDS has become a "wastebasket" for a number of disorders that can occur in patients with renal failure and may affect the CNS. It should be stressed that the diagnosis of DDS should be one of exclusion [50].

The pathogenesis of DDS has been extensively studied [14, 65, 78, 80]. Although it was previously felt that the symptoms of DDS were primarily due to the reverse urea effect, this does not appear to be the case [31, 69, 70]. It was felt that during rapid hemodialysis, urea was cleared less well from the brain than it was from plasma, and as a result, an osmotic gradient between brain and plasma was created because of the increased brain urea, resulting in cerebral edema [70]. Subsequent studies have shown that during dialysis, urea is cleared from brain at the same rate as from plasma [31, 69]. In recent studies with more sophisticated techniques, transport of urea in brain was quite rapid and was not different in normal and uremic brain [141]. Although patients with DDS do have increased brain osmolality compared to plasma, and symptoms are usually due to cerebral edema, the osmolar gap is one due primarily to unmeasured organic acids (idiogenic osmoles).

The management of DDS can be divided into preventative modalities and therapeutic maneuvers. In several studies, this syndrome has been treated by addition of osmotically active solute (glucose, glycerol, albumin, urea, fructose, sodium chloride, mannitol) to the dialysate or by substitution of sodium bicarbonate for sodium lactate (or acetate) in the dialysate [12, 50, 80, 120]. Recently, a new technique called "pure ultrafiltration" has been developed [127]. By this technique, the patient is subjected to ultrafiltration without dialysis. The net result is loss of fluid without the patient's undergoing dialysis. This procedure can then be followed by conventional dialysis without ultrafiltration. The role of ultrafiltration followed by dialysis in prevention of DDS is currently being evaluated [127]. In both humans and experimental animals, the occurrence of DDS can best be prevented by use of "slow" dialysis, that is, low blood flow rates (less than 4 hours) at frequent intervals (every 1–2 days). Until additional therapy becomes available, DDS can probably best be prevented by employing short, frequent dialyses at low blood flow rates in patients who are at risk [50].

Dialysis Dementia

Dialysis dementia (also called dialysis encephalopathy) is a progressive, frequently fatal neurologic disease, which was first described in the early 1970s [2, 4, 94]. The disease is seen almost exclusively in patients being treated with chronic hemodialysis. Although the early literature focused on the distinctive neurologic findings [2, 94], more recent reports from both Europe and the United States have suggested that some forms of dialysis dementia may be a part of a multisystem disease that includes encephalopathy, osteomalacic bone disease, proximal myopathy, and anemia [118–121, 142].

Although an increase in brain aluminum content has been strongly implicated in some cases of dialysis dementia, the evidence is less convincing in others. Dialysis dementia most likely represents a syndrome complex that is the final common pathway for a variety of etiologic agents. At this stage of our knowledge it seems useful to subdivide dialysis dementia into three categories [50] (Table 8-3): (1) an epidemic form that is related to contamination of the dialysate, often with aluminum; (2) a sporadic endemic form, in which aluminum intoxication is less likely to be a contributory factor; and (3) dementia associated with congenital or early childhood renal disease. The last condition has been reported in several children who were never dialyzed or exposed to aluminum compounds. These early childhood cases may represent developmental neurologic defects resulting from exposure of the growing brain to a uremic environment [6, 18, 126].

Table 8-3. Subgroups of dialysis dementia

Sporadic endemic
No clear relation to aluminum
Worldwide distribution
No known therapy
Epidemic
Geographic clusters
Often related to aluminum in dialysis water
Epidemic usually stops with treatment of water supply
Probably related to other trace elements in water (tin, manganese, cobalt, magnesium, iron)
Childhood
May be due to nonspecific effect of uremia on immature brain
No clear association with aluminum

The initial reports in 1972–1973 of dialysis dementia were soon followed by reports throughout the world [50]. These patients all had the endemic form and usually had been on chronic hemodialysis for more than 2 years before the onset of symptoms. Early symptoms consisted of a mixed dysarthria-apraxia of speech with slurring, stuttering, and hesitancy. Other findings included personality changes, psychoses, myoclonus, seizures, and finally dementia. Initial symptoms were usually intermittent and were often worse during dialysis. However, with time they generally became constant. In most cases, the disease progressed to death within 6 months [7]. Speech disturbances were found in 90 percent of patients, affective disorders culminating in dementia in 80 percent, motor disturbances, in 75 percent, and convulsions in 60 to 90 percent. In contrast to this fairly distinct clinical picture, brain histology is either normal or nonspecific.

Early in the disease, the EEG shows multifocal bursts of high-amplitude delta activity with spikes and sharp waves, intermixed with runs of more normal appearing background activity. These EEG abnormalities may precede overt clinical symptoms by 6 months. As the disease progresses, the normal background activity also deteriorates to slow frequencies [4, 10, 105]. The EEG changes, though pathognomic, are similar to those seen in other metabolic encephalopathies. Thus the diagnosis of DDS depends on the presence of the typical clinical picture described and can be confirmed by the characteristic EEG pattern [50].

Role of Aluminum in Dialysis Dementia

Aluminum intoxication was first implicated in this disorder by Mahurkar, Alfrey, and their associates in 1972 and 1973 [2, 94]. Aluminum content of brain gray matter was reported to be 11 times the normal value in patients with dialysis dementia (see Fig. 8-13). This value was approximately three times greater than that observed in patients who were on chronic hemodialysis, but without dialysis dementia. Aluminum content was also found to be increased in bone and other soft tissue in patients with dialysis dementia [2, 4].

Although significant absorption of oral aluminum can occur in patients with CRF, the weight of evidence is against oral aluminum as the major source of brain aluminum. The use of such compounds has been fairly universal, yet many cases of dialysis dementia have occurred in an epidemic form with geographic clusters. Epidemiologic studies have shown a strong association between aluminum in the water used to prepare dialysate and both the epidemic form of dialysis dementia and fracture from renal osteodystrophy [118, 121, 142]. In a survey by the European Dialysis and Transplant Association, 92 percent of patients with dialysis dementia had used untreated or softened water, as opposed to only 6 percent who had used deionized water [91]. The strongest evidence that aluminum may be directly responsible for some cases of dialysis dementia comes from an outbreak in Eindhoven, Holland. Two dialysis units used the same untreated municipal water supply and the same dialysate concentrate, and while one unit had six cases of dialysis dementia in a 9-month period, the other unit was unaffected. Investigation revealed that a corroding aluminum anode in the water heating system of the affected unit was adding aluminum to the dialysate of the affected unit [91].

Even low levels of aluminum in the dialysate will result in a net retention of aluminum in the body. Aluminum transferred across the dialyzer binds to a nondialyzable plasma constituent, resulting in higher levels in plasma than in the dialysate. It has been estimated that a dialysate aluminum concentration of only 70 μg/liter results in a minimum positive aluminum balance of 300 μg/day [53, 60]. Significant amounts of aluminum are also absorbed from the gastrointestinal tract after oral administration of aluminum hydroxide [75]. Since aluminum is normally excreted by the kidney, this can lead to significant aluminum retention in patients with renal insufficiency. It is also important to note that the solubility of aluminum is a function of pH; thus the environment in which the aluminum exists and the type of aluminum used by the patient will determine the toxicity of aluminum [64, 74, 91].

Most of the controversy surrounding the etiology of dialysis dementia has involved those cases that occur sporadically. As stated previously, dialysate aluminum levels are not always elevated, the use of aluminum-containing antacids is not different from that in unaffected patients, and brain aluminum levels in patients with dialysis dementia may overlap with those of unaffected patients. A large group of "sporadic cases" has been reported from Nashville [43]. In earlier studies the reported incidence of dialysis dementia in the area was 5 percent. This incidence persisted despite the use of deionized water with aluminum levels below 5 μg/liter in the dialysate. Bone disease was not clinically apparent in this group. Serum aluminum levels in the encephalopathic group were three to four times higher than in other dialyzed patients. These results suggest greater absorption or retention of aluminum in the group of encephalopathic patients. No other metals were measured in the Nashville study.

Despite these unresolved questions, most outbreaks of the epidemic form of dialysis dementia have been associated with high levels of aluminum in dialysate water. Reducing water aluminum levels to below 20 μg/liter appears to prevent the onset of the disease in patients who have just started dialysis. New cases may continue to appear in those patients who were previously exposed to the high aluminum dialysate. In patients with overt disease, eliminating the source of aluminum has resulted in improvement in only a few patients. Transplantation has generally not been helpful in patients with advanced disease. Diazepam or clonazepam is useful in controlling seizure activity associated with the disease, but is ineffective later and does not alter the final fatal outcome [105, 124].

Other Possible Causes of Dialysis Dementia

In addition to aluminum, many other conditions have been proposed as the cause of dialysis dementia. These include other trace elements, normal pressure hydrocephalus, and slow virus infection of the CNS [4, 33, 35, 57, 95, 99, 114, 128]. It has been suggested that some patients with dialysis dementia have altered cerebrospinal fluid dynamics, which is consistent with normal pressure hydrocephalus. Some patients with dialysis dementia were found to have normal cerebrospinal fluid dynamics but mild dilatation of the cerebral ventricles [78]. It is difficult to interpret these results, however, since it has been shown that many patients with end-stage renal disease without dialysis dementia also had ventricular dilatation with cerebral atrophy [114]. Furthermore, there is a poor correlation between ventricular dilatation, cerebral atrophy, and the presence of dementia.

Slow virus infection of the nervous system may also be a cause of dialysis dementia. The clinical manifestations of dialysis dementia resemble those of slow virus infections, such as kuru or Creutzfeldt-Jakob disease. In at least one instance, a slow virus (foamy virus) was isolated from the brains of patients who died with dialysis dementia [131].

Therapy of Dialysis Dementia

Deionization of the water used to prepare dialysate is now standard procedure in most dialysis units. However, deionization may be beneficial because it removes a number of agents in addition to aluminum. Other trace elements present in water may result in CNS toxicity. Such elements include cadmium, mercury, lead, manganese, copper, nickel, thallium, boron, and tin (see Fig. 8-14)[4, 143]. Manganese was increased in cortical white matter in eight encephalopathic patients in whom it was measured [35]. These patients also had elevated levels of aluminum in their gray matter. It is important to realize that tin was the first heavy metal found to be elevated in the brains of patients with dialysis dementia [4]. In patients with overt disease, eliminating the source of aluminum has only rarely resulted in improvement. However, improvement in symptoms has recently been reported in patients who were treated with deferoxamine [97]. However, some studies have suggested that deferoxamine without diazepam may lead to worsening of symptoms [68], and deferoxamine administration has been associated with neurotoxicity in other situations [109]. Thus, this mode of therapy may lead to problems of its own.

Treatment of sporadic cases of dialysis dementia, in which the etiology is not clear, is more difficult. As such, dialysis dementia must be differentiated from other metabolic encephalopathies, such as hypercalcemia, hypophosphatemia, hyperparathyroidism, acute heavy metal intoxications, and structural neurologic lesions such as subdural hematoma (Table 8-4). Because of the low incidence of dialysis dementia, the uncertain etiology of the disorder, and the poor correlation of plasma with tissue aluminum levels, a useful screening test has not been developed. Presently, a screening EEG and neurologic examination with emphasis on speech disturbances might be the only useful way for early detection of encephalopathy in affected patients.

At this time, the etiology of dialysis encephalopathy is uncertain. There are data, however, to indicate a possible role of aluminum in the epidemic form of dementia. There is no known satisfactory treatment for this condition, and all patients reported in the literature thus far have not survived. The patients usually die within 18 months of the time of diagnosis. The syndrome is not alleviated by increased frequency of dialysis, removal of aluminum from the dialysate, re-

Table 8-4. Differential diagnosis of nervous system complications of dialysis

Dialysis dementia
Metabolic encephalopathies
Hypercalcemia
Hypophosphatemia
Wernicke's encephalopathy
Hyperosmolarity
Hyponatremia
Encephalopathy
Drug intoxications
Trace element intoxications: manganese, mercury, lead, nickel, thallium, boron, vanadium, chromium, tin, cadmium
Hyperparathyroidism
Hypertensive encephalopathy
Structural lesions
Subdural hematoma
Normal pressure hydroencephalus
Stroke
Dialysis disequilibrium syndrome
Acute trace element intoxication (copper, nickel)
Subdural hematoma
Uremia
Nonketotic hyperosmolar coma
Cerebral embolus secondary to shunt declotting
Acute cerebrovascular accident
Cardiac arrhythmia
Depletion syndrome
Malfunction of fluid proportioning system
Excessive ultrafiltration
Hypoglycemia

nal transplantation, or treatment with deferoxamine.

Impairment of Intellectual Function

The impairment of intellectual function is another frequently recognized complication in patients who are on dialysis. There is no anatomic lesion that correlates with intellectual deterioration, and there are also no associated neurologic abnormalities. Although some studies suggest that the overall intellectual level in CRF patients does not differ significantly from normal, most studies have suggested that the IQ in dialysis patients is below that of the general population [50]. There also appears to be impairment of intellectual level as represented by the Wescher deterioration quotient; however, various learning tests did not indicate any gross learning abnormalities. Thus, based on psychological testing, it appears that CRF is frequently associated with organ-like losses of intellectual function, particularly information processing capacities. Based on the available evidence, the etiology of these abnormalities is not clear [9, 47, 110, 139].

PERIPHERAL NEUROPATHY

In general, there are two broad categories of peripheral neuropathy. These are described in terms of the pattern of involvement of the peripheral nervous system [15, 107, 133]. First, there are processes that result in a bilaterally symmetric disturbance of function and are called polyneuropathies. Polyneuropathy tends to be associated with exposure to toxic substances, metabolic disorders (uremia, diabetes, deficiency states), and some immune reactions that act diffusely on the peripheral nervous system. The second category comprises isolated lesions of peripheral nerves (mononeuropathy) or multiple isolated lesions (multiple mononeuropathy). In severe symmetric polyneuropathies, a generalized loss of peripheral nerve function may occur, and although this can be true of milder cases, the impairment is usually maximal distally in the limbs. A mixed motor and sensory polyneuropathy with a distal distribution results in weakness and wasting that is most frequently observed peripherally in the arms and legs. There are also distal sensory changes of "glove and stocking" distribution. In those neuropathies that involve "dying back" of the axons from the periphery, it appears that the neurons with the longest axons are first to be affected [15, 107].

Neuropathy associated with uremia is a distal, symmetric, mixed polyneuropathy. Motor and sensory nerves are usually both affected, and the lower extremities are more severely involved than are the upper [15, 22]. Clinically, uremic neuropathy cannot be distinguished from the neuropathies associated with many other metabolic disorders such as diabetes mellitus, chronic alcoholism, and various deficiency states. The occurrence of neuropathy bears no relationship to the type of underlying disease process, that is, glomerulonephritis or pyelonephritis. However, certain diseases that can lead to renal failure may simultaneously affect peripheral nerve function in a manner separate from the manifestations of uremia. Such diseases include amyloidosis, multiple myeloma, systemic lupus erythematosis, polyarteritis nodosa, diabetes mellitus, and hepatic failure [15].

The clinical manifestations of uremic neuropathy are characterized by several different stages. It appears that when the GFR is above 12 to 15 ml/minute, clinical evidence of neuropathy is generally absent [50, 137].

Peripheral Nerves

The restless legs syndrome is a common early manifestation of CFR [50]. Clinically, patients experience sensations in lower extremities such as crawling, prickling, and pruritus. The sensations are worse distally than proximally and are generally more prominent in the evening. The restless legs syndrome may initially be present in up to 40 percent of patients with CRF [15, 122]. Another symptom experienced by patients with early uremic neuropathy is the burning feet syndrome, which is present in less than 10 percent of patients with CRF [15, 106, 122]. Rather than "burning," the actual symptoms consist of swelling sensations, constriction, and tenderness of the distal lower extremities. Muscle irritability is also a frequent complaint in undialyzed patients with CRF. Any muscle can be affected, including those of the abdomen. The symptoms of muscle dysfunction may include increased muscle fatigability, weakness, atrophy, cramps, and increased irritability. Hemodialysis may also induce functional abnormalities in skeletal muscle, but their pathogenesis is not fully understood [15, 50, 136].

The physical signs of peripheral nerve dysfunction often begin with loss of deep tendon reflexes, particularly knee and ankle jerks, and impaired vibratory sensation. Loss of sensation in the lower leg is common and often takes the form of "stocking glove" anesthesia of the lower leg. The sensory losses include pain, light touch, vibration, and pressure [15, 106, 107, 122, 137].

Uremic Toxins and Nerve Conduction

Several "uremic toxins" have been identified based on correlation with depression of motor nerve conduction velocity (MNCV) in laboratory animals [59, 60, 67, 89, 124]. However, it must be taken into account that (1) depressed MNCV is cyclic, with abnormal low values one day and normal values the next, (2) there is a day-to-day variation in MNCV, which approaches 20 percent, and (3) the finding of depressed MNCV in laboratory animals associated with high plasma levels of potential "uremic neurotoxins" has generally not been confirmed in human subjects with renal failure [9, 51, 72, 86, 106].

Other compounds are said to be uremic toxins because their levels in blood correlated with depression of MNCV in patients with renal failure. These include urea, creatinine, PTH, myoinositol, transketolase, guanidine derivatives, and middle molecules [51]. Although it is possible to relate impairment in MNCV with levels in blood of various substances, the best correlation has been obtained between reduction in GFR and reduced MNCV [106, 107].

Parathyroid Hormone as a Possible Peripheral Nerve Toxin

Among the potential uremic neurotoxins, a substance that has probably received a disproportionate amount of attention is PTH [9, 98]. It has been suggested that PTH was a uremic neurotoxin, based on patients and dogs with CRF [17, 98, 130]. One way to evaluate the effects of PTH on nerve function is to evaluate nerve function in patients who have primary or secondary hyperparathyroidism without renal failure. In a study of 16 patients with primary hyperparathyroidism, MNCV was reported to be normal, and following parathyroidectomy there was no change in MNCV [114]. In another study of six patients with secondary hyperparathyroidism, MNCV was also found to be normal and did not appear to be affected by medical treatment of secondary hyperparathyroidism [96]. In a study of 12 patients with ARF, PTH levels were found to be more than three times the normal value [38], yet MNCV was normal in all patients despite elevated PTH levels [38, 60].

In a study of 35 uremic patients who were on chronic hemodialysis, the MNCV was 36 meters/second. Following parathyroidectomy by intervals of 3, 6, 9, and 12 months, no change in MNCV was observed [114]. A similar pattern was suggested by the studies of Teschan and co-workers [137]. They followed 72 patients for periods of up to 12 years. These patients had normal predialysis MNCVs, which were unaffected by dialysis. Thus, in patients with either acute or chronic renal failure, nerve conduction velocities remained normal, despite high plasma levels of PTH. There was no change in MNCV as a result of either recovery of renal function, chronic hemodialysis, or parathyroidectomy [38, 60, 96, 114, 137].

It was previously reported that in dogs with ARF, there was a decrement in the MNCV [61]. When the dogs were subjected to parathyroidectomy before the onset of uremia, the decline in MNCV was prevented. The study also showed that when normal dogs were infused with PTH, MNCV also decreased. However, other studies showed conflicting results [92, 116]. Thus, the preponderance of evidence does not suggest a role for PTH in the pathophysiology of uremia neuropathy.

Effects of Uremia on Autonomic and Cranial Nerve Dysfunction

Autonomic dysfunction commonly occurs in patients who are on dialysis. It is associated with postural hypotension, intestinal disorder, impaired sweating, and abnormal Valsalva maneuver [15, 34, 82]. The cranial nerves are also often affected in uremic patients. Transient nystagmus, miosis, heterophoria, sixth nerve palsy, vertigo, and facial asymmetry have been observed [87]. The most commonly affected cranial nerve is the eighth, with involvement of both auditory and vestibular divisions. Varying degrees of hearing loss, with occasional complete deafness, is also well described [87]. In such cases, it is important to distinguish deafness due to uremia from that associated with hereditary nephropathies and ototoxic drugs. Deafness associated with uremia may be reversible with dialysis or renal transplantation [51].

Effects of Therapy for Renal Failure on Uremic Neuropathy

Dialysis Therapy

There is a general consensus that in most patients with end-stage renal disease and neuropathy, the neuropathy will either stabilize or improve with regular dialysis therapy [15]. In patients with mild neuropathy, dialysis may result in apparent recovery. When patients have severe neuropathy prior to starting dialysis, recovery may be only partial, even after several years of dialysis. In some patients, there will be an initial worsening of MNCV over a period of several months, followed by gradual improvement. The most important parameter that determines the effects of dialysis on nerve function seems to be the condition of the patient prior to the initiation of dialysis. When dialysis is started with GFR in excess of 10 ml/minute, clinical neuropathy and associated disability are rare [137], since dialysis usually prevents further progression of neuropathy. It should be noted that in uremic diabetic subjects, it is difficult to distinguish between uremic and diabetic neuropathy. Following initiation of dialytic therapy, many diabetic patients will have a worsening of their neuropathy rather than an improvement, whereas successful renal transplantation seems to improve the neuropathy [51].

Renal Transplantation

The beneficial effects of successful renal transplantation on uremic neuropathy are more consistent than are those of dialysis. Transplanted patients usually show progressive improvement in peripheral nerve function over a period of 6 months to a year. The clinical remission appears to have a biphasic course, with an early phase of rapid (1–3 months) remission followed by a slow gradual improvement [29]. In general, sensory symptoms and signs disappear almost completely within days to weeks. Mild and moderate motor disturbances (weakness and wasting) improve rapidly during the first 3 to 6 months and more slowly after the first year. In some patients deep reflexes returned only late after transplantation. The same pattern was demonstrable in the most severely affected patients, who also showed considerable and rapid improvement of most peripheral neurologic disturbances. However, in these patients the remission was only partial. The limited data that are available suggest that impotence, autonomic neuropathy, and nerve deafness secondary to uremia are largely reversible within 2 years of renal transplantation [29, 34, 82, 86].

The reasons for the improvement in uremic neuropathy after transplantation are not clear. Electrophysiologic studies show normalization of MNCV. There is also a shortening of both proximal and distal latencies [16], segmental remyelination of distal nerve segments, and nerve axon regeneration after renal transplantation [29]. Nielsen [106–108] has formulated certain prognostic criteria to apply to patients who receive a successful renal transplant: Patients with mild or moderate neuropathy generally recover completely within 6 to 12 months, and patients with neuropathy also improve considerably, but isolated sensory-motor disturbances that have shown no evidence of improvement during the first 6 months tend to become permanent sequelae.

REFERENCES

1. Alfrey, A. C., LeGendre, G. R., and Kaehney, W. D. The dialysis encephalopathy syndrome: Possible aluminum intoxication. *N. Engl. J. Med.* 294:184, 1976.
2. Alfrey, A. C., Mishell, J. M., Burks, J., et al. Syndrome of dyspraxia and multifocal seizures associated with chronic hemodialysis. *Trans. Am. Soc. Artif. Intern. Organs* 18:257, 1972.
3. Ali, F., Tayeb, O., and Attallah, A. Plasma and brain cathecholamines in experimental uremia: Acute and chronic studies. *Life Sci.* 37:1757, 1985.
4. Andreoli, S. P., Bergstein, J. M., Sherrard, D. J., et al. Aluminum intoxication from aluminum-containing phosphate binders in children with azotemia not undergoing dialysis. *N. Engl. J. Med.* 310:1079, 1984.
5. Altmann, P., Al-Salihi, F., Butter, K., et al. Serum aluminum levels and erythrocyte dihydropteridine reductase activity in patients on hemodialysis. *N. Engl. J. Med.* 317:80, 1987.
6. Altmann, P., Hamon, C., Blair, J., et al. Disturbance of cerebral function by aluminum in haemodialysis patients without overt aluminum toxicity. *Lancet* 2:7, 1989.
7. Arieff, A. I. Effects of Water, Electrolyte and Acid Base Disorders on the Central Nervous System. In A. I. Arieff and R. A. DeFronzo (eds.), *Fluid, Electrolyte and Acid Base Disorders.* New York: Churchill Livingstone, 1985. Pp. 969–1040.
8. Arieff, A. I. Acid-Base Balance in Specialized Tissues: Central Nervous System. In D. W. Seldin and G. Giebish (eds.), *The Regulation of Acid-Base Balance.* New York: Raven, 1989. Pp. 107–122.
9. Arieff, A. I., and Armstrong, D. K. Parathyroid hormone and uremic neurotoxicity: An unproven association. *Contrib. Nephrol.* 20:56, 1980.
10. Arieff, A. I., Cooper, J. D., Armstrong, D., et al. Dementia, renal failure and brain aluminum. *Ann. Intern. Med.* 90:741, 1979.
11. Arieff, A. I., Guisado, R., Massry, S. G., et al. Central nervous system pH in uremia and the effects of hemodialysis. *J. Clin. Invest.* 58:306, 1977.
12. Arieff, A. I., Lazarowitz, V. C., and Guisado, R. Experimental dialysis disequilibrium syndrome: Prevention with glycerol. *Kidney Int.* 14:270, 1978.
13. Arieff, A. I., and Massry, S. G. Calcium metabolism of brain in acute renal failure: Effects of uremia, hemodialysis and parathyroid hormone. *J. Clin. Invest.* 53:387, 1974.
14. Arieff, A. I., Massry, S. G., Barrientos, A., et al. Brain water and electrolyte metabolism in uremia: Effects of slow and rapid hemodialysis. *Kidney Int.* 4:177, 1973.
15. Asbury, A. K. Uremic Neuropathy. In P. J. Dyck, P. K. Thomas, and E. H. Lambert (eds.), *Peripheral Neuropathy.* Philadelphia: Saunders, 1975. Vol. 2, pp. 982–992.
16. Aurbach, G. D. Neuromuscular disease in primary hyperparathyroidism. *Ann. Intern. Med.* 80:182, 1974.
17. Avram, M. M., Feingold, D. A., and Huatuco, A. H. Search for the uremic toxin: Decreased motor-nerve conduction velocity and elevated parathyroid hormone in uremia. *N. Engl. J. Med.* 298:1000, 1978.
18. Baluarate, H. R., Gruskin, A. B., Hlner, L. B., et al. Encephalopathy in children with chronic renal failure. *Clin. Dial. Transplant Forum* 7:95, 1977.
19. Berkseth, R. O., and Shapiro, F. L. An Epidemic of Dialysis Encephalopathy and Exposure to High Aluminum Dialysate. In G. E. Schreiner and J. F. Winchester (eds.), *Controversies in*

Nephrology. Washington, D.C.: Georgetown University Press, 1980. Pp. 42–51.
20. Berlyne, G. M., Ari, J. B., Knopf, E., et al. Aluminum toxicity in rats. *Lancet* 1:564, 1972.
21. Berti, F., and Shore, P. A. A kinetic analysis of drugs that inhibit the adrenergic neuronal membrane amine pump. *Biochem. Pharmacol.* 16:2091, 1967.
22. Blagg, C. R., Kemple, F., and Taverner, D. Nerve conduction velocity in relationship to the severity of renal disease. *Nephron* 5:290, 1968.
23. Blaustein, M. P. The relationship between sodium and calcium fluxes across cell membranes. *Rev. Physiol. Biochem. Pharmacol.* 70:33, 1974.
24. Bogdanski, T. P., Blaszkowski, T. P., and Tissari, A. H. Mechanism of storage and transport of biogenic amines: III. Effects of sodium and potassium on kinetics of 5-hydroxytryptamine and norepinephrine transport by rabbit synaptosomes. *Biochim. Biophys. Acta* 219:189, 1970.
25. Bogdanski, T. P., Blaszkowski, T. P., and Tissari, A. H. Mechanisms of biogenic amine transport and storage: IV. Relationship between K^+ and Na^+ requirement for transport and storage of 5-hydroxy tryptamine and norepinephrine in synaptosomes. *Biochim. Biophys. Acta* 211:521, 1970.
26. Bogdanski, D. F., and Brodie, B. B. Role of sodium and potassium ions in storage of norepinephrine by synaptic nerve endings. *Life Sci.* 5:1563, 1966.
27. Bogdanski, D. F., and Brodie, B. B. The effects of inorganic ions on the storage and uptake of ^3H norepinephrine by rat heart slices. *J. Pharm. Exp. Ther.* 165:181, 1969.
28. Bogdanski, D. F., Tissari, A. H., and Brodie, B. B. Role of sodium, potassium, ouabain and reserpine in uptake, storage and metabolism of biogenic amines in synaptosomes. *Life Sci.* 7:419, 1968.
29. Bolton, C. F., Baltzan, M. A., and Baltzan, R. B. Effects of renal transplantation on uremic neuropathy. *N. Engl. J. Med.* 284:1170, 1971.
30. Booth, R. F., and Clark, J. B. A rapid method for the preparation of relatively pure metabolically competent synaptosomes from rat brain. *Biochem. J.* 176:365, 1978.
31. Bowling, P. S., and Bourn, J. R. Discriminant analysis of electroencephalograms recorded from renal patients. *I.E.E.E. Trans. Biomed. Engin.* 25:12, 1978.
32. Boyer, J., Gill, G. N., and Epstein, F. H. Hyperglycemia and hyperosmolality complicating peritoneal dialysis. *Ann. Intern. Med.* 67:568, 1967.
33. Cajal, S. R. La fine structure des cewtres nervux. *Proc. R. Soc. Lond.* 55:444, 1984.
34. Carafoli, E., and Longoni, S. The Plasma Membrane in the Control of the Signaling Function of Calcium. In L. J. Mandel and D. C. Easton (eds.), *Cell Calcium and the Control of Membrane Transport.* New York: Rockefeller University Press, 1987. Vol. 42, p. 21.
35. Cartier, F., Allain, P., Gary, J., et al. Progressive myoclonic encephalopathy in dialysis patients. *Nouv. Presse Med.* 7:97, 1978.
36. Cogan, M., Covey, C., Arieff, A. I., et al. Central nervous system manifestations of hyperparathyroidism. *Am. J. Med.* 65:963, 1978.
37. Colburn, R. W., Goodwin, K. F., Murphy, D. L., et al. Quantitative studies of norepinephrine uptake by synaptosomes. *Biochem. Pharmacol.* 17:957, 1968.
38. Cooper, J. D., Lazarowitz, V. C., and Arieff, A. I. Neurodiagnostic abnormalities in patients with acute renal failure: Evidence for neurotoxicity of parathyroid hormone. *J. Clin. Invest.* 61:1448, 1978.
39. Coyle, J. T., and Snyder, S. H. Catecholamine uptake by synaptosomes in homogenates of rat brain: Stereospecificity in different areas. *J. Pharmacol. Exp. Ther.* 170:221, 1969.
40. Crapper, D. R., Dalton, A. J., Karlik, S. J., et al. Role of Aluminum in Alzheimer's Disease. In P. E. Alexander (ed.), *Electrolyte and Neuropsychiatric Disorders.* New York: S.P. Medical & Scientific Books, 1981. Pp. 89–111.
41. Crapper, D. R., Krishnan, S. S., and Quittkat, S. Aluminum, neurofibrillary degeneration and Alzheimer's disease. *Brain* 99:67, 1976.
42. Deferrari, G., Garibotto, G., Robaudo, C., et al. Brain metabolism of amino acids and ammonia in patients with chronic renal insufficiency. *Kidney Int.* 20:505, 1981.
43. Dewberry, F. L., McKinney, T. D., and Stone, W. J. The dialysis dementia syndrome: Report of fourteen cases and review of the literature. *A.S.A.I.O. J.* 3:102, 1980.
44. Dunea, G., Mahurkar, S. D., Mamdami, B., et al. Role of aluminum in dialysis dementia. *Ann. Intern. Med.* 88:502, 1978.
45. Eccles, J. C. The Physiology of synaptosomes. Berlin: Springer Verlag, 1964.
46. Editorial: Wernicke's preventable encephalopathy. *Lancet* 1:1122, 1979.
47. English, A., Savage, R. D., Britton, P. G., et al. Intellectual impairment in chronic renal failure. *Br. Med. J.* 1:888, 1978.
48. Flendrig, J. A., Kruis, H., and Das, H. A. Aluminum and dialysis dementia. *Lancet* 1:1235, 1976.
49. Fraser, C. L., and Arieff, A. I. Hepatic encephalopathy. *N. Engl. J. Med.* 313:865, 1985.
50. Fraser, C. L., and Arieff, A. I. Nervous system complications in uremia. *Ann. Intern. Med.* 109:143, 1988.
51. Fraser, C. L., and Arieff, A. I. Nervous System Manifestations of Renal Failure. In R. W.

Schrier and C. W. Gottschalk, *Diseases of the Kidney* (4th ed.). Boston: Little, Brown, 1988. Pp. 3063–3092.
52. Fraser, C. L., and Sarnacki, P. Parathyroid hormone mediates changes in calcium transport in uremic rat brain synaptosomes. *Am. J. Physiol.* 254:F837, 1988.
53. Fraser, C. L., Sarnacki, P., and Arieff, A. I. Abnormal sodium transport in synaptosomes from brain of uremic rats. *J. Clin. Invest.* 75:2014, 1985.
54. Fraser, C. L., Sarnacki, P., and Arieff, A. I. Calcium transport abnormality in uremic rat brain synaptosomes. *J. Clin. Invest.* 76:1789, 1985.
55. Fraser, C. L., Sarnacki, P., and Budayr, A. Evidence that parathyroid hormone-mediated calcium transport in rat brain synaptosomes is independent of cyclic adenosine monophosphate. *J. Clin. Invest.* 81:982, 1988.
56. Gatewood, J. W., Organ, C. H., and Mead, B. T. Mental changes associated with hyperparathyroidism. *Am. J. Psychiatry* 123:129, 1975.
57. Gibbs, C. J., and Gajdusek, D. C. Isolation and characterization of the subacute spongiform encephalopathies in man: Kuru and Creutzfeldt-Jacob disease. *J. Clin. Pathol.* 25:84, 1970.
58. Gillis, C. N., and Paton, D. M. Cation dependence of sympathetic transmitter retention by slices of rat ventricle. *Br. J. Pharmacol. Chemother.* 39:309, 1967.
59. Giovannetti, S., Balestri, P. L., and Barsotti, G. Methylguanidine in uremia. *Arch. Intern. Med.* 131:709, 1973.
60. Giulio, S. D., Chkoff, N., Lhoste, F., et al. Parathormone as a nerve poison in uremia. *N. Engl. J. Med.* 299:1134, 1978.
61. Goldstein, D. A., Chui, L. A., and Massry, S. G. Effect of parathyroid hormone and uremia on peripheral nerve calcium and motor nerve conduction velocity. *J. Clin. Invest.* 62:88, 1978.
62. Goldstein, D. A., Feinstein, E. I., Chiu, L. A., et al. The relationship between the abnormalities in EEG and blood levels of parathyroid hormone in dialysis patients. *J. Clin. Endocrinol. Metab.* 51:130, 1980.
63. Goldstein, D. A., and Massry, S. G. Effect of parathyroid hormone and its withdrawal on brain calcium and electroencephalogram. *Miner. Electrolyte Metab.* 1:84, 1978.
64. Graf, H., Stummvoll, H. K., Meisinger, V., et al. Aluminum removal by hemodialysis. *Kidney Int.* 19:587, 1981.
65. Grushkin, C. M., Korsch, B., and Fine, R. N. Hemodialysis in small children. *J.A.M.A.* 221:869, 1972.
66. Guisado, R., Arieff, A. I., and Massry, S. G. Changes in the electroencephalogram in acute uremia: Effects of parathyroid hormone and brain electrolytes. *J. Clin. Invest.* 55:738, 1975.
67. Gutman, R. A., Blumenkrantz, M. J., Chan, Y. K., et al. Controlled comparison of hemodialysis and peritoneal dialysis: Veterans Administration multicenter study. *Kidney Int.* 26:459, 1984.
68. Hagstam, K. E. EEG frequency content related to chemical blood parameters in chronic uremia. *Scand. J. Urol. Nephrol.* 7(Suppl.):1, 1971.
69. Heath, H., Hodgson, S. F., and Kennedy, M. A. Primary hyperparathyroidism. *N. Engl. J. Med.* 303:189, 1980.
70. Hennemann, H., Hevendehl, G., Horler, E., et al. Toxic sympathicopathy in uraemia. *Proc. Eur. Dialysis Transplant Assoc.* 10:166, 1973.
71. Hodgkin, A. L., and Keynes, R. D. Movements of labelled calcium in squid giant axons. *J. Physiol. (Lond.)* 138:253, 1957.
72. Iqbal, Z., and Ochs, S. Fast azoplasmic transport of a calcium-binding protein in mammalian nerve. *J. Neurochem.* 31:409, 1978.
73. Iversen, L. L., and Kravitz, E. A. Sodium dependence of transmitter uptake at adrenergic nerve terminals. *Mol. Pharmacol.* 2:360, 1966.
74. Kaehney, W. D., Alfrey, A. C., Holman, R. E., et al. Aluminum transfer during hemodialysis. *Kidney Int.* 12:361, 1977.
75. Kaehny, W. D., Hegg, A. P., and Alfrey, A. C. Gastrointestinal absorption of aluminum from aluminum-containing antacids. *N. Engl. J. Med.* 296:1389, 1977.
76. Katz, B., and Miledi, R. The timing of calcium action during neuromuscular transmission. *J. Physiol. (Lond.)* 189:535, 1967.
77. Katz, B., and Miledi, R. A study of synaptic transmission in the absence of nerve impulses. *J. Physiol. (Lond.)* 192:407, 1969.
78. Kennedy, A. C., Linton, A. L., and Eaton, J. C. Urea levels in cerebrospinal fluid after hemodialysis. *Lancet* 1:410, 1962.
79. Kennedy, A. C., Linton, A. L., Luke, R. G., et al. Electroencephalographic changes during hemodialysis. *Lancet* 1:408, 1963.
80. Kennedy, A. C., Linton, A. L., Renfrew, S., et al. The pathogenesis and prevention of cerebral dysfunction during dialysis. *Lancet* 1:790, 1964.
81. Kennedy, A. C., Luke, R. G., and Linton, A. L. Dialysis Disequilibrium Syndrome. In S. Shaldon and G. C. Cook (eds.), *Acute Renal Failure.* Oxford: Blackwell, 1964. Pp. 66–79.
82. Kersh, E. S., Kronfield, S. J., Unger, A., et al. Autonomic insufficiency in uremia as a cause of hemodialysis induced hypotension. *N. Engl. J. Med.* 290:650, 1974.
83. Kiley, J. E., Woodruff, M. W., and Pratt, K. L. Evaluation of encephalopathy by EEG frequency analysis in chronic dialysis patients. *Clin. Nephrol.* 5:245, 1976.
84. Kliger, A. S. Complications of Dialysis: Hemodi-

alysis, Peritoneal Dialysis, CAPD. In A. I. Arieff and R. A. DeFronzo (eds.), *Fluid, Electrolyte and Acid-Base Disorders.* New York: Churchill Livingstone, 1985. Pp. 777–825.

85. Kometiani, Z. P., Tsakadze, L. G., and Jariashvilli, R. Functional significance of the effects of neurotransmitters on the Na-K ATPase system. *J. Neurochem.* 42:1246, 1984.
86. Kopeloff, L. M., Barrera, S. E., and Kopeloff, N. Recurrent convulsive seizures in animals produced by immunologic and chemical means. *Am. J. Psychiatry* 98:881, 1942.
87. Kusakari, J., Kobayashi, T., Rokugmo, M., et al. The inner ear dysfunction in hemodialysis patients. *Tohoku J. Exp. Med.* 135:359, 1981.
88. Locke, S. J., Merrill, J. P., and Tyler, H. R. Neurological complications of acute uremia. *Arch. Intern. Med.* 108:75, 1961.
89. Lonergan, E. T., Semar, M., Sterzel, R. B., et al. Erythrocyte transketolase activity in dialyzed patients: A reversible metabolic lesion in uremia. *N. Engl. J. Med.* 284:1399, 1971.
90. Nadias, N. E., and Kraut, J. A. Uremic Acidosis. In D. W. Seldin and G. Giebish (eds.), *The Regulation of Acid-Base Balance.* New York: Raven, 1989. Pp. 285–318.
91. Mahoney, C. A., and Arieff, A. I. Uremic encephalopathies: Clinical, biochemical and experimental features. *Am. J. Kidney Dis.* 2:324, 1982.
92. Mahoney, C. A., and Arieff, A. I. Central and peripheral nervous system effects of chronic renal failure. *Kidney Int.* 24:170, 1983.
93. Mahoney, C. A., Sarnacki, P., and Arieff, A. I. Uremic encephalopathy: Role of brain energy metabolism. *Am. J. Physiol. (Renal Fluid Electrolyte Physiol.)* 247:F527, 1984.
94. Mahurkar, S. D., Dhar, S. K., Salta, R., et al. Dialysis dementia. *Lancet* 1:1412, 1973.
95. Makowski, L., Casper, D. L. D., Phillips, N. C., et al. Gap junction structures: II. Analysis of the x-ray diffraction data. *J. Cell Biol.* 74:629, 1977.
96. Mallette, L. E., Patten, B. M., and Engle, W. K. Neuromuscular disease in secondary hyperparathyroidism. *Ann. Intern. Med.* 82:474, 1975.
97. Malluche, H. H., Smith, A. J., Abreo, I., et al. The use of deferoxamine in the management of aluminum accumulation in bone in patients with renal failure. *N. Engl. J. Med.* 311:140, 1984.
98. Massry, S. G. Current status of the role of parathyroid hormone in uremic toxicity. *Contrib. Nephrol.* 49:1, 1985.
99. Mathew, R. J., Rabin, P., Stone, W. J., et al. Regional cerebral blood flow in dialysis encephalopathy and primary degenerative dementia. *Kidney Int.* 28:64, 1985.
100. Mayor, G. H., and Burnatowska-Hledin, M. A. Impaired renal function and aluminum metabolism. *Fed. Proc.* 42:2979, 1983.
101. Mayor, G. H., Sprague, S. M., Hourani, M. R., et al. Parathyroid hormone mediated aluminum deposition and egress in the rat. *Kidney Int.* 17:40, 1980.
102. McDermott, J. R., Smith, A. I., Ward, M. K., et al. Brain aluminum concentration in dialysis encephalopathy. *Lancet* 1:901, 1978.
103. McDermott, J. R., Smith, A. I., and Wisniewski, H. M. Brain aluminum in aging and Alzheimer disease. *Neurology* 29:809, 1979.
104. Minkoff, L., Gertner, G., Darawb, M., et al. Inhibition of brain sodium-potassium ATPase in uremic rats. *J. Lab. Clin. Med.* 80:71, 1972.
105. Nadel, A. M., and Wilson, W. P. Dialysis encephalopathy: A possible seizure disorder. *Neurology* 26:1130, 1976.
106. Nielsen, V. K. The peripheral nerve function in chronic renal failure: VI. The relationship between sensory and motor nerve conduction and kidney function, azotemia, age, sex and clinical neuropathy. *Acta Med. Scand.* 194:455, 1973.
107. Nielsen, V. K. The peripheral nerve function in chronic renal failure: VII. Longitudinal course during terminal renal failure and regular hemodialysis. *Acta Med. Scand.* 195:155, 1974.
108. Nielsen, V. K. The peripheral nerve function in chronic renal failure: A survey. *Acta Med. Scand. [Suppl.]* 573:7, 1974.
109. Ochs, S., Worth, R., and Chan, S. Y. Calcium requirement for axoplasmic transport in mammalian nerve. *Nature (Lond.)* 270:748, 1977.
110. Osberg, J. W., Meares, G. J., McKee, D. C., et al. Intellectual functioning in renal failure and chronic dialysis. *J. Chronic Dis.* 35:445, 1982.
111. Pagel, M. D., Ahmad, S., Vizzo, J. E., et al. Acetate and bicarbonate fluctuations and acetate intolerance during dialysis. *Kidney Int.* 21:513, 1982.
112. Papadakis, M. A., and Arieff, A. I. Unpredictability of clinical evaluation of renal function in cirrhosis: A prospective study. *Am. J. Med.* 82:945, 1987.
113. Paton, D. M. Cations and metabolic requirements for retention of metarminol by rat uterine horns. *Br. J. Pharmacol. Chemother.* 33:277, 1968.
114. Patten, B. M., Bilezikian, J. P., Mallette, L. E., et al. Neuromuscular disease in primary hyperparathyroidism. *Ann. Intern. Med.* 80:182, 1974.
115. Pauli, H. G., Vorburger, C., and Reubi, F. Chronic derangements of cerebrospinal fluid acid-base components in man. *J. Appl. Physiol.* 17:993, 1962.
116. Perry, T. L., Yong, V. W., Kish, S. J., et al. Neurochemical abnormalities in brains of renal fail-

ure patients treated by repeated hemodialysis. *J. Neurochem.* 45:1043, 1985.
117. Peterson, P. Psychiatric disorders in primary hyperparathyroidism. *J. Clin. Endocrinol.* 28:1491, 1968.
118. Pierides, A. M., Edwards, W. G., Cullum, U. X., et al. Hemodialysis encephalopathy with osteomalacic fractures and muscle weakness. *Kidney Int.* 18:115, 1980.
119. Pierides, A. M., Ward, M. K. and Kerr, D. N. S. Haemodialysis encephalopathy: Possible role of phosphate depletion. *Lancet* 1:1234, 1976.
120. Porte, F. K., Johnson, W. J., and Klass, D. W. Prevention of dialysis disequilibrium syndrome by use of high sodium concentration in the dialysate. *Kidney Int.* 3:327, 1973.
121. Prior, J. C., Cameron, E. C., Knickerbocker, W. J., et al. Dialysis encephalopathy and osteomalacic bone disease. *Am. J. Med.* 72:33, 1982.
122. Raskin, N. H., and Fishman, R. A. Neurologic disorders in renal failure. *N. Engl. J. Med.* 294:143, 1976.
123. Rasmussen, H. The calcium messenger system. *N. Engl. J. Med.* 314:1094, 1986.
124. Reznek, R. H., Salway, J. G., and Thomas, P. K. Plasma myoinositol concentrations in uraemic neuropathy. *Lancet* 1:675, 1977.
125. Rodrigo, F., Shideman, J., McHugh, R., et al. Osmolality changes during hemodialysis. *Ann. Intern. Med.* 86:554, 1977.
126. Rotundo, A., Nevins, T. E., Lipton, M., et al. Progressive encephalopathy in children with chronic renal insufficiency in infancy. *Kidney Int.* 21:486, 1982.
127. Rouby, J. J., Rottenbourg, J., and Durande, J. P. Hemodynamic changes induced by regular hemodialysis and sequential ultrafiltration hemodialysis: A comparative study. *Kidney Int.* 17:801, 1980.
128. Schaumberg, H. H., and Spencer, P. S. Toxic neuropathies. Neurology 29:429, 1979.
129. Scheinberg, D. Effects of uremia on cerebral blood flow and metabolism. *Neurology* 4:101, 1954.
130. Slatopolsky, E., Martin, K., and Hruska, K. Parathyroid hormone metabolism and its potential as a uremic toxin. *Am. J. Physiol.* 239:F1, 1980.
131. Smith, J. S. The investigation of dementia: Results in 200 consecutive admissions. *Lancet* 1:824, 1981.
132. Smogorzewski, M., Campese, V., and Massry, S. G. Abnormal norepinephrine uptake and release in brain synaptosomes of rats with chronic renal failure. *Kidney Int.* 36:458, 1989.
133. Spencer, P. S., Sabri, M., Schaumberg, H. H., et al. Does a defect of energy metabolism in the nerve fiber underlie axonal degeneration in polyneuropathies? *Ann. Neurol.* 5:501, 1979.
134. Teschan, P. E., and Arieff, A. I. Uremic and dialysis encephalopathies. In D. W. McCandless (ed.), *Cerebral Energy Metabolism and Metabolic Encephalopathy.* New York: Plenum, 1985. Pp. 263–286.
135. Teschan, P. E., Bourne, J. R., Reed, R. B., et al. Electrophysiological and neurobehavioral responses to therapy: The National Cooperative Dialysis Study. *Kidney Int.* 23:S58, 1983.
136. Teschan, P. E., and Ginn, H. E. The Nervous System. In S. G. Massry and A. L. Sellers (eds.), *Clinical Aspects of Uremia and Dialysis.* Springfield, IL: Thomas, 1976. Pp. 3–33.
137. Teschan, P. E., Ginn, H. E., Bourne, J. R., et al. Quantitative indices of clinical uremia. *Kidney Int.* 15:676, 1979.
138. Tissari, A. H., Schonhoffer, P. S., Bogdanski, D. F., et al. Mechanism of biogenic transport: II. Relationship between sodium and the mechanism of ouabain blockade of the accumulation of serotonin and norepinephrine by synaptosomes. *Mol. Pharmacol.* 5:593, 1969.
139. Treischmann, R. B., and Sand, P. L. WAIS and MMPI correlates of increasing renal failure in adult and medical patients. *Psychol. Rep.* 29:1251, 1971.
140. Van den Noort, S., Eckel, R. E., Brine, K., et al. Brain metabolism in uremic and adenosine-infused rats. *J. Clin. Invest.* 47:2133, 1968.
141. Verkman, A. S., and Fraser, C. L. Water and non-electrolyte permeability in brain synaptosomes isolated from normal and uremic rats. *Am. J. Physiol.* 250:R306, 1986.
142. Ward, M. K., Feest, T. G., Ellis, H. A., et al. Osteomalacic dialysis osteodystrophy: Evidence for a water-borne aetiological agent probably aluminum. *Lancet* 1:841, 1978.
143. Weiss, B. The behavioral toxicology of metals. *Fed. Proc.* 37:22, 1978.
144. Whittaker, V. P. The Synaptosome. In A. Lajtha (ed.), *Handbook of Neurochemistry.* New York: Plenum, 1969. Vol. 11, pp. 327–364.
145. Whittaker, V. P., Michaelson, I. A., Jeanette, R., et al. The separation of synaptic vesicles from nerve-endings particles (synaptosomes). *Biochem. J.* 90:293, 1964.

9 Hepatic Encephalopathy

Alan H. Lockwood

Although there are reports in older medical writings that may describe hepatic encephalopathy, the first clear descriptions of the cerebral disorder accompanying what is now called fulminant hepatic failure are found in Frerich's treatise on liver diseases [12]:

> In most cases we can distinguish two stages, that of excitement and depression, the former of which is characterized by delirium and convulsions, and the latter of which is characterized by progressively increasing coma. . . . In most cases, the nervous system derangements appeared simultaneously with jaundice; and they usually attracted the attention of the observer sooner than the slight jaundiced tint of conjuctivae. . . . Toward the termination of the disease the delirium and convulsions gave place to stupor, which in a short time has merged into the deepest coma, from which no shaking could rouse the patient.

This was an invariably fatal syndrome, and Frerichs did not describe recoveries, or what we now recognize as portal-systemic encephalopathy that attends chronic liver disease. The beginning of the contemporary era of hepatic encephalopathy thought probably dates to the review by Adams and Foley [1] in which they described additional clinical features, the basic neuropathology of hepatic encephalopathy, and the classic electroencephalographic features and speculated that the etiology was due to a disorder of metabolism, more specifically ammonia metabolism.

In spite of the many advances in our understanding of the pathophysiology and improvements in treatments of the disorder, this is still a common and underdiagnosed condition. Liver disease is the fifth ranked cause of lost years of life in Americans. In patients who die of liver disease, encephalopathy becomes a progressively more important cause of morbidity and mortality as the terminal stages of acute or chronic liver failure are reached.

Recent evidence, summarized in this chapter, suggests that there are aspects of the pathophysiology of hepatic encephalopathy that may make the disorder self-perpetuating. This phenomenon may be the result of time-dependent increases in the sensitivity of the brain to toxins that produce hepatic encephalopathy, especially ammonia, and direct effects of toxins on the brain that lead to the impairment of the body to metabolize toxins via extrahepatic pathways, particularly ammonia detoxification by skeletal muscle. For these reasons, it is essential that hepatic encephalopathy be diagnosed promptly and accurately and that aggressive medical therapy be instituted to terminate the encephalopathic state.

CLINICAL MANIFESTATIONS

The hepatic encephalopathy literature is made more confusing than it needs to be by problems with nomenclature. In this chapter, *hepatic encephalopathy* will be used synonymously with the term *portal-systemic encephalopathy.* This is a disorder of cerebral function with the potential for complete reversibility that is due to the failure of the liver to eliminate one or more toxins that affect brain function without producing permanent deficits of brain injury, other than the production of Alzheimer II astrocytes. *Chronic hepatic encephalopathy* or *chronic portal-systemic encephalopathy* is a term that should be reserved for the persistent form of the disorder and should not be used to include patients with hepatocerebral degeneration (discussed later). Since this latter disorder is, by definition, associated with additional pathologic features and the emergence of irreversible deficits, it is important to distinguish between these two syndromes. Unfortunately, this may be very difficult on clinical grounds alone, since there may be an overlap between the signs and symptoms associated with chronic encephalopathy and hepatocerebral degeneration. *Fulminant hepatic failure* is a less common syndrome characterized by massive necrosis of hepatocytes in which signs of encephalopathy are evident within 8 weeks of the onset of liver failure in patients with previously normal livers.

Hepatic encephalopathy is a clinical diagnosis that must be based on history, physical findings, and laboratory data. It is difficult to improve on the clinical descriptions of Adams and Foley [1]. They reported a reduced state of awareness that may be described as delirium (as recognized by Frerichs), stupor, or coma along with other abnormalities. Epileptic seizures are occasionally encountered. Seizures are more commonly due to alcohol withdrawal and may not be a part of the hepatic encephalopathy syndrome.

An alteration in the mental status is the hallmark of this disorder, and the diagnosis cannot be sustained without this finding. Disorders in alertness, orientation, memory, affect, perception, attention, and judgment may all be present. Mesulam and Geschwind [19] contend that disorders in selective attention underlie most of these abnormalities. According to this hypothesis, abnormalities of memory, judgment, and so on are the result of an impaired ability to devote sufficient mental energy to a task. Failure to perform follows. Patients and observers may report an inability to concentrate and on examination may be unable to complete thought processes. These inappropriate shifts of attention to irrelevant stimuli are characteristic of delirium. Additional evidence suggests that impaired central information processing is critical, along with disordered attention, perception, thought processes, and memory.

Because of the importance of the abnormality in the mental state in the diagnosis of this and other metabolic encephalopathies, early detection is important. Unfortunately, most patients at risk for the development of hepatic encephalopathy are not cared for by physicians with special skills and training in detecting abnormalities of mental function; this may lead to delay or failure to establish the diagnosis. There are a number of screening tests that can be administered quickly and easily to patients for whom this diagnosis should be considered. The mini mental state examination, developed by Folstein, Folstein, and McHugh [11], is well suited to this purpose. It is short and requires only a few minutes to administer, and it is simple and can therefore be given after very brief training. Performance is not affected by practice, and it can be used in a serial fashion to quantify improvement or regression of symptoms.

The cranial nerves are invariably intact, unless the patient is moribund due to cerebral edema, which may accompany fulminant hepatic failure or the multiple metabolic abnormalities, including renal failure and disorders of acid-base balance that are common in the terminal phases of hepatic encephalopathy. The pupils are usually somewhat smaller than normal, and the reaction to light may be blunted. Oculovestibular reflexes are intact, and usually passive head movement will produce eye movement attributable to third and sixth nerve function; occasionally ice-water caloric testing may be required.

There may be a variety of motor abnormalities, including the flapping tremor, or asterixis, which is a sudden complete lapse in postural tone. Asterixis was initially thought to be a specific finding indicative of hepatic encephalopathy. However, experience has shown that this helpful clinical sign is associated with uremia [26], other encephalopathies, and structural lesions of the brain. Electrophysiologic studies have shown that the postural lapses follow sudden, unexplained electrical silence in skeletal muscle. Asterixis may be observed in any voluntary muscle, including arm and hand extensors, flexors of the leg on the thigh, and protruders of the tongue. Abnormalities of muscle tone, hyperreflexia, and extensor plantar signs are all common. Unusual movements may be encountered; these usually clear with successful treatment.

Laboratory tests may be very helpful in establishing the diagnosis. Liver function tests are frequently abnormal, but the abnormalities may not be as severe as the clinical status would suggest. Chronic, severe liver disease may be associated with relatively normal serum enzyme levels and modest hyperbilirubinemia. Severe hypoalbuminemia and impaired clotting mechanisms are common. The blood ammonia level is frequently very helpful in establishing the diagnosis. Sherlock [25] reported a good correlation between the arterial ammonia level and impairments in consciousness, and Lockwood and co-workers [18] demonstrated significant correlations between elevations in the arterial ammonia concentration, the uptake and metabolism of ammonia by the brain, and the presence of encephalopathy. Several precautions must be taken to ensure an accurate result. Blood samples *must* be arterial. Ammonia levels may be reduced or elevated in venous blood due to unpredictable interactions between ammonia extraction and release by skeletal muscle. The development of toxin hypersensitivity (discussed later) may explain why some patients with "normal" ammonia levels are comatose.

Electrophysiologic studies are also helpful. Bickford and Butt [3] described three stages in the evolution of the EEG: a theta stage characterized by diffuse 4- to 7-Hz waves; a triphasic stage with surface-positive maximum deflections; and a delta stage with random, nonrhythmic slowing with little bilateral synchrony. Brenner's review [4] describes bursts of moderate to high amplitude activity (100–300 microvolts) with low frequencies (1.5–2.5 Hz) as being most characteristic. Abnormalities of visual evoked potentials have suggested abnormalities in gamma-aminobutyric acid (GABA)-ergic neurotransmission. However, failure to find similar abnormalities in patients treated with gamma-vinyl-GABA, a GABA transaminase inhibitor, makes this hypothesis tenuous.

Imaging studies of the brain are useful to exclude structural lesions such as subdural hematomas, which may occur in the population of patients at risk for the development of hepatic encephalopathy. Magnetic resonance imaging is an unexplored modality for the investigation of these patients, and it is possible that the microvacuolar changes in the brains of patients with chronic hepatocerebral degeneration, a complication of chronic hepatic encephalopathy, could be manifested by abnormal signal intensities in T2-weighted images.

The Alzheimer II astrocyte is the pathologic hallmark of hepatic encephalopathy. An account of the original description of this abnormality is provided, in translation, by Adams and Foley [1]. These abnormal astrocytes are present in the cerebral cortex and the lenticular, lateral thalamic, dentate, and red nuclei. Adams and Foley [1] speculated that the length of coma might correlate with the severity of the alteration. Constant infusions of ammonium ion produce this astrocyte change in primates. In rats with portacaval shunt-induced hyperammonemia, Alzheimer II astrocyte changes become evident about 5 weeks after shunt surgery. Ultrastructurally, these cells appear to be metabolically hyperactive; they have increased numbers of mitochondria, and there is proliferation of the endoplasmic reticulum. Immunohistochemical staining techniques have shown that Alzheimer II astrocytes have increases in stainable glutamine synthetase and glutamate dehydrogenase. In his review of the role of the astrocyte in hepatic encephalopathy, Norenberg [20] suggests that the clinical syndrome is secondary to astrocyte dysfunction.

Clincial Course and Complications of Hepatic Encephalopathy

Although mild, uncomplicated hepatic encephalopathy usually responds to treatment and complete recovery can be anticipated, patients with liver function that is severe enough to permit the emergence of encephalopathy are by definition severely ill, and it is common for patients to fail to do as well as hoped. Each episode of encephalopathy is associated with the risks of complications, the development of permanent neurologic deficits, the development of toxin hypersensitivity, and the emergence of a syndrome of self-perpetuating chronic encephalopathy. Therefore, in order to institute appropriate therapy, it is imperative that the diagnosis be established promptly.

Fulminant hepatic failure carries a poor prognosis, with an expected mortality rate of 80 to 85 percent. As with all cases of hepatic encephalopathy, the ultimate prognosis in this group most closely correlates with the course of the liver disease but can be strongly influenced (usually adversely) by intercurrent illnesses, such as infections or gastrointestinal hemorrhage.

Very severe hepatic coma carries a substantial risk of death or leaving the patient with permanent neurologic disability. In a prospective study of 500 patients with nontraumatic coma of at least 6 hours' duration, Levy and colleagues [15] identified 51 patients with hepatic coma. They assessed the best level of function within 1 year following the onset of coma as the outcome, since any decline after recovery could be considered preventable. In that group, 49 percent made no recovery. A good recovery with preservation of an ability to live independently was seen in only 27 percent, with a 2 percent incidence of the vegetative state and 14 and 8 percent exhibiting severe or moderate levels of neurologic disability respectively. Since this series required that patients be completely unresponsive for 6 hours or longer to be enrolled, it probably represents a worst-case outcome and emphasizes the importance of prompt appropriate therapy.

Hepatocerebral Degeneration

Although hepatic encephalopathy is usually completely reversible, a small number of patients are left with permanent deficits. This group of patients was most carefully studied by Victor, Adams, and Cole [28] in a comprehensive report describing the clinical and pathologic features of what they called chronic hepatocerebral degeneration unassociated with Wilson's disease. They reported 27 patients who had been followed for many years, including 17 who died and came to autopsy. Discrete episodes of hepatic encephalopathy were observed in 23 of the 27 patients. Surgically constructed portacaval shunts were present in 12. One patient was shunted during the course of surgery for carcinoma of the pancreas, had no liver disease, and developed the neurologic syndrome without having had prior episodes of encephalopathy. Although recurrent encephalopathy usually antedated the onset of the syndrome, there were exceptions. However, all patients had hyperammonemia or an abnormal ammonia tolerance. Clinically, these patients had dementia of varying severity; dysarthria and other signs attributable to cerebellar dysfunction, including limb and truncal ataxia; choreoathetosis; mild pyramidal tract signs; and tremor (not asterixis) while sustaining a prescribed position. Diffuse rigidity, positive grasp reflexes, nystagmus, and resting tremors were less common. On neuropathologic examination, these patients had polymicrocavitary degeneration in layers 5 and 6 of the cortex, the underlying white matter, the basal ganglia, and the cerebellum. Three patients had abnormalities of the spinal cord.

Other Central Nervous System Complications

In addition to the myelopathy described in association with hepatocerebral degeneration, evidence of cord dysfunction may appear without other stigmata of hepatocerebral degeneration [2,21,22]. These patients typically have severe liver disease that has required portacaval shunting to relieve pressure in varices and have experienced one or more episodes of hepatic encephalopathy followed by a progressive spastic paraparesis. Pathologic examinations have shown demyelination of the corticospinal tracts and a loss of Betz cells. Since brisk tendon reflexes and extensor plantar signs are usually seen in patients with reversible and chronic encephalopathy, early diagnosis of this syndrome is difficult.

Since patients with hepatic encephalopathy are often seriously ill with other problems, it is not surprising that other complications may develop during the course of the treatment of these individuals. While most of these can be easily attributed to the appropriate mechanisms and pathogenetic factors, the development of central pontine myelinolysis deserves mention. This syndrome was initially described in alcoholics and was believed to be a complication of alcoholism. Many of these patients have liver disease as well. More recent studies of this condition suggest that it is caused by rapid correction of hyponatremia, and experimental models of demyelination have been developed that replicate some of the findings observed in humans.

PATHOPHYSIOLOGY

The development of successful treatments for hepatic encephalopathy depends on understanding the mechanisms that operate to produce the disorder. Frerichs' insight into this aspect of liver disease was prescient [12]:

> Abnormal nervous symptoms must be referred to changes in the blood. I attribute the cause of the blood-intoxication to the complete arrest of the hepatic functions, [and] also [to] the cessation of the powerful influence which the liver exerts over the processes of metamorphosis of matter.

Much of the progress made since then consists of providing some details to this statement. Because of the complexity of the metabolic processes in the liver, a large number of hypotheses have been advanced to explain the development of the disorder. Suspected factors include hyperammonemia and its multiple neurochemical and neurophysiologic consequences; altered amino acid and neurotransmitter function, especially GABA; altered short-chain fatty acid metabolism; and high levels of mercaptans.

The Role of Ammonia

The recognition of the role of ammonia in the production of hepatic encephalopathy dates to studies of Gabuzda, Phillips, and Davidson [13], who observed encephalopathy as a complication of attempts to treat ascites in patients with cirrhosis with resins that exchanged sodium for ammonium ions; coma was a frequent complication. Further studies correlated changes in the mental status with the development of hyperammonemia and recommendations that ammonia-containing compounds be avoided. Somewhat later, Sherlock [25] correlated the fasting arterial ammonia concentration with the severity of encephalopathy. Subsequently, a number of publications and reviews have emphasized and strengthened this link [8,17,18]. Although the ammonia hypothesis is not without its detractors, the evidence to support the theory that it plays a central role in the production of hepatic encephalopathy is strong. There is a good correlation between blood ammonia levels and the severity of encephalopathy; this correlation is strengthened when the ammonia metabolites glutamine and alpha-ketoglutaramate are measured in cerebrospinal fluid (CSF) and correlated with the clinical status; patients with encephalopathy have higher brain uptake and metabolic rates for ammonia than nonencephalopathic patients with liver disease; ammonia reproducibly precipitates coma in animals and humans; and the most effective treatment strategies are those designed to reduce blood ammonia levels.

Ammonia is normally produced in the gastrointestinal tract and carried to the liver via the hepatic portal vein. In the liver, enzymes of the urea cycle convert ammonia to urea for subsequent excretion by the kidney. This detoxification pathway is supplemented by the ability of skeletal muscle to convert ammonia to the amide group of glutamine. The glutamine thus formed is then transported via the systemic circulation to the liver, where the amide group is used in urea synthesis [18]. In patients with portal hypertension and "natural" or surgical portacaval shunts, ammonia-laden blood enters the systemic circulation directly and is then pumped to the various organs as determined by blood flow. In patients with all or most of the portal blood shunted into the systemic vascular pool, skeletal muscle may become the single most important organ in the maintenance of ammonia homeostasis [18]. This scheme is depicted in Figure 9-1.

Studies of cerebral blood flow and metabolism in patients with hepatic coma have shown the reductions expected in patients with compromised levels of consciousness. After successful treatment, flow and metabolism are normalized.

Studies of flow and metabolism in animals have provided significant insights into poten-

Fig. 9-1. The general scheme for the metabolism of ammonia (and possibly other toxins). Ammonia is formed in the colon by enzymatic action and carried to the liver, where it is converted to urea for subsequent excretion. An enterohepatic urea circulation exists. In patients with portal-systemic shunts, natural or surgical, ammonia bypasses the liver and is carried to various body organs in proportion to their total blood flow. In the brain, ammonia is converted to glutamine and disrupts a number of cellular mechanisms, producing encephalopathy, and may stimulate satiety centers, leading to cachexia. Since skeletal muscle metabolizes large amounts of ammonia, muscle loss may predispose a patient to the development of further episodes of encephalopathy. (From Lockwood et al. [18] by copyright permission of the American Society for Clinical Investigation.)

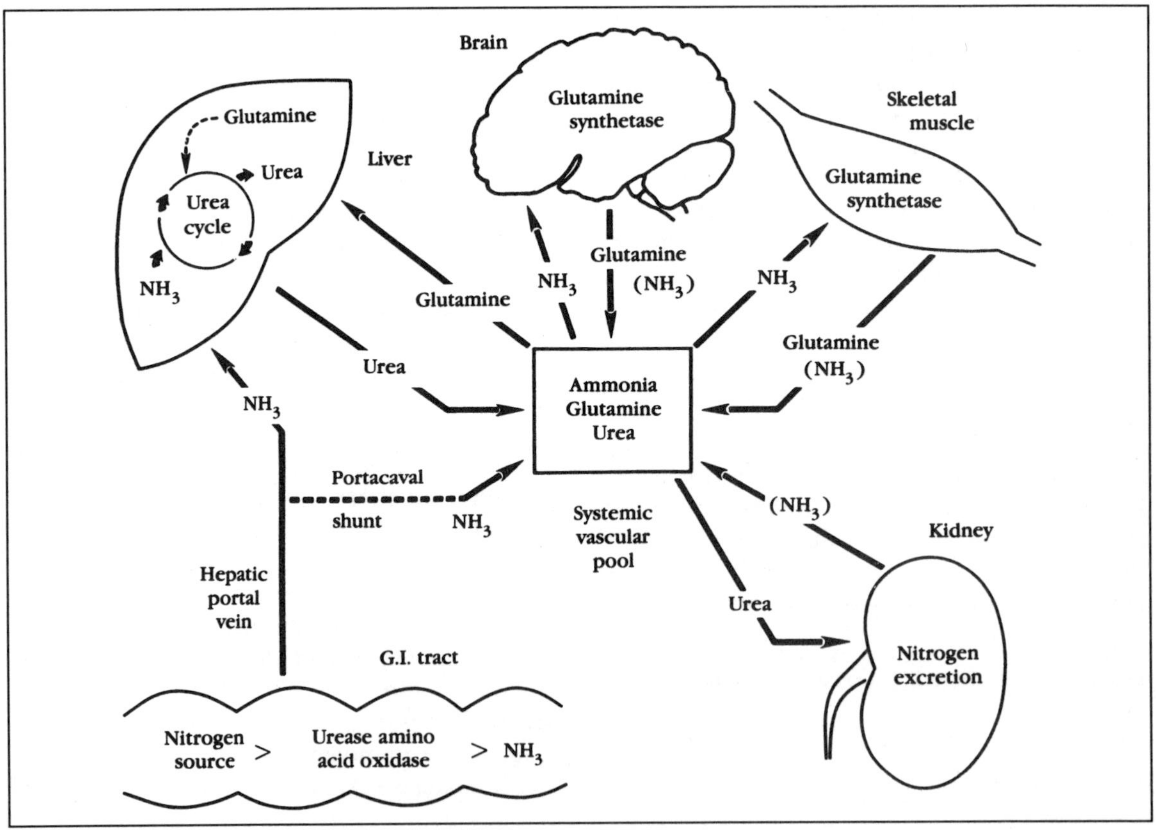

tially important mechanisms that lead to encephalopathy. Gjedde and associates [14] measured blood flow and oxygen metabolism in rats with portacaval shunts. They found that an ammonia challenge had very little effect 4 weeks after shunting but produced significant reductions 8 weeks after shunting. It is during this period of time that neuropathologic changes become evident. These data support the clinical impression that toxin hypersensitivity develops as liver disease progresses [29]. It is therefore possible, perhaps likely, that patients reported by Sherlock [25] who were comatose yet had "normal" arterial ammonia levels could still be toxic if the dose-response relationship for ammonia was altered.

Ammonia metabolism studies have been facilitated greatly by the use of the cyclotron-produced isotope ^{13}N, which can be used to produce high specific activity labeled ammonia. The use of ^{13}N-ammonia has led to substantial improvements in our understanding of the cerebral metabolism of this compound. Ammonia enters the brain by passive diffusion. Although both the ammonium ion and NH_3 gas can cross the blood-brain barrier, the barrier is about 200 times less permeable to the ion. Over the physiologic pH range, the cerebral uptake of ammonia is highly dependent on the blood-brain pH gradient. As blood pH falls, ammonia becomes more highly ionized and less able to diffuse across the barrier into the brain. At any given pH gradient value, cerebral blood flow determines the fractional extraction of ammonia [16]. Flow and extraction are reciprocally related: When flow is high, the period of time that a cohort of ammonia molecules is in contact with the barrier is short, and extraction is low; as flow falls, the contact time and the extraction rise. Normally, the brain extracts about half of the ammonia that is delivered by arterial blood [18]. In a study of ammonia metabolism, the whole brain ammonia metabolic rate was a linear function of the arterial concentration [18]. When patients were grouped according to the presence or absence of encephalopathy, the encephalopathic group had higher ammonia metabolic rates than the nonencephalopathic controls.

The metabolism of ammonia in the brain is highly compartmentalized. After the administration of tracer amounts of ^{13}N-ammonia, label can be in glutamate, the amino group of glutamine, and the amide group of glutamine in ratios of 1 : 5 : 400, confirming earlier studies that suggested that ammonia entering the brain is converted to glutamine in a highly compartmentalized system [7]. This explains the finding of high glutamine levels found in the brain and CSF of patients and animals with hepatic encephalopathy or experimental hyperammonemia. The concentration of glutamine, and its transamination product alpha-ketoglutaramate, can be measured in CSF and is a reliable indicator of the presence of hepatic encephalopathy. Technical considerations have prevented widespread use of these measures in the clinical setting.

A number of hypotheses speculating on the metabolic origin of hepatic encephalopathy have centered on the effects of ammonia on glucose metabolism. Early data suggested that the formation of glutamate, required for glutamine synthesis, would lead to depletion of the Krebs' cycle intermediate alpha-ketoglutarate. This hypothesis has been tested repeatedly, and convincing support has not been found. Hyperammonemia does appear to lead to adenosine triphosphate (ATP) depletion. After rapid brain fixation by microwave brain irradiation, neurochemical analysis confirmed ATP depletion in the midbrain reticular formation, but not in the immediately adjacent colliculus. This, coupled with other data showing ATP depletion at the onset of coma, makes it seem likely that there are impairments in energy metabolism during experimentally induced coma.

In a study of cerebral glucose metabolism after portacaval shunt construction, Lockwood and co-workers [17] reported evidence for global increases in metabolism that were least prominent in cortex and most prominent in the deeper gray structures, especially the reticular activating system, where metabolism was increased by about 75 percent. These authors speculated that these varied increases reflected a restructuring of functional interactions in the brain and were possibly responsible for the protean nature of the symptoms of hepatic encephalopathy. In that same study, the effect of small intracarotid infusions of ammonia was reported. The dorsal medical nucleus of the thalamus was among the regions stimulated by ammonia. Electrical stimulation of this nucleus causes satiety. This suggested the following self-perpetuating sequence: Hyperammonemic satiety leads to the weight loss and cachexia that is common in patients with severe liver disease and repeated episodes of encephalopathy. The reduction in skeletal muscle mass impairs the body's ability to detoxify ammonia, especially in patients with extensive portal-systemic shunts, and perpetuates hyperammonemia. This sequence, coupled with increases in the sensitivity to ammonia and perhaps other toxins, leads to the development of intractable encephalopathy due to the alterations in the metabolic anatomy of the brain produced by ammonia.

In addition to affecting metabolism, ammonia also exerts powerful effects of neurophysiologic mechanisms. Ammonium ions will substitute for sodium and potassium, with lower permeabilities, in giant squid axons. Ammonia also exerts potent inhibitory effect on chloride extrusion and produces a reversible depolarizing shift in the inhibitory postsynaptic potential toward the resting potential. Chloride pump inhibition can be shown to occur in hyperammonemic cats at ammonia concentrations encountered in symptomatic patients, suggesting that this may be an important mechanism affecting the brain.

Abnormalities of Neurotransmission

Because of the recognized central role that neurotransmitters play in the normal function of the brain and the clear evidence that abnormalities of neurotransmission affect the brain (e.g., ideopathic and drug-induced Parkinson's disease), a number of hypotheses have been advanced that suggest that altered neurotransmission is important in the pathogenesis of hepatic encephalopathy.

Glutamic Acid

A recognition of the link between glutamic acid and the conversion of ammonia to urea, often present at reduced levels in patients with liver disease, led to unsuccessful attempts to treat encephalopathy with glutamate infusions. There are small, but significant, decreases in brain glutamate levels after an ammonia challenge, leading to renewed speculation that a deficiency in a specific pool of this excitatory neurotransmitter might be implicated in the pathogenesis of hepatic encephalopathy. Other data have led to speculations that the inhibition of glutaminase leads to a lowering of synaptosomal glutamate content. In addition, glutamate release from hippocampal slices is enhanced by ammonia, a change not present in slices obtained from rats with portacaval shunts. Although the link between ammonia and glutamic acid metabolism is close, the evidence for a cause-and-effect relationship between alterations in glutamate metabolism and the production of encephalopathy is highly speculative.

Acetylcholine

Brain acetylcholine levels after the induction of acute and subacute ammonia intoxication are not altered, suggesting that abnormalities of acetylcholine are not involved in the production of hepatic encephalopathy.

Biogenic Amines and False Neurotransmitters

The false neurotransmitter hypothesis was advanced by Fischer and Baldasarini in 1971 [10]. They suggested that reductions in the metabolism and clearance of phenylalanine, tyrosine, and their amines, due to hepatocellular disease or portacaval shunting, lead to an increase in their cerebral uptake. Since tyrosine hydroxylase is the rate-limiting step in the cerebral metabolism of phenylalanine, increases in the size of the precursor pool were hypothesized to lead to an increase in octopamine and phenylethanolamine. Octopamine and phenylethanolamine are low-potency neurotransmitters and were present in increased concentration in the brains and hearts of animals made comatose by a two-stage ligation of the hepatic artery. These observations, combined with uncontrolled studies reporting improvement in hepatic encephalopathy after L-dopa administration and partial resolution of the hepatorenal syndrome after metaraminol infusions, strengthened the hypothesis that these "false" neurotransmitters were responsible for behavioral and circulatory problems associated with liver failure by competitively displacing true neurotransmitters from postsynaptic sites. These data, combined with earlier and reconfirmed reports of altered plasma amino acid profiles associated with liver failure, led to the hypothesis that proposed that the ratio of (valine + leucine + isoleucine)/(phenylalanine + tyrosine) was a useful predictor of encephalopathy, and that normalization of the ratio by the infusion of branched-chain amino acids (BCAA) (the numerator of the above ratio) would be a useful therapy that would normalize the brain neurotransmitter profile. A subsequent refinement of the hypothesis suggested that the increased brain levels of glutamine, formed from ammonia, acted as the driving force behind the uptake of aromatic amino acids (for review, see Lockwood [16]).

These reports, combined with uncontrolled, open clinical trials suggesting improvement after BCAA infusions or the administration of L-dopa, led to the commercial development and controlled clinical trials of amino acid mixtures and L-dopa. This latter treatment was shown to be ineffective and has been abandoned. Improvement in cerebral blood flow and metabolism after treatment with the dopamine agonist bromocriptine has been reported. Treatment strategies based on direct attempts to affect dopamine neurotransmission have been accordingly abandoned. The results of controlled trials of BCAAs are conflicting. One suggested deterioration, two showed no effect, and a fourth showed improved survival and cerebral function. All of these studies report that the amino acid ratio, defined above, was normalized during treatment, but there was no correlation between amino acid normalization and electroencephalographic or clinical improvement. In summary, the results of BCAA trials have been disappointing. The potential benefit is not clear-cut, and it seems imprudent at this time to rely on BCAAs as an exclusive treatment for this disorder (for review, see Lockwood [16]).

In addition to the disappointing results of the BCAA trials, the false neurotransmitter hypothesis has been weakened by reports that the treatment of animals with monoamine oxidase inhibitors or imipramine causes an increase in brain octopamine, without encephalopathy, and the study of Zieve and Olsen [33] in which intracerebral injections of octopamine at 20,000 times the normal concentration failed to produce an effect.

Gamma-Aminobutyric Acid

In recent years, there have been a number of reports suggesting that hepatic encephalopathy is caused by increases in brain GABA, the most abundant inhibitory neurotransmitter [16,24].

Normally, the brain is isolated from plasma and its amino acids, including GABA, by the blood-brain barrier, which is impermeable to compounds that have neurotransmitter action. GABA is present in the blood due to its formation by enteric bacteria. GABA is present in portal blood at concentrations twice that in systemic blood, attesting to the efficiency of hepatic GABA transaminase and its ability to metabolize 80 percent of noncerebral GABA. Thus, in a fashion that is completely analogous to the ammonia hypothesis, hepatic failure and portacaval shunting lead to increases in plasma GABA levels in animals and humans. Studies of the blood-brain barrier using alpha-aminoisobutyric acid in animals treated with the hepatotoxin galactosamine have shown an increase in the flux of this amino acid across the barrier. Additionally, there are numerous reports suggesting that liver disease in a variety of models alters GABA receptors in a fashion that may make the brain more susceptible to the effects of GABA. Thus it is postulated that a blood-brain barriers defect in patients with liver disease permits the influx of exogenous GABA, which in turn binds to neuronal GABA receptors, increasing neural inhibition, and causing encephalopathy (for reviews, see Lockwood [16] and Schafer and Jones [24]).

In the normal brain, GABA is sequestered in vesicles and is pharmacologically inactive until it is released into the synaptic cleft and binds to the GABA receptor. The GABA receptor is a highly specific complex molecule that contains at least five specific components: a GABA recognition site; a GABA modulin; a chloride ion channel; a benzodiazepine binding protein; and a protein that couples GABA recognition and ion channels. In addition to specific GABA binding sites, there are also nonspecific binding sites that exhibit lower affinities for GABA than shown by the specific sites. There are also GABA autoreceptors, which are GABA-sensitive sites on GABA-ergic terminals that bind GABA and inhibit GABA release and GABA sensitivity of sites in the nervous system, that do not have direct GABA input. This complexity and the system's capacity for multiple actions have caused problems in the interpretation of pharmacologic studies of GABA action in the brain. Similar caution should be applied to the analysis of the GABA hypothesis.

In addition to hesitations based on the complexity of the GABA system, there are data that are inconsistent with the GABA hypothesis. Mice given massive doses of GABA were unaffected, which suggests that it is extremely difficult to manipulate central GABA-ergic mechanisms by peripheral infusions. Even after complete peripheral GABA transaminase inhibition, labeled GABA does not cross the blood-brain barrier. GABA transaminase treatment does, however, cause a rapid and sustained increase in brain and CSF GABA levels, but gamma-vinyl-GABA, a GABA transaminase inhibitor that has been widely tested as an anticonvulsant, does not cause encephalopathy in humans and does not produce abnormalities in visual evoked potentials, including the type of abnormality that has been associated with experimental hepatic encephalopathy. Finally, no evidence for regional alterations in brain GABA levels has been found in animals given a portacaval shunt, and no abnormalities in brain GABA levels have been found in patients who died of cirrhosis of the liver.

In summary, there are facets of the GABA hypothesis that are deserving of further investigations [23], but there are also substantial weaknesses in the hypothesis and reasons to doubt its validity. From a clinical perspective, the debate about the GABA hypothesis may be unimportant, since proven treatment strategies shown to work by affecting the GABA system have not been developed.

Mercaptans

Mercaptans are organic thio alcohols, or thiols, that contain –SH groups instead of the –OH groups that are characteristic of typical alcohols. Mercaptans, especially methanethiol, have been implicated in the pathogenesis of hepatic encephalopathy [31].

Methanethiol is the most important mercaptan in humans and is presumably formed by the catabolism of methionine in the gastrointestinal tract. Methanethiol levels are elevated in patients with hepatic coma. Methanethiol levels, measured in end-tidal air samples and blood, correlate the clinical state, suggesting that they may contribute to the production of the clinical syndrome. In addition, animals develop coma when they are given various mercaptans in inspired air or by injection. Zieve, Doizaki, and Zieve [32] report that mercaptans act synergistically with ammonia or fatty acids to produce coma. They found that the coma-producing dose of either toxin was lowered when ammonia was given in non-coma-producing amounts.

This hypothesis has been challenged in a study that used improved chromatographic methods to measure blood methanethiol. Although the level was elevated in patients with encephalopathy, the correlation between the concentration and the severity of symptoms was poor. There were also problems precipitating coma in animals with reliability, even when doses were used that produced blood levels 10 times greater than those observed in patients. These observations led to a questioning of the importance of this class of compounds in the production of encephalopathy.

The place of mercaptans in the hierarchy of toxins implicated in the production of coma is thus somewhat uncertain. No study to date has measured levels of *all* putative toxins simultaneously and sequentially over the course of episodes of encephalopathy. Until such time, it is unreasonable to discard the mercaptan hypothesis completely, especially in view of the reports of synergism and the possibility of toxin hypersensitivity.

Short-Chain Fatty Acids (SCFA)

Fatty acids affect a wide variety of metabolic processes that may contribute to or cause the development of encephalopathy [16,30]. Coma was produced in animals by the intraperitoneal injection of short- and medium-chain fatty acids. Elevations in hexanoic and valeric acid blood levels have been found in patients with hepatic coma, leading to speculations that SCFAs may contribute to coma production either alone or acting synergistically with other toxins as previously described. There are several metabolic mechanisms that may explain coma production. Uncoupling of oxidative phosphorylation has been suggested, as has inhibition of hepatic urea formation, which could precipitate or exacerbate the development of hyperammonemia. There may also be an alteration of the mitochondrial respiratory state and state-control mechanisms.

Conclusions

A huge amount of clinical and experimental literature attests to the complexity of the pathophysiology of hepatic encephalopathy. Because of the central position of the liver in intermediate metabolism, it is quite reasonable to expect that liver disease will lead to a complex metabolic disorder. The term *metabolic chaos* has been used to describe fulminant hepatic failure and the myriad of associated secondary problems. Part of the problem centers on the probable need to differentiate between the neurologic disorder associated with fulminant hepatic failure and the disorders associated with chronic liver disease and portacaval shunt formation. Many of the experimental models of hepatic encephalopathy produce an acute syndrome of liver failure, whether caused by staged hepatic artery ligation or the administration of toxins, such as galactosamine or others. The pathophysiologic disturbances following these maneuvers are probably more relevant to fulminant hepatic failure syndromes, which, by definition, may evolve over 8 weeks. These paradigms should be contrasted with long-term portacaval shunt models, which may be more relevant to most cases of hepatic encephalopathy.

It seems naive, given the list of toxins and putative disease mechanisms, to pick only one factor as being responsible for all cases of encephalopathy associated with liver disease. This seems particularly relevant given reports of toxin synergism. Luckily, there are patients with reasonably well compensated liver disease who develop relatively uncomplicated encephalopathy. It may be through the study of this highly selected group of patients that we may learn the most about mechanisms. From the vantage point of published, well-controlled trials involving encephalopathic patients, this is the group who responds best to treatment strategies that lower blood ammonia levels. Clinically, it therefore seems prudent to attempt to lower the arterial ammonia level in every patient with hepatic encephalopathy while at the same time employing additional strategies that are designed to treat additional proven metabolic abnormalities.

TREATMENT

The treatment of the encephalopathic patient with liver disease may be very difficult. Success depends on the correct determination of the cause and treatment of the liver disease itself, in addition to the identification and treatment of factors that precipitated the episode of encephalopathy. This process may be accompanied by a large number of serious complications of liver failure and coma.

While it may seem redundant to state that successful treatment can only follow a correct diagnosis, this is worth emphasizing because of the high frequency with which relatively subtle alterations of mental capacity may be missed, unless thorough examinations are conducted or screening examinations such as the mini mental state are employed. Decrements in mental capacity may be subtle and range from slight inattentiveness in a high-level executive to failure to eat usual meals at a shelter in a destitute homeless alcoholic. Once the diagnosis is made, or in many cases suspected, a variety of proven therapeutic steps can be taken.

In planning therapy, it is important to differentiate patients with acute fulminant hepatic failure from patients with chronic liver failure with encephalopathy. Because of the extensive and severe hepatocellular necrosis that characterizes the former disorder, the metabolic abnormalities and impacts on other organs are much more severe and therapies correspondingly less effective. Success in the treatment of fulminant hepatic failure depends on sustaining the patient until hepatic regeneration occurs or until transplantation can be accomplished, depending on the individual circumstances. A variety of therapies, including exchange transfusion, the use of various columns designed to trap toxins, perfusion through cadaver livers, and hemodialysis, have all been tried with disappointing results. Terminally, these patients may lapse into coma with signs indicative of cerebral edema. Since therapies for portal-systemic or hepatic encephalopathy are better characterized and more effective than those for fulminant hepatic necrosis, the majority of this portion of the chapter will deal with this latter disorder.

In evaluating the results of any of the multitude of open or controlled trials of the various forms of treatment that have been applied to control hepatic encephalopathy, it is important to remember that it is likely that the very act of being included in an investigation will be therapeutic. Even patients receiving placebos will be removed from an environment or life-style that is hepatotoxic, and exacerbating medical problems will be treated. Therefore, treatments that are reported to be helpful in open trials, that is, those in which everyone receives the investigational agent, will lead to an improvement in a significant number of patients, even if the agent being evaluated is ineffective.

Since most advances in the treatment of hepatic encephalopathy have followed the improvements in our understanding of the pathophysiology of the disorder, it is useful to take a mechanistic approach to treatment. The hypothesis that hyperammonemia is a central factor in the pathogenesis of this disorder has led to the greatest therapeutic advances, and measures that are designed to lower ammonia levels will be considered first.

Since the majority of the ammonia in the hepatic portal vein, and in many cases the systemic circulation, is derived from colonic contents, a variety of strategies have been developed and tested that are specifically designed to eliminate or minimize colonic ammonia production. The treatment of acute encephalopathy should include a number of measures, some of which tend to be ignored in the practice of high-technology medicine. Initially there should be an immediate institution of a zero- or reduced-protein diet, followed by liberalization as indicated by the clinical course. This step is designed to reduce the nitrogenous load delivered to the colon, where amino acid oxidases and ureases cleave ammonia from precursor molecules. Since blood is high in protein, aggressive measures to diagnose and control gastrointestinal hemorrhage are warranted under the same rationale. The colon should be cleansed with laxatives or enemas to remove contents that give rise to ammonia. In some patients, fecal impaction may be sufficient to cause encephalopathy. More aggressive measures, such as colonic exclusion, are not warranted since the morbidity and mortality of the treatment exceed that of the disease.

Lactulose

Oral lactulose is the mainstay of treatment for both acute and chronic forms of hepatic encephalopathy, having replaced oral neomycin, because of potential renal and ototoxicity due to the absorption of small amounts of this antibiotic. Lactulose therapy is associated with reductions in the arterial ammonia concentration and clinical improvement, but the mechanisms behind these observations are not understood completely. Since this synthetic disaccharide is split in the gastrointestinal tract to produce acid and an osmotic diarrhea, both factors have been evaluated in terms of potential mechanisms that reduce the ammonia burden.

Lactulose was first used with the hope that acidification of the gastrointestinal tract would lead to a recolonization of the colon with non-urease-containing species, which would in turn reduce blood ammonia levels. Success in this and uncontrolled trials led to more systematic and carefully controlled studies.

The efficacy of oral lactulose was first shown in a double-blind crossover study of seven patients with cirrhosis and chronic hepatic encephalopathy who were given lactulose or sorbitol [9]. Lactulose treatment caused improvement in five patients and was associated with a reduction in arterial ammonia concentrations and improvements in the electroencephalogram. In all seven, chronic lactulose therapy was judged to be effective in preventing or reducing the severity of exacerbations of the encephalopathy. Sorbitol was without any discernible effect. The most definitive study did not appear for almost another 10 years [5]. In this multicenter trial, 33 patients were treated with lactulose and neomycin using a crossover design. Placebos were used in place of neomycin (1.5 gm 4 times daily) and sorbitol in place of lactulose (25 ml 4 times daily, advancing to induce two to three bowel movements per day). Dietary protein was maintained at about 40 gm/day in most patients. Lactulose was effective in 90 percent of all courses of therapy, as compared with 83 percent effectiveness of the neomycin plus sorbitol treatment, a difference that was not significantly different. Some individuals appeared to respond selectively to one form of treatment but not the other. The authors concluded that lactulose was an effective form of therapy and potentially less toxic than neomycin when chronic use is necessary.

The dosage of lactulose varies somewhat from patient to patient; however, 20 to 30 gm 4 times daily will usually be effective and should cause no more than two or three bowel movements per day without unacceptable side effects. Patients presenting with coma should receive hourly doses of 20 to 30 gm of lactulose until a catharsis is induced. The dosage should then be reduced. Adverse reactions to lactulose most frequently include abdominal bloating and diarrhea. These symptoms are dose related and usually subside to acceptable levels that permit the continuation of therapy when the daily dose is reduced. Since many patients with hepatic coma have coexisting and often severe electrolyte disturbances, care must be taken to avoid a further deterioration in electrolyte balance due to diarrhea. Conn and Lieberthal [6] have written a comprehensive review of the use of lactulose for the treatment of hepatic encephalopathy.

Although lactulose is clearly effective in treating hepatic encephalopathy, its mechanism of action is still not completely characterized. The initial mechanism, which is still widely cited, centers on the acidification of the stools caused by the hydrolysis of lactulose. It is clear that lactulose does cause an acidification of the entire gastrointestinal tract, as was shown in studies of patients given lactulose who then swallowed small pH meters that telemetered their data to external receivers as the device moved through the gastrointestinal tract. The acidified contents then presumably trap ammonia gas, which is highly diffusible, as the ammonium ion, which is much less diffusible. Theory then holds that the trapped ammonium ions are removed from the body in the feces. This theory has been challenged on the basis of studies that report a failure to measure an increase in the amount of ammonia excreted. This led to speculation that lactulose serves as a metabolic substrate for ammonia-fixing reactions catalyzed by intestinal bacteria, or alternatively, it may suppress deamidation of nitrogenous compounds. This uncertainty led Conn [6] to refer to lactulose as "a drug in search of a modus operandi." The hypothesis that lactulose works by fixing nitrogen in the colon has been supported by a study in which the nitrogen contents of various fecal fractions was measured during lactulose and lactulose plus neomycin therapy. Feces were examined, and it was found that the nitrogen content of the bacterial fraction and the soluble nitrogen fraction increased to 165 and 135 percent of control, respectively, during lactulose therapy. The bacterial nitrogen content fell by 28 percent during neomycin therapy. These investigators also measured the urea production rate and found a 23 percent reduction during lactulose therapy, which was attributed to the increases in bacterial and soluble nitrogen excretion.

Neomycin

Ironically, although oral neomycin was commonly used in the treatment of hepatic encephalopathy for years before lactulose was introduced, confirmation of its utility came with the same data showing the utility of lactulose [5]. In this study, patients were allocated to either a lactulose or neomycin plus sorbitol treatment that was preceded by a control period when neither treatment was given. There was a second treatment-free control period in the interval when the crossover was made. An analysis of these data, and other data, provided the needed evidence to support the "common knowledge" that neomycin is an effective treatment for this disorder. For acute encephalopathy, the usual dosage ranges between 4 and 12 gm daily in divided doses. Chronic therapy usually requires 2 to 3 gm/day. When neomycin must be used on a chronic basis, otologic and renal monitoring should be performed to detect early toxicity that may be irreversible. The simultaneous development of the hepatorenal syndrome may make this task very difficult and, except for extraordinary circumstances, is an indication for the discontinuation of neomycin therapy. Neomycin therapy may also be complicated by the development of diarrhea, malabsorption, or the overgrowth of the colon by resistant microorganisms.

Neomycin appears to act by killing bacteria in the colon that cleave urea into ammonia and carbon dioxide. This hypothesis has been supported by studies that report that although oral neomycin reduces bacterial nitrogen loss in the stool by 28 percent, this is more than compensated for by a 36 percent reduction in daily urea synthesis.

Lactitol

Recently there have been several reports comparing lactitol to lactulose. Lactitol, like lactulose, is a synthetic disaccharide. Lactitol and lactulose are equally effective for the treatment of acute portal-systemic encephalopathy and chronic encephalopathy.

Diet Therapy

Protein restriction has long been recognized as an important and effective means of therapy. While short-term protein restriction can be tolerated by most patients without complications, long-term restriction must be approached with great care. On one hand, there is a clear association between excessive protein ingestion and the precipitation or prolongation of encephalopathy, while on the other, there is a recognition that many patients with encephalopathy are malnourished and require protein to promote hepatocellular regeneration and prevent the development of cachexia.

The prevention of cachexia may become a primary goal in the therapy of these patients because of the importance of skeletal muscle in the detoxification of ammonia and the positive feedback cycle described above. It is possible that a therapeutic effect of the branched-chain amino acid therapy may lie in an ability to prevent the development of a negative nitrogen balance and avoidance of cachexia.

Diet therapy of patients with liver failure may be sufficient to control encephalopathy. Uribe and colleagues [27] compared a number of regimens, including 40 gm of meat protein plus neomycin, 40 gm of vegetable protein, and 80 gm of vegetable protein. They found both vegetable diets to be superior to the meat plus neomycin diet. They urged some caution in the use of the vegetable diets after observing two episodes of hypoglycemia and noting the large volume of food that must be ingested to maintain the 80-gm vegetable protein diet. These diets may work by avoiding methionine, a potential source of both ammonia and mercaptans, and by the cathartic effect of the bulk involved.

Agents Affecting Neurotransmission

The use of drugs and other compounds that may alter neurotransmitter levels in the brain for the treatment of hepatic encephalopathy has been fostered by the numerous hypotheses that propose that encephalopathy is caused, at least in part, by deranged neurotransmission. Because these treatment strategies have been so closely allied with the hypothetical pathophysiologic mechanisms presented earlier in this chapter, and since none of these treatments has been shown to be effective, only a brief summary will be presented. Attempts to alter dopaminergic function with L-dopa and bromocriptine have not been shown to be effective in controlled studies, in spite of earlier, anecdotal reports of almost miraculous recoveries after L-dopa administration. Similarly, amino acid therapy, given in attempts to influence the neurotransmitter profile by altering the concentrations of plasma amino acids that serve as precursors to neurotransmitters, has not been successful in reversing encephalopathy. GABA-benzodiazepine antagonist therapy is likely to be tried in the near future, but controlled studies have not been reported as of yet.

Miscellaneous Therapies

Because of the complexity of the metabolic disorder associated with liver disease, the fact that no single form of therapy works for all patients, and an absence of a complete understanding of the pathophysiology of hepatic encephalopathy, it is not surprising that many treatment strategies have been attempted. Conn and Lieberthal [6] have classified most of these therapies in terms of a presumed effect on ammonia metabolism. Therapies include administration of alpha-keto analogues of amino acids, colonic bypass or exclusion, use of antibiotics other than neomycin, acidification of the gastrointestinal tract, recolonization of the gastrointestinal tract with nonproteolytic bacteria, inhibition of or immunization against urease, increasing hepatic extraction of ammonia by obliterating portal-systemic anastomoses and the use of less comagenic portal-systemic surgical shunts such as the distal splenorenal shunt, promotion of the conversion of ammonia to less toxic compounds inducing hexamethylenetetraamine, and supportive measures designed to avoid anemia, hypoxemia, alkalosis, and electrolyte imbalance. Sedative hypnotics must be avoided. Hepatic transplantation may be employed in selected cases but lies outside the scope of this chapter.

FUTURE DIRECTIONS

The treatment of hepatic encephalopathy and related disorders has improved considerably since the descriptions of neurologic dysfunction in Frerich's monograph. For the most part, these improvements have followed the development of a rational basis for therapy based on an understanding of the pathophysiology of the neurologic dysfunction associated with various toxins and now, potentially, changes in neurotransmitter systems. It is likely that further improvements will follow refinements and testing of new hypotheses. Two new tools for neurologic research, positron emission tomography and magnetic resonance spectroscopy, are likely to play an important role in this process. Both of these techniques can be applied to the study of patients with the syndrome itself, rather than imperfect animal models, and both can acquire biologic information noninvasively and sequentially. The combination of these two techniques may facilitate the unraveling of many of the problems associated with studies of toxins and their metabolism as well as possible alterations in neurotransmitter function.

REFERENCES

1. Adams, R. D., and Foley, J. S. The neurological disorder associated with liver disease. *Res. Publ. Assoc. Nerv. Ment. Dis.* 32:198, 1953.
2. Bechar, M., Freud, M., Kott, E., et al. Hepatic cirrhosis with post-shunt myelopathy. *J. Neurol. Sci.* 11:101, 1970.
3. Bickford, R. G., and Butt, H. R. Hepatic coma: The electroencephalographic pattern. *J. Clin. Invest.* 34:790, 1955.
4. Brenner, R. P. The electroencephalogram in altered states of consciousness. *Neurol. Clin.* 3:615, 1985.
5. Conn, H. O., Leevy, C. M., Vlahcevic, Z. R., et al. Comparison of lactulose and neomycin in the treatment of chronic portal-systemic encephalopathy: A double blind controlled trial. *Gastroenterology* 72:573, 1977.
6. Conn, H. O., and Lieberthal, M. M. *The Hepatic Coma Syndromes and Lactulose.* Baltimore: Williams & Wilkins, 1979.
7. Cooper, A. J. L., McDonald, J. M., Gelbard, A. S., et al. The metabolic fate of N-13 labeled ammonia in rat brain. *J. Biol. Chem.* 254:4982, 1979.
8. Cooper, A. J. L., and Plum, F. Biochemistry and physiology of brain ammonia. *Physiol. Rev.* 67:440, 1987.
9. Elkington, J. G., Floch, M. H., and Conn, H. O. Lactulose in the treatment of chronic portal-systemic encephalopathy: A double blind clinical trial. *N. Engl. J. Med.* 281:408, 1969.
10. Fischer, J. E., and Baldasarini, R. J. False neurotransmitters and hepatic failure. *Lancet* 2:75, 1971.
11. Folstein, M. F., Folstein, S. E., and McHugh, P. R. Mini mental status: A practical method for grading the cognitive state of patients for the clinician. *J. Psychiatr. Res.* 12:189, 1975.
12. Frerichs, F. T. A clinical treatise on liver disease 1858. Translated by C. Murcheson. New York: Wood, 1879.
13. Gabuzda, G., Jr., Phillips, G. B., and Davidson, C. S. Reversible toxic manifestations in patients with cirrhosis of the liver given cation-exchange resins. *N. Engl. J. Med.* 246:124, 1952.
14. Gjedde, A., Lockwood, A. H., Duffy, T. E., et al. Cerebral blood flow and metabolism in

chronically hyperammonemic rats: Effect of an acute ammonia challenge. *Ann. Neurol.* 3:325, 1978.

15. Levy, D. E., Bates, D., Caronna, J. J., et al. Prognosis in non-traumatic coma. *Ann. Intern. Med.* 94:293, 1981.
16. Lockwood, A. H. Hepatic encephalopathy: Experimental approaches to human metabolic encephalopathy. *CRC Crit. Rev. Neurobiol.* 3:105, 1987.
17. Lockwood, A. H., Ginsberg, M. D., Rhoades, H. M., et al. Cerebral glucose metabolism after portcaval shunting in the rat: Patterns of metabolism and implication for the pathogenesis of hepatic encephalopathy. *J. Clin. Invest.* 78:86, 1986.
18. Lockwood, A. H., McDonald, J. M., Reiman, R. E., et al. The dynamics of ammonia metabolism in man: Effects of liver disease and hyperammonemia. *J. Clin. Invest.* 63:449, 1979.
19. Mesulam, M. M., and Geschwind, N. Disordered state in the postoperative period. *Urol. Clin. North Am.* 3:199, 1976.
20. Norenberg, M. D. The astrocyte in liver disease. *Adv. Cell. Neurobiol.* 2:303, 1981.
21. Pant, S. S., Rebeiz, J. J., and Richardson, E. P., Jr. Spastic paraparesis following portacaval shunts. *Neurology* 18:135, 1968.
22. Read, A. E., Sherlock, S., Laidlaw, J., et al. The neuropsychiatric syndromes associated with chronic liver disease and an extensive portalsystemic circulation. *Q. J. Med.* 36:135, 1967.
23. Roberts, E. Editorial: The γ-aminobutyric acid (GABA) system and hepatic encephalopathy. *Hepatology* 4:342, 1984.
24. Schafer, D. F., and Jones, E. A. Potential Neural Mechanisms in the Pathogenesis of Hepatic Encephalopathy. In H. Popper and F. Schaffer (eds.), *Progress in Liver Diseases.* New York: Grune & Stratton, 1982.
25. Sherlock, S. Pathogenesis and management of hepatic coma. *Am. J. Med.* 24:805, 1958.
26. Tyler, H. R. Neurologic disorders in renal failure. *Am. J. Med.* 44:737, 1968.
27. Uribe, M., Marquez, M. A., Ramos, G. G., et al. Treatment of chronic portal-systemic encephalopathy with vegetable and animal protein diets: A controlled crossover study. *Dig. Dis. Sci.* 27:1109, 1982.
28. Victor, M., Adams, R. D., and Cole, M. The acquired (non-Wilsonian) type of chronic hepatocerebral degeneration. *Medicine* 44:345, 1965.
29. Walker, C., and Schenker, S. Pathogenesis of hepatic encephalopathy with special reference to the role of ammonia. *Am. J. Clin. Nutr.* 23:619, 1970.
30. Zieve, L. Encephalopathy Due to Short- and Medium-Chain Fatty Acids. In D. W. McCandless (ed.), *Cerebral Energy Metabolism and Metabolic Encephalopathy.* New York: Plenum, 1985.
31. Zieve, L., and Brunner, G. Encephalopathy Due to Mercaptans and Phenols. In D. W. McCandless (ed.), *Cerebral Energy Metabolism and Metabolic Encephalopathy.* New York: Plenum, 1985.
32. Zieve, L., Doizaki, W., and Zieve, F. J. Synergism between mercaptans and ammonia or fatty acids in the production of coma: A possible role for mercaptans in the pathogenesis of hepatic coma. *J. Lab. Clin. Med.* 83:16, 1974.
33. Zieve, L., and Olsen, R. L., Can hepatic encephalopathy be caused by a reduction of brain noradrenalin or dopamine? *Gut* 18:688, 1977.

10 Central Nervous System Manifestations of Hypophosphatemia and Phosphorus Depletion

James P. Knochel and Alberto Montanari

Central nervous system dysfunction is the most important consequence of severe phosphorus deficiency and hypophosphatemia. It usually occurs in persons being refed or hyperalimented as treatment for severe weight loss as a consequence of starvation, gastrointestinal disease, or chronic respiratory acidosis. In nearly all instances, profound muscular weakness is a concurrent event. This potentially fatal illness is predictable and preventable and, when recognized early in its course, responds favorably to correction of hypophosphatemia with phosphate salts. As will be discussed, alcoholic subjects with hypophosphatemia generally do not develop hypophosphatemic encephalopathy.

PHOSPHORUS METABOLISM

The total phosphorus content of a normal 70-kg adult is about 23 mol (700 gm). Of this, 80 percent is contained in bone, 9 percent in skeletal muscle, and the remainder in viscera and extracellular fluid [106].

A normal adult ingests about 1 gm of phosphorus each day. This value varies widely and tends to be higher in those who consume large quantities of soluble phosphates such as those found in meat or dairy products. Phosphates in meat or milk are almost completely absorbed from the midjejunum, and approximately 90 percent of this quantity will be excreted into the urine. In contrast, larger fractions of phosphate compounds contained in certain vegetable fibers are not soluble and thus may not be absorbed. As a result, persons ingesting normal mixed diets excrete from 60 to 90 percent of the ingested phosphorus in the urine.

Regulation of phosphorus balance occurs by variation of renal tubular reabsorption. In the normal subject, the kidneys retain approximately 80 percent of phosphate filtered by the glomerulus. The major factors affecting renal phosphorus reabsorption include glomerular filtration rate per se, parathyroid hormone, effective arterial volume, and arterial tension of carbon dioxide. Parathyroid hormone decreases phosphate reabsorption, as does an expanded arterial volume and hypercarbia. Systemic acidosis per se increases phosphate excretion predominantly by reducing glycolysis, which allows phosphorus leakage from cells, which in turn causes hyperphosphatemia. The usual renal response to hyperphosphatemia is phosphaturia.

Inorganic plasma phosphate at pH 7.4 exists as HPO_4^{-2} and $H_2PO_4^{-1}$ in a ratio of approximately 4:1. These two species of inorganic phosphate exist in a pH-dependent equilibrium. The pKa of the reaction $H_2PO_4^{-1} \leftrightarrows H^+ + HPO_4^{-2}$ is 6.8. Due to their extremely low and high pKa respectively, the undissociated phosphoric acid and fully dissociated trivalent phosphate ion concentrations are very small and can be neglected for clinical purposes [71].

Plasma phosphorus is determined as the inorganic phosphate but in almost all laboratories is reported as elemental phosphorus in milligrams per deciliter. The normal concentration of elemental phosphorus in human plasma is 3.0 to 4.5 mg/dl. Since the atomic weight for phosphorus is 31, this normal concentration represents between 1.0 and 1.5 mM. The average valence of phosphate is 1.8 at pH 7.4 (i.e., $[4 \times HPO_4^{-2}] + [1 \times H_2PO_4^{-1}]/4 + 1$). Thus, normal plasma concentrations of phosphate, expressed as milliequivalents per liter, range from 1.7 to 2.6 mEq/liter.

Most intracellular phosphorus exists as organic phosphate compounds such as creatine phosphate and adenosine mono- and triphosphates. In red cells the predominant intracellular phosphate compound is 2,3-diphosphoglycerate (2,3-DPG). While total intracellular phosphate content is quite high, free inorganic phosphate concentration is only about 1 mM [53,84]. Although the free inorganic phosphate concentration in intracellular water is lower than that in extracellular fluid, phosphate-containing molecules do make up a major component of intracellular anions. Phosphate groups in organic compounds such as adenosine triphosphate (ATP) are ionized and behave as anions at normal intracellular pH such that ATP for example, possessing a valence of −3.5, constitutes between 10 and 30 mEq/liter of intracellular anion [65]. Inorganic phosphate in the cell is also partially bound (complexed) to other anions such as calcium and magnesium and consequently is non-ionized. Much of this fraction is effectively sequestered within intracellular organelles such as mitochondria. This moiety is in equilibrium with both the extracellular phosphate and the intracellular glyceraldehyde-3-phosphate, with which it reacts to form 1,3-diphosphoglycerate, and it participates in the generation of ATP. Phosphate, like potassium, tends to have a relatively constant relationship to total body nitrogen. Thus, if one excludes the changes in the balance of phosphorus in bone, significant accumulation or loss of whole body phosphorus is generally proportional to gains or losses of nitrogen. For muscle the molar ratio of phosphorus to nitrogen is 0.03, and with significant muscle wasting both phosphorus and nitrogen are lost from muscle cells proportionately [1,7].

THE CAUSES AND SIGNIFICANCE OF HYPOPHOSPHATEMIA

Hypophosphatemia is especially common among hospitalized patients. The prevalence of hypophosphatemia in hospitalized patients varies depending on the type of cases one encounters. It is common in severe alcoholics [96]. The prevalence in a general hospital population varies between 0.24 to 2.15 percent [89]. A single measurement of serum phosphorus on the first hospital day often underestimates its prevalence. In patients with alcoholism, a characteristic pattern is progressive lowering of serum phosphorus over the course of several days [55].

Hypophosphatemia is arbitrarily defined as serum inorganic phosphorus concentration less than 2.5 mg/dl (0.83 mM). It does not always indicate the existence of phosphorus deficiency. Similarly, phosphorus deficiency may be associated with normal or even elevated levels of serum phosphorus, for example, in severe, prolonged diabetic ketoacidosis. In some instances, hypophosphatemia of itself may be of no importance, while in others it may have important implications. The causes of hypophosphatemia are shown in Table 10-1.

In most instances, hypophosphatemia reflects either inadequate intake, decreased intestinal absorption, shifts from serum into cells, or decreased reabsorption by the kidney. Starvation alone does not ordinarily lead to pronounced reductions of serum phosphate. Hypophosphatemia tends to occur more often in malnourished or starved patients who then ingest a diet containing absorbable nutrients, such as carbohydrate, that is deficient in phosphorus [59]. In humans and adult animals, administration of a phosphorus-deficient but otherwise normal diet results in only a modest depression of serum phosphorus concentration [56]. It is not until phosphate-binding antacids are added to the diet that severe hypophosphatemia occurs.

Perhaps the most common cause of modest hypophosphatemia in hospitalized patients is respiratory alkalosis [55,56]. Upon admission to hospitals, many patients are in pain or may be frightened and as a result hyperventilate sufficiently to reduce arterial PCO_2 and elevate their arterial pH. Severe hyperventilation may occur with bacteremia and sepsis, heat stroke, neuroleptic malignant syndrome, panic attacks, psychiatric depression, alcoholic withdrawal, hepatic coma, salicylate poisoning, or painful attacks of gout. By such means, respiratory alkalosis and hypophosphatemia are exceptionally common findings in patients who are ill with a large variety of disorders. In many instances, modest hypokalemia occurs simultaneously.

Administration of glucose and the consequent release of insulin may also cause moderate hypophosphatemia. Insulin increases the cellular uptake of glucose and phosphorus, mostly in liver and skeletal muscle. In normal individuals, the decline in serum phosphorus as a result of glucose or, independently, insulin administration does not exceed 0.5 mg/dl. However, when glucose is administered to a starving individual or a patient with hepatic cirrhosis, the hypophosphatemic response may be much more pronounced [18,24]. Such a response is associated with virtual disappearance of phosphorus from the urine. Consequently, the acute reduction of serum phosphorus in the face of a markedly

Table 10-1. Causes of hypophosphatemia

- Decreased dietary intake
- Decreased intestinal absorption
  - Vitamin D deficiency
  - Malabsorption
  - Steatorrhea
  - Secretory diarrhea
  - Vomiting
  - PO_4-binding antacids
- Shifts from serum into cells
  - Respiratory alkalosis
    - Sepsis
    - Heat stroke
    - Neuroleptic malignant syndrome
    - Hepatic coma
    - Salicylate poisoning
    - Gout
    - Panic attacks
    - Psychiatric depression
  - Hormonal effects
    - Insulin
    - Glucagon
    - Epinephrine
    - Androgens
    - Cortisol
    - Anovulatory hormones
  - Nutrient effects
    - Glucose
    - Fructose
    - Glycerol
    - Lactate
    - Amino acids
    - Xylitol
  - Cellular uptake syndromes
    - Recovery from hypothermia
    - Burkitt's lymphoma
    - Histiocytic lymphoma
    - Acute myelomonocytic leukemia
    - Acute myelogenous leukemia
    - Treatment of pernicious anemia
    - Hungry bone syndrome
      - Following parathyroidectomy
      - Acute leukemia
- Increased excretion into the urine
  - Hyperparathyroidism
  - Renal tubular defects
    - Renal rickets
    - Polyostotic fibrous dysplasia
    - Postrenal transplantation
    - Oncogenic osteomalacia
  - Aldosteronism
  - Licorice ingestion
  - Volume expansion
  - Inappropriate secretion of ADH
  - Mineralocorticoid administration
  - Corticosteroid therapy
  - Diuretics

reduced phosphorus excretion implies an intracellular shift.

Accelerated phosphorus uptake by rapidly proliferating malignant cells causes acute hypophosphatemia in patients with Burkitt's lymphoma cell leukemia [109], histiocytic lymphoma in leukemic transformation [72], acute myelogenous leukemia, and acute myelomonocytic leukemia [113]. In these cases, phosphorus excretion was minimal, indicating that cellular uptake was probably responsible for the hypophosphatemia.

Moderate hypophosphatemia as a result of increased urinary losses is common and has many explanations. Parathyroid hormone reduces phosphorus reabsorption by the renal tubule. Nevertheless, patients with primary hyperparathyroidism seldom show serum phosphorus concentrations below 2 mg/dl unless their intake of phosphorus is low or they simultaneously ingest phosphate-binding antacids.

Oncogenic osteomalacia is a disorder characterized by bone pain and sometimes disabling muscular weakness associated with either benign mesenchymal tumors or malignant disease of the prostate or lung [88]. Biochemically, it is associated with malabsorption of calcium and phosphorus, hypophosphatemia, and phosphaturia. Measurements of vitamin D metabolites show normal concentrations of 25-hydroxycholecalciferol but low values for the 1,25-dihydroxy metabolite, thus suggesting that the tumor produces an inhibitor of 25-hydroxy vitamin D 1α-hydroxylase. Indeed, Drezner and associates [30] have elicited direct support for the existence of such a substance that results in impaired phosphorus reabsorption.

Administration of diuretics may also be associated with reduction in serum phosphate concentration [62]. The most phosphaturic is acetazolamide, followed by thiazides and furosemide.

THE CAUSES OF SEVERE HYPOPHOSPHATEMIA

Severe hypophosphatemia, defined as a serum phosphorus concentration between 0.1 and 1.5 mg/dl, occurs in a limited number of circumstances. These are listed in Table 10-2.

Table 10-2. Causes of severe hypophosphatemia

Chronic alcoholism and alcoholic withdrawal
Dietary deficiency and phosphate-binding antacids
Severe thermal burns
Recovery from diabetic ketoacidosis
Hyperalimentation
Nutritional recovery syndrome
Respiratory alkalosis
Therapeutic hyperthermia
Neuroleptic malignant syndrome
Recovery from exhaustive exercise
Renal transplantation
Acute renal failure

Chronic Alcoholism and Alcohol Withdrawal

Chronic alcoholism and alcohol withdrawal are the most common causes of severe hypophosphatemia. That hypophosphatemia occurs in as many as 50 percent of hospitalized alcoholics is widely appreciated [96]. Most chronic alcoholics who are not acutely ill show either a normal or slightly depressed serum phosphorus concentration. It is commonly observed that hospitalized alcoholic patients have been unable to eat for a period of days before admission to the hospital or, alternatively, enter a state of alcohol withdrawal. Two important factors generally explain hypophosphatemia in such patients. First, administration of intravenous fluids containing nutrients without phosphorus may cause cellular uptake. Second, the usual hyperventilation and respiratory alkalosis that prevail in withdrawing alcoholics may also result in hypophosphatemia due to cellular uptake. Before withdrawal occurs, ketoacidosis may cause heavy phosphorus losses in urine [73].

Some alcoholic patients become hypomagnesemic and show modest total body deficits of magnesium [50]. In animals, magnesium depletion causes an elevation of serum phosphorus, phosphaturia, and severe phosphorus deficiency in skeletal muscle [21,105]. Thus, in experimental magnesium deficiency, phosphorus deficiency occurs despite an abundant dietary phosphorus intake [24].

Table 10-3. Muscle cell composition*

	P	*Mg*	*Ca*	*Na*	*Cl*	*K*
Normal subjects (n = 12)	28.7	8.1	1.8	9.9	7.5	42.8
Alcholic patients (n = 23)	20.4	6.0	6.2	25.1	12.0	35.8
Normal dogs (n = 11)	29.1	8.9	1.8	13.2	5.8	42.7
Alcoholic dogs (n = 12)	21.3	7.8	3.1	24.5	10.8	31.1

* mmol (P) or mEq/100 gm fat-free dry weight.

Although the foregoing events would adequately explain the development of hypophosphatemia in the hospitalized alcoholic, the underlying causes are much more complicated. Measurement of muscle composition in severe chronic alcoholics discloses a complex derangement in which total phosphorus and magnesium are abnormally low and sodium, chloride, and calcium contents are abnormally elevated [2,75]. In some patients, potassium content of skeletal muscle is also low. Potassium deficiency in skeletal muscle of alcoholics is seldom severe and when it exists, it is nearly always discovered that dietary potassium intake has been inadequate, or the patient has received diuretics or has experienced diarrhea or vomiting. Clearly, some hypokalemic alcoholics show normal values for muscle potassium content, indicating that their hypokalemia is probably the result of respiratory alkalosis. As indicated in Table 10-3, while the average value for total skeletal muscle phosphorus content in alcoholic patients was 20.4 mmol/100 gm, some patients demonstrate values as low as 12 mmol/100 gm. If one assumes that all muscle tissue is uniformly affected and that skeletal muscle occupies 40 percent of the body mass, the total deficiency of phosphorus in skeletal muscle alone extrapolates to a value of 1800 mmol in those patients with the lower values. Although one can speculate that a poor phosphorus intake and perhaps the associated use of phosphate-binding antacids, magnesium deficiency, vomiting, or diarrhea might have caused such a deficit of phosphorus, we have shown that chronic administration of intoxicating quantities of ethanol to dogs causes equally severe phosphorus deficiency in skeletal muscle despite a generous intake of all essential nutrients, including phosphorus [12,31]. The values we observed in dogs under control conditions and following administration of intoxicating doses of ethanol twice daily for 2 months are also shown in Table 10-3. Our observations suggest that alcohol per se somehow exerts toxicity on the muscle cell and is responsible for disorganization of muscle composition, despite a nutritious diet. The precise cause whereby these effects occur is unknown. Since phosphate transport in nearly all tissues examined is dependent on normal sodium transport [13], perhaps deranged sodium transport is somehow related to loss of phosphate from muscle.

Dietary Deficiency and Phosphate-Binding Antacids

Phosphorus is sufficiently abundant in natural foods that deficiency resulting from an inadequate food intake in normal humans is virtually impossible. To develop phosphorus deficiency as a result of poor dietary intake usually requires that a person also consume large quantities of phosphate-binding antacids. Alternatively, feeding a child or growing animal a phosphorus-deficient diet will cause phosphorus deficiency because new protoplasm will be synthesized without adequate phosphorus to maintain proper tissue stores. A notable exception to this is the chronic alcoholic subject who obtains most of his caloric intake from alcoholic beverages. Ethanol is 7 calories/gm and is generally phosphate free.

Feeding human volunteers a diet selectively deficient in phosphorus along with large quantities of phosphate-binding antacids may in time lead to a rather distinct clinical syndrome. It consists of anorexia, paresthesias, muscular weakness, and bone pain [70]. These symptoms usually do not appear until serum phosphorus concentration falls below 1.0 mg/dl. They improve rapidly when phosphorus is restored to the diet. Of interest, hypercalciuria also occurs. The excess urinary calcium is derived from bone, mobilized from that site as hydroxyapatite (Ca, P, CO_3), perhaps representing an attempt to maintain a normal concentration of phosphorus in serum. Under these conditions, phosphorus virtually disappears from the urine.

Severe Thermal Burns

Patients with extensive third-degree burns whose kidney function remains intact often become hypophosphatemic by the second to the tenth day after their injury. Hypophosphatemia may become severe [67]. According to most observers, as serum phosphorus declines, phosphorus excretion into the urine usually falls to very low levels. Most patients with burns hyperventilate, and consequently respiratory alkalosis may be responsible for the hypophosphatemia.

Phosphorus Deficiency in Diabetes Mellitus

Severe hypophosphatemia is commonly observed in patients undergoing treatment for diabetic ketoacidosis. Untreated patients generally show hyperphosphatemia even though phosphorus deficiency may coexist. Insulin deficiency and acidosis reduce phosphorylation, cellular uptake of glucose, and glycolysis, so that net phosphorus balance by the cell is negative. Deficiency of insulin and excess of glucagon may also contribute to the marked catabolism in DKA.

A number of studies have shown that diabetic ketoacidosis causes net phosphorus losses into the urine [4,45]. Ditzel [27] speculated that phosphate deficiency may be responsible for impaired oxygen release to tissues and hypothetically may play a role in diabetic retinopathy or neuropathy. Because of the assertions that phosphorus deficiency may increase morbidity and since virtually all patients become hypophosphatemic during treatment of diabetic ketoacidosis, it was implicitly assumed that phosphate therapy during management of diabetic ketoacidosis was not only appropriate but effective as well. However, it is to be emphasized that subsequent reevaluation of the foregoing notion has raised a great deal of doubt about the efficacy of phosphate therapy in most patients with diabetic ketoacidosis. In fact, to date there have been six publications [8,36,52,54,63,108] showing clearly that in the majority of patients with diabetic ketoacidosis, total insulin requirements, glucose utilization, time required to correct pH, repair of anion gaps, recovery of red cell organic phosphates and adenine nucleotides to normal, and time required to return to mental alertness are not materially affected by phosphate therapy. A limited number of studies on patients with diabetes mellitus whose disease is well controlled shows no evidence for phosphorus deficiency before they develop ketoacidosis. Most patients with ketoacidosis are admitted to a hospital for treatment within 2 or 3 days after becoming ill, and even though they are wasting phosphorus into the urine, the total body loss does not usually attain a level of importance. When untreated, the serum phosphorus value in these patients is normal or frankly elevated. Although it falls rapidly following treatment with fluids and insulin, provision of sufficient phosphate salts to prevent hypophosphatemia has no apparent salutary effect on the outcome of treatment. For these reasons, blanket recommendations for phosphate therapy for all patients with diabetic ketoacidosis are losing favor.

Seldin and Tarail [91] reported phosphorus excretion rates averaging 80 mg/hour in patients with diabetic ketoacidosis before treatment. If an adult of average size were sick for 3 days, this would produce a total phosphorus deficiency of only 193 mmoles or 0.84 percent of total body phosphorus.

While the foregoing data indicate that net phosphorus deficiency is rather trivial in the majority of patients with diabetic ketoacidosis, a small number, perhaps about 5 percent of patients, will have substantial phosphorus deficiency, and in nearly all of these, it will be clearly evident at the time the diagnosis of ketoacidosis is made. *The evidence for severe phosphorus deficiency in this small number of pa-*

tients consists of a serum phosphorus level that is found to be inappropriately low despite the coexistence of severe metabolic acidosis. In addition, hypophosphatemia is found before treatment with insulin and fluids has been initiated. If phosphate salts are not administered to these patients, their serum phosphorus levels will fall further and perhaps reach levels as low as 0.1 mg/dl. At this level, especially if allowed to persist, several important complications of hypophosphatemia may well appear. In the more common type of patient described earlier in whom phosphate salts are not required, it is common to see serum phosphorus fall from elevated values before treatment to concentrations ranging between 1.5 and 2.4 mg/dl. It is in this group of patients that treatment does not appear to be beneficial. On the other hand, in those patients who have severe phosphorus deficiency at the time when the diagnosis of diabetic ketoacidosis is made, as evidenced by very severe hypophosphatemia, it is assumed that treatment *is* necessary. Several characteristic features will help the clinician predict the existence of severe hypophosphatemia in these patients. Usually, such patients are young type I diabetics. Characteristically, vomiting has not been a pronounced component of their illness. The absence of vomiting permits continued ingestion of large amounts of fluids, which in turn aggravates the usual degree of polyuria. Because of the lack of vomiting and the ability to maintain fluid balance better, the prodrome of diabetic ketoacidosis may be measurable in weeks rather than the usual 2 or 3 days and, accordingly, the opportunity to excrete greater quantities of intracellular ions will be proportionately greater. In addition, many of these patients have hypokalemia at the time of admission despite the coexistence of metabolic acidosis. Generally speaking, a depression of blood pH will usually serve to elevate both serum phosphorus and serum potassium concentrations. When both of these values are either normal or low in the presence of severe untreated diabetic ketoacidosis, one should suspect that their relative deficiencies are proportionately severe.

In summary, modest hypophosphatemia occurs in nearly all patients undergoing treatment for diabetic ketoacidosis. However, it does not consistently indicate an important degree of phosphorus deficiency. This explains the inability to demonstrate any useful benefit in routinely using phosphate supplements for most patients. In contrast, some patients, usually young persons, may develop diabetic ketoacidosis more slowly, which permits development of severe phosphorus depletion. Such patients should receive phosphorus salts during treatment of diabetic ketoacidosis.

Hyperalimentation

Administration of nutrients in large quantities either intravenously or via the gut may cause severe hypophosphatemia. This requires (1) an inadequate quantity of phosphorus in the diet in comparison to total calories and other nutrients and (2) a cellular mass that is shrunken but yet capable of an anabolic response. Most clinical instances of hyperalimentation-induced hypophosphatemia occur in patients with severe weight loss or with gastrointestinal disorders who are unable to consume or absorb adequate nutrients. As will be pointed out subsequently, some of the most convincing cause-and-effect relationships between hypophosphatemia, erythrocyte dysfunction, and central nervous system dysfunction have been described in this setting.

Nutritional Recovery Syndrome

The nutritional recovery or refeeding syndrome represents a constellation of findings consisting of heart failure and a variety of electrolyte derangements observed during treatment of patients with severe protein-calorie malnutrition or starvation. In contrast to hyperalimentation, hypophosphatemia may occur during administration of calories in normally required quantities.

This syndrome can be reproduced in experimental animals and is commonly seen during overzealous feeding of patients who have lost marked quantities of weight as the result of food fadism or anorexia nervosa [57,103]. Based on clinical descriptions, such patients present many of the complications observed in starved prisoners encountered after World War II. In addition to hypophosphatemia provoked by nutrients, such patients show other serious disturbances such as hypokalemia, hypomagnesemia, metabolic acidosis, and severe glucose intolerance. The observation that feeding with small quantities of skim milk rather than pure carbohydrates causes less morbidity is very likely ascribable to the reduced calories and the higher phosphorus and potassium content of skim milk.

Respiratory Alkalosis

Mild hyperventilation induces a slight decline of phosphorus concentration. However, that prolonged, intense hyperventilation may lead to a decline of serum phosphorus to values in the vicinity of 0.5 mg/dl is well known [76]. This could have an important bearing on the appearance of severe hypophosphatemia in patients withdrawing from alcohol and in patients who hyperventilate because of various metabolic encephalopathies.

Acute panic disorder [20] represents a constellation of symptoms including headache, a perception of dyspnea, paresthesias, and a sensation of impending doom that occurs in clusters. It is clearly associated with hyperventilation and respiratory alkalosis. As one would expect, hypophosphatemia and hypokalemia are common. Of interest, certain persons with this poorly understood syndrome show clearly reproducible attacks during infusion with sodium lactate [42]. Compared to control subjects, patients with panic attacks have low resting values for phosphorus and after administration of 350 mmol of sodium lactate over a period of 20 minutes show a fall from an average of 2.4 mg/dl to 1.7 mg/dl. Some of the patients had values as low as 0.8 mg/dl. In normal subjects, serum phosphorus values did not fall below 2.5 mg/dl.

Hyperthermia

Guntupalli and co-workers [46] have observed that patients undergoing induced hyperthermia as treatment for malignancy show a fall of serum phosphorus from 3.5 ± 0.18 to 0.6 ± 0.1 mg/dl ($p < .001$). Severe hypophosphatemia also occurs in acute heat stroke [60], in which it is thought to be the result of respiratory alkalosis.

Neuroleptic Malignant Syndrome

The neuroleptic malignant syndrome, characterized by autonomic instability, muscular rigidity, dystonia, and hyperpyrexia, occurs in some patients medicated with haloperidol and a variety of dopamine-blocking drugs. Certain neuromuscular components of this disorder, such as rigidity, dystonia, and extrapyramidal signs, sharply differentiate it from heat stroke. In nine patients described by Harsch [48], two developed major rhabdomyolysis and acute renal failure. It was notable that of the nine, only these two showed severe hypophosphatemia (levels were 0.7 and 1.1 mg/dl) early in the illness. Although there is no evidence that hypophosphatemia plays an etiologic role in the neuroleptic malignant syndrome, the relationship between hypophosphatemia and rhabdomyolysis appears to be well established, as will be described later in this chapter.

Hypophosphatemia After Running

Severe hypophosphatemia (0.1 mg/dl) has also been observed in competitive runners after completing a "half" marathon [22, 23]. In fact, it appears to be lower in those who collapse. Measurements of serum phosphorus later showed spontaneous recovery. Unfortunately, body temperature or pH data were not available. It was suggested [107] that rapid cellular uptake of phosphorus to resynthesize phosphocreatine following the run was the likely explanation [26].

THE EFFECT OF ACUTE HYPOPHOSPHATEMIA WITHOUT PHOSPHORUS DEFICIENCY IN NORMAL SUBJECTS

Whether severe hypophosphatemia has any adverse effects when it occurs in a healthy person is an unsettled issue. Patients with neurotic hyperventilation may show serum phosphorus values less than 1.0 mg/dl when they experience paresthesias, tetany, and light-headedness. Nonetheless, no specific disorders related to hypophosphatemia have been described in such patients. Similarly, there has been no indication that voluntary hyperventilation of sufficient magnitude to reduce serum phosphorus to such levels has caused any harmful effects. In studies [61] of underweight but normal dogs made hypophosphatemic by hyperalimentation (serum P $<$ 1.0 mg/dl), no chemical evidence of tissue injury was observed.

Many investigators have found that feeding a diet deficient in phosphorus results in immediate mobilization of bone apatite so as to provide a source of phosphorus to maintain serum levels within a normal range (see below). Our own studies [61] suggest that acute hypophosphatemia also rapidly mobilizes phosphorus from muscle.

Balance studies were performed by Montanari and colleagues [74] in previously normal humans with coma due to head injury. Their serum phosphorus declined from normal to severely depressed values (0.2–0.4 mmol/liter) during 11 days of total parenteral nutrition. Mean negative cumulative balance of phosphorus did not exceed 50 mmol, and skeletal muscle content of phosphorus showed a small, but distinct decline of about 10 percent of baseline values. These human studies agree with those in animals suggesting that internal redistribution of phosphorus from blood and skeletal muscle to other tissues takes place during phosphorus-deficient parenteral nutrition, resulting in hypophosphatemia.

The foregoing studies suggest that hypophosphatemia of itself, and of short duration, apparently causes no harmful effects to the muscle cell. This would explain why evidence of cellular injury is generally lacking in patients with simple hyperventilation-induced respiratory alkalosis and the large number of clinical conditions associated with modest degrees of hypophosphatemia in which phosphorus deficiency apparently does not coexist. In contrast, if cell injury caused by actual phosphorus deficiency [59] or chronic alcoholism [58] preexists, then induction of acute hypophosphatemia by hyperalimentation may be associated with evidence of frank cellular destruction.

Progressive, severe phosphorus depletion associated with hypophosphatemia is a well-recognized cause of acute rhabdomyolysis, especially in the setting of alcoholic withdrawal [2, 38, 55, 58, 59] or less commonly in total parenteral nutrition [74, 75]. Cardiomyopathy has also been well characterized [25, 39, 40, 79, 102].

HYPOPHOSPHATEMIC SYNDROMES

Respiratory Insufficiency

A rather distinctive syndrome of progressive respiratory insufficiency has been described in patients with hypophosphatemia that may be caused by diaphragmatic weakness or neurologic impairment or both.

Several clinical reports have described patients treated with total parenteral nutrition (TPN) who have developed acute hypophosphatemia associated with respiratory failure.[17, 35, 41, 49, 64, 77, 80, 82, 112]. A number of these patients became seriously ill because of respiratory acidosis and hypoxia. Most were in intensive care unit settings and were desperately ill, and some were also receiving large amounts of glucose or amino acids intravenously. Some of the patients demonstrated abnormalities of central nervous system function or peripheral neuropathy. Although profound weakness and muscle paralysis in some of the patients suggested the Guillain-Barré syndrome, the cerebrospinal fluid was usually normal. In many instances, patients could not be weaned from respirators at the anticipated time.

Nearly all patients who have developed acute respiratory failure in the presence of hypophosphatemia induced by TPN had preexisting conditions that would be expected to cause abnormalities of muscle cell ion transport and element composition. Reported instances of this interesting phenomenon have occurred in patients with chronic intestinal fistulas, malabsorption syndrome, Crohn's disease, ulcerative colitis, small bowel resecton, exocrine pancreatic insufficiency, chronic alcoholism associated with malnutrition, and gastrointestinal cancer. Others have suffered from chronic respiratory acidosis or cor pulmonale [98]. In each instance, serum phosphorus concentrations have been less than 1.0 mg/dl when respiratory failure occurred. In some cases, the patients were also hypokalemic. However, as in the report of Newman, Neff, and Ziporin [77], respiratory failure persisted despite correction of hypokalemia, apparently responding to subsequent administration of phosphate salts and correction of hypophosphatemia. Experimental studies of phosphorus-deficient dogs also showed diminished diaphragm function as a result of muscular weakness [81]. In the patient described by Ritz [85], it is doubtful that a serum potassium value of 3.1 mEq/liter could be responsible for the advanced state of neuromuscular dysfunction.

Oddly enough, *frank clinically evident rhabdomyolysis almost never occurs in patients who slowly become hypophosphatemic during hyperalimentation.* More subtle degrees of rhabdomyolysis in patients with respiratory failure and muscular paralysis could occur, but this is difficult to ascertain since muscle enzyme data are missing from nearly all reports. In line with the cases described by Newman, Neff, and Ziporin [77, 78] in which creatine phosphokinase values were normal, rhabdomyolysis in this setting is probably absent or mild. This speculation is based on the fact that serum phosphorus in such patients remains profoundly depressed day after day and does not follow the usual course of spontaneous correction as ordinarily seen in acute rhabdomyolysis [59]. That serum phosphorus may be within normal limits or even elevated in the presence of acute rhabdomyolysis induced by phosphorus depletion and hypophosphatemia has been recognized in studies of both humans [59] and animals [39]. In such instances, the initial hypophosphatemia is presumably missed, and it is assumed that the residual phosphorus content of skeletal muscle is released in sufficient quantities to correct the preexistent hypophosphatemia. In fact, in our previously reported clinical studies [59], the serum phosphorus concentration was higher and the muscle phosphorus content lower in those patients with the greatest clinical degree of rhabdomyolysis. The "masking" of phosphorus deficiency as the cause of muscle injury in such instances might also explain the report by Stewart and Hensley [97], who described acute rhabdomyolysis during the course of TPN in a woman with long-standing celiac disease and esophageal carcinoma. Her symptoms appeared on the twentieth day of TPN, and according to their report, hypophosphatemia was excluded. In such cases, muscle phosphorus measurements might have proved the cause to be phosphorus deficiency. Because of such observations, namely, that acute rhabdomyolysis may spontaneously correct hypophosphatemia, the possibility arises that rhabdomyolysis might sometimes be a useful biologic event intended to cure hypophosphatemia endogenously so as to provide inorganic phosphate to sustain energy metabolism in vital organs. Rhabdomyolysis apparently does not occur as a consequence of acute hypophosphatemia unless muscle cell injury preexists. Thus, almost all cases of hypophosphatemic rhabdomyolysis occur in alcoholics, who probably all have preexistent muscle cell damage [59]. This relationship may also explain the observation that the respiratory insufficiency syndrome and the hypophosphatemic neurologic syndromes are hardly ever seen in alcoholics because rhabdomyolysis usually corrects their hypophosphatemia spontaneously. It must be appreciated that the extent of rhabdomyolysis may be minimal, and acute renal failure is not inevitable [9].

As reported by several authors [5, 43, 98], acute hypophosphatemia may supervene in patients with preexisting chronic pulmonary disease and respiratory insufficiency. This may occur as a consequence of artificial ventilation, intravenous nutrient administration, or both. Respiratory muscle weakness, which is a well-known component of respiratory insufficiency in such patients, may be exacerbated further by hypophosphatemia. Thus, weaning these patients from mechanical ventilation may become difficult. Conversely, phosphorus administration is able to improve ventilatory function significantly, as demonstrated by measuring diaphragm contractility [5] or inspiratory and expiratory pressures [43].

Fiaccadori and colleagues [33, 34] observed

that patients with chronic obstructive pulmonary disease and acute respiratory failure show alterations in muscle cell composition surprisingly similar to those demonstrated in chronically phosphorus-depleted animals (elevated sodium and water, low potassium and magnesium, depressed ATP content and energy charge potential). Also muscle phosphorus was reduced both in quadriceps femoris and, more importantly, in intercostal muscles [32]. Thus it would be expected that superimposition of acute hypophosphatemia results not only in worsening of respiratory failure, but also in skeletal muscle injury. However, in spite of such muscle changes conceivably predisposing to muscle cell necrosis, frank rhabdomyolysis has never been reported in respiratory insufficiency with hyposphosphatemia. This might extend further the previously described concept that alcohol-induced severe muscle damage may be in some way a specific prerequisite for clinically evident rhabdomyolysis in hypophosphatemia.

In nonalcoholic patients with respiratory insufficiency, muscle cells have presumably not been damaged sufficiently that hypophosphatemic rhabdomyolysis could occur.

It should be kept in mind that respiratory failure appearing during the course of TPN is not always the result of hypophosphatemia. Covelli and associates [19] described three patients who developed respiratory acidosis that was not apparently associated with hypophosphatemia or other recognizable element disturbance. Rather, it occurred as the patients received increased carbohydrate loads. In these patients, ventilatory capacity was not sufficient to remove the increased quantity of carbon dioxide produced by metabolism. It is well known that patients who are debilitated or starved show depression of the hypoxic ventilatory response [16, 29].

Erythrocyte Dysfunction in Phosphorus Deficiency and Hypophosphatemia

Erythrocyte dysfunction specifically impairing release of oxygen from oxyhemoglobin may play a critical role in central nervous system dysfunction in hypophosphatemia. For this reason, the following discussion will consider the clinical settings associated with hypophosphatemia that affect 2,3-DPG.

Two important abnormalities of red cells may occur in phosphorus deficiency: impairment of oxygen release and, in rare instances, hemolysis. The red cell is unique in that it is the only tissue in the body that produces 2,3-DPG [44]. 2,3-DPG becomes bound to hemoglobin and serves to enhance dissociation of oxygen from the hemoglobin molecule. ATP also has this effect, but to a much lesser extent. The interaction of 2,3-DPG with oxyhemoglobin has been well characterized [10, 66]. Its functional status may be expressed quantitatively by the term P_{50}, which refers to the oxygen tension at which hemoglobin is 50 percent saturated. The normal value for P_{50} is about 27 ± 1.2 mm Hg. Severe phosphorus deficiency may reduce P_{50} to the vicinity of 16 mm Hg. In studies in which red cells were depleted of ATP and 2,3-DPG, it has been observed that either when phosphorus is restored to previously hypophosphatemic cells or when adenosine is added in the presence of phosphorus, the recovery rate of 2,3-DPG exceeds that of ATP [83, 99].

Diabetic Ketoacidosis

Both metabolic acidosis [3] and severe phosphorus deficiency reduce red cell 2,3-DPG. Ditzel [28] postulated that impaired red cell delivery of oxygen to critical tissues such as the brain might be implicated in diabetic ketoacidosis with coma. He also proposed that subtle abnormalities of oxygen release in peripheral tissues could be implicated in such complications as diabetic neuropathy, retinopathy, endothelial injury, or other vascular complications in longstanding diabetes mellitus. Although certain older studies on patients with diabetic ketoacidosis reported many years ago [14, 44, 47] suggested that severe phosphorus deficiency was the rule in all cases of diabetic ketoacidosis, this was not confirmed by others [4, 91]. As pointed out before, the vast majority of patients with diabetic ketoacidosis develop this complication over just a few days, so that there has not been adequate time to permit development of severe phosphorus deficiency. On the other hand, newly discovered diabetics who have been out of control for prolonged periods have had more opportunity to develop serious phosphorus depletion.

In diabetic ketoacidosis, measurements of red cell 2,3-DPG content are most often only slightly depressed and show a pattern of rapid recovery during treatment despite the almost invariable occurrence of transient hypophosphatemia. Keller and Berger [54] compared 12 patients with diabetic ketoacidosis who were not treated with phosphate and 12 patients who were treated with phosphate. Red cell 2,3-DPG was depressed in both groups initially, and although the rate of recovery was slightly more rapid in those treated with phosphate, recovery also progressed rapidly in the untreated group. In practical terms, the difference was probably not sufficient to be important clinically. In addition, this study also indicates that 2,3-DPG levels in red cells can be restored despite worsening hypophosphatemia.

Kono, Kuwajima, and Tarui [63] examined red cell glycolytic compounds and adenine nucleotides in six patients with diabetic ketoacidosis. Although hypophosphatemia appeared in each patient during treatment, red cell 2,3-DPG was reconstituted despite a progressive fall of serum phosphorus concentration. Data from a representative patient in this report are shown in Figure 10-1. This was a 45-year-old man whose plasma glucose concentration was 583 mg/dl. His arterial pH on admission was 7.06, PCO_2 was 12.6 mm Hg, and bicarbonate concentration 3.3 mEq/liter. Large concentrations of ketones were present in both blood and urine. As arterial pH was corrected, his serum phosphorus values fell from greater than 10 to a value less than 1 mg/dl. As serum phosphorus

Fig. 10-1. Biochemical data on patient with diabetic ketoacidosis. For explanation, refer to text. F-6-P = fructose 6-phosphate; F-D-P = fructose-diphosphate; 2,3-DPG = 2,3-diphosphoglycerate; ATP = adenosine triphosphate; AMP = adenosine monophosphate; ADP = adenosine diphosphate. (Reprinted with permission from N. Kono, M. Kuwajima, and S. Tarui, *Diabetes* 30:346. Copyright © 1981 by the American Diabetes Association.)

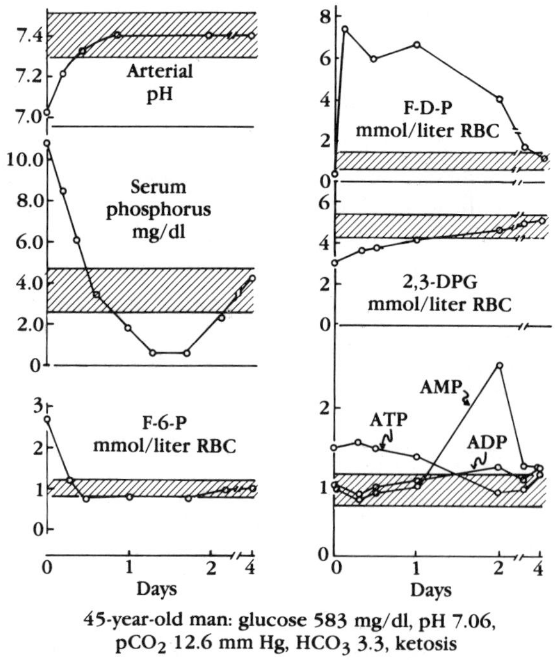

fell and pH was corrected, the value for fructose 6-phosphate, initially elevated, rapidly fell to a normal range. On the other hand, the initial fructose diphosphate values were abnormally low but increased rapidly in response to improvement of acidosis and remained elevated until treatment was underway for a period of 2 days. Of interest, his value for 2,3-DPG was slightly depressed but rose to normal within 24 hours with correction of pH and without treatment with phosphate. It is notable that his red cell content of ATP was slightly elevated on admission.

This patient is probably representative of the great majority of diabetics with ketoacidosis as they are admitted to the hospital. Phosphorus deficiency had not become so severe as to result in gross distortions of red cell glycolytic products or adenine nucleotides. One of the most important regulators of phosphofructokinase (PFK) activity is pH. The studies by Kono, Kuwajima, and Tarui [63] suggest that the bulk of glycolytic abnormalities in diabetic ketoacidosis result from inhibition of PFK activity because of metabolic acidosis. This effect is independent of hypophosphatemia or depletion of intracellular stores of phosphorus. Thus, simple correction of acidosis is usually sufficient to correct these abnormalities. Such findings cast doubt upon Ditzel's hypothesis [28] that vascular disease or perhaps retinopathy could have resulted from repeated bouts of cellular hypoxia related to deficient 2,3-DPG in red cells in poorly controlled diabetics. Of practical importance, such information clearly indicates that the majority of patients with diabetic ketoacidosis do not require treatment with phosphorus.

Hyperalimentation

In contrast to diabetic ketoacidosis, in which phosphorus deficiency is ordinarily mild, severe deficiency may occur in other conditions. Indeed, patients treated for inanition or anorexia nervosa by TPN have developed some of the most remarkable and most serious complications of hypophosphatemia [69].

Travis and associates [99] measured intermediary glycolytic products in red cells from five patients whose serum phosphorus concentration fell to 1 mg/dl or less during the course of intravenous hyperalimentation. The sum of dihydroxyacetone phosphate and glyceraldahyde 3-phosphate (together referred to as triose phosphates) is about 8 μmol/ml in normal red cells. In patients with severe phosphorus deficiency, this value rises enormously to a range of 200 to 600 μmol/ml. This piling up of triose phosphates in red cells occurs because inorganic phosphate is a cofactor necessary for activity of glyceraldehyde-3-phosphate dehydrogenase, which facilitates conversion of triose phosphates to 1,3-diphosphoglycerate. As a consequence, erythrocyte glycolysis after this step is suppressed. Thereby, both 2,3-DPG and ATP synthesis may be severely compromised.

According to Travis and colleagues [99], the decline of ATP has two additional important effects. First, low ATP decreases red cell hexokinase activity and thus retards formation of glucose phosphate. Thereby, the supply of precursor for all glycolytic organic products in the cell is reduced. Second, low ATP increases the activity of PFK. Thereby, conversion of fructose 6-phosphate to fructose diphosphate and, in turn, triose phosphates increases. Administration of intravenous phosphate for 2 days was associated with a prompt recovery of 2,3-DPG to normal despite a simultaneous decline of serum phosphorus from 0.9 to 0.6 mg/dl. The important studies by Travis and colleagues [99] and Kono, Kuwajima, and Tarui [63] point out clearly that red cell glycolytic products and adenine nucleotides depend not only on inorganic phosphate stores but, of equal importance, on the pH status of the cell. The contrasting effects of these two clinical states are shown in Figure 10-2.

Sodium concentration and transmembrane transport were measured in erythrocytes of patients with acute hypophosphatemia by Borghi and co-workers [15]. They found an 80 percent increase in red cell sodium concentration and a marked reduction in the ouabain-sensitive component of sodium efflux rate constant (sodium-potassium pump). The relationship of sodium efflux to the pump rate constant was altered, indicating impairment of the response of the pump to changes in red cell sodium concentration. These abnormalities of the red cell sodium pump may be reliably attributed to the low ATP

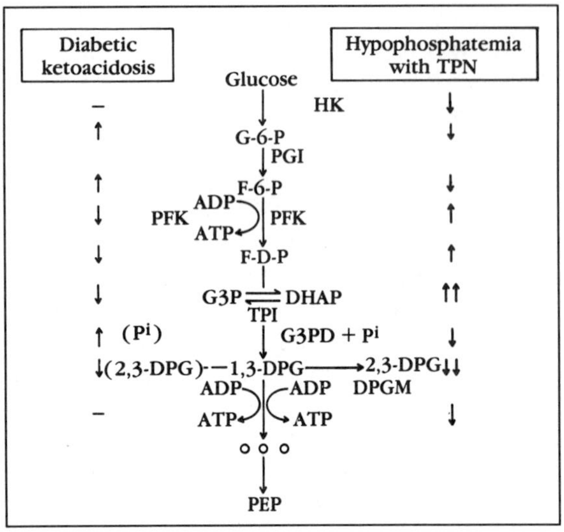

Fig. 10-2. The arrows indicate the deviation of red blood cell metabolite concentrations from normal, in patients with hypophosphatemia during treatment of diabetic ketoacidosis and in patients with hypophosphatemia induced by total parenteral hyperalimentation (TPN). For detailed explanation, see text. HK = hexakinase; G-6-P = glyceraldehyde 6-phosphate; F-6-P = fructose 6-phosphate; ADP = adenosine diphosphate; ATP = adenosine triphosphate; PFK = phosphofructokinase; F-D-P = fructose diphosphate; G3P = glyceraldehyde -3-phosphate; DHAP = dihydroxyacetone phosphate; TPI = triose phosphate; G3PD = glyceraldehyde-3-phosphate dehydrogenase; P^i = inorganic phosphate; 2,3-DPG = 2,3-diphosphoglycerate; 1,3-DPG = 1,3 diphosphoglycerate; DPGM = diphosphoglycerate mutase; PEP = phospherolpyruvate.

content of hypophosphatemic erythrocytes [69, 99], although ATP was not measured in that study. The role of such an abnormality of cation transport in the red cell is uncertain. Rather, the hypothesis may be advanced that the hypophosphatemia-induced defect in sodium-potassium pump rate found in the red cell reflects a more generalized ion transport disturbance equally affecting more complex tissues such as skeletal muscle and the nervous system. Actually, changes in intra/extracellular cation distribution compatible with defective sodium-potassium pump occur in acutely hypophosphatemic animals [58] and humans [75]. In addition, elevated muscle sodium with low resting membrane potential [38] and reduced ATP content [61] have been found in experimental chronically phosphorus-depleted dogs.

Nervous System Dysfunction in Hypophosphatemia

Dysfunction of the central nervous system has been well characterized in severe hypophosphatemia, especially during the course of hyperalimentation in patients with disease causing severe weight loss. A sequence of symptoms compatible with a metabolic encephalopathy has been described by Silvis and colleagues [93, 94]. In such patients, hypophosphatemia usually occurs after approximately 1 week or more of hyperalimentation with solutions of glucose and/or amino acids not containing enough phosphorus to prevent hypophosphatemia. The sequence of abnormalities consists of irritability, apprehension, muscular weakness, numbness, paresthesias, dysarthria, confusion, obtundation, convulsive seizures, coma, and death. Although such a clinical state could be confused with that of delirium tremens in the alcoholic, the lucid visual and auditory hallucinations in the alcoholic usually do not occur in the patient with hypophosphatemia. Obviously both conditions may coexist. Travis and associates [99] described paresthesias about the mouth and the limbs, mental obtundation, and hyperventilation in three of eight patients who became hypophosphatemic during hyperalimentation. At the same time, these patients displayed a sharp drop in red cell 2,3-DPG content and a marked drop in their hemoglobin P_{50} values. These findings were correlated with an abnormality of the electroencephalogram. Both abnormalities disappeared and the patients recovered symptomatically as hypophosphatemia was corrected. Indeed, red cell 2,3-DPG returned to normal during supplementation with phosphorus despite worsening hypophosphatemia reflecting cellular uptake of phosphorus. Most notably, such symptoms do not occur when adequate phosphorus is provided to prevent hypophosphatemia during hyperalimentation.

Emphasis has been placed on the importance of central nervous system complications in patients who slowly develop severe hypophosphatemia during the course of hyperalimentation induced by TPN [17, 85, 93, 94, 99, 111]. However, symptoms and findings more recently emphasized include ptosis, amblyopia, distortions of color perception, dysphagia, dysphonia, impairment in the ability to swallow secretions, respiratory weakness, and hypercarbia in a setting of profound muscle weakness and diminished deep tendon reflexes. As pointed out in the section dealing with respiratory insufficiency, some patients with slowly developing hypophosphatemia develop all clinical features of the Guillain-Barré syndrome with ascending paralysis, areflexia, and respiratory muscle paralysis [87]. Obviously a patient with this complication who also displays ophthalmoplegia and bulbar dysfunction must have the diagnosis of botulism excluded. Such a case was described in a patient with anorexia nervosa treated by TPN [6]. Other cases closely resemble Wernicke's encephalopathy [101], in which dramatic improvement has been observed following correction of hypophosphatemia. Asterixis has also been described [95]. Peripheral neuropathy documented by nerve conduction studies has also been reported [110]. A syndrome resembling encephalitis has been described in children with malnutrition who became ill after 1 week of refeeding [51]. Although phosphorus levels were not measured, the possibility of hypophosphatemia seems likely. These children developed coarse tremors resembling parkinsonism, mainly involving the upper extremities, but also the legs, neck, and tongue. They remained alert. Freiman, Pettifor, and Moodley [37] described hypotonia in infants undergoing treatment for protein-calorie malnutrition. They also described a markedly positive correlation between hypophosphatemia and the occurrence of death during treatment. Obviously, all levels of nervous system dysfunction may be seen. As one might suspect, smooth muscle function is also apparently affected by severe hypophosphatemia as evidenced by ileus.

Table 10-4. Neuromuscular manifestations associated with hypophosphatemia and phosphorus deficiency

Anorexia
Tremors
Irritability
Apprehension
Numbness
Confusion
Disorientation
Obtundation
Anisocoria
Lethargy
Hyperventilation
Seizures
Abnormal electroencephalogram
Coma
Death
Athetosis
Myoclonus
Ballismus
Asterixis
Dysarthria
Nasal speech
Ptosis
Swallowing disturbances
Amblyopia
Color distortion
Ataxia
Paresthesias
Hyporeflexia
Peripheral neuropathy
Muscle paralysis
Abnormal nerve conduction velocity
Abnormal resting membrane potential
Guillian-Barré-Strohl-like syndrome
Wernicke-like syndrome
Hypotonia in infants
Encephalitis-like syndrome in infants (?)
Generalized muscle weakness
Rhabdomyolysis

As listed in Table 10-4, all levels of nervous system dysfunction may be seen in association with hypophosphatemia. Obviously, different regions of central and peripheral nervous system may be unpredictably affected. Polyneuroradicular symptoms are consistent with prominent impairment of cranial or spinal nerves. Partial bulbar palsy may be suspected when ptosis, dysarthria, and difficulty in swallowing are associated with alveolar hypoventilation. Other findings such as ataxia suggest pontocerebellar dysfunction. Basal ganglia seem to be affected when hypophosphatemic patients develop asterixis or tremors.

Symptoms of hypophosphatemic metabolic encephalopathy suggest a generalized impairment of brain function. An attractive but unproven hypothesis may be that this latter condition reflects a prominent effect of impairment in brain oxygenation resulting from red cell dysfunction [93, 94, 99].

It is worth reemphasizing that in patients who develop syndromes of central or peripheral nervous system dysfunction, and also in those who develop respiratory failure as a result of hypophosphatemia, rhabdomyolysis is virtually nonexistent. Presumably, the apparent prerequisite for ongoing skeletal muscle injury is missing. The failure to develop rhabdomyolysis results in inexorable and progressive hypophosphatemia and thus permits full expression of nervous system failure. In addition, it is noteworthy that most of these patients are not alcoholics. Ironically, the alcoholic, probably because of preexisting muscle injury, rapidly develops rhabdomyolysis with hypophosphatemia and thereby spontaneously corrects the hypophosphatemia without developing nervous system syndromes or respiratory failure. In this sense, chronic alcoholism may have a protective effect.

Malnourished dogs treated with hyperalimentation so as to deliberately induce hypophosphatemia develop ataxia, convulsions, and death [86, 111]. In both our studies [58] and others [86], animals deprived of phosphorus during hyperalimentation developed pronounced weakness, fasciculations, and profound anorexia and would usually die after about 5 to 7 days. Their serum phosphorus values were well below 1 mg/dl. In contrast, animals fed the same diet containing phosphorus did not have to be gavage fed and displayed no symptoms whatsoever except apparent hunger.

Although central nervous system manifestations of phosphorus deficiency appear to occur with regularity in experimental animals and in patients hyperalimented without adequate phosphorus who become hypophosphatemic, to date there has been only one single study of brain chemical composition or histology to characterize this important complication of hypophosphatemia.

Bhaskaran, Massry, and Campese [11] showed marked alterations in catecholamine content of the brain with reduced norepinephrine, epinephrine, and dopamine levels in several regions of central nervous system in rats submitted to phosphorus depletion for 8 weeks. They suggested that such changes may play a role in the brain dysfunction of the phosphate-depleted state. However, an 8-week period of phosphate depletion is able to reduce blood pressure substantially in rats [90]. Thus, it could not be excluded that abnormalities in brain catecholamines were secondary to hypotension in this rat model of phosphate depletion.

TREATMENT OF HYPOPHOSPHATEMIA

Any patient under treatment for severe weight loss by oral refeeding and most especially TPN should be observed very carefully for central or peripheral nervous system dysfunction, cardiopulmonary failure, and a number of acute metabolic disturbances. The last include hypophosphatemia, hypokalemia, hypomagnesemia, metabolic acidosis, and disturbances of blood glucose concentration. Excellent examples illustrating the potentially tragic consequences of refeeding have been published by Weinsier and Krumdieck [104] and Sheridan and Collins [92]. All of these complications are preventable.

The major question in the evaluation of a patient with hypophosphatemia is whether the low serum phosphorus concentration is indicative of a true phosphorus deficiency syndrome. It is reemphasized that less than 0.5 percent of total body phosphorus is present in the extracellular fluid pool; accordingly, hypophosphatemia does not necessarily denote phosphorus deficiency, since it may be consequent to no more than an intracellular shift. For example, in a previously healthy subject, acute hyperventilation, which induces an acute and transient shift of extracellular fluid phosphorus to the intracellular space, can cause a similar degree of hypophosphatemia to that observed after prolonged nausea and vomiting in a chronic alcoholic patient with alcoholic ketoacidosis. The hypophosphatemia in the previously healthy subject with acute hyperventilation, however, is associated with normal body phosphorus stores and does not require treatment, whereas the same degree of hypophosphatemia in the alcoholic patient or the patient undergoing nutritional replacement most likely represents phosphorus deficiency and requires phosphate replacement therapy.

In most cases of hypophosphatemia, the need for phosphate supplementation can be determined as follows. First, a careful history, physical examination, and review of the medications and intravenous fluid therapy, combined with the laboratory data, which include arterial blood gases, urinary phosphorus, and creatinine (for calculation of fractional excretion of phosphorus) can help establish the cause of the hypophosphatemia. The patient's need for phosphate replacement therapy can then be determined from the results of these investigations.

In patients with moderate hypophosphatemia (1.0–2.5 mg/dl), if there is no history of previous renal or gastrointestinal losses, and if there is no evidence of the expected consequences of phosphorus depletion, then there is no need for phosphate replacement. This is especially the case if the hypophosphatemia is caused by hyperventilation or nutrient administration that results in transient shifts of phosphorus from extracellular to intracellular sites. In most of these cases, the identification and treatment of the primary cause usually results in restoration of blood phosphorus concentration to normal. On the other hand, if the hypophosphatemia occurs in wasted patients who are suspected of having previous renal and gastrointestinal phosphorus losses, or in those who have evidence of alcoholism, malnutrition, or increased catabolism, or most importantly, if there is evidence of a phosphorus depletion syndrome, then careful replacement of phosphorus deficiency is indicated.

If the patient is able to tolerate oral intake, the safest and most efficient mode of therapy is the administration of skim or low-fat (0.5% fat) milk, which contains approximately 0.9 mg of phosphorus per milliliter. Milk is also a rich source for calcium, potassium, magnesium, and protein, and its use is ideal in malnourished patients. In severely wasted patients, total fluid volume on the first day should probably not exceed 1.5 liters, of which 0.5 to 1.0 liter could be low-fat milk. This may be gradually increased depending on observation of cardiopulmonary status and laboratory measurements. A typical patient with severe hypophosphatemia would require between 32 to 64 ounces (about 1–2 liters) of milk per day, as each serving of 250 ml contains approximately 235 mg of elemental phosphorus and the average patient requires 1000 to 2000 mg of phosphorus per day to have body stores repleted within 7 to 10 days.

Patients who are unable to tolerate milk can be given any of the oral preparations listed in Table 10-5. Intravenous administration of phosphorus is usually reserved for patients with se-

Table 10-5. Phosphate preparations for intravenous use

Preparation	*Composition (mg/ml)*	*Phosphate (mmol/ml)*	*Sodium (mEq/ml)*	*Potassium (mEq/ml)*
K phosphate	236 mg K_2HPO_4 224 mg KH_2PO_4	3.0	0	4.4
Na phosphate	142 mg Na_2HPO_4 276 mg $NaH_2PO_4 \cdot H_2O$	3.0	4.0	0
Neutral Na phosphate	10.0 mg Na_2HPO_4 2.7 mg $NaH_2PO_4 \cdot H_2O$	0.09	0.2	0
Neutral Na, K phosphate	11.5 mg Na_2HPO_4 2.6 mg KH_2PO_4	1.10	0.2	0.02

vere hypophosphatemia who cannot take milk or tablets, or who are overtly symptomatic and have evidence of erythrocyte, platelet, and leukocyte dysfunction, cardiomyopathy, respiratory muscle weakness, or altered mental status as a result of the severe hypophosphatemia. Since we do not have a practical means to determine the degree of intracellular phosphorus depletion, we cannot calculate the exact amount of phosphorus that needs to be replaced. An earlier study suggested 2.5 to 5.0 mg of elemental phosphorus per kilogram of body weight be administered intravenously every 6 hours to replete phosphorus in patients with severe hypophosphatemia [68], although the efficacy of this therapy was not validated. A more recent study administered 9 mmol of phosphorus in 77 mM NaCl intravenously as a continuous infusion over 12 hours, which corresponds to approximately 2 mg/kg body weight every 6 hours [100]. Employing this regimen, mean serum phosphorus concentration increased from a baseline value of 0.81 mg/dl to 1.27 mg/dl in 12 hours, to 1.67 mg/dl in 24 hours, 2.07 mg/dl in 36 hours, and 2.80 mg/dl in 48 hours. Once a serum phosphorus concentration of 2.0 to 2.5 mg/dl is achieved, it would be safe to switch to oral replacement therapy.

An important factor that should also be considered in the treatment of patients with hypophosphatemia is that some of them may also have low serum magnesium levels. Of note, phosphorus deficiency may result in increased urinary magnesium excretion, and magnesium deficiency may also result in increased urinary phosphorus excretion. Therefore, in selected patients, the hypomagnesemia, if present, may need to be corrected for the successful correction of the hypophosphatemia. In this regard, milk is also a good source for magnesium, as each 250 ml of milk contains 34 mg of this element.

SIDE EFFECTS AND COMPLICATIONS OF TREATMENT OF HYPOPHOSPHATEMIA

The major side effects of phosphorus replacement therapy are diarrhea, especially with oral preparations, and hyperphosphatemia, hypocalcemia, hyperkalemia (if potassium phosphate salts are employed), metabolic acidosis, and volume excess, especially with intravenous preparations.

The diarrhea is a dose-related phenomenon, and it can generally be avoided if phosphorus tablets are given in divided doses and if the total dose is limited to 4 tablets a day.

The hyperphosphatemia is a direct consequence of excessive phosphorus administration, especially if the patient has renal insufficiency. Since intracellular phosphorus depletion cannot be accurately estimated, and since the initial serum concentration response to intravenous phosphorus replacement does not indicate the degree of depletion and also does not predict the serum concentration response to further therapy, one has to monitor the serum phosphorus concentration carefully every 12 to 24 hours during intravenous replacement therapy. One of the consequences of hyperphosphatemia is that it causes hypocalcemia and can result in metastatic calcification and hypotension and impair renal function. Pulmonary vascular calcification with hypoxia due to a diffusion block may be a fatal complication.

Hyperkalemia may occur in patients with decreased renal function and oliguria, since most of the phosphorus preparations contain potassium. Therefore, serum potassium should also be closely monitored during phosphorus administration.

Finally, some of the phosphorus preparations including oral phosphosoda (pH 4.8), acid sodium phosphate (pH 4.9), intravenous sodium phosphate (pH 5.7), and potassium phosphate (pH 6.6) are acidic and when administered in large doses may result in metabolic acidosis.

REFERENCES

1. Albright, F., and Reifenstein, E. C. *The Parathyroid Glands and Metabolic Bone Disease.* Baltimore: Williams & Wilkins, 1948.
2. Anderson, R., Cohen, M., Haller, R., et al. Skeletal muscle phosphorus and magnesium deficiency in alcoholic myopathy. *Miner. Electrolyte Metab.* 4:106, 1980.
3. Astrup, P. Relationship of pH to red cell 2,3-DPG content. *Adv. Exp. Med. Biol.* 6:67, 1970.

4. Atchley, D. W., Loeb, R. F., and Richards, D. W. On diabetic acidosis: A detailed study of electrolyte balances following the withdrawal and reestablishment of insulin therapy. *J. Clin. Invest.* 12:297, 1933.
5. Aubier, M., Murciano, D., Lecocguic, Y., et al. Effect of hypophosphatemia on diaphragmatic contractility in patients with acute respiratory failure. *N. Engl. J. Med.* 313:420, 1985.
6. Backmund, H., and Gerlinghoff, M. Anorexia nervosa: Bedrohlicheneurologische Komplikationen durch hypophosphatemie. *Nervenartz* 57:542, 1986.
7. Baldwin, D., Robinson, P. K., Zierler, K. L., and Libenthal, J. C. Interrelations of magnesium, potassium, phosphorus, and creatinine in skeletal muscle of man. *J. Clin. Invest.* 31:850, 1952.
8. Becker, D. J., Brown, D. R., Steranka, B. H., and Drash, A. L. Phosphate replacement during treatment of diabetic ketosis. *Am. J. Dis. Child.* 137:241, 1983.
9. Better, O. S., and Stein, J. H. Early management of shock and prophylaxis of acute renal failure in traumatic rhabdomyolysis. *N. Engl. J. Med.* 322:825, 1990.
10. Benesch, R., and Benesch, R. E. Intracellular organic phosphates as regulators of oxygen release by hemoglobin. *Biochem. Biophys. Res. Commun.* 26:162, 1967.
11. Bhaskaran, D., Massry, S. G., and Campese, V. M. Effect of hypophosphatemia on brain catecholamines content in the rat. *Miner. Electrolyte Metab.* 13:469, 1987.
12. Blachley, J. D., Ferguson, E. R., Carter, N. W., and Knochel, J. P. Chronic alcohol ingestion induces phosphorus deficiency and myopathy in the dog. *Trans. Assoc. Am. Physicians* 93:110, 1980.
13. Blachley, J. D., Johnson, J. H., and Knochel, J. P. The harmful effects of ethanol on ion transport and cellular respiration. *Am. J. Med. Sci.* 289:22, 1985.
14. Bolger, H. A., and Peters, J. P. The concentration of the blood and of the urine in diabetic toxemia. *Arch. Intern. Med.* 36:857, 1925.
15. Borghi, L., Canali, M., Sani, E., et al. Erythrocyte sodium transport in acute hypophosphatemia in man. *Miner. Electrolyte Metab.* 10:26, 1984.
16. Canham, M. Respiratory acidosis, intermittent ventilation and parenteral nutrition (letter). *Ann. Intern. Med.* 96:254, 1982.
17. Chudley, A., Ninan, A., and Young, G. B. Neurologic signs and hypophosphatemia with total parenteral nutrition. *Can. Med. Assoc. J.* 125:604, 1981.
18. Corredor, D. G., Sabeh, G., Mendelsohn, L. D., et al. Enhanced post glucose hypophosphatemia during starvation therapy of obesity. *Metabolism* 18:754, 1969.
19. Covelli, H. D., Black, J. W., Olsen, M. S., and Beekman, J. F. Respiratory failure precipitated by high carbohydrate loads. *Ann. Intern. Med.* 95:579, 1981.
20. Cowley, D. S., and Roy-Byrne, P. P. Hyperventilation and pain. *Am. J. Med.* 83:929, 1987.
21. Cronin, R. E., Ferguson, E. R., Shannon, W. A., Jr., and Knochel, J. P. Skeletal muscle injury after magnesium depletion in the dog. *Am. J. Physiol.* 243:F113, 1982.
22. Dale, G., and Fleetwood, J. A. Profound hypophosphatemia in patients collapsing after a "fun run." *Br. Med. J.* 292:447, 1986.
23. Dale, G., Fleetwood, J. A., Weddell, A., and Ellis, R. D. Fitness, unfitness, and phosphate. *Br. Med. J.* 294:939, 1987.
24. Danowski, T. S., Gillespie, H. K., Fergus, E. B., and Puntereri, A. J. Significance of blood sugar and serum electrolyte changes in cirrhosis following glucose, insulin, glucagon, or epinephrine. *Yale J. Biol. Med.* 29:361, 1956–1957.
25. Davis, S. V., Olichwier, K. K., and Chakko, S. C. Reversible depression of myocardial performance in hypophosphatemia. *Am. J. Med. Sci.* 295:183, 1988.
26. Dawson, M. J., Gadian, D. J., and Wilkie, D. R. Contraction and recovery of living muscles studied by ^{31}P nuclear magnetic resonance. *Physiol. J.* 267:703, 1977.
27. Ditzel, J. Impaired oxygen release caused by alterations of the metabolism in the erythrocytes in diabetes. *Lancet* 1:721, 1972.
28. Ditzel, J. Importance of plasma inorganic phosphate on tissue oxygenation during recovery from diabetic ketoacidosis. *Horm. Metab. Res.* 5:471, 1973.
29. Doekel, R. C., Jr., Swillich, C. W., Coggin, C. H., et al. Clinical semi-starvation depression of hypoxic ventilatory response. *N. Engl. J. Med.* 295:358, 1976.
30. Drezner, M. K., Lobaugh, B., Lyles, K. W., et al. The Pathogenesis and Treatment of Tumor-Induced Osteomalacia. In A. W. Norman, K. Schaefer, D. Herrath, and H. G. Grigoleit (eds.), *Vitamin D Chemical, Biochemical and Clinical Endocrinology of Calcium Metabolism.* Berlin: Walter de Gruyter, 1982. Pp. 949–954.
31. Ferguson, E. R., Blachley, J. D., Carter, N. W., and Knochel, J. P. Derangements of muscle composition, ion transport and oxygen consumption in chronically alcoholic dogs. *Am. J. Physiol.* 246 (*Renal Fluid Electrolyte Physiol.*) 15:F700, 1984.
32. Fiaccadori, E., Coffrini, E., Vitali, P., et al. Phosphorus Depletion in Axial and Respiratory Muscles of Patients with COPD: A preliminary report. In A. Grasino, C. Rampulla, and N. Ambrosino (eds.), *Chronic Pulmonary Hyperinflation.* New York: Springer-Verlag, 1989.
33. Fiaccadori, E., Del Canale, S., Arduini, U., et al.

Intracellular acid-base and electrolyte metabolism in skeletal muscle of patients with chronic obstructive lung disease and acute respiratory failure. *Clin. Sci.* 71:703, 1986.
34. Fiaccadori, E., Del Canale, S., Vitali, P., et al. Skeletal muscle energetics, acid-base equilibrium and lactate metabolism in patients with severe hypercapnia and hypoxemia. *Chest* 92:883, 1987.
35. Finck, G. A., Mai, C., and Gregor, M. Passagere polyneuropathie mit hirnnervenbeteiligung durch hypophosphatamie. *Nervenarzt* 50:778, 1979.
36. Fisher, J. N., and Kitabachi, A. E. A randomized study of phosphate therapy in the treatment of diabetic ketoacidosis. *J. Clin. Endocrinol. Metab.* 57:177–180, 1983.
37. Freiman, I., Pettifor, J. M., and Moodley, G. M. Serum phosphorus in protein energy malnutrition. *J. Pediatr. Gastroenterol. Nutr.* 1:547, 1982.
38. Fuller, T. J., Carter, N. W., Barcenas, C., and Knochel, J. P. Reversible experimental myopathy associated with phosphorus depletion. *J. Clin. Invest.* 57:1019, 1976.
39. Fuller, T. J., Nichols, W. W., Brenner, B. J., and Peterson, J. C. Effects of phosphorus depletion on left ventricular energy generation. *Adv. Exp. Biol. Med.* 103:395, 1977.
40. Fuller, T. J., Nichols, W. W., Brenner, B. J., et al. Reversible depression in myocardial performance in dogs with experimental phosphorus deficiency. *J. Clin. Invest.* 62:1194, 1978.
41. Furlan, A. J., Hanson, M., Cooperman, A., and Farmer, R. G. Acute areflexic paralysis. *Arch. Neurol.* 32:706, 1975.
42. Gorman, J. M., Cohen, B. S., Liebowicz, M. R., et al. Blood gas changes and hypophosphatemia in lactate-induced panic. *Arch. Gen. Psychiatry* 43:1067, 1986.
43. Gravelyn, T. R., Brophy, N., Siegert, C., and Peters-Golden, P. Hypophosphatemia-associated respiratory muscle weakness in a general inpatient population. *Am. J. Med.* 84:870, 1988.
44. Guest, G. M., and Rapoport, S. Role of acid-soluble phosphorus compounds in red blood cells. *Am. J. Dis. Child.* 58:1072, 1939.
45. Guest, G. M., and Rapoport, S. Clinical studies of the organic acid-soluble phosphorus of red blood cells in different acidotic states. *J. Lab. Clin. Med.* 26:190, 1940.
46. Guntupalli, K. K., Sladen, A., Selker, R. G., et al. Effects of induced total-body hyperthermia on phosphorus metabolism in humans. *Am. J. Med.* 77:250, 1984.
47. Haldane, J. B. S., Wigglesworth, D. B., and Woodrow, C. E. The effect of reaction changes on human inorganic metabolism. *Proc. R. Soc. Med. [Biol.]* 96:1, 1924.
48. Harsch, H. Neuroleptic malignant syndrome: Physiological and laboratory findings in a series of 9 cases. *J. Clin. Psychiatry* 48:328, 1987.
49. Hasselstrøm, L., Wimberley, P. D., and Nielsen, V. G. Hypophosphatemia and acute respiratory failure in a diabetic patient. *Intensive Care Med.* 12:429, 1986.
50. Jones, J. E., Shane, S. R., and Jacobs, W. H. Magnesium balance studies in chronic alcoholism. *Ann. N. Y. Acad. Sci.* 252:274, 1975.
51. Kahn, E., and Falcke, H. C. A syndrome simulating encephalitis affecting children recovering from malnutrition (kwashiorkor). *J. Pediatrics* 49:37, 1956.
52. Kanter, Y., Gerson, J. R., and Bessman, A. N. 2,3-Diphosphoglycerate, nucleotide phosphate, and organic and inorganic phosphate levels during the early phases of diabetic ketoacidosis. *Diabetes* 26:429, 1977.
53. Keitt, A. S. Changes in the content and ^{32}P incorporation of glycolytic intermediates during incubation of normal and hereditary spherocytosis erythrocytes. *Br. J. Haemotol.* 11:177, 1965.
54. Keller, U., and Berger, W. Prevention of hypophosphatemia by phosphate infusion during treatment of diabetic ketoacidosis and hyperosmolar coma. *Diabetes* 29:87, 1980.
55. Knochel, J. P. The pathophysiology and clinical characteristics of severe hypophosphatemia. *Arch. Intern. Med.* 137:203, 1977.
56. Knochel, J. P. Hypophosphatemia in the alcoholic. *Arch. Intern. Med.* 140:613, 1980.
57. Knochel, J. P. Complications of total parenteral nutrition. *Kidney Int.* 27:489, 1985.
58. Knochel, J. P., Barcenas, C., Cotton, J. R., et al. Hypophosphatemia and rhabdomyolysis. *Trans. Assoc. Am. Physicians* 91:156, 1978.
59. Knochel, J. P., Bilbrey, G. L., Fuller, T. J., and Carter, N. W. The muscle cell in chronic alcoholism: The possible role of phosphate depletion in alcoholic myopathy. *Ann. N. Y. Acad. Sci.* 252:274, 1975.
60. Knochel, J. P., and Caskey, J. H. The mechanism of hypophosphatemia in acute heat stroke. *J.A.M.A.* 238:425, 1977.
61. Knochel, J. P., Haller, R., and Ferguson, E. Selective Phosphorus Deficiency in the Hyperalimented Hypophosphatemic Dog and Phosphorylation Potentials in the Muscle Cell. In S. G. Massry, E. Ritz, and H. Jahn (eds.), *Advances in Experimental Medicine and Biology.* Vol. 128: Phosphate and Minerals in Health and Disease. New York: Plenum, 1980. Pp. 323–334.
62. Knox, F., and Haramati, A. Renal Regulation of Phosphate Excretion. D. W. Seldin and G. Giebisch (eds.), The Kidney: Physiology and Pathophysiology. New York: Raven, 1985. Pp. 1390–1391.

63. Kono, N., Kuwajima, M., and Tarui, S. Alteration of glycolytic intermediary metabolism in erythrocytes during diabetic ketoacidosis and its recovery phase. *Diabetes* 30:346, 1981.
64. Lee, K. L., Sibbald, W. J., Holliday, R. L., and Linton, A. L. Hypophosphatemia associated with coma. *Can. Med. Assoc. J.* 119:143, 1978.
65. Lehninger, A. L. *Biochemistry.* New York: Worth, 1975.
66. Lenfant, C., Torrance, J. F., Woodson, R. D., et al. Role of organic phosphates in the adaptation of man to hypoxia. *Fed. Proc.* 29:1115, 1970.
67. Lennquist, S., Lindell, B., Nordstrom, H., and Sjoberg, H. E. Hypophosphatemia in severe burns: A prospective study. *Acta Chir. Scand.* 145:1, 1979.
68. Lentz, R. D., Brown, D. M., and Kjellstrand, C. M. Treatment of severe hypophosphatemia. *Ann. Intern. Med.* 89:941, 1978.
69. Lichtman, M. A., Miller, D. R., Cohen, J., and Waterhouse, C. Reduced red cell glycolysis, 2,3-diphosphoglycerate and adenosine triphosphate concentration, and increased hemoglobin oxygen affinity caused by hypophosphatemia. *Ann. Intern. Med.* 74:562, 1971.
70. Lotz, M., Zisman, E., and Bartter, F. C. Evidence for a phosphorus depletion syndrome in man. *N. Engl. J. Med.* 278:409, 1968.
71. Marshall, R. W. Plasma Fractions. In B. E. C. Nordin, (ed.), *Calcium, Phosphate, and Magnesium Metabolism.* New York: Longman, 1976.
72. Matzner, Y., Prococimer, M., Polliack, A., et al. Hypophosphatemia in a patient with lymphoma in leukemic phase. *Arch. Intern. Med.* 141:805, 1981.
73. Miller, P. D., Heinig, R. E., and Waterhouse, C. Treatment of alcoholic acidosis: The role of dextrose and phosphorus. *Arch. Intern. Med.* 138:67, 1978.
74. Montanari, A., Borghi, L., Curti, A., et al. Acute hypophosphatemia during total parenteral nutrition in man: Its effect on muscle cell composition. *Adv. Exp. Med. Biol.* 151:229, 1982.
75. Montanari, A., Borghi, L., Curti, A., et al. Skeletal muscle cell abnormalities in acute hypophosphatemia during total parenteral nutrition. *Miner. Electrolyte Metab.* 10:52, 1984.
76. Mostellar, M. E., and Tuttle, E. P., Jr. Effects of alkalosis on plasma concentration and urinary excretion of inorganic phosphate in man. *J. Clin. Invest.* 43:138, 1964.
77. Newman, J. H., Neff, T. A., and Ziporin, P. Acute respiratory failure associated with hypophosphatemia. *N. Engl. J. Med.* 296:1101, 1977.
78. Newman, J. H., Neff, T. A., and Ziporin, P. Acute respiratory failure associated with hypophosphatemia (letter). *N. Engl. J. Med.* 297:336, 1977.
79. O'Connor, L. R., Klein, K. L., and Bethune, J. E. Effect of hypophosphatemia on myocardial performance in man. *N. Engl. J. Med.* 297:901, 1977.
80. Oster, P., Rieben, F. W., Schmidt-Gayk, H., and Schlierf, G. Lahmungen bei hypophosphatamie. *Dtsch. Med. Wochenschr.* 102:1422, 1977.
81. Planas, R. F., McBrayer, R. H., and Koen, P. A. Effects of hypophosphatemia on pulmonary muscle performance. *Adv. Exp. Med. Biol.* 151:283, 1982.
82. Prins, J. G., Schrijver, H., and Staghouwer, J. H. Hyperalimentation, hypophosphatemia and coma. *Lancet* 1:1253, 1973.
83. Rapoport, S., Dietz, F., and Sauer, G. Quantitative Aspekte des phosphoglyceratzyklus in roten blutzellen. *Acta Biol. Med. Germ.* 13:693, 1964.
84. Rasmussen, H., and Bordier, P. J. *The Physiological and Cellular Basis of Metabolic Bone Disease.* Baltimore: Williams & Wilkins, 1974.
85. Ritz, E. Acute hypophosphatemia. *Kidney Int.* 22:84, 1982.
86. Rosen, R. A., Leach, W., and Arieff, A. I. Central nervous system dysfunction and hypophosphatemia. *Kidney Int.* 12:460, 1977.
87. Rosenberg, M., McCarten, J. R., Snyder, B. D., and Tulloch, J. W. Hypophosphatemia with reversible ataxia and quadriparesis. *Am. J. Med. Sci.* 93:261, 1987.
88. Ryan, E. A., and Reiss, E. Oncogenous osteomalacia. *Am. J. Med.* 77:501, 1984.
89. Ryback, R. S., Eckardt, M. H., and Pautler, C. P. Clinical relationships between serum phosphorus and other blood chemistry values in alcoholics. *Arch. Intern. Med.* 140:673, 1980.
90. Saglikes, Y., Massry, S. G., Iseki, K., et al. Effect of phosphate depletion on blood pressure and vascular reactivity to norepinephrine and angiotensin II in the rat. *Am. J. Physiol.* 248:F93, 1985.
91. Seldin, D. W., and Tarail, R. The metabolism of glucose and electrolytes in diabetic acidosis. *J. Clin. Invest.* 29:552, 1950.
92. Sheridan, P. H., and Collins, M. Potentially life-threatening hypophosphatemia in anorexia nervosa. *J. Adolesc. Health Care* 4:44, 1983.
93. Silvis, S. E., DiBartolomeo, A. G., and Aaker, H. M. Hypophosphatemia and neurological changes secondary to oral caloric intake. *Am. J. Gastroenterol.* 73:215, 1980.
94. Silvis, S. E., and Paragas, P. D. Paresthesias, weakness, seizures and hypophosphatemia in patients receiving hyperalimentation. *J. Lab. Clin. Med.* 62:513, 1972.
95. Sobrevia, R. S., and Tey, A. D. Asterixis como manifestacion neurologica de hipofosforemia. *Med. Clin. (Barc.)* 83:651, 1984.
96. Stein, J. H., Smith, W. O., and Ginn, H. E. Hypo-

phosphatemia in acute alcoholism. *Am. J. Med. Sci.* 252:78, 1966.
97. Stewart, P. M., and Hensley, W. Acute polymyopathy during total parenteral nutrition. *Br. Med. J.* 283:1578, 1981.
98. Storm, T. L. Severe hypophosphatemia during recovery from acute respiratory acidosis. *Br. Med. J.* 289:456, 1984.
99. Travis, S. F., Sugerman, H. J., Ruberg, R. L., et al. Alterations of red cell glycolytic intermediates and oxygen transport as a consequence of hypophosphatemia in patients receiving intravenous hyperalimentation. *N. Engl. J. Med.* 285: 763, 1971.
100. Vannatta, J. B., Whang, R., and Papper, S. Efficacy of intravenous phosphate therapy in the severely hypophosphatemic patient. *Arch. Intern. Med.* 141:885, 1981.
101. Vanneste, J., and Huge, J. Acute severe hypophosphatemia mimicking Wernicke's encephalopathy. *Lancet* 1:44, 1986.
102. Vered, Z., Battler, A., Motro, M., et al. Left ventricular function in patients with chronic hypophosphatemia. *Am. Heart J.* 107:796, 1984.
103. Weinsier, R. L., and Krumdieck, C. L. Death resulting from overzealous total parenteral nutrition: The refeeding syndrome revisited. *Am. J. Clin. Nutr.* 34:393, 1980.
104. Weinsier, R. L., and Krumdieck, C. L. Death resulting from overzealous total parenteral nutrition: The refeeding syndrome revisited. *Am. J. Clin. Nutr.* 34:393, 1981.
105. Whang, R., and Welt, L. G. Observations in experimental magnesium depletion. *J. Clin. Invest.* 42:305, 1963.
106. Widdowson, E. M., McCance, R. A., and Spray, C. M. The chemial composition of the human body. *Clin. Sci.* 10:113, 1951.
107. Wilkie, D. R. Profound hypophosphatemia in patients collapsing after a "fun run" (letter). *Br. Med. J.* 292:692, 1986.
108. Winter, R. J., Harris, C. J., Phillips, L. S., and Green, O. C. Diabetic ketoacidosis: Induction of hypocalcemia and hypomagnesemia by phosphate therapy. *Am. J. Med.* 67:897, 1979.
109. Wollner, A., Shalit, M., and Brezis, M. Tumor genesis syndrome: Hypophosphatemia accompanying Burkitt's lymphoma cell leukemia. *Miner. Electrolyte Metab.* 12:173, 1986.
110. Yagnik, P., Singh, N., and Burns, R. Peripheral neuropathy with hypophosphatemia in a patient receiving intravenous hyperalimentation. *Southern Med. J.* 78:1381, 1985.
111. Yawata, Y., Craddock, P., Hebbel, R., et al. Hyperalimentation hypophosphatemia: Hematologic and neurologic dysfunction due to ATP depletion. *Clin. Res.* 31:729, 1973.
112. Youssef, H. A. E. Hypophosphatemic respiratory failure complicating total parenteral nutrition: A potentially lethal iatrogenic. *Int. Surg.* 67:371, 1982.
113. Zamkoff, K. W., and Kirschner, J. J. Marked hypophosphatemia associated with acute myelomonocytic leukemia. *Arch. Intern. Med.* 140:1523, 1980.

11 Neurologic Manifestations of Endocrine Dysfunction

Robert C. Griggs

Neurologic abnormalities can occur in most endocrine disorders. Most endocrinopathies can now be recognized early and treated more successfully than in the past. As a result, the fully developed clinical picture of hormonal excess or deficiency is seen only infrequently. The major exception is that, with the continued and even increased use of high-dose corticosteroids, severe exogenous Cushing's syndrome remains frequent, and the neurologic effects of adrenocorticotropic hormone (ACTH) or corticosteroids are a common clinical problem. This chapter will consider disorders related to adrenal, thyroid, and gonadal dysfuction.

GENERAL MECHANISMS OF NEUROLOGIC DYSFUNCTION IN ENDOCRINE DISEASE

The clinical manifestations of endocrinopathies result from the individual or combined effects of (1) altered whole-body electrolyte or substrate milieu, (2) direct effect of the hormone (or its lack) on brain metabolic-electrical activity, and (3) action of the hormone as neurotransmitter. Thus, the major neurologic manifestations of hypoadrenalism are usually the consequence of disordered electrolyte balance, hypotension, or both. Thyroid hormone deficiency, on the other hand, can produce both severe electrolyte imbalance and the direct effect of thyroid hormone deficiency on brain function. As a final example, ACTH has at least three actions that can alter brain function: a direct effect on neurons as a neurotransmitter, a direct effect on cellular actions, and indirect effects produced by changes in electrolyte balance. Thus, excess ACTH appears likely to produce severe, specfic brain dysfunction. However, excess ACTH in turn results in hypercortisolism, which acts both to modulate cell membrane potentials directly and then to activate cortisol receptors in the cell nucleus. Glucocorticoids can also affect the nervous system by their effect on electrolytes.

There is increasing evidence for direct cell membrane or cell nucleus binding of hormones, which then presumably act either to produce a second messenger or to activate or inhibit the rate of transcription of genetic information directly. Such effects on the genome then regulate the synthesis of neurotransmitters or their receptors. Corticosteroids, thyroid hormone, parathyroid hormone, insulin, calcitonin, estrogens, androgens, and many other hormones bind to various sites in the central and peripheral nervous system. The availability of techniques for studying their tissue localization and their genetic activation (or inhibition) should expand our understanding of the behavioral and neurologic effects of numerous hormones in the not-too-distant future.

Abnormal endocrine function can be the result of, rather than the cause of, brain dysfunction. Thus developmental brain anomalies can alter gonadal function [59]; seizure disorders produce neuroendocrine abnormalities [29]; depression is associated with elevations of plasma cortisol and a pseudo-Cushing's syndrome [19]; and a number of multisystemic disorders produce endocrine disease: Myotonic dystrophy causes gonadal atrophy [21] and the adrenoleukodystrophies adrenal insufficiency [45].

Table 11-1. Neurologic complications of ACTH and corticosteroid excess

Brain
Psychosis: manic-depressive; schizophreniform
Suicide: ideation and attempts
Insomnia
Hypomania, euphoria
Impaired consciousness (infrequent)
Spinal cord, root
Compression by epidural fat
Skeletal muscle
Atrophy
Necrotizing myopathy (secondary to hypokalemia)
Other
Proptosis and limitation of ocular motility
Pseudotumor cerebri
Carney complex: associated schwannomas, myxomas

ADRENAL DISORDERS

Excess ACTH and Corticosteroids (Table 11-1)

The majority of patients with endogenous hypercortisolism show mental changes [64]. Depression and hypomania are the most common abnormalities [64]. Psychosis and suicide attempts are common. The mental status changes can occur before other signs of hypercortisolism, although the diagnosis is seldom suspected at this time. Disturbances of cognitive function, confusional states, and rarely alteration of sensorium occur [4]. Exogenous corticosteroids tend to produce euphoria and insomnia. When severe, the clinical neuropsychiatric picture is usually that of hypomania. In contrast, endogenous ACTH or corticosteroid excess is associated with a broader spectrum of abnormalities [63].

The incidence of psychosis attributable to prednisone is minimal ($< 1\%$) in patients receiving less than 40 mg of the drug but rises to nearly 20 percent in patients taking ove 80 mg/day [3]. Alternate-day regimens of prednisone are less likely to produce psychosis than daily therapy but can produce dramatic mood swings between hypomanic and depressive behaviors [60]. Studies comparing the incidence of behavioral abnormalities in patients with ACTH-producing as opposed to adrenocortical tumors suggest that ACTH is more likely to cause neuropsychiatric signs than corticosteroids alone [36,40]. A similarly greater degree of central nervous system toxicity for exogenous ACTH has also been noted [44].

Neurologic abnormalities other than behavioral disturbances attributable to corticosteroids include muscle weakness and atrophy as well as the effects of corticosteroids to increase epidural and retroorbital fat with resulting mass effects (Table 11-1). Pseudotumor cerebri can occur with high-dose corticosteroids but is more likely to occur as steroids are tapered.

The muscle atrophy caused by corticosteroids is usually proximal and shows features of myopathy by electromyography. Biopsy of muscle shows atrophy, especially of type 2 muscle fibers. The creatine kinase level is usually normal [23]. Muscle weakness in patients with Cushing's syndrome can occasionally be the result of hypokalemia and resulting muscle necrosis [53]. In most instances, however, the muscle weakness results from atrophy. The atrophy is in all likelihood the result of a decrease in muscle protein synthesis [51]; muscle destruction is actually diminished [46]. Cushing's syndrome can be associated with a multisystemic tumor syndrome (Carney complex) that produces neurologic disease by means not directly related to hypercortisolism. Schwannomas of peripheral nerve, pituitary tumors, and atrial myxomas can all eventuate in neurologic signs and symptoms [71].

Pathogenesis of Corticosteroid-Induced Neuropsychiatric Abnormalities

While the precise basis for corticosteroid effects on the brain is not completely understood, there is convincing evidence for specific glucocorticoid receptors on neuronal membranes [9]. Such receptors can mediate rapid effects of corticosteroids such as the inhibition of ACTH release. Many other effects of corticosteroids are delayed and attributable to a cascade of events. Binding of corticoid to cytosolic receptors is followed by release of a second messenger such as 3′,5′-cyclic adenosine monophosphate (AMP) or by formation of a complex that then activates nuclear receptors [58]. Receptor-binding of glucocorticoids is concentrated in limbic system neurons [62]. While there are no data on humans, various manipulations of these cell's receptor activity in animals have modified the behavioral effects of corticosteroids [9]. There is also strongly positive glucocorticoid receptor imunoreactivity in the neurons of the paraventricular parvocellular nucleus, the anterior periventricular nucleus, and the mediobasal portions of the hypothalamus [18]. More widespread binding is present in cortex, thalamus, and anterior horn cells.

The possibility that synthetic corticosteroids such as dexamethasone may have a different action on the central nervous system is suggested by the paucity of dexamethasone receptors in the limbic system. Binding is much greater in endothelial cells of blood vessels and choroid plexus and in epithelial cells of the ventricles [19].

Ideally, studies of the central nervous system effects of exogenous corticosteroids and ACTH would be based on observations of their effects in patients with diseases that spare the nervous system. On the other hand, since there is evidence that antecedent psychiatric disease [3] or neurologic disease [44] may predispose patients to psychotic reactions during administration of ACTH or prednisone, the pathobiology may require an *anlage* of neurologic disease. Patients with multiple sclerosis have as high as a 20 percent incidence of hypomanic reactions to ACTH and prednisone. As with endogenous hypercorticism, ACTH appears more likely than prednisone to result in psychosis [44]. In fact, in one series, only patients with Cushing's disease and high levels of ACTH had neuropsychiatric abnormalities [63].

The higher incidence of neuropsychiatric symptoms in patients with endogenously [36,40] or exogenously [44] elevated levels of ACTH may relate to the known effects of ACTH on brain function. DeWied and van Ree [11] have shown that ACTH, and more specifically a small polypeptide portion of the ACTH molecule (the $ACTH_{4-9}$ analogue), produces striking behavioral changes in animals. These polypeptides, unlike ACTH, have no effect on the adrenal gland. An analogous peptide, melanocyte-stimulating hormone (MSH), produces similar effects on behavior in humans. Alterations in other neuroactive peptides such as beta-endorphin are also present in patients with Cushing's syndrome and have been postulated to be related to mental changes. On the other hand, the effect of ACTH on adrenal steroid production could result in elevated levels of hormones with different effects than prednisone. For example, there is evidence for a greater androgen production and greater mineralocorticoid production in patients given ACTH.

Management of Corticosteroid- or ACTH-Related Psychosis

Correction of Cushing's syndrome often results in dramatic improvement in mental state. Patients developing an acute psychosis in the context of corticosteroid therapy of systemic illness often remit spontaneously or may improve with increased corticosteroid, which suggests that underlying disease may account for the "steroid psychosis." Dosage reduction or, in the case of ACTH-induced psychosis, switching to a corticosteroid is often effective (Table 11-2). Various medications have been used to treat or prevent steroid-induced manic episodes or hypomania. Lithium is the agent most widely reported to be effective [14,30]; clonazepam has been used successfully in patients unable to take or unresponsive to lithium [69]. Patients do not necessarily become psychotic with reintroduction of ACTH or prednisone [3]. In rare instances of steroid psychosis attributable to ectopic ACTH secretion or to adrenocortical carcinoma, treatment has proved virtually impossible. A recent report suggests that the cortisol-receptor antagonist mifepristone may rapidly alleviate psychosis in such patients [68].

Addison's Disease

Most patients with severe deficiency of adrenal corticosteroids manifest behavioral disturbances. Apathy, lethargy, depression, fatigue, and cognitive disturbances are frequent [5]. Addisonian crisis includes coma as a severe manifestation. Many such patients may have other severe metabolic disturbances including hyponatremia, hypoglycemia, reduced cardiac output, or disturbed temperature regulation. Patients with Addison's disease are also sensitive to sedative drugs and may develop encephalopathy when given standard doses of narcotics, barbiturates, or phenothiazines. Muscle weakness occurs in patients with severe corticosteroid deficiency, and muscle destruction is occasionally demonstrable.

Table 11-2. Management of ACTH and corticosteroid mental status changes

Exclude coincidental or alternative diagnoses, especially:
Sepsis
Meningitis
Electrolyte disturbance
ACTH-induced psychosis:
Substitute daily prednisone (at a maximum of 40 mg/day if possible)
Discontinue ACTH
Corticosteroid-induced changes:
Dosage reduction (if possible) to 40 mg/day
Change dosage schedule to once daily and then to alternate-day regimen
Neuroleptic use
Lithium (caution if diuretics or salt restriction prescribed)
Clonazepam

The high incidence (~50%) of clinically inapparent adrenoleukodystrophy in boys with adrenal insufficiency [57] suggests that this disorder must be considered in such patients even when neurologic abnormalities are lacking. It is possible that some early cases of Addison's disease–related neurologic dysfunction could have had this disease. Although adrenoleukodystrophy is an X-linked disorder, carriers often manifiest signs of moderate severity: spasticity, gait disturbance, and ataxia [45]. Peripheral neuropathy also occurs. Any patient with adrenal insufficiency and neurologic abnormalities should have appropriate serum studies for long-chain fatty acids to look for these peroxisomal disorders [45]. Another factor that could account for neurologic disease in patients with Addison's disease is the finding that many patients with adrenal failure have secondarily elevated ACTH levels; neuropsychiatric abnormalities could relate to this hormone.

The ability of corticosteroids to alter brain sensory function has been demonstrated by the studies of Henkin and associates [27]. Audition, taste, and smell are all hyperacute in patients with adrenal cortical insufficiency. Thresholds return to normal in 24 to 48 hours after replacement therapy. These data provide some of the best evidence for a specific role for corticosteroids in neurologic function.

Corticosteroid Withdrawal

Neurologic abnormalities often occur as corticosteroids are tapered. When the disease being treated is characterized by neurologic disease (e.g., multiple sclerosis, systemic lupus erythematosus), reactivation of the underlying disease is likely. Occasional patients manifest rheumatic complaints and can have evidence of arthropathy, splenomegaly, fever, and mental status changes (so-called Slocumb's pseudorheumatism). Pseudotumor cerebri also occasionally occurs as long-term steroids are being tapered.

THYROID DISORDERS

Hyperthyroidism

Severe thyrotoxicosis is usually associated with behavioral abnormalities (Table 11-3). Hypomanic or agitated behavior is common. A spectrum of other changes including psychosis can occur, although in certain instances premorbid behavioral disturbances were present. In older patients, particularly those with severe, apathetic thyrotoxicosis, thyroid storm can develop and be associated with obtundation [48]. Most such severely ill patients have multiple other reasons for obtundation, including heart failure, infection, malnutrition, or atrial fibrillation and cerebral embolism.

Tremor is present in over 90 percent of patients with thyrotoxicosis and is often severe, particularly in younger patients. The tremor is maximal with sustention and is absent at rest. At times tremor is so marked that it suggests chorea; occasional patients actually manifest severe chorea, athetosis, or dystonia [16,25]. Meige syndrome (blepharospasm with oromandibular tremor) has also been reported in thyrotoxicosis [49].

Reflexes are usually hyperactive in patients with thyrotoxicosis. Occasionally patients have leg weakness accompanied by spasticity and pathologic reflexes. The constellation of findings in such patients has been termed Basedow's paraplegia [15]. It is possible that myopathy is the cause of weakness in such patients and their upper motor neuron signs simply the effect of the central nervous system changes of thyrotoxicosis. Myelopathy may not be present, and there is no definite documentation of spinal cord pathology in thyrotoxicosis.

Ophthalmoplegia occurs as a complication of an infiltrative ophthalmopathy but can also occur as the result of ocular muscle disease. Bulbar paralysis and other features of amyotrophic lateral sclerosis including fasciculations have been reported [17]. Thyrotoxic myopathy is seen in nearly 100 percent of patients with thyrotoxicosis. Muscle atrophy can be profound. Electromyography shows signs of myopathy; biopsy shows atrophy; the creatine kinase is often normal or low [53]. Since joint pain (particularly of the shoulders and hips) is occasionally seen with thyrotoxicosis, a diagnosis of polymyalgia rheumatica or polymyositis is often considered.

The neurologic manifestations of thyrotoxicosis usually resolve with treatment. Instances where recovery is incomplete may reflect coincidental disease.

Table 11-3. Neurologic manifestations of thyrotoxicosis

Central nervous system
Psychosis: mania, schizophreniform
Hypomania, euphoria
Depression, apathy (especially older patients)
Coma (only in thyroid storm)
Tremor
Chorea, athetosis, dystonia, Meige syndrome
Myelopathy (Basedow's paraplegia)
Neuromuscular
Amyotrophic lateral sclerosis-like illness
Peripheral neuropathy
Muscle atrophy
Bulbar palsy
Periodic paralysis
Ophthalmopathy

Pathogenesis of Thyrotoxic Neurologic Dysfunction

There is no clear understanding of how thyroid hormone or its excess affects brain. Cerebral oxygen consumption is not increased in thyrotoxicosis, and brain mitochondria do not undergo the changes that occur in other tissues. There is some evidence that thyrotoxicosis increases the sensitivity of adrenergic receptors, leading to a state of sympathetic overactivity [42]. The dramatic benefit of catecholamine beta-receptor anatagonists is strong support for this postulate. However, the spectrum of neurologic changes seen with thyrotoxicosis is far greater than that seen in conditions associated with an excess of catecholamines. Moreover, a recent study found no augmentation of response of thyrotoxic patients to infused isoproterenol; it is necessary to develop additional hypotheses to account for the peripheral manifestations of hyperthyroidism and its response to beta-adrenergeic blocking agents [42].

Neurons have receptors for both thyroxine (T_4) and triiodothyronine (T_3) [50]. There is considerable evidence that T_4 is converted to T_3 in brain as it is in other tissues [34] and that T_3 is the biologically active hormone [34]. There is a high concentration of T_3 receptors in the adult brain [50]. However, while thyroid hormone is clearly of major importance in brain development [8], the basis for its effect on adult brain remains uncertain.

Treatment of Thyrotoxic Neurologic Dysfunction

In general, treatment consists of the appropriate management of the underlying thyroid disorder. Patients with severe psychiatric disorders usually require both beta blockers and phenothiazines, often in high dosages, while antithyroid medication is being initiated and thyrotoxicosis controlled. Where psychiatric disturbance was coincidental or related to antecedent illness, long-term neuroleptic therapy may be necessary. The possibility that certain personality types predispose patients to thyrotoxicosis has even been suggested [41].

Beta blockade improves or reverses most neuromuscular manifestations as well as tremor [70]. It even prevents attacks of hypokalemic periodic paralysis. It is helpful to recall that beta blockade acts to raise T_4 levels but does not actually affect thyroid function. Acetazolamide (the usual treatment for periodic paralysis) is contraindicated in thyrotoxic periodic paralysis and has caused severe side effects [56].

The frequent association of thyrotoxicosis with pernicious anemia and the occasional association with adrenal insufficiency bear consideration in the management of all patients. Unless it is clear that adrenal corticoid levels are appropriate, severely ill patients with thyrotoxicosis should probably be given corticosteroids.

Hypothyroidism

The majority of patients with myxedema have somnolence or lethargy (Table 11-4). Where myxedema is severe, coma can develop, although in most if not all cases, the obtundation occurs in the setting of infection, injudicious sedative or analgestic use, or other coincidental factors [43]. The most severe mentation abnormalities often occur in association with hypoxia, and the reported abnormalities of hypoxic ventilatory drive in myxedema [72] may result in a predisposition to severe hypoxia.

Table 11-4. Neurologic manifestations of hypothyroidism

Central nervous system
Alternations in consciousness: lethargy, stupor, coma
Psychomotor retardation, intellectual impairment, dementia
Seizures (infrequent)
Psychosis, agitation
Ataxia
Deafness
Ophthalmoparesis, ptosis
Neuromuscular disease
Peripheral neuropathy
Generalized
Compressive (e.g., carpal tunnel syndrome)
Myasthenic syndrome
Myopathy

A spectrum of other central nervous system manifestations are frequent in patients with myxedema. Dementia or more subtle intellectual impairment often precedes the diagnosis by many years. All patients with dementia deserve tests of thyroid function, both T_4 and thyroid-stimulating hormone (TSH). The latter is important because of the rare instances (usually on a pharmacologic or hereditary basis) where T_4 may be spuriously elevated and result in apparent normal levels. Free thyroxine levels will also be helpful in these circumstances.

Other, less common neurologic manifestations that occur with myxedema are ataxia, deafness, and generalized peripheral neuropathy [7]. The presence of subtle, subclinical generalized neuropathy may predispose patients to the frequent occurrence of entrapment neuropathies such as the carpal tunnel syndrome.

Muscle involvement occurs in the majority of patients with myxedema. Furthermore, the reduced clearance of creatine tissue seen in hypothyroid patients frequently results in very high creatine kinase levels [20] and leads to the suspicion of a primary myopathy in many patients. Muscle enlargement, muscle cramps, weakness, and fatigue are all frequent in myxedema [35].

It is worth noting that subclinical hypothyroidism is a frequent occurrence in the elderly (3–7% in some series). Thyroid replacement is doubtless indicated in most patients but unless there are non-neurologic signs of myxedema, symptoms should not necessarily be attributed to hypothyroidism. Futhermore, in critically ill patients, T_4 levels are often depressed, the so-called euthyroid sick patient. TSH levels are normal in this setting, and thyroid replacement is not indicated.

Pathogenesis of Neurologic Manifestations of Hypothyroidism

Thyroid hormone is critical for neuronal development, and its lack in infancy leads to the severe mental retardation of the cretin. The basis for the signs in adult patients is poorly defined. Both structural and functional enzymatic changes have been noted in skeletal muscle [12,32], but equally severe findings occur in patients without such findings.

Most patients with myxedema who present with obtundation have one or more factors other than hypothyroidism to account for encephalopathy, including hyponatremia, acidosis, hypoxia, hypercarbia, hypothermia, or infection [43]. Drug metabolism is impaired in hypothyroidism; sedatives, phenothiazines, or opiates may accumulate in toxic amounts [43]. The extreme sensitivity of hypothyroid patients to neuroleptics such as phenothiazines [39] suggests that dopaminergic function is compromised in the thyroid-deficient brain. Cerebral blood flow and metabolism are reduced, usually in proportion to clinical manifestations and electroencephalographic slowing.

Treatment of Hypothyroid Neurologic Disease

Thyroid replacement with thyroxine (T_4) in gradually increasing doses is sufficient for most patients. Myxedema coma, however, may require intravenous administration of hormone; T_3 is the biologically active hormone and its use may produce more rapid recovery [6]. Since the mortality remains high in myxedema coma [2], aggressive treatment is indicated. Corticosteroid treatment is advisable in patients suspected of severe myxedema, in part because of the association of adrenal insufficiency in patients whose hypothyroidism results from hypopituitarism. Autoimmune hypothyroidism can also be associated with a similar, autoimmune adrenal insufficiency. As a general rule, the severely ill patient with myxedema should receive corticosteroids as well as thyroid replacement.

Hypothyroidism itself causes a megaloblastic anemia [30], but coincidental pernicious anemia should always be considered as a cause of neurologic signs even if hematologic function is normal. Vitamin B_{12} should be given to anemic patients with hypothyroidism until B_{12} levels have been shown to be normal.

Encephalopathy in Hashimoto's Disease

Hashimoto's thyroiditis is an inflammatory disease of the thyroid gland associated with autoantibodies to specific hormonal and cellular antigens within the thyroid gland. A number of central nervous system abnormalities occur in patients with Hashimoto's thyroiditis: stupor or coma, generalized seizures, myoclonic seizures, tremor, athetosis, and focal signs suggesting stroke [26,61]. Patients respond to corticosteroids but may require other immunosuppressive treatment [26,61,66]. In certain patients, the stroke-like character of the episodes has suggested vasculitis as the basis for the syndrome, but there is no convincing evidence that an inflammatory vasculopathy is present.

Recognizing the encephalopathy of patients with Hashimoto's thyroiditis may assume importance when considering the neurologic abnormalities of hyperthyroid patients. Many patients with thyroiditis are hypothyroid, and the neurologic abnormalities might be attributable simply to low T_4 levels. Most patients with the encephalopathy of Hashimoto's thyroiditis have had only slightly low T_4 levels and slight elevations of TSH [61]. It is likely that cases of myxedema resulting from Hashimoto's disease will have features of both severe hypothyroid brain dysfunction and the immune-mediated syndrome of neurologic dysfunction. Such cases have not yet been recognized.

Gonadal Steroids

Alterations of androgens, estrogens, and prolactin as well as their controlling releasing or inhibiting hormones have major effects on neuropsychiatric function as well as on sexuality. Studies over the past two decades suggest that many common behavioral disorders and variations can be explained, at least in part, by the changing hormonal milieu of the brain.

Female Sexual Function

Estrogens, androgen, and progesterone have complex interactions important in female sex drive as well as in behavioral and physical manifestations of menarche, the premenstrual syndrome, and the menopause. Female sex drive is clearly androgen dependent [52], but proceptivity for sexual activity is also related to changes in the estrogen and progesterone levels of the menstrual cycle [67]. In addition to hormonal effects on sexual behavior, it is clear that estrogen deficiency is responsible for a panoply of behavioral disturbances that occur with menopause. Depression, social withdrawal, and isolation accompany estrogen deficiency and respond to its administration [18]. While there is a concern about the oncogenic potential of long-term estrogen replacement, it is important to recognize that the physiologic "hot flashes" are a sign of estrogen deficiency and indicate a likelihood that new neuropsyhchiatric symptoms are based on that deficiency [41].

Premenstrual Syndrome

The premenstrual syndrome (PMS) affects up to 30 percent of women and is associated with variations in mood and irritable behavior [55]. Major disability and behavioral abnormalities ranging from hypomania to severe depression or agitation are seen in a small percentage of women. The PMS should be defined as rigorously as possible to avoid attributing vague symptoms to a poorly delineated condition. PMS consists of weight gain, acneiform rash, breast swelling and tenderness, leg edema, and abdominal bloating and is accompanied by depression, anxiety, fatigue, irritability, and interference with customary activities. The PMS must recur regularly and be predictable [55]. Although symptoms of PMS usually begin prior to menstruation, they often continue throughout menses and may not become maximal until 2 to 4 days after onset of menstruation. Various treatment strategies are indicated for severe dysphoria. Gonadotropin-releasing hormone [47] and progesterone [10] have both been effective.

Male Sexual Function

The effects of androgens on psychological and physiologic aspects of male sexual function have been carefully studied. A deficiency of testosterone decreases libido and diminishes reflex penile erectile function [38]. Androgens exert an important effect on prenatal brain development in animals [1]. A similar effect is likely in humans [31], in whom behavioral data suggest that not only sexual orientation, but also aggression, energy expenditure, and other masculine behavioral attributes are androgen dependent [37].

Androgen deficiency results in a decrease in muscle mass, which is reversed by androgen administration. The effect of supraphysiologic levels of testosterone is less clear. While testosterone increases muscle mass and muscle protein synthesis [22], it is not established that muscle function or strength is improved [24]. There is some evidence that a combination of exercise training and androgen administration will produce an increase in muscle strength greater than exercise training alone [28]. Compounding the difficulty in separating the effects of exercise from those of androgens is the fact that exercise elevates testosterone levels. Current evidence suggests that androgen deficiency results in weakness in hypogonadal men but that androgens do not have any clear benefit in supraphysiologic amounts.

REFERENCES

1. Berlin, F. S., and Meinecke, C. F. Treatment of sex offenders with antiandrogenic medication: Conceptualization, review of treatment modalities, and preliminary findings. *Am. J. Psychiatry* 138:601, 1981.

2. Blum, M. Myxedema coma. *Am. J. Med. Sci.* 264:432, 1972.
3. Boston Collaborative Drug Surveillance Program. Acute adverse reactions to prednisone in relation to dosage. *Clin. Pharmacol. Ther.* 13:694, 1972.
4. Brown, G. M. Psychiatric and Neurologic Aspects of Endocrine Disease. In Krieger, D. T. and J. C. Hughes (eds.), *Neuropsychiatry in Endocrine Diseases.* Sunderland, MA: Sinauer Associates, 1981. Pp. 185–193.
5. Cleghorn, R. A. Adrenal cortical insufficiency: Psychological and neurological observation. *Can. Med. Assoc. J.* 65:449, 1951.
6. Cook, D. M., and Boyle, P. J. Rapid reversal of myxedema madness with triiodothyronine. *Ann. Intern. Med.* 104:893, 1986.
7. Cremer, G. M., Goldstein, N. P., and Paris, J. Myxedema and ataxia. *Neurology* 19:37, 1969.
8. DeGroot, L. J. Larsen, P. R., Refetoff, S., and Stanbury, J. B. *The Thyroid and Its Diseases.* New York: Wiley, 1984.
9. deKloet, E. R. Function of steroid receptor systems in the central nervous system. *Clin. Neuropharmacol.* 7:272, 1984.
10. Dennerstein, L., Spencer-Gardner, C., Gotts, G., et al. Progesterone and the premenstrual syndrome: A double blind crossover trial. *Br. Med. J.* 290:1617, 1985.
11. de Wied, D., and van Ree, J. M. Neuropeptides, mental performance and aging. *Life Sci.* 31:709, 1982.
12. Edwards, R. H. T., Khaleeli, A. A., and Mills, K. R. Muscle function in endocrine and metabolic myopathy. *Semin. Neuro.* 3:294, 1983.
13. Ehrhardt, A. A., and Meyer-Bahlburg, H. F. L. Prenatal sex hormones and the developing brain: Effects on psychosexual differentiation and cognitive function. *Ann. Rev. Med.* 30:417, 1979.
14. Falk, W. E., Mahnke, M. W., and Poskanzer, D. C. Lithium prophylaxis of corticotropin-induced psychosis. *J.A.M.A.* 241:1011, 1979.
15. Feibel, J. H., and Campa, J. F. Thyrotoxic neuropathy (Basedow's paraplegia). *J. Neurol. Neurosurg. Psychiatry* 39:491, 1976.
16. Fidler, S. M., O'Rourke, R. A., and Buchsbaum, H. W. Choreoathetosis as a manifestation of thyrotoxicosis. *Neurology* 21:55, 1971.
17. Fisher, M., Mateer, J. E., Ullrich, I., and Gutrecht, J. A. Pyramidal tract deficits and polyneuropathy and hyperthyroidism: Combination clinically mimicking amyotrophic lateral sclerosis. *Am. J. Med.* 78:1041, 1985.
18. Fuxe, K., Wikström, A. C., Okret, S., et al. Mapping of glucocorticoid receptor immunoreactive neurons in the rat tel- and diencephalon using a monoclonal antibody against rat liver glucocorticoid receptor. *Endocrinology* 117: 1803, 1985.
19. Gold, P. W., Loriaux, L., Roy, A., et al. Responses to corticotropin-releasing hormone in the hypercortisolism of depression and Cushing's disease. *N. Engl. J. Med.* 314:1329, 1986.
20. Goldman, J., Matz, R., Mortimer, R., and Freeman, R. High elevations of creatine phosphokinase in hypothyroidism. *J.A.M.A.* 238:325, 1977.
21. Griggs, R. C., Kingston W., Herr, B. E., et al. Lack of relationship of hypogonadism to muscle wasting in myotonic dystrophy. *Arch. Neurol.* 42:881, 1985.
22. Griggs, R. C., Kingston, W., Jozefowicz, R. F., et al. Effect of testosterone on muscle mass and muscle protein synthesis. *J. Appl. Physiol.* 66:498, 1989.
23. Griggs, R. C., Mendell, J., and Miller, R. Myopathies in Systemic Diseases. In *Evaluation and Management of Myopathies.* Philadelphia: Davis, 1992.
24. Griggs, R. C., Pandya, S., Florence, J. M., et al. Randomized controlled trial of testosterone in myotonic dystrophy. *Neurology* 39:219, 1989.
25. Heffron, W., and Eaton, R. P. Thyrotoxicosis presenting as choreoathetosis. *Ann. Intern. Med.* 73:425, 1970.
26. Henderson, L. M., Behan, P. O., Aarli, J., et al. Hashimoto's encephalopathy: A new neuroimmunological syndrome. *Ann. Neurol.* 22:140, 1987.
27. Henkin, R. I., McGlone, R. E., Daly, R., and Bartter, F. C. Studies on auditory thresholds in normal man and in patients with adrenal cortical insufficiency: The role of adrenal cortical steroids. *J. Clin. Invest.* 46:429, 1967.
28. Hervey, G. R., Knibbs, A. V., Burkinshaw, L., et al. Effects of methandienone on the performance and body composition of men undergoing athletic training. *Clin. Sci.* 60:457, 1981.
29. Herzog, A. G., Russell, V., Vaitukaitis, J. L., and Geschwind, N. Neuroendocrine dysfunction in temporal lobe epilepsy. *Arch. Neurol.* 39:133, 1982.
30. Hines, J. D., Halsted, C. H., Griggs, R. C., and Harris, J. W. Megaloblastic anemia secondary to folate deficiency associated with hypothyroidism. *Ann. Intern. Med.* 68:792, 1968.
31. Huffer, V., Scott, W. H., Connor, T. B., and Lovice, H. Psychological studies of adult male patients with sexual infantilism before and after androgen therapy. *Ann. Intern. Med.* 61:255, 1964.
32. Hurwitz, L. J., McCormick, D., and Allen I. V. Reduced muscle α glucosidase (acid-maltase) activity in the hypothyroid myopathy. *Lancet* 1:67, 1970.
33. Jeffcoate, W. J., Silverstone, J. T., Edwards, C. R. W., and Besser, M. Psychiatric manifestations of Cushing's syndrome: Response to lowering of plasma cortisol. *Q. J. Med.* 48:465, 1979.
34. Kaplan, M. M. The role of thyroid hormone deio-

dination in the regulation of hypothalamo-pituitary function. *Neuroendocrinology* 38:254, 1984.
35. Khaleeli, A. A., Griffith, D. G., and Edwards, R. H. T. The clinical presentation of hypothyroid myopathy and its relationship to abnormalities in structure and function of skeletal muscle. *Clin. Endocrinol.* 19:365, 1983.
36. Krauthammer, C., and Klerman, G. L. Secondary mania: Manic syndromes associated with antecedent physical illness or drugs. *Arch. Gen. Psychiatry* 35:1333, 1978.
37. Kreuz, L. E., and Rose, R. M. Assessment of aggressive behavior and plasma testosterone in a young criminal population. *Psychosom. Med.* 34:321, 1972.
38. Kwan, M., Greenleaf, W. J., Mann, J., et al. The nature of androgen action on male sexuality: A combined laboratory–self-report study on hypogonadal men. *J. Clin. Endocrinol. Metab.* 57:557, 1983.
39. Levander, S., and Rosenqvist, U. Cerebral function in hypothyroid patients. *Neuropsychobiology* 5:274, 1979.
40. Ling, M. H. M., Perry, P. J., and Tsuang, M. T. Side effects of corticosteroid therapy. *Arch. Gen. Psychiatry* 38:471, 1981.
41. Martin, J. B., Reichlin, S., and Brown, G. M. *Clinical Neuroendocrinology* (2nd ed.). Philadelphia: Davis, 1987. Pp. 650–652.
42. McDevitt, D. G., Riddell, J. G., Hadden, D. R., and Montgomery, D. A. D. Catecholamine sensitivity in hyperthyroidism and hypothyroidism. *Br. J. Clin. Pharmacol.* 6:297, 1978.
43. Menendez, C. E., and Rivlin, R. S. Thyrotoxic crisis and myxedema coma. *Med. Clin. North Am.* 57:1463, 1973.
44. Minden, S. L., Orav, J., and Schildkraut, J. J. Hypomanic reactions to ACTH and prednisone treatment for multiple sclerosis. *Neurology* 38:1631, 1988.
45. Moser, H. W., Moser, A. E., Singh, I., and O'Neill, B. P. Adrenoleukodystrophy: Survey of 303 cases. Biochemistry, diagnosis and therapy. *Ann. Neurol.* 16:628, 1984.
46. Moxley, R. T., Lorenson, M., Griggs, R. C., et al. Decreased breakdown of muscle protein after prednisone therapy in Duchenne dystrophy (DD). VII International Congress on Neuromuscular Diseases, September 16–21, 1990, Munich, West Germany. *J. Neurol. Sci.* 98:419, 1990.
47. Muse, K. N., Cetel, N. S., Futterman, L. A., and Yen, S. S. C. The premenstrual syndrome: Effects of "Medical Ovariectomy." *N. Engl. J. Med.* 311:1345, 1984.
48. Newcomer, J., Haire, W., and Hartman, C. R. Coma and thyrotoxicosis. *Ann. Neurol.* 14:689, 1983.
49. Nutt, J. G., Carter, J., DeGarmo, P., and Hammerstad, J. P. Meige syndrome and thyroid dysfunction. *Neurology* 34(Suppl. 1):222, 1984.
50. Oppenheimer, J. H. The Nuclear Receptor-Triiodothyronine Complex: Relationship to Thyroid Hormone Distribution, Metabolism, and Biological Action. In J. H. Oppenheimer and H. H. Samuels (eds.), *The Molecular Basis of Thyroid Hormone Action.* New York: Academic Press. Pp. 1–35. 1983.
51. Pacy, P. J., and Halliday, D. Muscle protein synthesis in steroid-induced proximal myopathy: A case report. *Muscle Nerve* 12:378, 1989.
52. Pardridge, W. M., Gorski, R. A., Lippe, B. M., and Green, R. Androgens and sexual behavior. *Ann. Intern. Med.* 96:488, 1982.
53. Pleasure, D. E., Walsh, G. O., and Engel, W. K. Atrophy of skeletal muscle in patients with Cushing's syndrome. *Arch. Neurol.* 22:118, 1970.
54. Ramsay, I. Thyrotoxic muscle disease. *Postgrad. Med. J.* 44:385, 1968.
55. Reid, R. L., and Yen, S. S. C. Premenstrual syndrome. *Am. J. Obstet. Gynecol.* 139:85, 1981.
56. Riggs, J. E., and Griggs, R. C. Diagnosis and treatment of the periodic paralysis. *Clin. Neuropharmacol.* 4:123, 1976.
57. Sadeghi-Nejad, A., and Senior, B. Adrenomyeloneuropathy presenting as Addison's disease in childhood. *N. Engl. J. Med.* 322:13, 1990.
58. Sakly, M., and Koch, B. Ontogenesis of glucocorticoid receptors in anterior pituitary gland: Transient dissociation among cytoplasmic receptor density, nuclear uptake and regulation of corticotropic activity. *Endocrinology* 108:591, 1981.
59. Schwankhaus, J. D., Currie, J., Jaffe, M. J., et al. Neurologic findings in men with isolated hypogonadotropic hypogonadism. *Neurology* 39:223, 1989.
60. Sharfstein, S. S., Sack, D. S., and Fauci, A. S. Relationship between alternate-day corticosteroid therapy and behavioral abnormalities. *J.A.M.A.* 248:2987, 1982.
61. Shaw, P. J., Walls, T. J., Newman, P. K., et al. Hashimoto's encephalopathy: A steroid-responsive disorder associated with high antithyroid antibody titers—report of 5 cases. *Neurology* 41:228, 1991.
62. Sheridan, P. J. Autoradiographic localization of steroid receptors in the brain. *Clin. Neuropharmacol.* 7:281, 1984.
63. Starkman, M. N., and Schteingart, D. E. Neuropsychiatric manifestations of patients with Cushing's syndrome. *Arch. Intern. Med.* 141:215, 1981.
64. Starkman, M. N., Schteingart, D. E., and Schork, M. A. Depressed mood and other psychiatric manifestations of Cushing's syndrome: Relation-

ship to hormone levels. *Psychosom. Med.* 43:3, 1981.

65. Swanson, J. W., Kelly, J. J., and McConahey, W. M. Neurologic aspects of thyroid dysfunction. *Mayo Clin. Proc.* 56:504, 1981.
66. Thrush, D. C., and Boddie, H. G. Episodic encephalopathy associated with thyroid disorders. *J. Neurol. Neurosurg. Psychiatry* 37:696, 1974.
67. Udry, J. R., and Morris, M. N. Distribution of coitus in the menstrual cycle. *Nature* 220:593, 1968.
68. van der Lely, A. J., Foeken, K., van der Mast, R. C., and Lamberts, S. W. J. Rapid reversal of acute psychosis in the cushing syndrome with the cortisol-receptor antagonist mifepristone (RU 486). *Ann. Intern. Med.* 114:143, 1991.
69. Viswanathan, R., and Glickman, L. Clonazepam in the treatment of steroid-induced mania in a patient after renal transplantation. *N. Engl. J. Med.* 320:319, 1989.
70. Weinstein, R., Schwartzman, R., and Levey, G. S. Propranolol reversal of bulbar dysfunction and proximal myopathy in hyperthyroidism. *Ann. Intern. Med.* 82:540, 1975.
71. Young, W. F., Carney, J. A., Musa, B. U., et al. Familial Cushing's syndrome due to primary pigmented nodular adrenocortical disease. *N. Engl. J. Med.* 321:1659, 1989.
72. Zwillich, C. W., Pierson, D. J., Hofeldt, F. D., et al. Ventilatory control in myxedema and hypothyroidism. *N. Engl. J. Med.* 292:662, 1975.

12 Neurologic Manifestations of Hypothermia

David M. Holtzman and Roger P. Simon

Accidental hypothermia constitutes a major health problem not only in the United States but worldwide. It causes a variety of systemic manifestations as well as significant morbidity and mortality. In the 13-year period from 1968 to 1980, 6460 deaths in the United States alone were attributed to the effects of cold [15]. Mortality rates vary according to a number of factors, a few of which are shown in Table 12-1. Because of the magnitude of this problem, it is important to understand the way in which the nervous system reacts to cold in order to evaluate hypothermic patients appropriately. In addition, there are a number of disease states that affect the ability of either the central (CNS) or peripheral (PNS) nervous system to regulate core temperature and hence lead to hypothermia. In this chapter, temperature-regulating mechanisms in normal and pathologic states will be reviewed. Emphasis will be placed on clinical neurologic manifestations of hypothermia with a brief review of systemic manifestations. Pathophysiology and laboratory abnormalities will be discussed as well as current recommendations for treatment.

There have been numerous accounts throughout history documenting the CNS effects of hypothermia. Because of the gradual appearance of a death-like state, many reports have emphasized both the protective yet sedative effect of hypothermia on the brain.

On March 23, 1756, a Swedish peasant intoxicated with brandy was bowled over by the wind and fell asleep in the snow. He was found the next morning frozen stiff, and was put into a coffin ready for burial. Later in the day a physician arrived unexpectedly and examined the body. The face and extremities were ice-cold, the joints immovable, the eyes fixed open, and there were no signs of breathing or heartbeat. However, the physician, S. Naucler, thought that there was some warmth at the pit of the stomach and ordered the arms and legs to be rubbed while he applied hot fomentations to the trunk. As a result, the patient gradually revived and, next day, was recovering. [49].

Table 12-1. Hypothermia mortality rates* by age and sex: United States, 1968–1980.

Age group (years)	*Rate*		*Rate ratio (male/female)*
	Males	*Females*	
<1	1.61	0.99	1.6
1	0.09	0.18	0.5
2–4	0.24	0.20	1.2
5–9	0.09	0.03	2.6
10–14	0.34	0.04	8.8
15–24	1.31	0.34	3.8
25–34	1.73	0.33	5.2
35–44	3.31	0.62	5.3
45–54	5.81	1.48	3.7
55–64	8.63	1.76	4.9
65–74	11.68	2.41	4.9
≥75	23.71	7.30	3.2

* Deaths per 1,000,000 persons.
Source: CDC [15].

Because of the diffuse effects of hypothermia on the CNS, it is important to understand the spectrum of the "normal" neurologic examination in this state and in addition its limitations in regard to assessing other clinical and laboratory findings relevant to overall patient care.

TEMPERATURE REGULATION

Humans are homeotherms. They maintain their body temperature within a range of ± 2 degrees Celsius (2°C) despite larger variations in ambient temperature. This is in contrast to poikilothermic species, which assume the temperature of their environs. Hypothermia is defined as a core temperature (rectal, esophageal, tympanic) less than 35°C [44]. Because of the importance in mammals of maintaining strict control of temperature, a complex monitoring system has evolved that is governed by the hypothalamus. Receptors in the skin, spinal cord, brain stem, and diencephalon act as major system inputs, while the central and peripherally generated processes governing shivering, vasomotor control, sweating, basal metabolic rate, and behavior act as outputs (Fig. 12-1). This system may be disrupted because of malfunction at specific points in the overall network of temperature regulation or because of diffuse abnormalities (Table 12-2).

The skin has cutaneous thermoreceptors, which have a variety of properties. These include one or more of the following, which differ depending on the neuron involved: (1) static discharge at constant temperature (T), (2) dynamic response to temperature changes—dT/dt, and (3) no dependence on mechanical stimuli [26]. Both cold and warm receptors have been identified in mammals (Fig. 12-2). Many of these neuronal fibers are probably unmyelinated. Their axons travel from the skin to the dorsal root ganglion and then synapse at the corresponding dermatomal level in the spinal cord. A second neuron then sends its axon up the contralateral spinothalamic tract to the thalamus. After a third synapse, a thalamic neuron then projects to the cortex. At a skin temperature of 33°C, both cold and warm sensitive neurons are active, but there is a thermally neutral sensation [26].

Both vasomotor and sudomotor responses to temperature variation are exquisitely sensitive to local skin changes. These responses also vary depending on body location. Whereas many cholinergic fibers that are involved in vasodilatation project to the trunk and proximal limbs, sympathetic noradrenergic fibers that are in-

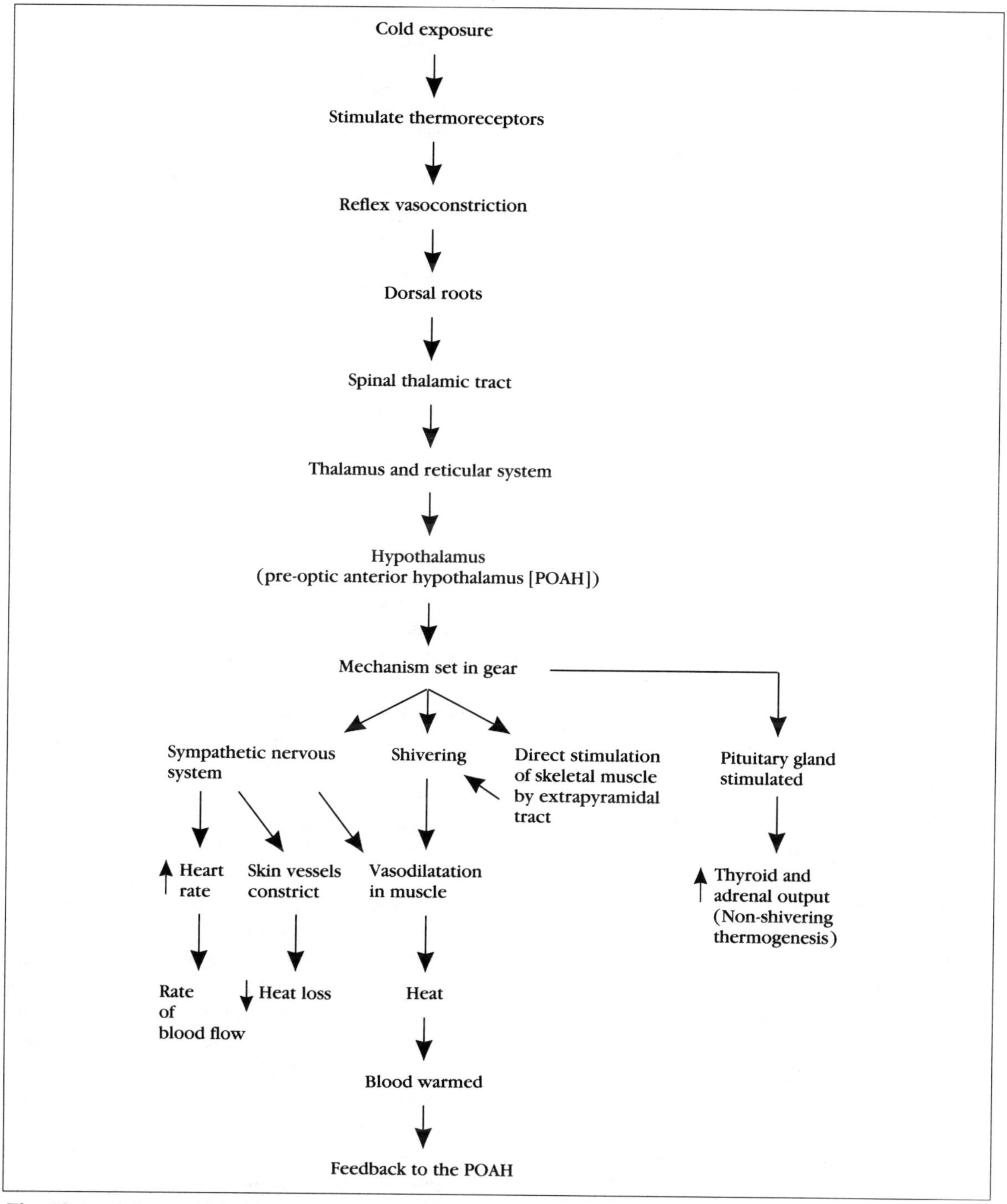

Fig. 12-1. Schema of thermoregulation. (Reproduced, with permission, from J. B. Reuler, Hypothemia: Pathophysiology, clinical settings, and management. *Ann. Intern. Med.* 89:519, 1978.)

Table 12-2. Causes of hypothermia

CNS disorders
Hypothalamic: trauma, tumor, vascular abnormalities, inflammatory process, Wernicke's encephalopathy
Midbrain: tumors, vascular abnormalities, Wernicke's encephalopathy
Spinal cord: tumors, trauma
Metabolic disorders
Hypothryroidism, hypopituitarism, hypoadrenalism, hypoglycemia
Skin disorders
Erythrodermas, burns, vasodilatation secondary to drugs
Diffuse effect on thermoregulatory system
Drugs (alcohol, phenothiazines, sedatives, anesthetic agents), sepsis, malnutrition, exposure, overall debilitated state (infants, elderly), uremia, liver failure, controlled hypothermia, anorexia nervosa

volved in vasoconstriction are abundant in the head and brow region [26]. Different anatomic contributions to overall sweat production have been noted: face—21 percent, chest and back—21 percent, abdomen—17 percent, upper legs—15 percent, lower legs—8 percent, upper arms—12 percent, and lower arms—6 percent [40]. Although core temperature sensors can override local skin responses, certain diseases of the skin can overwhelm body defenses and induce hypothermia. These include certain erythrodermas and severe burns.

The locus of greatest temperature sensitivity in mammals seems to be the preoptic-anterior hypothalamus. Cold and warm stimulation studies have also revealed the spinal cord and midbrain to be temperature-sensitive CNS structures [25]. Cooling the hypothalamus in dogs causes a series of responses including shivering, vasoconstriction, increasing basal metabolic rate (BMR), and activation of the sympatheticoadrenal system [26]. Neurotransmitters have also been shown to affect temperature regulation. Intraventricular injections of norepinephrine (NE) in cats, dogs, and monkeys activated heat loss and lowered body temperature, while 5-hydroxytryptamine (5-HT) had the opposite effect [26]. There appear to be specific grouped cells in the anterior hypothalamus that respond to local injections of NE and 5-HT in the same way as to intraventricular injections. Acetylcholine-responsive cells are also present within the hypothalamus but do not seem to be grouped [39]. Because humans maintain a near constant temperature, the concept of a set point has been discussed for many years. There are, however, a number of natural phenomenon that involve day-to-day temperature fluctuation. The hypothalamus is clearly associated with the daily periodic 1.0 to 1.5°C temperature changes of the diurnal rhythm, as well as the hyperthermic response secondary to endogenous or exogenous pyrogens that may alter the physiologic "set point."

A number of pathologic processes can directly involve the hypothalamus and could theoretically result in hypothermia. Abnormalities can include neoplasms, particularly craniopharyngiomas and astrocytomas. In infants, intracranial hemorrhage may occur in this area [27]. Lesions in this region are often accompanied by signs of hypothalamic dysfunction such as precocious puberty, diabetes insipidus, somnolence, and obesity. Other neurologic abnormalities are also common because of the proximity of the hypothalamus to neighboring structures. Pyramidal, cerebellar, sensory, and ophthalmologic findings are often present. Both trauma and idiopathic gliosis in this region have been reported to cause hypothermia [23]. Other disease entities involving the hypothalamus can result in hypothermia, which in itself may be one of the only clues to the underlying diagnosis.

Hypothermia has been noted in association with Wernicke's encephalopathy as well as in patients with hypoglycemia. Kedes and Field [30] reported five patients with mild hypothermia (all with temperature about 35°C) who had serum glucose levels less than 30 mg/dl. One of the five had no other symptoms of hypoglycemia. It has been shown that lowered core temperature occurs via intracellular depletion of glucose. It is unclear whether this is a direct or secondary effect of glucose on the hypothalamus [24]. A patient with Wernicke's encephalopathy has been described with persistent hypothermia without other known cause [31]. On autopsy, pathology showed necrosis of the dorso and ventromedial hypothalamic nuclei as

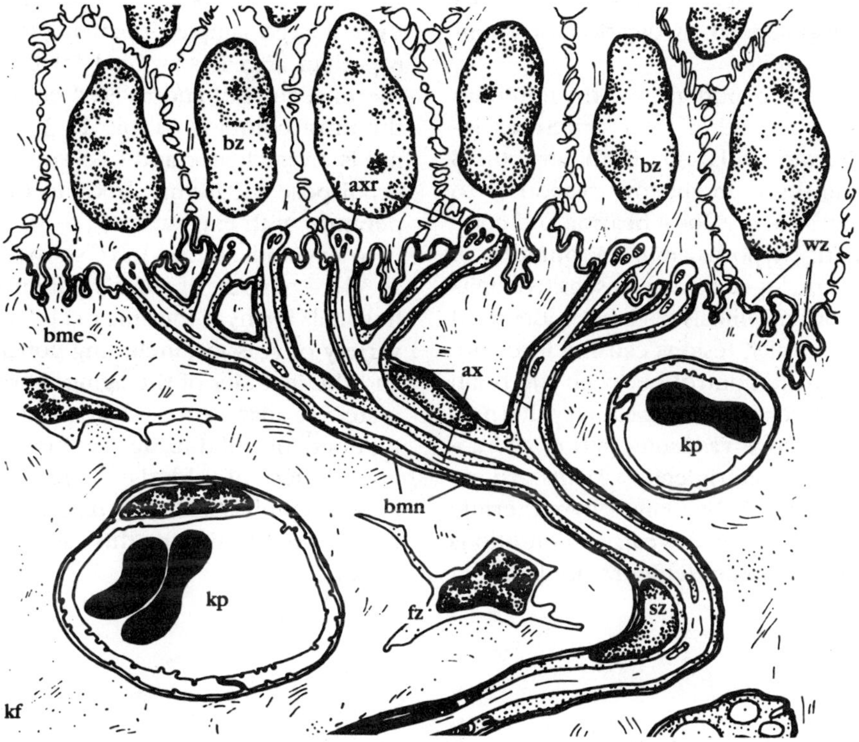

Fig. 12-2. Semischematic diagram of nerve endings at the site of an electrophysiologically identified cold receptor in the hairy skin of a cat's nose. ms = myelin sheath of afferent nerve; sz = nonmyelinated Schwann cell accompanying terminal axons (ax) to basement membrane (bme) of epidermis; bmn = basement membrane of nerve terminals; axr = receptive endings with mitochondria; bz = basal epidermal cells; wz = root feet of basal cells; kp = capillaries; fz = fibrocyte; kf = collagen fibrils of stratum papillare. (From H. Hensel, Cutaneous Thermoreceptors. In: *Handbook of Sensory Physiology.* Heidelberg: Springer, 1972. Vol. II, pp. 79–110.)

well as gliosis and capillary overgrowth, findings characteristic of this disease. The mammillary bodies and periventricular areas of the midbrain were also involved. There are a few other cases in the literature of Wernicke's disease associated with hypothermia, although none have pathologic correlation. One patient with clinical Wernicke's encephalopathy had baseline hypothermia and inappropriate response to heating and cooling, which normalized after thiamine therapy [34]. Because of the possible absence of a febrile response, infections should be looked for carefully in any patient suspected of having Wernicke's disease.

Approximately 20 cases of recurrent idiopathic spontaneous hypothermia have been reported in the literature [33]. It has been reported with an age of onset from infancy to adulthood. Ten of the reported cases had the clinical triad of recurrent hypothermia, episodic hyperhidrosis, and agenesis of the corpus callosum known as Shapiro's syndrome [48]. The fundamental pathophysiology in cases with or without agenesis of the corpus callosum remains to be determined. Although some patients have other evidence of hypothalamic dysfunction, this is not universal [33]. Because of the abrupt disturbance of autonomic mechanisms in some clinical cases, the term *diencephalic epilepsy* has been used to describe some of these patients [42]. There is no clinical or experimental evidence that there are actual epileptic events. A few patients have improved after anticonvulsant therapy [33]. It is unclear whether these cases represent a response to medication or spontaneous improvement.

In addition to the hypothalamus, the midbrain and spinal cord are other CNS structures involved in thermoregulation. Both structures elicit the same thermoregulatory responses to artificial changes such as local heating and cooling as does the hypothalamus. A number of "cold"- and "warm"-specific thermosensitive units in the spinal cord of animals have been identified (Fig. 12-3). Clinically, lesions causing interruption of temperature control between the brain stem and spinal cord can lead to hypothermia. Because of ineffective vasoconstriction and abnormal shivering, quadriplegic patients are extremely susceptible to becoming hypothermic during periods of adverse weather conditions with lowering of ambient temperature [1].

Defective temperature regulation can occur because of very specific CNS lesions. If, however, a large sample of patients from a U.S. metropolitan area is surveyed for causes of hypothermia, alcohol and related complications are the most common (Table 12-3). Because ethanol is a vasodilator and CNS suppressant, it can predispose the human body to decreased temperature with exposure.

In England, studies have shown that as many as 3 to 4 percent of elderly patients admitted to hospitals are hypothermic [41]. This occurs for a variety of reasons, including concurrent illness and the inability of the aging thermoregulatory system to adapt to a cold environment. Despite a number of modifiable factors found in the households of elderly patients, one recent report emphasized the difficulty of preventing hypothermia in this age group (Table 12-4).

Fig. 12-3. Average static discharge of thermosensitive units in spinal cord and skin. (Adapted from E. Simon and M. Iriki, Sensory transmission of spinal heat and cold sensitivity in ascending spinal neurons. *Arch. Ges. Physiol.* 328:103, 1971, and H. Hensel and D. R. Kenshalo, Warm receptors in the nasal region of cats. *J. Physiol.* (London) 204:99, 1969.)

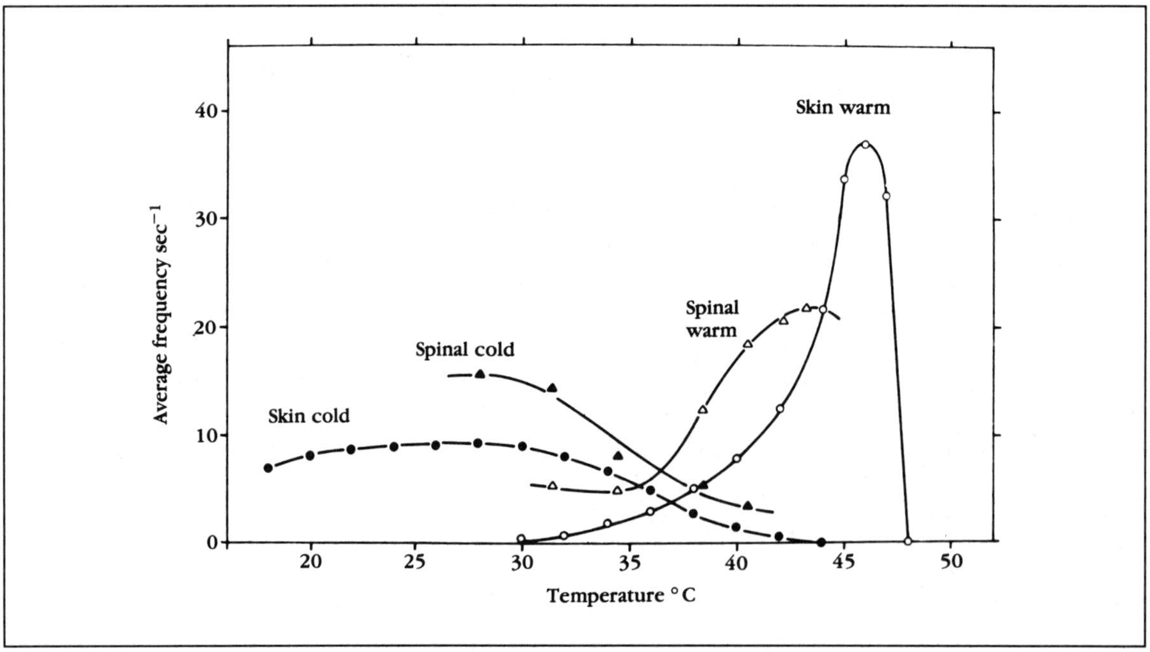

Table 12-3. Causes of hypothermia in 148 cases[a]

Cause	*No. of Patients*
Alcohol Abuse	63(43%)
Wernicke's encephalopathy[b]	26(18%)
Sepsis	28(19%)
Exposure only	21(14%)
Hypoglycemia	18(12%)
Sedative overdose	15(10%)
Hepatic encephalopathy	10(7%)
Shock due to heart failure or gastrointestinal bleeding	9(6%)
Structural brain lesion or infarct[c]	8(5%)
Head trauma	5(3%)
Hypothyroidism	5(3%)
Diabetic ketoacidosis	4(3%)
Renal failure	2(1%)
Ethylene glycol poisoning	1(1%)

[a] Percentage total is greater than 100% because 35 patients had more than one contributing factor.
[b] Diagnosed by eye movement abnormalities or autopsy findings.
[c] Includes 4 patients with subdural or intracerebral hemorrhage, 1 with a brain tumor, 1 with a ventricular shunt obstruction, 1 with a brainstem stroke, and 1 with fat emboli.
Source: Fischbeck and Simon [21].

CLINICAL MANIFESTATIONS OF HYPOTHERMIA

The initial clinical picture of patients with hypothermia is dominated by their neurologic signs and symptoms. Under controlled conditions, these findings remain very predictable. In a hospital setting in which multiple medical abnormalities come into play, neurologic findings correlate with the degree of hypothermia but have a greater degree of variability. Dugid, Simpson, and Stowers [18] offer some general observations of the major clinical and neurologic findings seen as hypothermic patients progress from 35 to 24°C. They noted that shivering ceases and is followed by muscular rigidity between 32.0 and 29.5°C. This is accompanied by a fine tremor, which can be detected on the electrocardiogram. Consciousness is often impaired, and the skin is pale, cold, dry, and corpse-like; a variable degree of subcutaneous edema is present. Below 29.5°C, the pupils react poorly to light, and the tendon reflexes may be delayed and sluggish. The respiratory rate and heart rate are depressed, and the blood pressure is low or unrecordable [18].

Pulse, blood pressure, and respirations go through two general phases. From 35 to 32°C, there is a responsive phase in which blood pressure and pulse tend to increase as volume increases in the central circulation, and diuresis ensues. This is followed by a slowing phase from 32 to 24°C in which blood pressure, pulse, and respiration decrease [22]. In an acute care setting, these parameters also follow this basic pattern but in a less uniform way. In 97 patients from San Francisco General Hospital with accidental hypothermia, pulse and blood pressure decreased with declining temperature [21]. The pulse was less than 60 in most patients, with a temperature less than 27°C (80°F), whereas blood pressure drop was not as regular (Figs. 12-4A and B). Rate of respiration did not vary significantly as temperature dropped, although at temperatures below 27°C, 50 percent of patients had respiratory rates of less than 12 per minute (Fig. 12-4C).

Table 12-4. Number of elderly patients with inadequate heating

Heating Inadequacies	*First Visit*	*Second Visit*
No heating in bedroom	10	3
No heating in bathroom or toilet	16	16
No heating in corridor	18	18
Windows open at night	10	2
Inadequate clothing	1	1

Source: Otty and Roland [41].

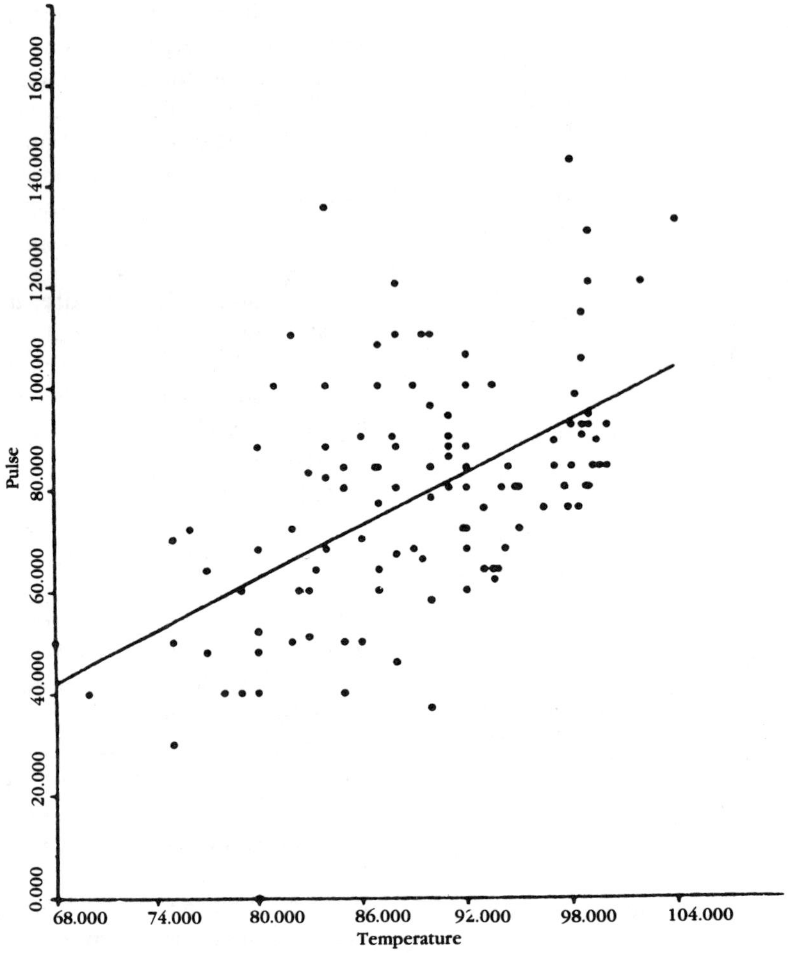

A

Fig. 12-4. Temperature versus pulse (A), temperature versus blood pressure (B), temperature versus respirations (C) in 97 hospitalized patients with hypothermia.

Neurologic observations in a controlled setting were perfomed on 42 patients during prolonged periods of human refrigeration by Fay and Smith [20] in 1940. They noted that with a rectal temperature as low as 34°C, thought processes were unaltered and patients showed no memory loss or emotional instability. As temperatures were further lowered, psychomotor retardation slowly increased with perseveration of speech. Dysarthria developed below 33.5°C, and between 27 and 28°C, most patients were unable to say a word. Four patients had their temperatures lowered to below 27°C. Vocal response was elicited with difficulty, but in one of four conversation did persist to 23.5°C. Of note is that all patients regardless of the degree of hypothermia had retrograde amnesia for the period of refrigeration, despite normal memory and reasoning during part of the experience.

Pupillary size remained regular at all temperatures. Pupillary reaction to light was noted to be sluggish in all refrigerated patients with temperatures below 32°C. All four with temperatures below 27°C had no reaction to light. Radial, biceps, triceps, knee, and ankle reflexes actually increased between 37.0 and 29.5°C, with reflexes often becoming depressed with temperatures less than 29.5°C. Four of four patients with

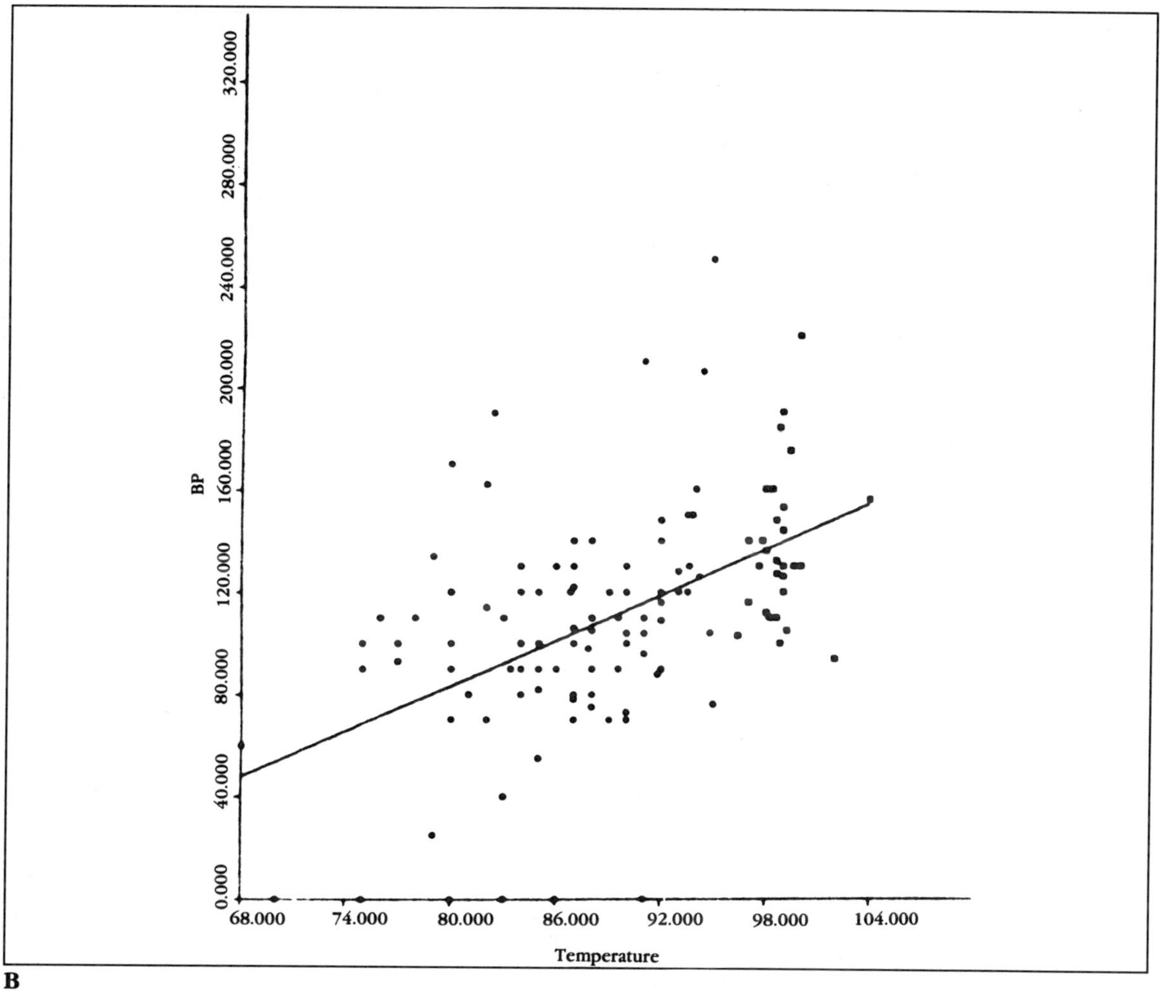

B

temperatures below 27°C had absent reflexes. Muscle stiffness was noted to occur universally, with myotonia often elicitable in all 42 refrigerated patients. Spontaneous myokymia was observed with temperatures as low as 29°C. Characteristic postures were noted in "cold" patients, with the limbs held close to the torso along with the upper and lower extremities assuming a flexed position. There were no athetotic, dystonic, or choreatic movements noted in any of the refrigerated patients.

In general, the results of Faye and Smith correlate with observations made by Fischbeck and Simon [21] in 97 patients with accidental hypothermia (Table 12-5). In this group, consciousness also progressively declined with temperature. Only 2 patients with temperatures as low as 31°C were still described as alert. All 20 patients with temperatures between 27.0 and 29.5° C were confused or only responded purposefully to pain. Surprisingly, 6 of 18 patients with a temperature between 20 and 27°C were described as lethargic or confused but remained verbal, one with a temperature of 20°C. Only 2 of 20 had slight or no response to pain, showing it is unusual for a patient to appear "dead," even with severe hypthermia. In accidental hypothermia, the range in level of consciousness was broader than in the controlled environment.

Fifty percent of those patients with a temperature between 27 and 32°C and 41 percent of those with a temperature below 27°C had nor-

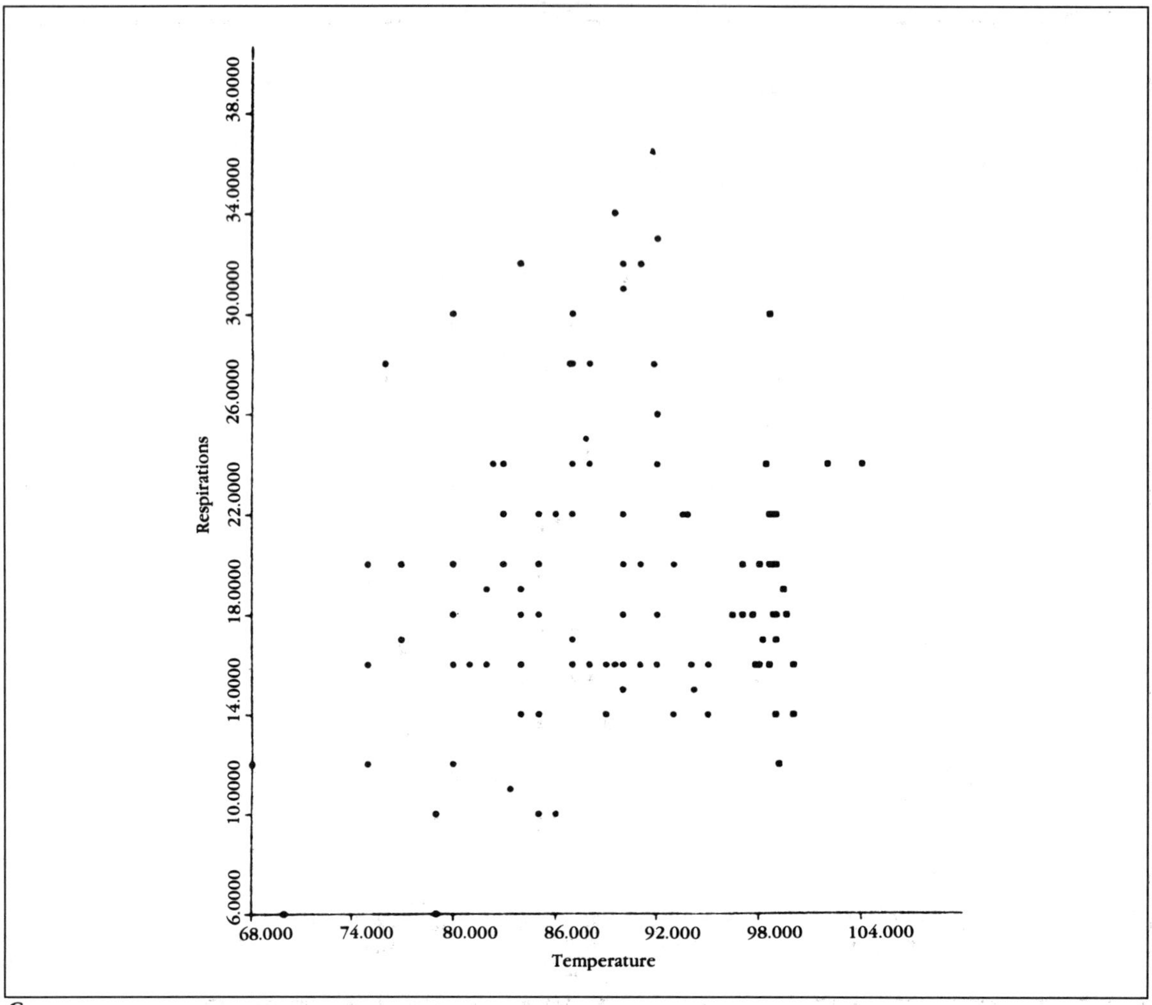

C

Fig. 12-4. (*Continued.*)

mally reactive pupils. Eighteen percent of those with a temperature below 27°C had "fixed" pupils. Four patients initially had unequal pupils, which returned to normal after rewarming. Although there was a clear trend for response to light to become more sluggish with decreasing temperature, even at less than 27°C there was no predictable response. The amplitude of deep tendon reflexes showed a progressive decrease with temperature ($p < .0001$). Fourteen of 40 (45%) patients with temperature below 29.5°C had diminished or absent reflexes, yet 10 of 17 (59%) retained normal reflexes with a temperature below 27°C. Nine of 9 patients with temperature less than 29.5°C had increased muscle tone, as did 7 of 11 with temperature between 29.5 and 32.0°C. Increased muscle tone was by far the most sensitive though nonspecific clinical sign indicating temperature below 29.5°C, as compared to diminished reflexes, sluggish pupils, or eye movement abnormalities. Abnormal eye movements (nystagmus, decreased motility, impaired oculovestibular reflexes) were frequent but did not correlate with temperature. Because of increased muscle tone, neck stiffness was often present. In 46 patients whose cerebrospinal fluid was sampled, none had a pleocytosis. One patient was noted to have dysto-

Table 12-5. Neurologic findings in 97 selected hypothermic patients

Determination	*Severe Hypothermia: 20° to 27°C (68° to 80°F)*	*Moderate Hypothermia: 27° to 29.5°C (80° to 85°F)*	*Moderate Hypothermia: 29.5° to 32°C (85° to 90°F)*	*Mild Hypothermia: 32° to 35°C (90° to 95°F)*
Level of consciousness[a]				
Alert	0	0	2(7%)	6(21%)
Lethargic or confused	6(33%)	14(67%)	20(69%)	18(64%)
Purposively responsive	9(50%)	7(33%)	7(24%)	4(14%)
Decorticate posturing	1(6%)	0	0	0
Unresponsive	2(11%)	0	0	0
Pupils[b]				
Normally reactive	7(41%)	11(58%)	20(67%)	17(71%)
Sluggish	7(41%)	7(37%)	6(20%)	6(25%)
Fixed	3(18%)	1(5%)	4(13%)	1(4%)
Deep trendon reflexes (best response elicitable)[a]				
Increased	0	0	0	2(8%)
Normal	10(59%)	11(61%)	28(93%)	21(84%)
Decreased	7(41%)	7(39%)	2(7%)	2(8%)
Muscle tone[b]				
Increased	6(100%)	3(100%)	7(64%)	4(57%)
Normal	0	0	4(36%)	3(43%)
Eye movements[c]				
Full without nystagmus	14(88%)	12(71%)	20(74%)	18(75%)
Full with nystagmus	0	2(12%)	2(7%)	3(13%)
Not full	2(13%)	3(18%)	5(19%)	3(13%)
Plantar response[c]				
Both flexor	10(83%)	13(81%)	20(83%)	21(100%)
One or both extensor	2(17%)	3(19%)	4(17%)	0

[a] Significant variation ($p < 0.0001$).
[b] Significant variation ($p < 0.01$).
[c] No significant variation ($p > 0.05$).
Source: Fischbeck and Simon [21].

nic movements at 27°C. The presence or absence of extensor plantar response did not correlate with hypothermia in either series.

Mental status depression, sluggish pupillary response to light, increased muscle tone, and diminished deep tendon reflexes correlate with degreee of hypothermia. The range of these changes is quite broad in accidental hypothermia. This variability may be accounted for by associated diseases, reliability of varied observers, or variability of circumstances and duration of hypothermia. Because the patient with accidental hypothermia often presents with such varied factors, these findings probably represent a realistic range to be expected in the neurologic examination in such a group. To summarize, in mild hypothermia, 32 to 35°C, the patient may be normal or confused, but reflexes will likely be normal to increased and pupillary response will be intact. In moderate hypothermia, 27 to 32°C, the patient may still respond verbally. Muscle tone will begin to increase, with reflexes being normal to diminished. Pupillary response will be normal or sluggish. In severe hypothermia, 20 to 27°C, the patient is unlikely to respond verbally, although it is uncommon to have no response to painful stimuli. Reflexes will be diminished, and muscle tone will be increased. Pupillary response will be sluggish or absent. Major deviations from this outline should prompt the search for factors other than hypothermia as a cause for altered nervous system function.

PATHOPHYSIOLOGY OF HYPOTHERMIA

Hypothermia induces a variety of complex physiologic changes that affect all aspects of bodily function. Many of the compensatory changes are protective in nature. The rate of chemical reactions decreases by approximately 50 percent per each 10°C decrease in temperature. Basal metabolic rate is similary affected, falling to 50 percent of normal at 28°C [10]. Because of the associated decrease in oxygen requirement, the tolerance of tissue to hypoxia is increased during clinical hypothermia. The clinical application of this fact stems chiefly from laboratory observations that suggested the feasibility of complete circulatory arrest to permit cardiac surgery in a bloodless field [6–9]. The main limiting factor in hypothermic surgery without continued perfusion of oxygenated blood is brain damage. Experiments have shown that even with deep hypothermia (17–20°C), CNS damage occurs after 60 minutes of circulatory arrest [45]. Individual hippocampal slices have been analyzed after deprivation of oxygen and glucose in the setting of hypothermia. The critical survival time with regard to complete recovery of neural activity and high-energy phosphates was 10 minutes at 37°C, 15 minutes at 28°C, and 45 minutes at 21°C [50]. The decrease in the rate of metabolism of individual organs with temperature reduction is not the same even if the temperature of each organ is held constant. If the initial sympathetic response to hypothermia is suppressed by anesthesia or drugs, total cardiac output decreases progressively with decreasing temperature [52]. Blood flow to liver, heart, and brain is reduced proportionally, whereas the kidney is seen as the most dispensable organ regarding blood flow as hypothermia ensues (Fig. 12-5). Urinary output, which is an important clinical sign of organ perfusion, usually decreases in states of hemorrhage or sepsis. Urine flow initially increases with decreasing temperatures secondary to both cutaneous vasoconstriction with subsequent increase in central blood volume as well as to depressed oxidative tubular activity with resulting decreased resorption of sodium and water [44,47]. This may result in hypovolemia. Hyperglycemia is frequently seen in the setting of hypothermia, which probably results from the inhibition of insulin release from the pancreas as well as decreased peripheral glucose utilization [17]. Since these changes revert with rewarming, insulin should not be used in this clinical setting.

Hypothermia has important effects on cardiovascular function and electrical activity in the myocardium. As noted previously, blood pressure and pulse progressively decline with temperature. The most important hemodynamic effect of cold is an increase in myocardial irritability. As body temperature falls, there is a progressive slowing of the sinus rate and prolon-

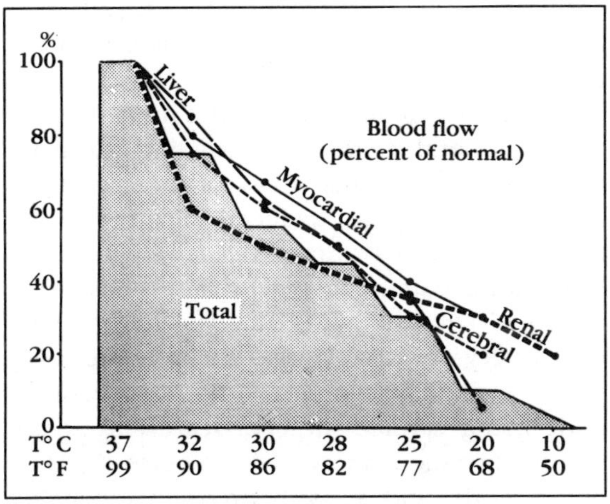

Fig. 12-5. Blood flow to the organs reduces with progressive hypothermia. The shaded area is total flow. The heart, liver, and brain maintain a higher level of flow in comparison with the kidneys to 27°C. However, at 25 to 20°C, renal and myocardial blood flows are sustained at 20 to 25 percent of normothermic levels, whereas cerebral and hepatic blood flow show greater decreases. (Reproduced with permission from E. Blair, *Clinical Hypothermia.* New York: McGraw Hill, 1964.)

gation of the P–R interval and Q–Tc intervals [16]. The most typical electrocardiographic abnormality associated with hypothermia is the J wave (also called the Osborn wave or camel hump sign). It is consistently found when the temperature is below 25°C (Fig. 12-6). Although atrial fibrillation is the most common rhythm disturbance in hypothermia, occurring in 50 to 60 percent of patients, ventricular fibrillation is the most dangerous rhythm [16]. In experimental animals, spontaneous ventricular fibrillation begins to occur at 24°C [4]. In the clinical setting of accidental hypothermia, where other medical problems frequently coexist, the fibrillation threshold is lowered and is an immediate hazard below 28°C [44].

Depression of the respiratory rate does occur with decreasing temperature (see Fig. 12-4C) but is not usually clinically significant. Bronchopneumonia, however, is quite common in elderly patients with hypothermia. This most likely occurs due to CNS depression (decreased cough reflex) and an increase in lung secretions.

Fig. 12-6. Hypothermia. The body temperature was 80°F. Note the J waves in all leads, with prolonged Q–T interval and low T waves. Intermittent baseline oscillation is present as a result of somatic muscle tremors. The heart rate is 32 beats per minute. (From Chou [16].)

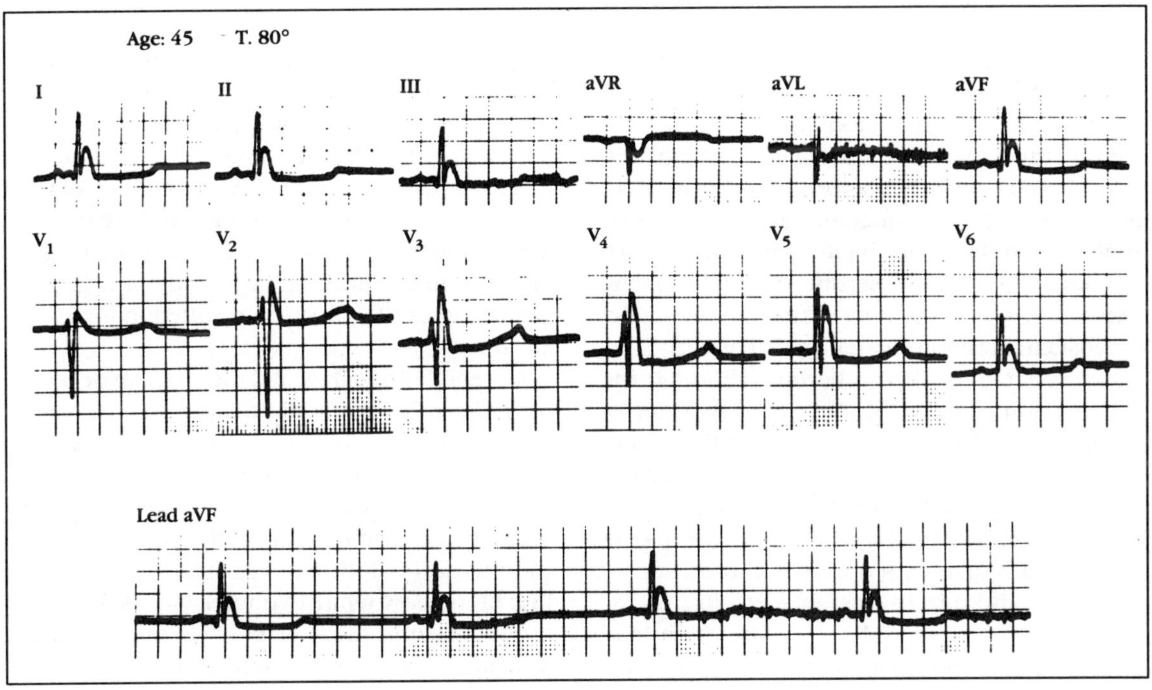

The mortality rate in this group of patients is quite high [36]. Hypothermia increases the affinity of oxygen to hemoglobin and shifts the oxyhemoglobin dissociation curve to the left. This is not clinically significant, however, because of the body's decrease in oxygen requirement. It is important to recognize the effect of hypothermia on blood gas measurements. With each 1°C decrease in body temperature, there is an increase in pH of .015, a decrease in PCO_2 of 4.4 percent, and a decrease in PO_2 of 7.2 percent [13,43]. This assumes that measurements of arterial blood gas (ABG) are made with the blood sample at the patient's body temperature. It is controversial as to whether the uncorrected ABG, measured at the patient's body temperature, represents a value that should be interpreted in the same manner as an ABG at 37°C. The alkalosis and hypocarbia during hypothermia are defended by physiologic mechanisms. Many authors feel that if acceptable blood gas values are measured at a temperature of 37°C, the temperature of the electrode, it is unnecessary to alter mechanical ventilation or inspired carbon dioxide and oxygen concentrations [52].

Hypothermia causes a decrease in bowel motility and clinically a rigid abdominal wall, which makes the abdominal examination difficult to interpret [22]. Hemorrhagic pancreatitis has been described in an autopsy study and attributed to microvascular sludging from lowered temperature [18,22]. Laboratory evidence of pancreatitis (increased amylase) in accidental hypothermia, even in a predominantly alcoholic population, is uncommon and has been reported to have an incidence of about 10 percent [53]. Other serum enzymes (lactic dehydrogenase, creatine kinase, glutamic-oxaloacetic transaminase) are frequently elevated in accidental hypothermia, although the relative contribution of skeletal muscle, myocardium, and liver is unclear from clinical studies [22,36,53]. Detoxification and conjugation abilities of the liver are decreased, which causes drugs to remain in the system longer and at higher levels than with otherwise normal doses [10]. Hypothermia causes an elevation of the hematocrit due to splenic contraction and plasma loss as well as an increase in blood viscosity at temperatures less than 27°C [28]. It is unclear as to the clinical importance of these factors.

There are a number of changes in the central and peripheral nervous system that normally occur in hypothermia. Many of these changes can be monitored. Reduced electroencephalographic activity may result in a burst-suppression pattern and finally, at less than 70°F, an isoelectric reading [10]. Hypothermia produces very regular changes in brain stem auditory evoked potentials (BAEP). In patients undergoing cardiac surgery, decreasing temperature produces increased latencies of BAEP waves I, III, and V, with prolongation being more severe for later components [37]. The temperature latency relationship is best expressed by an exponential curve (Figs. 12-7 and 12-8), with all BAEPs present above 23°C but absent below 20°C. It is probable that the combined effects of axonal slowing as well as impaired transmitter release resulting in slowed synaptic transmission produce the BAEP effects. [5].

Cerebrospinal fluid (CSF) pressure has been measured during induced hypothermia and in rewarming [11]. In 58 of 70 episodes of rewarming (most greater than 35 hours), there was an increase in drowsiness. It was most severe in patients actively rewarmed or following prolonged hypothermia. After rewarming, CSF pressure was often in the range of 300 mm of water, with one case up to 600 mm of water. Some patients with increased pressure had dramatic improvement of mentation with removal of CSF. In 30 cases, CSF was examined during cooling and rewarming, and in 14, CSF pressure increased on rewarming. In 9 of the 14, gradual reduction of CSF pressure resulted in increased alertness.

Cerebral blood flow and metabolism decrease progressively with decreasing temperatures secondary to both a decrease in mean arterial blood pressure and an increase in vascular resistance [10,52]. Cerebral blood flow has been measured in two patients with accidental hypothermia [19]. Both patients had reduced cerebral blood flow while hypothermic. As there was no decrease in mean arterial pressure in these patients, it seems that increased vascular resis-

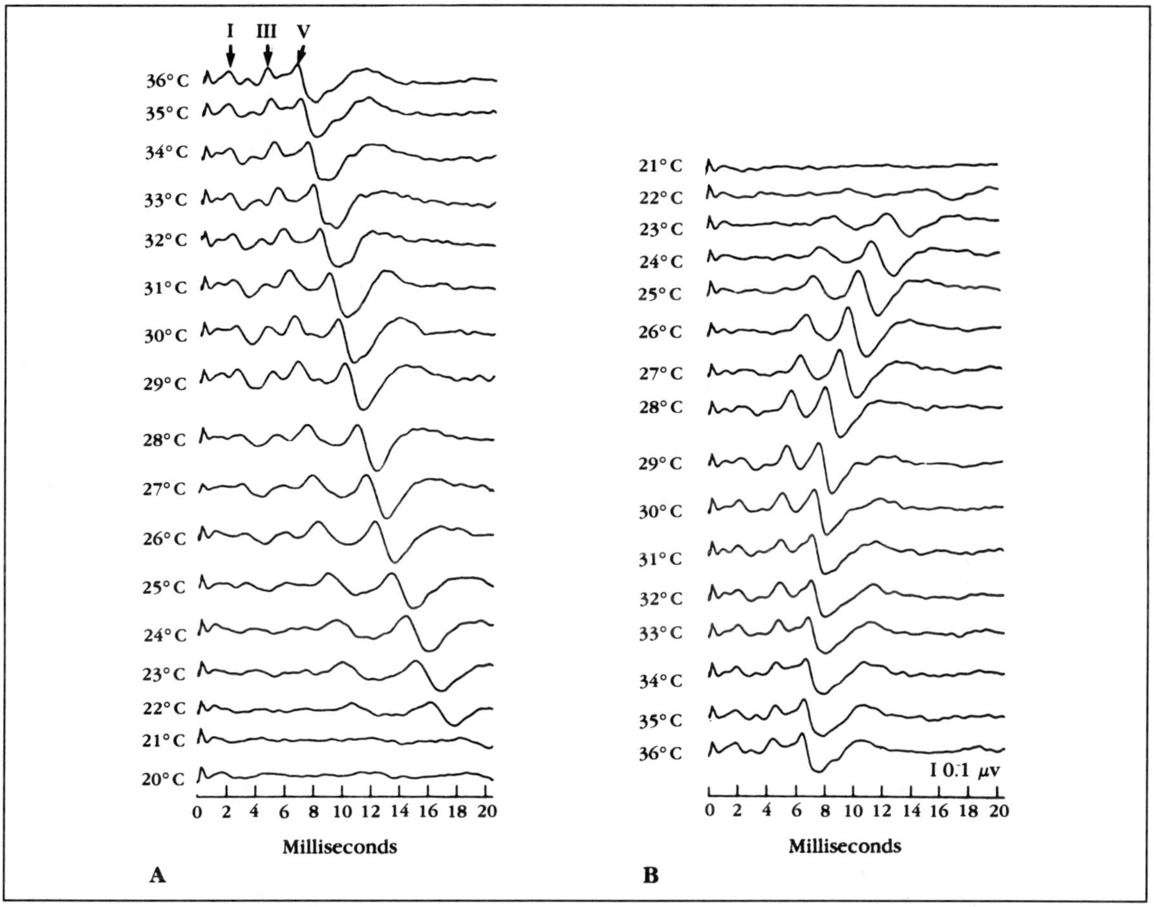

Fig. 12-7. Brain stem auditory potentials (BAEPs) in a 48-year-old man during hypothermia (A) and subsequent rewarming (B). Major peaks are identified with Roman numerals. There is a progressive prolongation of all components with decreasing temperature and the disappearance of BAEPs at 20°C. With rewarming, BAEPs returned to precooling status. (From Markand et al. [37])

tance accounted for the reduced blood flow in these cases. Increased blood viscosity and cerebral vasoconstriction may both play a role in increased vascular resistance.

Temperature has notable effects on the neuromuscular system. Results of electromyogram and nerve conduction studies are affected by hypothermia. Intramuscular temperature affects the parameters of motor unit potentials. Mean duration increases and mean amplitude declines as temperature falls. There is an increase in the number of polyphasic potentials, which presumably relates to increased temporal dispersion of individual muscle fiber action potentials with a reduction in temperature [3]. There is a 2.4 meter/second decrease in maximum motor conduction velocity of human ulnar nerve per each 1°C drop in temperature [12,14]. This emphasizes the importance of measuring skin temperature in clinical electromyography. Depending on the clinical disease process, slowed nerve conduction velocity may be erroneously interpreted as a demyelinating neuropathy in the presence of lowered skin temperature. The mechanical performance of muscle in response to temperature changes parallels that of chemical reactions, with an approximate 50 percent reduction in shortening velocity and power output per 10°C drop. It is interesting to note that the mechanical performance of frog sartorius muscle does not change after long-term exposure to different ambient temperatures, imply-

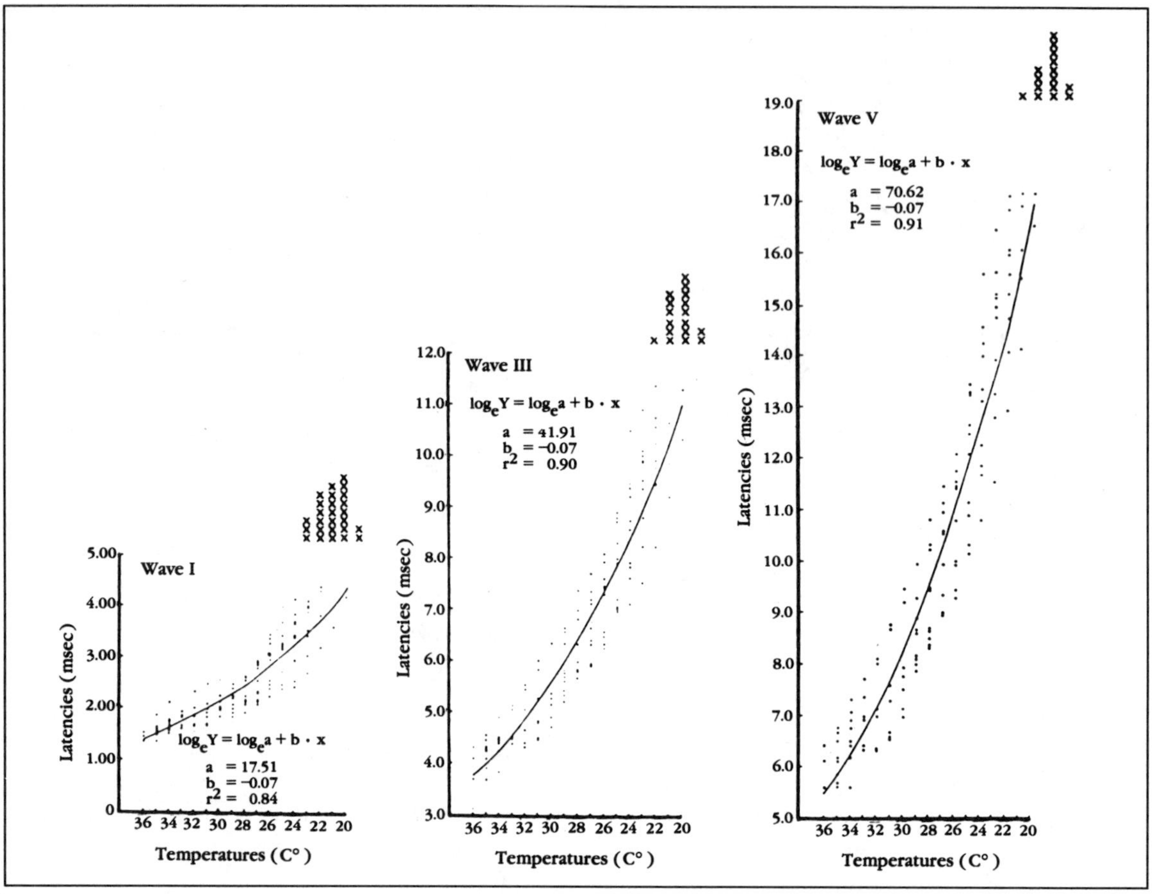

Fig. 12-8. Scatter plots showing the relationship of latencies of waves I, III, and V of brain stem auditory evoked potentials to nasopharyngeal temperature during cooling. Absence of a component is denoted by x. Note that the temperature-latency relationship, which is exponential, is denoted by the equation $\log_e Y = \log_e a + bx$, where Y = latency, a = Y intercept, b = regression coefficient, and x = temperature; r^2 = coefficient of determination. (From Markland et al. [37].)

ing that muscle does not have the ability to alter its mechanical properties secondary to prolonged hypothermia [46].

TREATMENT OF HYPOTHERMIA

The treatment of hypothermia is quite varied because of intercurrent disorders that often affect the clinical course of many patients. Treatment clearly must be tailored to the individual patient. There is a wide range in the ability of human beings to tolerate cold. For example, people immersed in water colder than 6°C after shipwreck usually die of hypothermia within 75 minutes [38]. There is, however, a single case report from Iceland in which a large man survived 5 to 6 hours swimming to shore in such water without ill effects [29]. The man was studied and found to have a much greater insulating ability secondary to a large amount of subcutaneous fat. This emphasizes the point that the tolerance of many patients is quite variable and that the first step in treatment of hypothermia is the alteration of modifiable factors that predispose to hypothermia. These include avoiding cold exposure, the use of appropriate garments in all individuals, and ensuring the proper home supervision of elderly or invalid patients who may be unable to contol their environment adequately [41].

There are a number of baseline studies that should be obtained on all hypothermic patients. After the history and physical examination and measurement of temperature with an appropriate low-registering thermometer, a number of blood tests should be performed and supportive therapy instituted (Table 12-6).

There are three major categories of rewarming techniques that are described in the literature. Active total rewarming involves placing the cold patient in warm surroundings such as heated water. This can be hazardous because of the danger of precipitating hypotension resulting from vasodilatation [35]. Active core rewarming emphasizes warming the trunk and leaving the extremities cold until the heart is warm. This has been accomplished by such methods as colonic irrigation, mediastinal irrigation via thoracotomy, hemodialysis, peritoneal dialysis, extracorporeal blood rewarming, and inhalation rewarming [34]. Passive rewarming involves removing the victim from the exposed environment, covering him with a blanket, and warming IV fluids to 37°C [22]. The choice of either passive or active rewarming should be individualized.

At low temperatures, it may be impossible to convert a fibrillating heart to a normal rhythm. Debrillation is often unsuccessful at body temperatures less than 86°F [2]. This is one of the clear-cut indications for the use of an active rewarming method such as mediastinal irrigation with open thoracotomy and external cardiac compression or even partial cardiopulmonary bypass with warmed extracorpeal blood [51]. Once the temperature increases toward normal, defibrillation may then be possible. It seems prudent to place all patients with a core temperature of less than 90°F in an intensive care unit with cardiac monitoring because of the risk of malignant dysrhythmias. Close monitoring should also be carried out on all patients with secondary potentially fatal complications such as acute pancreatitis or possible sepsis. It is important to avoid attempts at extensive manipulations (intubation, Swan-Ganz catheter) in stable patients who have not yet developed cardiac complications unless absolutely necessary [2]. Such maneuvers may precipitate cardiac rhythm disturbances.

Table 12-6. Therapy of Hypothermia

Diagnosis with low-reading rectal thermometer, history, physical examination
Initial laboratory evaluation: hematocrit, platelet count, white cell count, electrolytes, glucose, liver function tests, amylase, renal function testing, creatine kinase, blood cultures, chest x-ray, electrocardiogram, arterial blood gas (measured at 37°C)
Drug therapy: IV thiamine, oxygen, broad-spectrum antibiotics
Intensive care unit if temperature $< 32°C$ or other complications
Passive rewarming in most cases unless cardiovascular compromise

The mortality of hypothermia varies widely in the literature. In accidental hypothermia in which alcohol and exposure are the only two complicating variables, mortality is less than 10 percent [22,53]. Series in which many elderly patients with multiple medical problems are included have much higher mortality rates [18,36]. Although there have been reports of successful treatment of hypothermia utilizing active rewarming methods, a properly controlled and randomized comparison of aggressive and spontaneous rewarming has never been made [32,35]. It seems clear that no intervention other than passive external rewarming is necessary when the clinical course progresses favorably from the outset [35].

Because of the protective effect of hypothermia on the brain, cardiac resuscitation attempts despite a prolonged period of low cerebral blood flow may still have a good outcome. Some clinicans believe that patients who appear dead after a long exposure to cold temperature should not be considered dead until they are at near normal core temperature and are still unresponsive to cardiopulmonary resuscitation [2]. Obviously, clinical judgment is important in such cases when time of asystole is completely unknown.

CONCLUSIONS

Because of the dominant role that neurologic signs and symptoms play in clinically recognizing hypothermia, it is important that all clinicians be familiar with the normal physiology of this state. It remains a common problem throughout much of the temperate world with mortality rates being highest in the elderly population [15]. A number of factors such as drugs, central nervous system disease, and exposure should make the clinician wary of its existence, which can often go undetected without the use of low-reading thermometers. Hypothermia in itself can have a marked protective effect on organ systems and in a sense places patients in a state of suspended animation. Its possible cardiac complications make hypothermia important to recognize early so that immediate monitoring or treatment may commence. As the extreme neurologic state in hypothermia may resemble death, the phrase "no one is dead until they are warm and dead" should be remembered.

REFERENCES

1. Altus, P. A., Hickman, J. W., and Nord, J. Accidental hypothermia in a healthy quadriplegic patient. *Neurology* 35:427, 1985.
2. American Heart Association. Standards and guidelines for cardiopulmonary resuscitation (CPR) and emergency cardiac care (ECC). *J.A.M.A.* 255, 1986.
3. Aminoff, M. J. *Electromyography in Clinical Practice* (2nd ed.) New York: Churchill Livingstone, 1987.
4. Angelakos, E. T. Hypothermic ventricular fibrillation. *Ann. N. Y. Acad. Sci.* 80:353, 1959.
5. Benita, M., and Conde, H. Effects of local cooling upon conduction and synaptic transmission. *Brain Res.* 36:133, 1972.
6. Bigelow, W. G., Lindsay, W. K., and Greenwood, W. F. Hypothermia: Possible role in cardiac surgery, investigation of factors governing survival in dogs at low body temperature. *Ann. Surg.* 132:849, 1950.
7. Bigelow, W. G., Lindsay, W. K., and Harrison, R. C. Oxygen transport and utilization in dogs at low body temperatures. *Am. J. Physiol.* 160:125, 1950.
8. Bigelow, W. G., and McBirnie, J. E. Further experiences with hypothermia for intracardiac surgery in monkeys and ground hogs. *Ann. Surg.* 137:361, 1953.
9. Bigelow, W. G., Mustard, W. T., and Evans, J. G. some physiologic concepts of hypothermia and their applications to cardiac surgery. *J. Thorac. Surg.* 28:463, 1954.
10. Blair, E. *Clinical Hypothermia.* New York: McGraw-Hill, 1964.
11. Bloch, M. Cerebral effects of rewarming following prolonged hypothermia: Significance for the management of severe cranio-cerebral injury and acute pyrexia. *Brain* 90:769, 1967.
12. Bolton, C. F., Carter, K., and Koval, J. J. Temperature effects on conduction studies of normal and abnormal nerve. *Muscle Nerve* 5:S145, 1982.
13. Bradley, A. F., Stupfel, M., and Severinghaus, J. W. Effect of temperature on PCO_2 and PO_2 of blood in vitro. *J. Appl. Physiol.* 9:201, 1956.
14. Buchthal, F., and Rosenfalck, A. Evoked action potentials and conduction velocity in human sensory nerves. *Brain Res.* 3:1, 1966.
15. CDC. Hypothermia-associated deaths—United States, 1968–1980. *M.M.W.R.* 34:753, 1985.
16. Chou, T. C. *Electrocardiography in Clinical Practice.* New York: Grune & Stratton, 1979.
17. Curry, D. L., and Curry, K. P. Hypothermia and insulin secretion. *Endocrinology* 87:750, 1957.
18. Duguid, H., Simpson, R. G., and Stowers, J. M. Accidental hypothermia. *Lancet* 7214:1213, 1961.
19. Ehrmantraut, W. R., Ticktin, H. E., and Fazekas, J. F. Cerebral hemodynamics and metabolism in accidental hypothermia. *Arch. Intern. Med.* 99:57, 1957.
20. Fay, T., and Smith, G. W. Observations on reflex responses during prolonged periods of human refrigeration. *Arch. Neurol. Psychiatry.* 45:215, 1941.
21. Fischbeck, K. H., and Simon, R. P. Neurological manifestations of accidental hypothermia. *Ann. Neurol.* 10:384, 1981.
22. Fitzgerald, F. T., and Jessop, C. Accidental hypothermia: A report of 22 cases and review of the literature. *Adv. Intern. Med.* 27:127, 1982.
23. Fox, R. H., Davies, T. W., Marsh, F. P., and Urich, H. Hypothermia in a young man with an anterior hypothalamic lesion. *Lancet* 2:185, 1970.
24. Freinkel, N., Metzger, B. E., Harris, E., et al. The hypothermia of hypoglycemia: Studies with 2-deoxy-D-glucose in normal human subjects and mice. *N. Engl. J. Med.* 287:841, 1972.
25. Gale, C. C. Neuroendocrine aspects of thermoregulation. *Annu. Rev. Physiol.* 35:391, 1979.
26. Hensel, H. Neural processes in thermoregulation. *Physiol. Rev.* 53:948, 1973.
27. Johnson, R. H., and Lambie, D. G. Autonomic Function and Dysfunction. In A. K. Asbury, G. M. McKhann, and W. I. McDonald (eds.), *Diseases of the Nervous System.* Philadelphia: Saunders, 1986.

28. Kanter, G. S. Hypothermic hemoconcentration. *Am. J. Physiol.* 214:856, 1968.
29. Keatinge, W. R., Coleshaw, S. R. K., and Millard, C. E. Exceptional case of survival in cold water. *Br. Med. J.* 292:171, 1986.
30. Kedes, L. H., and Field, J. B. Hypothermia: A clue to hypoglycemia. *N. Engl. J. Med.* 271:785, 1964.
31. Koeppen, A. H., Daniels, J. C., and Barron, K. D. Subnormal body temperatures in Wernicke's encephalopathy. *Arch. Neurol.* 21:493, 1969.
32. Ledingham, I. M., and Mone, J. G. Treatment after exposure to cold. *Lancet* i:534, 1982.
33. LeWitt, P. A., Newman, R. P., Greenberg, H. S., et al. Episodic hyperhidrosis, hypothermia, and agenesis of corpus callosum. *Neurology* 33:1122, 1983.
34. Lipton, J. M., Payne, H., Garza, H. R., and Rosenberg, R. N. Thermolability in Wernicke's encephalopathy. *Arch. Neurol.* 35:750, 1978.
35. Maclean, D. Emergency management of accidental hypothermia: A review. *J. R. Soc. Med.* 79:528, 1986.
36. Maclean, D., Griffiths, P. D., and Emslie-Smith, D. Serum-enzymes in relation to electrocardiographic changes in accidental hypothermia. *Lancet* 2:1266, 1968.
37. Markand, O. N., Lee, B. I., Warren, C., et al. Effects of hypothermia on brainstem auditory evoked potentials in humans. *Ann. Neurol.* 22:507, 1987.
38. Molnar, G. W. Survival of hypothermia by men immersed in the ocean. *J.A.M.A.* 131:1046, 1946.
39. Myers, R. D., and Yaksh, T. L. Control of body temperature in the unanaesthetized monkey by cholinergic and aminergic systems in the hypothalamus. *J. Physiol.* 218:609, 1971.
40. Nadel, E. R., Mitchell, J. W., and Stolwijk, J. A. J. Control of local and total sweating during exercise transients. *Int. J. Biometeorol.* 15:201, 1971.
41. Otty, C. J., and Roland, M. O. Hypothemia in the elderly: Scope for prevention. *Br. Med. J.* 295:419, 1987.
42. Penfield, W. Diencephalic epilepsy. *Arch. Neurol. Psychiatry* 22:358, 1929.
43. Rahn, H., Reeves, R. B., and Howell, B. J. Hydrogen ion regulation, temperature, and evolution. *Am. Rev. Respir. Dis.* 112:165, 1975.
44. Reuler, J. B. Hypothermia: Pathophysiology, clinical settings, and management *Ann. Intern. Med.* 89:519, 1978.
45. Rittenhouse, E. A., Mohri, H., Dillard, D. H., and Merendino, K. A. Deep hypothermia in cardiovascular surgery. *Ann. Thorac. Surg.* 17:63, 1974.
46. Rome, L. C. The effect of long-term exposure to different temperatures on the mechanical performance of frog muscle. *Physiol. Zool.* 56:33, 1983.
47. Segar, W. E., Riley, P. A., and Barila, T. G. Urinary composition during hypothermia. *Am. J. Physiol.* 185:528, 1956.
48. Shapiro, W. R., and Plum, F. Paroxysmal hypothermia and mutism accompanying agenesis of the corpus callosum. *Neurology* 17:317, 1967.
49. Smith, A. U. Viability of supercooled and frozen mammals. *Ann. N.Y. Acad. Sci.* 80:291, 1959.
50. Tanimoto, M., and Okada, Y. The protective effect of hypothermia on hippocampal slices from guinea pig during deprivation of oxygen and glucose. *Brain Res.* 417:239, 1987.
51. Towne, W. D., Geiss, W. P., Yanes, H. O., and Rahimtoola, S. H. Intractable ventricular fibrillation associated with profound accidental hypothermia: Successful treatment with partial cardiopulmonary bypass. *N. Engl. J. Med.* 287:1135, 1972.
52. Wong, K. C. Physiology and pharmacology of hypothermia. *West. J. Med.* 138:227, 1983.
53. Weyman, A. E., Greenbaum, D. M., and Grace, W. J. Accidental hypothermia in an alcoholic population. *Am. J. Med.* 56:13, 1974.

13 Hyperthermia and Temperature Regulation

John R. Sutton

The maintenance of internal body temperature at approximately 37°C despite environmental temperature extremes is a characteristic of healthy humans. This feature has been unique to birds and mammals only during the past 70 million years, but it has conferred an important evolutionary advantage, making them independent of their environment; however, this is at the expense of a high metabolic rate. At 37°C, we are close to the ceiling of thermal viability compared with the lower end of the temperature scale. Thus, we have evolved much more elaborate temperature-regulating mechanisms to prevent overheating rather than overcooling. Figure 13-1 demonstrates how we adapt to changes in environmental temperature by increasing our heat loss above a certain limit and increasing our heat production below a certain limit.

THERMAL EXCHANGE

There are three bidirectional avenues of thermal exchange between the body and the environmental—conduction, convection, and radiation—and one unidirectional change—evaporation of heat lost from the body to the atmosphere. This is expressed in the heat storage equation of Winslow:

$$S = M \pm R \pm Cv \pm Cd - E$$

in which S is heat storage, M is metabolic heat production, R is heat gained or lost through radiation, Cv is heat gained or lost by convection, Cd is heat gained or lost by conduction, and E is heat lost from evaporation. Although one can respond physiologically to a hot or cold environment, it is important to emphasize that the most important factors enabling us to exercise under conditions of environmental extremes are behavioral, not physiologic. That is, we really depend on protecting ourselves with insulated clothing and seeking shelter from immoderate heat or cold; these measures have allowed us to survive and exercise in such situations.

In the cold, the two primary physiologic responses are the ability to regulate blood flow within the body and increasing skin blood flow when there is a need to dissipate heat from the core to the surface or restrict skin blood flow

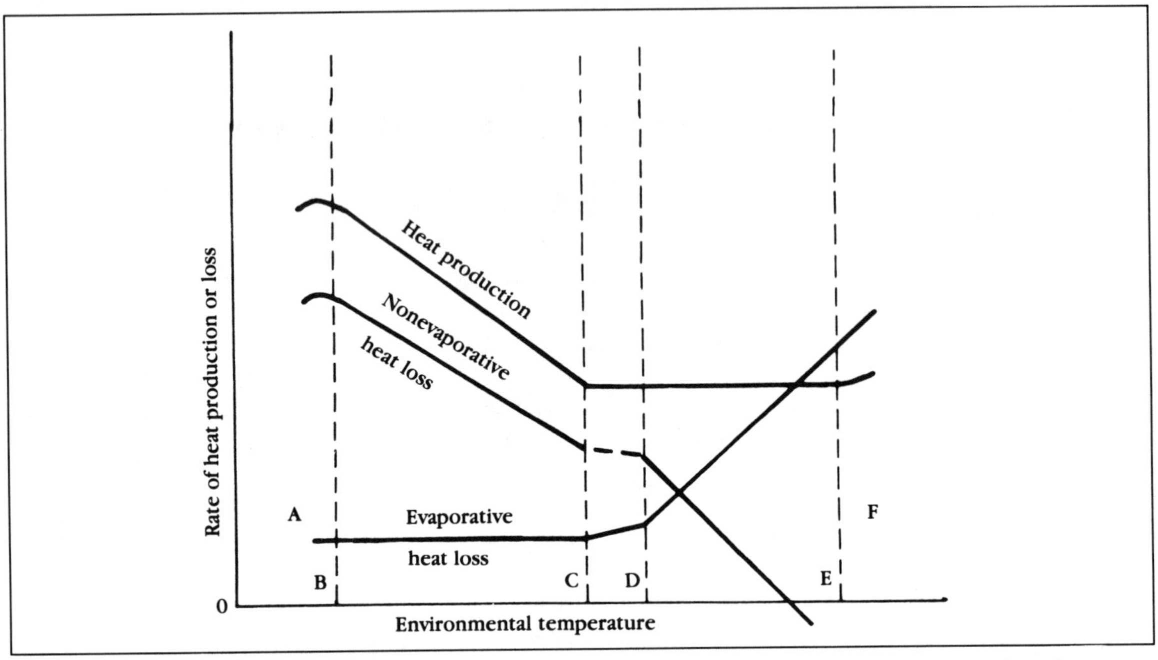

Fig. 13-1. Diagram of relationship between heat production, evaporative and nonevaporative heat loss, and deep body temperature in a homeothermic animal. A = zone of hypothermia; B = temperature of summit metabolism and incipient hypothermia; C = critical temperature; D = temperature of marked increase in evaporative loss; E = temperature of incipient hyperthermial rise; F = zone of hyperthermia; CD = zone of least thermoregulatory effort; CE = zone of minimum metabolism; BE = thermoregulatory range. These zones were defined by Mount (Mount, L. E. The Concept of Thermal Neutrality. In J. L. Monteith and L. E. Mount [eds.], *Heat Loss from Animals and Man.* London: Butterworth, 1974).

when it is necessary to reduce skin heat loss and maintain the body's core temperature. Additionally, we can increase heat production several-fold. Thus, we have a thermoregulatory system that appears to operate around a thermal set point, sensing information from the core and the skin. Hence, whenever the core temperature varies from that set point, the appropriate heat-producing or heat-losing mechanisms are stimulated during exercise or by a primary change in skin temperature at a constant core temperature if the heat load is external [21]. Changes in skin blood flow also alter the central circulation in both heat and cold. Training improves our adaptation to cold [1]. Rowell and colleagues [33] and Hales [14] have demonstrated that any increase in skin blood flow will be accompanied by decreases in renal and splanchnic blood flow. Exercising in the heat will also result in an increase in skin blood volume, a factor that will be clinically important in the production of syncope when people stop exercising at the end of a race but remain upright, develop venous pooling in the legs, and become syncopal.

The combination of heat acclimatization and increased physical fitness has been well demonstrated to enhance performance in the heat. Wyndham [40], Piwonka and Robinson [26], and Gisolfi and Robinson [12] showed that trained individuals had a greater heat-dissipating capacity than untrained. Part of this is due to the increased sensitivity of sweating mechanisms with training and a lowering of the sweating threshold [24]. An additionally important factor in the increased heat tolerance of the fit individual is the increased blood volume induced by training, recently demonstrated by Senay, Mitchell, and Wyndham [34], Convertino, Greenleaf, and Bernauer [6], Fortney and associates [10], and Green and co-workers [13]. This topic was well reviewed by Harrison [17].

Females have been considered to be at a disadvantage compared with males when exercising in the heat because of their substantially lower sweat rate [11,19,41]. A further sex difference is the greater surface area to weight ratio (A_D/Wt) of females. However, this issue is considerably more complex. When skin temperature is above ambient temperature, an increased A_D/Wt would be an advantage to females because of the relatively larger surface area available for heat loss in comparison to the mass available for heat production. Per unit of volume of sweat produced, women reach a lower body core temperature than men and have therefore been considered more efficient temperature regulators [9]. Differences in cardiorespiratory fitness between males and females may also be responsible for differences in thermal response [7,9,25,38]. The importance of cardiorespiratory fitness in determining the differences in temperature regulation between males and females was recently addressed by Avellini, Kamon, and Krajewski [4], who selected men and women with identical cardiorespiratory fitness, equal surface areas, and equal surface area-to-mass ratios. Although the numbers were small (four in each group), in an acute heat stress study, the women in the follicular phase of the menstrual cycle had lower sweat rates, rectal temperatures, and heart rates than the men. Following 10 days of acclimatization, the differences between the sexes were eliminated. The rectal temperatures and heart rates were similar. The sweat rate increased during exercise in both groups—but more so in the men, suggesting that sweating was more effective in the women.

HYPERTHERMIA AND FEVER

The key role of the hypothalamus in temperature regulation has been known for some time, and a distinction should be made between the simple elevation of body temperature as it occurs in hyperthermia associated with exercise when the hypothalamus is functioning normally and fever associated with a variety of infectious and noninfectious processes in which the body temperature is increased and the set point of the hypothalamus is also elevated. Thus, hyperthermia may be considered as a result of an imbalance between peripheral mechanisms of heat production and heat loss favoring increased heat storage, whereas in fever, although there must be an imbalance for body core temperature to rise, the set point is also increased.

The occurrence of fever with disease has been known since Hippocratic times, but it was Wunderlich who popularized the use of the clinical thermometer in 1868 and stated, "The more my obervations were multiplied, the more firmly rooted did my conviction become of the unparalleled value of this method of investigation, as giving an accurate and reliable insight into the condition of the sick" [39]. To this day, the use of clinical thermometry remains a valuable although increasingly less appreciated indication of an underlying disorder. While descriptions of fever such as intermittent fever, remittent fever, sustained fever, relapsing fever, Pel-Epstein fever, and rat bite fever probably are outdated, one cannot impress enough upon the student and new graduate the importance of an accurate and frequent measurement of body core temperature in people with a variety of disabilities. It might also be pointed out that if in doubt about body core temperature measurements, the rectal temperature is far superior to oral or axillary temperature measurements. This becomes particularly so when people tend to hyperventilate and the buccal mucosa may be considerably cooler than the body core temperature, as is commonly the case in respiratory infections and hyperthermia following exercise.

The frequent and accurate recording of temperature is important to determine whether in fact there is an organic illness. It may be helpful in the assessment of the severity and duration of the illness and certainly the response to treatment. Whether fever is beneficial to the organism is debatable. However, evidence from poikilotherms such as fish and lizards indicates that the survival rate following infection is increased with an elevated temperature. By contrast, humans who fail to develop a fever following an infectious process, particularly those who are already debilitated or aged, have a poor prognosis.

Exercise Hyperthermia

Hyperthermia is a normal concomitant of exercise and has been documented in marathons [27] and fun runs [36]. The problems related to an excessive body core temperature may occur when the environmental circumstances do not appear to be particularly extreme or even when the day is cold [36]. With exercise, there is a normal shift in the circulating fluid volume. Adolph [2] demonstrated that water was disproportionately lost from plasma compared with other body tissues. Moreover, if significant dehydration occurs, the heat-dissipating mechanisms will be compromised further. The competition between the skin and muscle for blood flow is a competition accentuated by exercise, and, for a comparable external heat stress, skin blood flow will be lower compared with the resting state [33]. Studies by Hales and colleagues [16] have demonstrated that during severe heat stress, skin blood flow begins to fall. The same situation pertains when central venous pressure is reduced by lower body negative pressure [23,42]. When these data are taken in concert, Rowell [32] concluded that the hierarchy of homeostatic mechanisms favors the maintenance of arterial pressure and circulation to the vital organs at the expense of skin vasodilatation and thermoregulation. In their recent publication concerning circulatory changes in collapsed fun runners, Hales and colleagues [16] have demonstrated a marked reduction in skin blood flow when compared to "control runners." They postulated that the reduction in skin blood flow occurred when right heart filling pressures were reduced. To date, no human data are available to support this hypothesis, although supportive animal data do exist [15].

Nonenvironmental Hyperthermia—The Fevers

Nonenvironmentally induced causes include direct involvement of the hypothalamus with a variety of neoplastic or infiltrative disorders such as tumors, sarcoidosis, intracranial hemorrhage, or thromboses that can give rise to hyperthermia. Also there have been abnormalities in thermoregulation reported in anorexia nervosa. The following disorders most commonly give rise to elevations in temperature:

1. Infectious processes by virus, bacteria, rickettsiae, and parasites.
2. Neoplastic disorders, often complicated by infection, but malignancies, particularly if they are metastatic, are frequently associated with febrile states, especially carcinoma of the lung, pancreas, liver, and the lymphomas. Sometimes a fever may be the only manifestation of the underlying neoplastic disorder.
3. Hemolytic disorders such as sickle cell crisis, collagen vascular disease, lupus erythromatosus, drug fevers, and serum sickness.
4. Trauma such as crushing injuries and large hematomas.
5. Acute metabolic and familial disorders such as gout, porphyria, thyrotoxic crises, and familial Mediterranean fever.
6. Thrombosis and infarction such as myocardial infarction and pulmonary embolus.
7. Malignant hyperthermia and malignant neuroleptic syndrome.

GENESIS OF FEVER AND THE ENDOGENOUS PYROGENS

The factors from leukocytes and their endogenous pyrogens have been studied for more than 30 years, but it now seems that there are several leukocyte-derived factors that can initiate fever when stimulated with viruses, endotoxin, or other inflammatory agents. These are interleukin-1-alpha, interleukin-1-beta, interferon, and tumor necrosis factor (cachectin) [8]. Much work has been done to characterize these endogenous pyrogens, and it is now appreciated that they are not produced exclusively by leukocytes. Dinarello, Cannon, and Wolff [8] suggest that they should be referred to as a special class of polypeptides and as cytokines that are intrinsically pyrogenic. A variety of other factors can stimulate the release of endogenous pyrogens. They include especially the antigen antibody complexes in the presence of pyrogen.

The mechanisms whereby endogenous pyrogens trigger the hypothalamus are not entirely clear, but activation of prostaglandin E_2 (PGE_2) is currently the most favored process, and injection of arachidonic acid into the hypothalamus will produce fever. Of all the cyclo-oxygenase products, PGE_2 is the most potent fever-producing agent. Furthermore, the efficacy of aspirin and other antipyretics to reduce fever appears to be directly related to their ability to block brain cyclo-oxygenase. For more details, the reader is referred to the excellent review by Dinarello, Cannon, and Wolff [8].

CLINICAL MANIFESTATIONS OF HEAT DISORDERS

Heat illness should be regarded as a continuum of hyperthermic states and is classified as such by the Medical Research Council of Great Britain and the World Health Organization. The terms ***heat exhaustion*** and ***heatstroke*** both fall within the general definition of heat illness and are the most severe forms of heat injury to afflict the exercising individual. Although differentiation between the two is often tenuous, it has been proposed that serious central nervous system dysfunction is the major distinguishing feature of heatstroke. In the original description, anhydrosis and a rectal temperature in excess of 41°C were both regarded as essential components of heatstroke. However, with the recent observations of hyperthermic states in fun runs and short-duration exercise events where dehydration is not a problem, insistence on the presence of all criteria before a diagnosis is made would frequently obscure the potentially life-threatening state of the patient and might result in delayed treatment.

Clinical manifestations of hyperthermia will depend predominantly on the circumstances and the underlying cause. Although in general the manifestations are more dramatic with higher temperatures, there is tremendous individual variation. The following are manifestations of exertional heat injury:

1. Heat cramps. These are classically brief, intermittent, and often excruciating and follow severe exercise. They are not specifically related to heat and are thought to be the result of sodium deficiency, often associated with excess water replacement following a dehydrating run.
2. Heat exhaustion/heatstroke. These should be considered as a continuum and should always be suspected in anyone who collapses after exertion in the heat. Of course, under extreme environmental conditions, the aged and the infirm may be at risk of developing heatstroke and heat exhaustion even without undue exertion. Sometimes there can be catastrophic numbers of victims, as in the Peking "epidemic" of 1743 during which 1100 people died during a prolonged heat wave. This has also been commonly reported during intensely hot summers in the southern United States and southern Europe. One of the most graphic descriptions of heatstroke was reported from the British frigate docked at Liverpool in 1841 when "the weather gradually became warmer; double awnings were spread, the decks were kept constantly wetted and every precaution used to prevent exposure of men. In one day, from a species of coup de soleil, three lieutenants and thirty men were lost." It was stated that at one time the decks resembled a slaughterhouse, so numerous were the bleeding patients. This was probably the first description of the coagulation problems that accompany severe heatstroke.

Classic exertional heat injury should be identified relatively easily. It has been increasingly reported in runners, military recruits during exercises, miners, cyclists, and football players. In its classic form, it presents with acute onset, has multiple organ pathology, and should be considered in anyone whose behavior is bizarre following exercise or when environmental conditions are extreme. However, as has been recently documented in fun runs and marathons, when severe exertion occurs, the environmental conditions do not need to be extreme for heatstroke to occur.

Neurologic Abnormalities

A variety of neurologic presentations may occur with heat exhaustion and heatstroke including impaired judgment, irritability, hallucinations, delirium, central nervous system depression with coma, and on occasion, status epilepticus with decerebrate rigidity, ocular gyric crises, and opisthotonus. Cerebellar syndromes with ataxia and also the chronic thalamic syndrome have been reported following heatstroke. The duration of unconsciousness in those who regain consciousness but then lapse back into coma carries a worse prognosis. The clinical manifestations of exertional heat injury are listed in Table 13-1.

PREVENTION AND MANAGEMENT OF HEATSTROKE, HEAT EXHAUSTION, AND HEAT SYNCOPE

Exertional heatstroke and other thermal illness are preventable, but the athletes and the organizers and medical directors of fun runs need to be aware that such possibilities exist. Futhermore, a simple understanding of the pathophysiologic mechanisms involved in the genesis of heatstroke will prevent tragedies such as army recruits running in wet suits and suc-

Table 13-1. The clinical manifestations of exertional heat injury

System	*Comment*
Cardiovascular	
Sinus tachycardia	Invariable finding
Transient hypertension	Rare
Hypotension and shock	Rare
Acute left heart failure	Rare; higher incidence in older population
Pulmonary	
Hyperventilation	Common finding
Pulmonary edema	Rare: present as final complication before death
Pulmonary infarction	Rare
Neurologic	
Delirium, hallucinations, status epilepticus, oculogyric crises, opisthotonus	Occur fairly commonly; manifestations of hyperirritability that often occur in association with nervous system depression
Coma	A feature of moderate to severe heat stroke
Cerebellar syndromes	Rare
Hemiplegic episodes	Rare
Renal	
Acute nephropathy	Occurs in 50% of patients who develop heat stroke
Chronic interstitial nephritis	Uncommon
Hematologic	
Purpura, conjunctival hemorrhage, manifestation of bleeding into lungs, kidneys, myocardium, liver or central nervous system	Occurs with bleeding diathesis. Rare, but when it occurs, prognosis is very poor.
Gastrointestinal	
Diarrhea and vomiting	Common, especially during first 24 hours
Hematemesis and melena	Rare; occur in association with bleeding diathesis
Endocrine	
Clinical signs of hypoglycemia (blood sugar levels of < 25 mg/dl)	Uncommon
Musculoskeletal	
Muscles rigid and contracted	Common finding; associated with elevation in serum enzymes and myoglobinuria

Source: Hart, L. E., and Sutton, J. R. Environmental considerations for exercise. *Clin. Cardiol.* 5:246, 1987.

cumbing to heatstroke [5]. The interaction of the susceptible runner with a given set of environmental circumstances sets the stage for heat illness and heatstroke. It is important to appreciate that high humidity with high solar radiation on a windless day reduces the body's ability to lose heat by the most effective means—evaporation. Evidence suggests that the most susceptible individuals include the young, the old, and those who are dehydrated, ill, obese, unfit, and lacking heat acclimatization [35]. Also, many fun runs are held in the spring when runners are as yet unacclimatized. They often train in the cool of the day in the morning or evening but compete when the environmental conditions are hottest. Also at this time of year, an unseasonably hot day following weeks of cold weather is not uncommon. Hughson and coworkers [20] have shown that many of the runners who collapse with heatstroke are trying to outdo themselves with their best-ever times and fail to heed the early warning signals of impending disaster.

Heat exhaustion and heatstroke are part of a continuum, the principal difference being the alteration of consciousness in heatstroke. Hyperthermia usually above 39.5°C and sometimes as high as 43°C is seen in both [30]. The most important point to emphasize is that treatment must begin on-site. This highlights organizational strategies and the need to be able to diagnose accurately with measurement of core temperature and institute cooling therapy including intravenous fluids at the race site. Delay can be fatal. Many race organizers indentify the nearest hospital emergency room facilities to be used for "collapsed" runners or casualties; however, this will postpone the onset of treatment and may jeopardize the patient unnecessarily. In an experience of several hundred thousands of runners, no serious sequelae have resulted when resuscitation and cooling have been instituted at the race site. The converse has not been the case [18,28,29,31]. We are aware of more than a dozen fatalities that have occurred when resuscitation facilities were not available immediately on-site. Furthermore, when the runner reaches the emergency room, the realization of a potentially life-threatening illness may not always be apparent to the attending staff; there may be a delay in establishing the correct diagnosis by measuring core temperature and a further lag in instituting treatment.

Having established the diagnosis, the essential features of treatment are intravenous therapy to reestablish the circulation and cooling. Cooling with a fan and a fine warm spray [37] was a method introduced to treat Mecca pilgrims, an approach that Keilblock [22] has shown to be the most effective means to reduce the elevated temperature when compared with several alternatives (Table 13-2).

It is important to appreciate that both hypothermia and hyperthermia can occur in the

Table 13-2. Efficacies of different body cooling procedures relative to passive cooling

Method of cooling	*Cooling rate* Relative*	*Cooling rate* $0°C\ min^{-1}$
Passive	—	0.054
Six ICPs on major arteries	−9	0.049
Body covered with ICPs	+35	0.074
Evaporative cooling	+50	0.081
Evaporative plus six ICPs	+59	0.086
Whole body immersion (25°C)	+39	0.075
Whole body immersion (12°C)	+385	0.262

ICP = "instant" cold packs.
* Percentage increase relative to passive cooling.
Source: Kielblock [22], p. 495.

same race. Hamiltion, Ontario's "Billy Sherring Round the Bay" race of 30 km is the oldest distance race in North America; it was established in 1894 and has been held annually at the end of March, when weather conditions are usually cool. Although the front runners will finish with an elevated temperature, the winds off the lake invariably cool the slower runners to the extent that some will be hypothermic. At this time of year, unseasonably hot days may also occur before any runner has had a chance to become acclimatized to heat. The medical directors of runs held in the spring and autumn must prepare to treat some casualties who are too hot as well as others who may be too cold. Accurate measurement of rectal (core) temperature with an "IVAC" or low-reading thermometer is essential to establish the diagnosis and follow the clinical progress of the patient following institution of the appropriate treatment.

In an attempt to educate organizers of fun runs to the potential hazards, the American College of Sports Medicine has issued a position stand, "Prevention of Thermal Injuries During Distance Running" [3]. This document has also been translated into language suitable for the lay public and is available from the American College of Sports Medicine.

REFERENCES

1. Adams, T., and Haberling, E. J. Effects of training on response to cold. *J. Appl. Physiol.* 13:226, 1958.
2. Adolph, E. F. Blood Changes in Dehydration. In E. F. Adolph (ed.), *Physiology of Man in the Desert.* New York: Interscience, 1947. Pp. 160–171.
3. American College of Sports Medicine. Position stand: Prevention of thermal injuries during distance running. *Med. Sci. Sports Exerc.* 16(5):ix, 1984.
4. Avellini, B. A., Kamon, E., and Krajewski, J. T. Physiological responses of physically fit men and women to acclimation to humid heat. *J. Appl. Physiol.* 49:254, 1980.
5. Brahams, D. Death of a soldier: Accident or neglect? *Lancet* i:485, 1988.
6. Convertino, V. A., Greenleaf, J. E., and Bernauer, E. M. Role of thermal and exercise factors in the mechanism of hypervolemia. *J. Appl. Physiol.* 48:657, 1980.
7. Dill, D. B., Soholt, L. F., McLean, D. C., et al. Capacity of young males and females for running in desert heat. *Med. Sci. Sports* 9:137, 1977.
8. Dinarello, C. A., Cannon, J. G., and Wolff, S. M. New concepts on the pathogenesis of fever. *Rev. Infect. Dis.* 10:168, 1988.
9. Drinkwater, B. L., Denton, J. E., Kupprat, I. C., et al. Aerobic power as a factor in women's response to work in hot environments. *J. Appl. Physiol.* 41:815, 1976.
10. Fortney, S. M., Wenger, C. B., Bove, J. R., and Nadel, E. R. Effect of blood volume on forearm venous and cardiac stroke volume during exercise. *J. Appl. Physiol.* 55:884, 1983.
11. Fox, R. H., Lofstedt, B. E., Woodward, P. M., et al. Comparison of thermoregulatory function in men and women. *J. Appl. Physiol.* 26:444, 1969.
12. Gisolfi, C., and Robinson, S. Relations between physical training, acclimatization and heat tolerance. *J. Appl. Physiol.* 26:530, 1969.
13. Green, H. J., Hughson, R. L., Thomson, J. A., and Sharratt, M. T. Supramaximal exercise after training-induced hypervolemia: I. Gas exchange and acid-base balance. *J. Appl. Physiol.* 62:1944, 1987.
14. Hales, J. R. S. Effects of exposure to hot environments on the regional distribution of blood flow and on cardiorespiratory function in sheep. *Pfluegers Arch.* 344:133, 1973.
15. Hales, J. R. S. A case supporting the proposal that cardiac filling pressure is the limiting factor in adjusting to heat stress. *Yale J. Biol. Med.* 59:237, 1986.
16. Hales, J. R. S., Stephens, F. R. N., Fawcett, A. A., et al. Lowered skin blood flow and erythrocyte sphering in collapsed fun-runners. *Lancet* 1:1494, 1986.
17. Harrison, M. H. Effect of thermal stress and exercise on blood volume in humans. *Physiol. Rev.* 65:149, 1985.
18. Hart, L. E., Egier, B. P., Shimizu, S. G., et al. Exertional heatstroke: The runner's nemesis. *Can. Med. Assoc. J.* 122:1144, 1980.
19. Hertig, B. A., and Sargent, F., II. Acclimatization of women during work in hot environments. *Fed. Proc.* 22:810, 1963.
20. Hughson, R. L., Green, H. J., Houston, M. E., et al. Heat injuries in Canadian mass participation runs. *Can. Med. Assoc. J.* 122:1141, 1980.
21. Jessens, C. Thermoregulatory Mechanisms in Severe Heat Stress with Exercise. In J. R. S. Hales and D. Richards (eds.), *Heat Stress.* Amsterdam: Excerpta Medica, 1987. Pp. 1–18.
22. Kielblock, A. J. Strategies for the Prevention of Heat Disorders with Particular Reference to the Efficacy of Body Cooling Procedures. In J. R. S. Hales and D. Richards (eds.), *Heat Stress.* Amsterdam: Excerpta Medica, 1987. Pp. 489–497.
23. Nadel, E. R., Mack, G. W., Nose, H., and Tripathi, A. Tolerance to Severe Heat and Exercise: Pe-

ripheral Vascular Responses to Body Fluid Changes. In J. R. S. Hales and D. Richards (eds.), *Heat Stress.* Amsterdam: Excerpta Medica, 1987. Pp. 117–131.
24. Nadel, E. R., Pandolf, K. B., Roberts, M. F., and Stolwijk, J. A. J. Mechanisms of thermal acclimatization to exercise and heat. *J. Appl. Physiol.* 37:515, 1974.
25. Pandolf, K. B., Sawka, M. N., and Gonzalez, R. R. *Human Performance Physiology and Environmental Medicine at Terrestrial Extremes.* Indianapolis: Benchmark, 1988.
26. Piwonka, R. W., and Robinson, S. Acclimatization of highly trained men to work in severe heat. *J. Appl. Physiol.* 22:9, 1967.
27. Pugh, L. G. C. E., Corbett, J. L., and Johnson, R. H. Rectal temperatures, weight losses, and sweat rates in marathon running. *J. Appl. Physiol.* 23:347, 1967.
28. Richards, C. R. B., and Richards, D. Prevention of Exercise-Induced Heat Stroke. In J. R. Sutton and R. M. Brock (eds.), *Sports Medicine for the Mature Athlete.* Indianapolis: Benchmark, 1986. Pp. 151–166.
29. Richards, R., and Richards, D. Medical Management of Fun Runs. In J. R. S. Hales and D. Richards (eds.), *Heat Stress.* Amsterdam: Excerpta Medica, 1987. Pp. 513–525.
30. Richards, R., Richards, D., Schofield, P., et al. Reducing the hazards in Sydney's *The Sun* "City-to-Surf" runs, 1971–1979. *Med. J. Aust.* 2:453, 1979.
31. Richards, R., Richards, D., Schofield, P., et al. Management of heat exhaustion in Sydney's *The Sun* "City-to-Surf" fun runners, 1971–1979. *Med. J. Aust.* 2:457, 1979.
32. Rowell, L. B. Human cardiovascular adjustments to exercise and thermal stress. *Physiol. Rev.* 54:75, 1974.
33. Rowell, L. B., Detry, J. M. R., Profant, G. R., and Wyss, C. Splanchnic vasoconstriciton in hyperthermic man: Role of falling blood pressure. *J. Appl. Physiol.* 31:864, 1971.
34. Senay, L. C., Jr., Mitchell, D., and Wyndham, C. H. Acclimatization in a hot, humid environment: Body fluid adjustments. *J. Appl. Physiol.* 40:786, 1976.
35. Sutton, J. R., and Bar-Or, O. Thermal illness in fun running. *Am. Heart J.* 100:778, 1980.
36. Sutton, J. R., Coleman, M. J., Millar, A. P., et al. The medical problems of mass participation in athletic competition: The "City-to-Surf" Race. *Med. J. Aust.* 2:127, 1972.
37. Weiner, J. S., and Khogali, M. Physiological body cooling unit for treatment of heat stroke. *Lancet* i: 507, 1980.
38. Weinman, K. P., Slabochova, Z., Bernauer, E. M. et al. Reactions of men and women to repeated exposures to humid heat. *J. Appl. Physiol.* 22:533, 1967.
39. Wunderlich, C. A. *On the Temperature in Diseases: A Manual of Medical Thermometry.* London: The New Sydenham Society, 1871. P.v.
40. Wyndham, C. H. The physiology of exercise under heat stress. *Ann. Rev. Physiol.* 35:193, 1973.
41. Wyndham, C. H., Morrison, J. F., and Williams, C. G. Heat reactions of male and female Caucasians. *J. Appl. Physiol.* 20:357, 1965.
42. Zoller, R. P., Mark, A. L., Abboud, F. M., et al. The role of low pressure baroreceptors in reflex vasoconstrictor responses in man. *J. Clin. Immunol.* 51:2967, 1972.

14 Systemic Disorders and Cerebral Demyelinating Lesions

Stephen Brennan and Juan Carlos Ayus

In 1959, Adams, Victor, and Mancall [3] reported a new neurologic syndrome associated with a previously undescribed pathologic lesion in the brain stem of four patients with alcoholism and/or malnutrition. Since that time, many more patients with so-called central pontine myelinolysis (CPM) have been described and the spectrum of the disease has become better understood. Early in the history of CPM, a possible association between the clinical syndrome and various electrolyte abnormalities was suggested. In the past 10 years, substantial controversy has been raised over the causal relationship between electrolyte disorders (principally hyponatremia) and central nervous system demyelinating disorders. One theory is that hyponatremia is the proximate cause of CPM in most patients with the syndrome [60]. Another hypothesis is that CPM is an iatrogenic disease, brought on by overzealous use of hypertonic saline, leading to correction of hyponatremia at excessive rates (i.e., > 1–2 mEq/liter/hour) [87]. Yet another school holds that the rate of correction itself is not the offender; rather, the absolute degree of change, particularly if the final serum sodium concentration rises to normal or hypernatremic levels, leads to the pathologic and clinical findings [15]. Lastly, another group of investigators [6] believes that the brain lesions associated with hyponatremia (hyponatremic encephalopathy) are largely due to a combination of hypoxia, herniation, and pressure necrosis. Demyelination is thought to usually be secondary to anoxia/hypoxia or increased intracranial pressure [40,95], and the clinical manifestations are sometimes delayed, giving a false appearance of some relationship to therapy.

The diversity of opinions on this subject is not yet resolved. Because of the rarity of clinical CPM, as well as the difficulty of achieving an antemortem diagnosis, it is difficult to collect a series of patients to examine prospectively. Indeed, the vast majority of cases of CPM reported in the literature are presented as case reports. It has not yet been possible to develop an animal model that is completely analogous to the human disease, so that further study in an experimental setting has been difficult. Finally, since most investigators in the field believe that theirs is the only correct approach, a randomized prospective clinical trial is likely to meet with substantial ethical objections.

Additionally, there is some apparent confusion in the literature over the use of the diagnostic term *central pontine myelinolysis* (CPM). Although originally described as a distinct pathologic entity where cerebral demyelinating lesions were confined to the pons [3], the term has recently been assigned somewhat arbitrarily to patients or laboratory animals who had demyelination of the brain that was either (a) pontine, (b) extrapontine, or (c) both pontine and extrapontine, or (d) had clinical manifestations similar to those of patients with CPM but without autopsy or radiologic confirmation of cerebral demyelination. In this chapter, the term *cerebral demyelinating lesions* will be used to mean any cerebral demyelination that is confirmed by autopsy, magnetic resonance imaging (MRI) or computed tomography (CT) scanning, regardless of the location of the lesions in the brain [15]. Such a description will include both pontine and extrapontine myelinolysis.

The purpose of this chapter is to try to synthesize the available data on the relationship between abnormalities in serum sodium and the development of cerebral demyelination in a balanced way. By presenting a balanced viewpoint, it is hoped that readers will develop for themselves a framework from which to derive their own conclusions.

CLINICAL FEATURES

Many authors have noted the relatively recent appearance of CPM into clinical medicine despite the long history of many of its antecedents (especially alcoholism) in society [67]. This is all the more remarkable given its dramatic clinical and pathologic presentation. There are four salient features of the disease. First and foremost are the motor abnormalities; second are cranial nerve abnormalities; third are alterations in the sensorium; and fourth are the distinctive histologic abnormalities seen in CPM. In a general sense, CPM has been considered a fatal disease. It is clear from autopsy-based studies, however, that the neurologic syndrome may at times be absent even in patients with clear-cut neuropathology [3,72]. Furthermore, there have been reports of patients with a classic clinical presentation of CPM who have shown substantial improvement or even total resolution of their deficits [43,52]. Thus, the natural history of the disease and the relationship between structural lesions in the brain stem and neurologic impairments await further clarification.

Additionally, it is now clear that demyelinating lesions associated with hypoxic insults, particularly cardiac arrest [57], carbon monoxide intoxication, anesthesia, accidents, certain drug intoxications, and attempted strangulation [44,45], can produce demyelinating lesions of the brain that are essentially identical to those that have often been labeled "central pontine myelinolysis" in the recent literature [65,87,98]. As is the case in those patients described as having "central pontine myelinolysis" in the literature, patients suffering hypoxic insults associated with the above clinical conditions may demonstrate cerebral demyelinating lesions in many different locations in the brain [44]. In the following discussion, use of the term *central pontine myelinolysis* (CPM) will imply that the diagnosis has been clearly established on radiologic or pathologic grounds.

Perhaps the most dramatic of the neurologic findings in patients with CPM is motor weakness of the extremities [3,65,98]. This usually begins in an insidious manner but can progress rapidly to a point where flaccid quadriplegia may be seen. Lower extremities may be affected more severely than upper extremities, usually but not invariably without lateralization. Asymmetric motor findings may reflect extrapontine lesions [46]. Deep tendon reflexes are commonly abnormal (perhaps the most common clinical finding in CPM) but nonspecific [65]. Ataxia of gait is frequently encountered in the early stages of the syndrome. Tremors, rigidity, and abnormal movements are remarkable for their absence. Pathologic reflexes are often noted. The motor weakness can be so severe that respiratory paralysis ensues, necessitating mechanical ventilation [23]. In patients in whom CPM has resolved significantly, the motor abnormalities are usually the most persistent and require months (at least) to ameliorate [43,52, 89,90].

Cranial nerve abnormalities also frequently occur, particularly as a pseudobulbar palsy pattern [3,23,89]. Most patients have dysarthria but are rarely aphonic. They are often able to understand and even follow commands; patients have been reported who can communicate by means of head movement or eye-blinking code [35]. This has led to a description of CPM as a "locked-in" syndrome in some cases [67]. Dysphagia has also been noted in some patients in the absence of odynophagia. The cranial nerves controlling ocular movements have also been afflicted in many patients. The isolated palsy of the muscles controlled by the abducens nerve has been suggested as a relatively specific finding for pontine disease in general and CPM in particular [72]. For the most part, the other cranial nerves are not involved.

Altered mental status is an early finding in most patients with CPM [74]. Deficits in short-term memory are common. Higher cognitive functions are almost invariably affected, but this may be difficult to test adequately in a paralyzed individual. Behavioral abnormalities including agitation and inappropriate acts have also been noted. In most patients, these latter usually give way to a depressed sensorium characterized by poor arousability, lethargy, and eventually coma. Seizures are the exception, and suggest an underlying toxic or metabolic encephalopathy (e.g., hyponatremia) or increased intracranial pressure. The recovery of mental status toward normal may suggest a better prognosis in those patients in whom it occurs.

The sine qua non of CPM, however, is the characteristic pathologic findings [3,65]. These consist of a symmetric, sharply delineated (though often irregular) demyelination in the central basis pontis, usually with dramatic sparing of axonal fibers. Histologically this is said to mimic the lesion of multiple sclerosis; only the anatomic distribution of the lesions in the two diseases is distinctive [20]. Extrapontine lesions are seen in about 10 percent of patients with CPM [98]. These are usually symetrical and occur mainly in the thalamus, basal ganglia, and internal capsule. The pathogenesis of these lesions as well as their predilection for a characteristic location is not known. It has been theorized that the demyelination results from selective ischemia due to basilar artery insufficiency, venous obstruction, or cerebral edema [58]. However it is difficult to rationalize the peculiar distribution of lesions on the basis of a single vascular abnormality [27] and almost equally difficult to explain the lack of axonal involvement.

CPM virtually never occurs in previously normal individuals. It was initially described as a disease of alcoholics and malnourished persons, but it has also been seen in patients with many other systemic diseases including nonalcoholic liver disease (e.g., Wilson's disease) and tumors (both leukemias and solid neoplasms). Whether or not CPM can occur as a consequence of electrolyte disorders or their treatment remains an unsettled issue at this time. One of the most interesting epidemiologic questions about the syndrome is why it suddenly appeared in the late 1950s. Most investigators believe that it did not simply occur unrecognized prior to that time; it is felt that CPM simply did not exist (or was unbelievably rare) until the second half of the twentieth century. Certainly many of the predisposing conditions existed and were well recognized for millenia prior to the recognition of CPM. Therefore it is believed that some technologic advance resulted in its appearance. Potential candidates have included the "plastic revolution" with a subsequent widespread availability of intravenous fluids, the increasing use of autoanalyzers with improved recognition (and consequent treatment) of electrolyte disorders, and the growing use of diuretic compounds (and their associated complications), all of which occurred at about this time. The reasons for the epidemic of CPM in the last 30 years remain obscure. For these reasons, we will review the possible relationships between electrolyte abnormalities and CPM in an attempt to put the controversy into perspective.

HUMAN STUDIES

One of the major difficulties confronting those who study the interactions between hyponatremia and CPM is that practically the entire literature on the subject is in the form of reviews or case reports with a paucity of well-controlled prospective observations. The reported incidence of CPM in autopsy-based studies is 0.25 to 5.8 percent [28,37,46]. The prevalence of hyponatremia in patients with CPM is not well known. Many of the early case reports either do not mention serum sodium levels or state that electrolytes were normal. Because of this, various reviewers have obtained widely discrepant values for the percentage of patients with CPM and hyponatremia, between 20 and 88 percent [37,67].

This seems to be related to whether the patients in whom electrolytes are unreported are excluded from analysis. In any event, it is clear that hyponatremia is neither necessary nor sufficient for the development of CPM. Many reported patients with CPM never had hyponatremia [66], and most hyponatremic patients do not develop CPM [15].

A certain fraction of individuals with CPM have had very good documentation of their serum sodium levels with no evidence of hyponatremia at any time in their course. In fact, some of these patients have been hypernatremic during the period in which clinical CPM developed and evolved [15,68,87]. These hypernatremic individuals have been mainly alcoholics and patients with severe thermal burns [66] in whom there seems to be a special predisposition to CPM independent of serum electrolytes. In these patients, strong diagnostic consideration is frequently given to the possibility of Wernicke's encephalopathy, especially if mental status abnormalities dominate the early picture of CPM. However, the pathologic lesion of CPM is definitely different from that seen in alcoholic CNS disease, both in its distribution and with respect to the degree of axonal involvement [49,70].

What is the pathogenesis of CPM in the normo- or hypernatremic patient? The answer to this question is unknown. It is seen that most such patients have an underlying disease process capable of causing CNS injury. This predisposing factor, whether it is alcoholic cirrhosis, an episode of severe hypoxia, or an intracranial tumor such as a craniopharyngioma, renders the brain more susceptible to injury caused by osmotic stress, perhaps due to increased blood-brain barrier permeability, as observed in some cases [21,83]. It is tempting to speculate that an acute change in serum sodium levels that would otherwise be well tolerated leads to an acute influx of solute into the brains of individuals at risk with consequent brain swelling and resultant injury. This scenario lacks experimental support at this stage. However, numerous investigations in animal systems (see next section) have demonstrated an acute decrease in brain water content and an increase in neuronal concentration of electrolytes in normal animals following treatment of severe hyponatremia with infusions of hypertonic NaCl sufficient to cause hypernatremia.

Hyponatremia if untreated leads to a constellation of neurologic findings culminating in lethargy, weakness, seizures, and death [14,56]. It is well accepted by all investigators that hyponatremia leading to these symptoms should be remedied in some fashion to avoid potentially disastrous neurologic outcomes. The problem of hyponatremia can be clearly separated from CPM in an etiologic sense. That is, hyponatremia alone does not cause either the clinical or histologic findings of CPM. The fundamental problem in this area is one of degree. Thus, virtually all physicians caring for a seizing patient with a sodium concentration of 100 mEq/liter would try to treat the hyponatremia in order to stop the seizures. However, is it sufficient simply to restrict fluid intake, knowing that this course alone is likely to take several days to raise the serum sodium substantially? Is it reasonable to raise the serum sodium aggressively at a rate of 1 mEq/liter/hour or more and thus run the theoretic risk of inducing CPM in a patient who might otherwise have had a relatively benign outcome? To answer these questions, one must know several things. First, what is the prognosis for a patient with severe symptomatic hyponatremia, and how does the rate of correction of the serum sodium affect outcome [11]? Second, is it possible to predict which patients will develop CPM if treated for hyponatremia? Third, does the rate of correction or the absolute change in serum sodium influence the development of CPM?

The outcome of hyponatremia is not known with certainty. Some investigators believe that even severe decreases in the serum sodium are relatively safe in most patients and that therefore most patients with hyponatremia do not warrant therapy with hypertonic saline solutions. In a retrospective study of patients identified from a computer search for all patients with severe hyponatremia, patient mortality and neurologic morbidity were extremely low [86]. However an approach of this type is looking at a much broader population than that in which treatment is likely to be most beneficial. In a prospective study of patients referred for symptomatic hyponatremia, another group was able to demonstrate significant morbidity and mortality from a conservative approach to treatment of hyponatremia [5]; in another report, more rapid correction of hyponatremia was associated with a better outcome (Fig. 14-1). None of the aforementioned studies take into account the age and sex of the individuals affected. Recent evidence suggests that such features may be very important in the pathogenesis of hyponatremic encephalopathy [40]. Nonetheless, these studies are probably representative of the patient population most likely to need (and benefit from) treatment of hyponatremia. It seems probable, therefore, that patients with active neurologic complaints related to hyponatremia deserve correction of their serum electrolytes. It is equally true that the asymptomatic patient with hyponatremia of practically any severity should not be treated aggressively; water restriction would probably suffice in such a case.

At the present time it is not possible to predict with certainty which patients will develop cerebral demyelination after inappropriate treatment of electrolyte disorders (even when treatment is clearly indicated) or in any of the other clinical settings in which the syndrome occurs. An emerging concept, however, is that some clinical scenarios are so often associated with the development of cerebral demyelination that the physican's awareness of the possibility of myelinolysis must be triggered to prevent the problem. The first is the patient with alcoholic

Fig. 14-1. Survival rates in patients with severe symptomatic hyponatremia treated with "rapid" correction (2 mmol/liter hour) versus "slow" correction (< 0.6 mmol/liter/hour). (From Ayus, Krothapalli, and Arieff [14].)

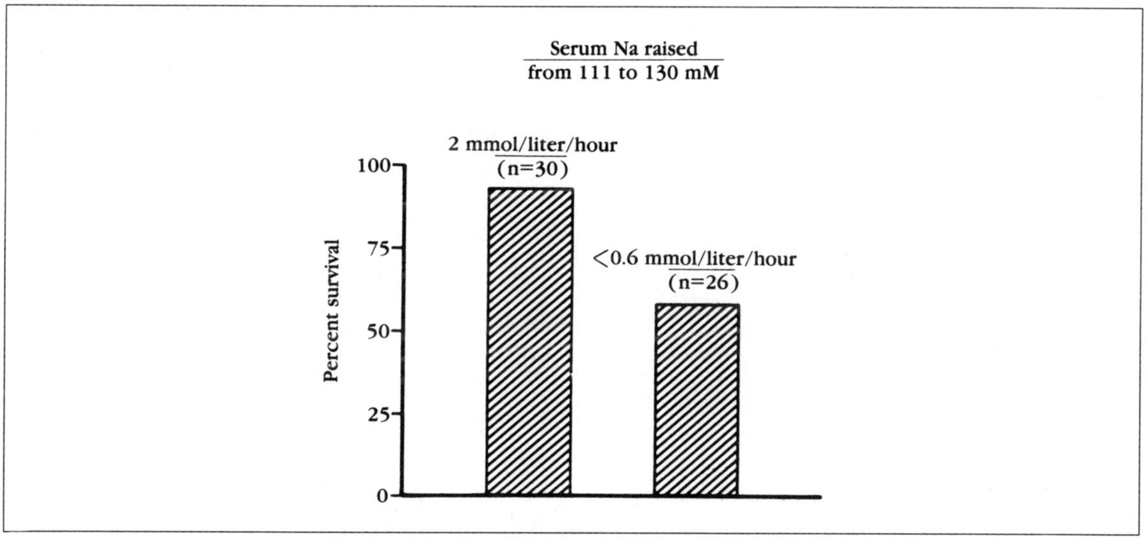

cirrhosis who develops hypernatremia, and another is the female patient who has been taking a thiazide diuretic and becomes severely hyponatremic with very mild symptomatology.

There is suggestive evidence that patients with the acute onset of hyponatremia are more likely to suffer a neurologic complication of the hyponatremia, and less likely to experience morbidity from cerebral demyelinating lesions, than are patients with a comparable degree of hyponatremia that develops chronically [5]. However, other pretreatment indices are generally not predictive of the development of cerebral demyelination. One important exception is the gender of the patient (Table 14-1). It has been found that many of the patients who develop hyponatremia and subsequent brain damage are women on therapeutic doses of thiazide diuretics [1,10,86]. These women are seen to develop significant hyponatremia over a period of days to weeks. Excessive correcting of hyponatremia in such patients is more likely to result in cerebral demyelination than the same degree of correction in men with comparable levels of serum sodium prior to treatment. The possible pathophysiologic basis for this sex difference is unclear but is being actively investigated (see next section) [41,42,76,85].

A major group of patients who seem to be at risk for the development of cerebral demyelinating lesions are alcoholics (Table 14-2). In these patients, it is common to see some hepatic dysfunction, which may take the form of micronodular cirrhosis or acute alcoholic hepatitis. There seems to be a higher percentage of males in this group; however, this may reflect a greater tendency for alcohol abuse in men as compared with women rather than an increased susceptibility in male alcoholics. In these patients, hyponatremia (serum sodium < 130 mEq/liter) seems to be a less constant finding. On the contrary, the majority of such patients in whom electrolytes have been reported have manifested a period of hypernatremia at some point in their course. Alcohol abuse is obviously a much more common disease than is CPM, and there must be many thousands of alcoholics in whom a period of hypernatremia is not followed by development of cerebral demyelinating lesions. The reasons why cerebral demyelinating lesions develop in only some of these patients are unknown but may be related to the underlying state of nutrition or preexisting alcoholic central nervous system disease. In any event, there is a definite predisposition to the development of cerebral demyelinating lesions in alcohol abusers, which is unrelated to the development or treatment of hyponatremia.

There are other patients who develop CPM without a history of either diuretic use or alcoholism (Table 14-3). However, these patients are not normal prior to the onset of cerebral demyelinating lesions. Often there is a history of malnutrition, metabolic diseases, or malignancies. Among the patients with tumors, there is a high incidence of cases in which a primary intra-

Table 14-1. Characteristics of patients with CPM and diuretic use*

	M	*F*
n (%)	6 (33.3)	12 (66.7)
Age (yrs)	50.8 ± 2.2	58.5 ± 3.5
Initial PNa	104.2 ± 2.4	107.6 ± 4.0
ΔNa 24°	22.8 ± 5.6	17.7 ± 3.3
ΔNa 48°	24.0 ± 2.0	26.5 ± 5.5
Highest PNa	138.7 ± 4.2	137.2 ± 3.2

n = number of patients; M = male; F = female; PNa = plasma sodium; ΔNa 24° = absolute change in sodium concentration 24 hours after therapy; ΔNa 48° = absolute change in sodium concentration 48 hours after therapy.

* Only patients in whom a change in serum sodium after 24 or 48 hours of therapy could be calculated are included. Results are expressed as mean ± SE.

Source: Data from references 2,4,12,13,23–27,29–31,34, 35,38,43,46–49,51,52,58,60–68,70,72–75,77,78,80–83, 87–90,92,93,98.

Table 14-2. Characteristics of patients with CPM and alcohol abuse*

	M	*F*
n (%)	20 (76.9)	6 (23.1)
Age (yrs)	48.8 ± 2.5	50.5 ± 4.1
Initial PNa	118.6 ± 3.7	107.5 ± 4.8
ΔNa 24°	17.8 ± 3.3	23.3 ± 4.9
ΔNa 48°	23.3 ± 4.3	27.3 ± 5.8
Highest PNa	144.3 ± 2.3	134.0 ± 2.7

* Patients with both alcohol abuse and diuretic use are included in Table 14-1. Only patients in whom a change in serum sodium after 24 or 48 hours of therapy could be calculated are included. Abbreviations and references as in Table 14-1.

Table 14-3. Characteristics of patients with CPM and miscellaneous underlying disorders*

	M	*F*
n (%)	7 (35.0)	13 (65.0)
Age (yrs)	24.9 ± 7.1	40.6 ± 5.2
Initial PNa	119.7 ± 4.6	110.9 ± 4.5
ΔNa 24°	19.3 ± 3.4	19.7 ± 2.8
ΔNa 48°	31.0 ± 10.0	27.7 ± 3.6
Highest PNa	157.8 ± 13.6	141.7 ± 3.9

* None of these patients had a history of either diuretic use or alcoholism. Only patients in whom a change in serum sodium after 24 or 48 hours of therapy could be calculated are included. Abbreviations and references as in Table 14-1.

cranial neoplasm (e.g., craniopharyngioma) is present. Several of the children reported with craniopharyngioma and subsequent cerebral demyelinating lesions developed this complication after surgical treatment of the tumor [53,64]. This raises the possibility that the neurosurgical procedure may be important etiologically in the development of cerebral demyelinating lesions in these patients, perhaps by causing neuronal swelling due to changes in intracranial pressure or alterations in blood-brain barrier permeability characteristics. However, the majority of patients in this miscellaneous group have no history of intracranial tumors or neurosurgery; thus, some other reason must be invoked for the onset of cerebral demyelinating lesions.

It has proved difficult to predict which members of an alcoholic population are at high risk for the development of cerebral demyelinating lesions. One group are those patients who are chronic alcoholics with end-stage liver disease, develop hepatic encephalopathy, and are treated with lactulose [15,39]. Hypernatremia may complicate such therapy [71]. Almost all cirrhotic patients with fulminant hepatic failure and hypernatremia have had a negative fluid balance, which appears to be secondary to osmotic loss of fluid, either from the gastrointestinal tract or kidney [39]. Among such patients, hypernatremia may develop after a loss of free water by means of either osmotic diarrhea or diuresis. Similarly, as many as 25 percent of such patients may develop hypernatremia secondary to osmotic diarrhea associated with lactulose therapy. The hyponatremia thus appears to be directly related to a negative fluid balance and is associated with a mortality in excess of 65 percent [40]. Therefore, a negative fluid balance should be avoided in alcoholic subjects with liver disease. Other measures to attempt to identify and protect at-risk patients have not been rewarding. Similarly, patients with the miscellaneous disorders associated with cerebral demyelinating lesions form such a large and heterogeneous group that identification and risk stratification are impossible in practical terms. Most of the present controversy surrounding CPM is centered on patients with hyponatremia who eventually develop the syndrome. In such patients, it is thought, the onset of cerebral demyelinating lesions may be predictable and, even more important, avoidable. If this is so, an iatrogenic disease may be prevented. Current research into CPM following hyponatremia is largely divided into two camps. On the one hand, some investigators believe that cerebral demyelinating lesions result from the rapid correction of hyponatremia and consequently that the serum sodium should be raised very gingerly in patients with symptomatic hyponatremia [87]. Conversely, other investigators believe that the potential consequences of symptomatic hyponatremia are so potentially catastrophic that immediate treatment sufficient to raise the serum sodium to a level that remedies the neurologic symptoms is necessary [15]. Each of these approaches will be discussed in turn.

Ever since the association was first noted between cerebral demyelination and hyponatremia, people have wondered whether the cure was worse than the disease [22]. Almost all patients who developed cerebral demyelination had been treated with hypertonic NaCl to raise the serum sodium rather precipitously (i.e., over a period of hours to days). Following a short-lived period of improvement, the patients deteriorated rapidly. In reviews of the patients' courses, it could be seen that many of these patients had rates of correction that approached or exceeded 1 to 2 mEq/liter/hour. Therefore, it was felt by some that rapid correction at rates above 0.5 to 1.0 mEq/liter/hour were potentially hazardous. It had been further noted that other hyponatremic patients whose serum sodiums were corrected at a more modest rate (< 0.5 mEq/liter/hour) did not seem to develop CPM. It had been suggested in one study, for example, that patients whose sodium levels were corrected at the faster rate uniformly developed cerebral demyelination, while those treated more slowly did not [68]. However, as the authors of that study noted, almost all the patients in the group that developed cerebral demyelination had a period of hypernatremia that could be demonstrated. Thus, the possibility existed that overcorrection rather than rate of correction was the culprit.

When one reviews all the case reports of cerebral demyelinating lesions complicating patients with hyponatremia, where sufficient information is presented to allow the reader to calculate the rate of correction and determine the presence or absence of hypernatremia, it becomes clear that rate of correction per se is relatively unimportant. The most important factors appear to be the final value for the serum sodium or the absolute change at the end of 24 or 48 hours of therapy (Fig. 14-2). There have been cases of cerebral demyelinating lesions developing in the face of correction rates of less than 0.4 mEq/liter/hour [48]; conversely, cerebral demyelinating lesions have not been noted in occasional cases of hyponatremia treated at rates of nearly 5 mEq/liter/hour [19,97]. However, the common denominator has been the final serum sodium at 48 to 72 hours of therapy. In patients in whom the serum sodium rises to nearly the normal range or above in this time frame, cerebral demyelination is frequently seen. However, if the ultimate level of serum sodium remains in the mildly hyponatremic range (120–130 mEq/liter) and the absolute change in serum sodium is less than about 25 mEq/liter, the rate at which this occurs is relatively inconsequential, and cerebral demyelination is seldom seen (Fig. 14-3). We therefore conclude that the development of cerebral demyelination is relatively insensitive to the rate of correction as long as neither hypernatremia nor eunatremia develops quickly and that the absolute change in serum sodium is controlled [15].

Recent studies reinforce the concept that cerebral hypoxia is the major factor leading to the development of cerebral demyelinating lesions in patients with symptomatic hyponatremia. Furthermore, development of such lesions is

Fig. 14-2. Absolute change in serum sodium concentration 24 and 48 hours after treatment in patients who developed CPM with a history of alcohol abuse (EtOH), current use of diuretics, or other conditions. (Data from references listed Table 14-1).

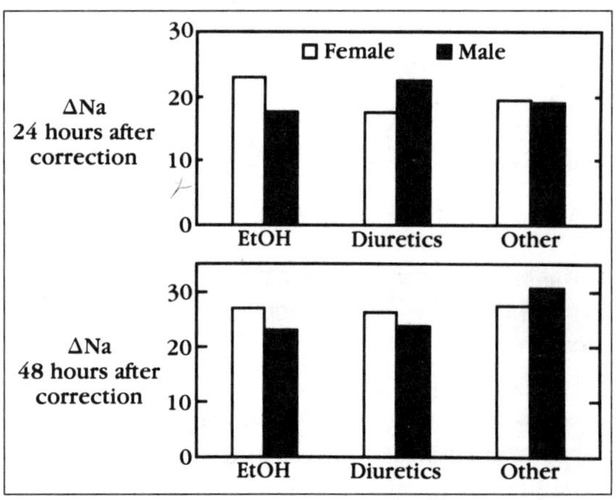

Fig. 14-3. Absolute change in serum sodium concentration in patients with and without cerebral demyelinating lesions. Group I patients (without demyelination) had lower absolute changes in sodium concentration immediately following hypertonic saline (A), at 24 hours (B), and at 48 hours (C) following treatment than did either a concurrent group of patients with demyelination (Group II, D) or patients reported in the literature (Group III, E) in whom demyelination was present and the rate of correction could be accurately determined. (From Ayus, Krothapalli, and Arieff [15].)

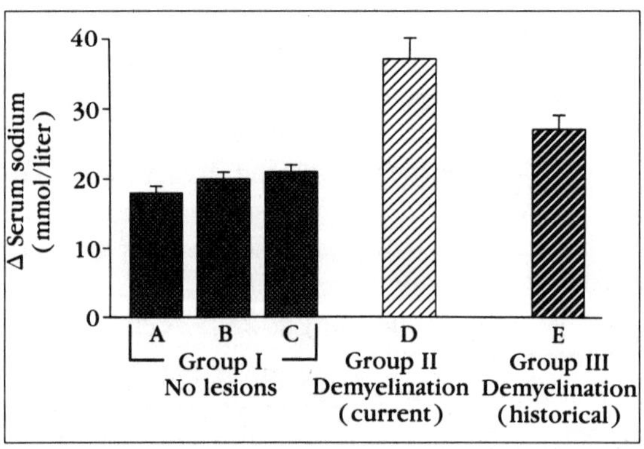

usually independent of therapy. In a recent series of 11 patients with symptomatic hyponatremia who presented with respiratory arrest, all who survived more than three days had diffuse cerebral demyelinating lesions at autopsy [40a]. Two clinical studies of more than 80 patients with symptomatic hyponatremia revealed that among those dying or suffering permanent brain damage, the mean arterial PO_2 was only 31 mm Hg in adults [16] and 45 mm Hg in children [7], levels known to cause cerebral demyelination in healthy subjects without hyponatremia. Among 20 patients with symptomatic hyponatremia who were diagnosed as having CPM, retrospective neuroradiologic evaluation demonstrated that only 3 of 20 patients (15%) actually had the disorder [91a]. Of these 3 patients, all were long-term chronic alcoholics, who may well have had CPM for reasons relating to their alcoholism. Of the 20 patients, 95 percent had a definite hypoxic episode prior to any therapy for their hyponatremia, and the distribution of brain lesions corresponded to that typically seen in hypoxic encephalopathy [44,45] (Fig. 14-4).

Thus, CPM is very uncommon among patients with symptomatic hyponatremia suffering permanent brain damage and is virtually always associated with chronic alcoholism when present [91a]. Severe systemic hypoxemia is usually present in such patients [7,16], many present with respiratory arrest [7,16,40a], and the distribution of brain lesions is similar to that of cerebral hypoxia (see Fig. 14-4).

ANIMAL STUDIES

It has been difficult to develop an animal model that is completely analogous to the human syndrome of CPM. In some systems, demyelination occurs in a different distribution than is seen in human disease [17,54]. In others, axonal involvement is more prominent than is typical in humans, although this may simply represent an earlier stage in the development of the disease [50,55,59]. Furthermore, the disease has been reproduced only in models of hyponatremic states; thus the spectrum of CPM related to alcoholism or other chronic diseases has not been studied in animal systems. However, some interesting work has been done in an attempt to understand the pathophysiology of cerebral demyelination and its relation to correction of hyponatremia. These can be divided into two broad categories of work. Some investigators have been studying mechanisms of brain water

Fig. 14-4. The distribution of brain lesions with 20 patients who had a preliminary diagnosis of central pontine myelinolysis (CPM). Only five patients had pontine lesions, and only three of 20 patients had anatomic criteria for the diagnosis of CPM. The distribution and morphology of the lesions, as well as the clinical histories, are compatible with hypoxic brain damage. (From Tien, R., et al. [91a].)

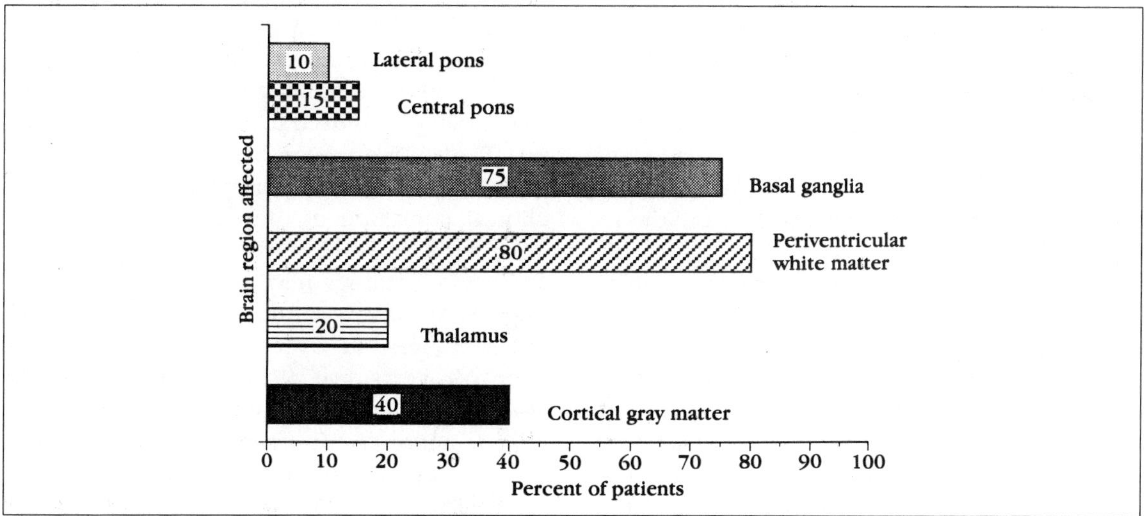

and solute homeostasis and their relation to cerebral demyelination. Others have looked directly at neurologic function and pathology following correction of hyponatremia under different conditions.

In the acute phase of hyponatremia, plasma osmolality is decreased. Since most cells are more or less freely permeable to water, the change in plasma osmolality leads to water entry and cell swelling in all body tissues, including the brain. All cells have the ability to regulate their volume by changing their solute content. Thus, as hyponatremia becomes chronic, the body's cells begin to adapt to their new swollen state, and active extrusion of solute takes place [84]. This allows the cell to regain its former volume at the expense of a lowered intracellular solute content. The opposite is true in hypernatremia. Cells shrink because of water extraction due to increased extracellular fluid tonicity, and active uptake of solute occurs to allow cell volume to expand [33]. It is of interest that different tissues accomplish this adaptation at very different rates.

It has been clearly shown that nervous system cells are remarkably resistant to changes in volume in the face of external osmotic stresses. Hyponatremia sufficient to cause a nearly 25 percent increase in water content of skeletal muscle or liver is barely capable of raising brain water content by a detectable amount [9,36,94,96]. Similarly, published studies of hypernatremia in animals have shown a significant decrease in water content in most tissues, but brain water content is well preserved [32]. The reasons why this occur are not entirely clear but probably relate at least in part to the rapidity with which the brain is able to adapt its solute content in response to an osmotic challenge. Thus, it has been shown that brain uptake of electrolytes and amino acids occurs rapidly in hypernatremic animals, and presumably this allows cell volume to remain reasonably constant [33]. Brain uptake of potassium and amino acids occurs in hyponatremic mice treated with hypertonic saline. It is also likely that the hydroosmotic water permeability of the central nervous system is low [94], so that changes in water content tend to occur slowly in the brain (compared with other cells exposed to the same change in tonicity). Eventually, these volume defense mechanisms in the brain act to protect it from acute changes that could otherwise adversely affect function.

For some reason, however, this elegant system sometimes fails. This may occur either because the limits of adaptation are breached (e.g., the cells may be simply unable to adapt to a serum sodium < 100 mEq/liter) or because osmolality is changing faster than the adaptive process can operate. In either event, the brain's function becomes compromised, and symptoms related to the changes in brain volume or solute composition become clinically evident. At this point, in both humans and animals, treatment becomes necessary to avoid death or permanent neurologic disability. It is also at this point that the hyponatremic patient becomes vulnerable to the possible development of cerebral demyelinating lesions.

To induce cerebral demyelination, the animal must first be made hyponatremic. This is usually done by parenteral administration of antidiuretic hormone (ADH) or one of its analogues combined with a water load [17,36,91,94,96]. This results in the development of severe hyponatremia (serum sodium usually < 110 mEq/liter) over several days. Although often referred to as a model of chronic hyponatremia, it must be remembered that the usual human patient with hyponatremia often develops and sustains the condition over a considerably longer time interval. At this time, in most series in the literature going back over 60 years, virtually all investigators have observed that a substantial percent of animals so treated will have died of hyponatremia, and most of the remainder will be symptomatic if ADH is used to induce the hyponatremia [8, 40]. Treatment is begun at this point with either water restriction or hypertonic NaCl. The clinical condition of the animals is observed, brain water and electrolytes are often measured, and brain histology may be examined. This sequence of investigation has been repeated, more or less, in over 30 studies beginning over 60 years ago [79]. Findings from the aforementioned animal model have resulted in several important observations. The first is that the development of demyelinating lesions is at least partly a function of the chronicity of the hyponatremia [69]. Animals with a longer duration of hyponatremia have been shown to be more susceptible to cerebral demyelination than animals with a comparable degree of depression in the serum sodium of only 1 to 2 days' duration. These animals are equally symptomatic while hyponatremic; therefore hyponatremia alone does not cause CPM, nor does its treatment. Other factors must be involved. Since, in the acute studies, there has been less time for an adaptive change in solute content of the brain to develop, it seems probable that in some way the volume regulatory efflux of solute during chronic hyponatremia (or its reverse during excessive correction) may be responsible for the onset of brain damage.

Another finding from animal studies has been the observation that hyponatremia alone in the absence of respiratory arrest does not cause cerebral demyelination [17,50,55,59]. It is clear that the demyelination seen in these animal models does not occur until treatment of serum sodium is begun. Thus, in addition to being clinically different, the pathologic findings associated with cerebral demyelination are not due solely to derangements in sodium levels in the plasma. It has also been noted in animal studies that the rate of correction of hyponatremia is less important than the absolute change in serum sodium. In most animal experiments, the final sodium concentration reaches normal or elevated levels in the animals in whom cerebral demyelination develops [17,50,54,55,59]. The absolute change in serum sodium also usually exceeds 20 to 30 mEq/liter [17,50,59,69]. In animals in whom the correction of serum sodium is not allowed to exceed mildly hyponatremic levels, or the change in sodium concentration is less than 20 to 30 mEq/liter, cerebral demyelination is much less likely to occur, regardless of the rate of correction in milliequivalents per liter per hour [17,50,59]. Hypertonic NaCl alone is not responsible for histologic lesions in animals treated for hyponatremia, since similarly rapid correction with fluid restriction alone can also cause myelinolysis [17].

The relationship between the severity of hyponatremia, the method of its correction, and the final sodium correction on the development of cerebral demyelinating lesions has recently been explicitly explored [18]. Overall survival was best in animals that underwent spontaneous correction of mild hyponatremia (85% survival) or rapid correction of severe hyponatremia to mildly hyponatremic levels (100% survival). On the other hand, rats with severe hyponatremia that underwent either spontaneous correction or rapid correction to normonatremic levels had much worse survival (32% and 12% survival, respectively). In addition, histopathologic examination of the brains of these animals revealed widespread structural damage consisting of evolving myelinolysis or acute cellular necrosis in the groups with the poorer outcome, whereas the groups that did well had no evidence of structural lesions.

One final point that often goes overlooked in these studies is the mortality of the animals. It is not unusual to read of 50 to 75 percent mortality rates among the animals with hyponatremia [50,59]. Although this mortality rate greatly exceeds that seen in human patients with hyponatremia, it emphasizes the potentially malignant nature of this electrolyte disturbance. The problem of hyponatremia is not solely one of its treatment; a low serum sodium can directly cause permanent disability or death [5,7,16].

It has been of interest that most patients with hyponatremia who go on to develop cerebral demyelination, especially after diuretic use, are women [86]. Some interesting studies have been conducted to determine if there is a constitutional difference between males and females in their ability to defend against an osmotic challenge. Although these experiments are still in progress, preliminary data suggest that there is indeed a difference in brain water and solute content between male and female animals with similar degrees of hyponatremia [16]. This is discussed in great detail in Chapter 4.

If the development of hypernatremia is indeed important to the pathogenesis of cerebral demyelination then it ought to be possible to cause the syndrome in normal animals by the simple expedient of making them hypernatremic. Unfortunately this has not been possible. Animal studies have shown that an acute increase in the serum sodium concentration to moderately hypernatremic levels does not result in the onset of cerebral demyelination [17,59]. This may mean that hypernatremia per se is not important in the pathogenesis of cerebral demyelination. However, the increases in serum sodium in these experiments are generally smaller than those induced by correction of hyponatremia, and the inability of hypernatremia to induce cerebral demyelination may thus be due to the smaller absolute change in serum sodium. Furthermore, normal animals without a preexisting metabolic or structural lesion of the central nervous system may be relatively resistant to the development of cerebral demyelination in any case.

A PATHOGENETIC MODEL FOR CEREBRAL DEMYELINATION

How then are we to find a common thread that can bind together all these diverse elements and explain the clinical, pathologic, and experimental findings that are associated with cerebral demyelination? We would propose that for cerebral demyelination to develop, at least three things must occur:

1. Preexisting abnormality of the central nervous system: Cerebral demyelination is not a disorder that affects normal people. Its prevalence in patients with tumors, malnutrition, alcoholism, hypoxia, or electrolyte disorders is low, but one of these things must be present as a backdrop for cerebral demyelination to develop. We believe that the underlying disease leads to an abnormality in brain structure or function, which sets the stage for the development of cerebral demyelination if the subsequent events allow it.
2. Loss of ability to regulate brain cell volume: In the setting of hyponatremia of long duration, the cell potassium and sodium levels are low because of active efflux of solutes from the cell. When a cell is then subjected to a hypertonic stress, solute gradients may abruptly change, and influx mechanisms may be unable to meet the rapidly changing needs of the organism.
3. Exposure to a volume regulatory stress: It is probably the case that even the damaged brain that has lost some of its ability to regulate its own cellular composition is still able to adapt within poorly defined limits. It is only when these limits are exceeded that cerebral demyelination develops. It appears that in most cases that limit is a rapid increase in plasma sodium of no more than about 25 mEq/liter. Whether that change takes place in 24 to 48 hours is of little consequence; however if the limit is exceeded, adaptation may no longer be possible and cerebral demyelination occurs. It may even be possible that this third condition alone is sufficient to cause cerebral demyelination to occur. However, it does not happen that way in clinical medicine because the magnitude of the volume stress may need to be so severe that other problems supervene and are treated before cerebral demyelinating lesions can develop.

CONCLUSIONS

CPM is a rare but dramatic clinical entity characterized by the development of progressive weakness leading to quadriparesis, pseudobulbar palsy, and mental status abnormalities. It is usually fatal, although rare instances of recovery have been recorded. The typical demyelinating lesion in the central basis pontis can be seen even in the absence of the clinical syndrome. Extrapontine lesions occur occasionally but are usually overshadowed clinically by the pontine manifestations. The syndrome is often unsuspected during life. CPM cannot be diagnosed in the absence of anatomic or radiologic confirmation, and the condition is often diagnosed incorrectly. CPM does not occur in previously normal individuals, and it must always be distinguished from cerebral demyelination from other causes, such as hypoxia. Three groups of patients seem to be at risk for the development of cerebral demyelinating lesions: women who become hyponatremic because of diuretic use, alcoholics, and a miscellaneous group whose major feature appears to be malnutrition or neoplastic disease. The appearance of the disorder in the mid to late 1950s has been taken as suggestive evidence that CPM is an iatrogenic disease that only developed as a result of rapidly advancing biotechnology and the ability to diagnose and treat fluid and electrolyte problems more easily.

Hyponatremia is by no means a universal finding in patients who develop cerebral demyelination and may even be present in only a minority of cases. However, the association between a low serum sodium and cerebral demyelinating lesions is important, since excessive correction of the sodium concentration is etiologically important in the development of such brain lesions. In the patients at risk for development of cerebral demyelinating lesions who are not hyponatremic (e.g., alcoholic and malnourished persons), it is difficult or impossible to predict the patients who will develop cerebral demyelinating lesions. Nevertheless, hypernatremia should be avoided in these patients, since it probably increases the risk.

The treatment of hyponatremia is controversial. Untreated, hyponatremia can lead to seizures, permanent disability, or death. On the other hand, the treatment of hyponatremia is thought by some to result in cerebral demyelination. There does not appear to be strong evidence that rapid correction of hyponatremia leads to cerebral demyelination as long as the patient's sodium level does not increase by more than about 25 mEq/liter by the end of 48 to 72 hours even if the entire correction takes place in the first 24 to 48 hours. Correction to normo- or hypernatremic levels is definitely associated with increased risk of development of demyelinating brain lesions.

Animal studies, while imperfect, tend to support this view. It is probably the case that cell volume regulation within the brain is inadequately adapted and responds inappropriately to osmotic stresses outside its regulatory range. The possible role of hormonal influences in the response to hyponatremia needs to be further investigated. Other factors, such as possible changes in blood-brain barrier permeability, could also play a role, but further research is needed.

A pathogenetic scheme for the development of cerebral demyelination has been proposed. According to this scheme, a structural, functional, or metabolic lesion is present in the brain. This leads to an inability of the brain to cope adequately with a broad range of cell volume regulatory needs. When presented with an osmotic challenge outside its regulatory range (e.g., hypernatremia), the increased permeability of the central nervous system leads to the development of myelinolysis. The molecular mechanism by which this occurs is unknown. However, it is safe and in the patient's interest to treat hyponatremia actively as long as the serum sodium does not rise above about 125 mEq/liter; under no circumstances should the absolute rise in serum sodium exceed 25 mEq/liter within the initial 48 hours of therapy.

These concepts have been expanded in recent literature on this topic [12,13,24]. One of the major problems in relation to hyponatremic encephalopathy is a delay in its recognition. This occurs in part because of the nonspecific nature of the symptoms, which can be mimicked by a number of other entities including narcosis, phenothiazine side effects, viral encephalitis, or intracranial hemorrhage. The treatment of hyponatremia depends on its severity, but prophylaxis is more desirable when possible (e.g., in the postoperative patient). When acute correction with hypertonic NaCl is necessary, the infusion should be terminated whenever the patient becomes totally asymptomatic or the serum sodium has either increased by 20 to 25 mEq/liter or reached a value of 120 to 125 mEq/liter. When these guidelines are followed, patient survival and neurologic outcome are both superior to results achieved with either more gradual or more excessive correction.

REFERENCES

1. Abramow, M., and Cogan, E. Clinical aspects and pathophysiology of diuretic-induced hyponatremia *Adv. Nephrol. (Paris)* 13:1, 1984.
2. Adams, J. H. Central pontine myelinolysis. In H. Jacobs (ed.), Proceedings of 4th International Congress of Neuropathology, vol. 3, Munchen, 1961, pp. 303–308.
3. Adams, R. D., Victor, M., and Mancall, E. L. Central pontine myelinolysis: A hitherto undescribed disease occurring in alcoholic and malnourished patients. *Arch. Neurol. Psychiatry* 81:154, 1959.

4. Aleu, F. P., and Terry, R. D. Central pontine myelinolysis. *Arch. Pathol.* 76:140, 1963.
5. Arieff, A. I. Hyponatremia, convulsions, respiratory arrest, and permanent brain damage after elective surgery in healthy women. *N. Engl. J. Med.* 314:1529, 1986.
6. Arieff, A. I. Hyponatremia associated with permanent brain damage. *Adv. Intern. Med.* 32:325, 1987.
7. Arieff, A. I., Ayus, J. C. and Fraser, C. L. Death or permanent brain damage in healthy children with hyponatremia. *Brit. Med. J.* (in press): 1992.
8. Arieff, A. I., and Guisado, R. Effects on the central nervous system of hypernatremic and hyponatremic states. *Kidney Int.* 10:104, 1976.
9. Arieff, A. I., Kleeman, C. R., Keushkerian, A., et al. Brain tissue osmolality: Method of determination and variations in hyper- and hypo-osmolar states. *J. Lab. Clin. Med.* 79:334, 1972.
10. Ashraf, N., Locksley, R., and Arieff, A. I. Thiazide-induced hyponatremia associated with death or neurologic damage in outpatients. *Am. J. Med.* 70:1163, 1981.
11. Ayus, J. C. Diuretic-induced hyponatremia. *Arch. Intern. Med.* 146:1295, 1986.
12. Ayus, J. C., and Arieff, A. I. Symptomatic hyponatremia: Correcting sodium deficits safely. *J. Crit. Illness* 5:905, 1990.
13. Ayus, J. C., and Arieff, A. I. Symptomatic hyponatremia: Making the diagnosis rapidly. *J. Crit. Illness* 45:846, 1990.
14. Ayus, J. C., Krothapalli, R. K., and Arieff, A. I. Changing concepts in treatment of severe symptomatic hyponatremia. *Am. J. Med.* 78:897, 1985.
15. Ayus, J. C., Krothapalli, R. K., and Arieff, A. I. Treatment of symptomatic hyponatremia and its relation to brain damage. *N. Engl. J. Med.* 317:1190, 1987.
16. Ayus, J. C. and Arieff, A. I. Effects of age and gender on outcome in patients with postoperative hyponatremia. *Ann. Intern. Med.:* (in press), 1992.
17. Ayus, J. C., Krothapalli, R. K., and Armstrong, D. L. Rapid correction of severe hyponatremia in the rat: Histopathological changes in the brain. *Am. J. Physiol.* 248:F711, 1985.
18. Ayus, J. C., Krothapalli, R. K., Armstrong, D. L., and Norton, H. J. Symptomatic hyponatremia in rats: Effect of treatment on mortality and brain lesions. *Am. J. Physiol.* 257 (*Renal Fluid Electrolyte Physiol.* 26):F18, 1989.
19. Ayus, J. C., Olivero, J. J., and Frommer, J. P. Rapid correction of severe hyponatremia with intravenous hypertonic saline solution. *Am. J. Med.* 72:43, 1982.
20. Bailey, O. T., Bruno, M. S., and Ober, W. B. Central pontine myelinolysis. *Am. J. Med.* 29:902, 1960.
21. Behar, A. Bental, E., and Aviram, A. Central pontine myelinolysis. *Acta Neuropathol.* 3:343, 1964.
22. Berl, T. Treating hyponatremia: Damned if we do and damned if we don't. *Kidney Int.* 37:1006, 1990.
23. Berry, K., and Olszewski, J. Central pontine myelinolysis: A case report. *Neurology* 13:531, 1963.
24. Brennan, S., and Ayus, J. C. Treatment of Hypoosmolar and Hyperosmolar States. In W. N. Suki and S. G. Massry (eds.), *Therapy of Renal Diseases and Related Disorders* (2nd ed.). Boston: Kluwer, 1991. Pp. 1–16.
25. Brunner, J. E., Redmond, J. M., Haggar, A. M., and Elias, S. B. Central pontine myelinolysis after rapid correction of hyponatremia: A magnetic resonance imaging study. *Ann. Neurol.* 23:389, 1988.
26. Burcar, P. J., Norenberg, M. D., and Yarnell, P. R. Hyponatremia and central pontine myelinolysis. *Neurology* 27:223, 1977.
27. Cadman, T. E., and Rorke, L. B. Central pontine myelinolysis in childhood and adolescence. *Arch. Dis. Child.* 44:342, 1969.
28. Chason, J. L., Landers, J. W., and Gonzalez, J. E. Central pontine myelinolysis. *J. Neurol. Neurosurg. Psychiatry* 27:317, 1964.
29. Chercover, D. J., and Norman, M. G. Central pontine myelinolysis in a 6-month-old infant with rapidly corrected hyponatremia. *Ann. Neurol.* 16:261, 1984.
30. Cole, M., Richardson, E. P., and Segarra, J. M. Central pontine myelinolysis: Further evidence relating the lesion to malnutrition. *Neurology* 14:165, 1964.
31. Conger, J. D., McIntyre, J. A., and Jacoby, W. J. Central pontine myelinolysis associated with inappropriate antidiuretic hormone secretion. *Am. J. Med.* 47:813, 1969.
32. Cserr, H. F., DePasquale, M., and Patlak, C. S. Regulation of brain water and electrolytes during acute hyperosmolarity in rats. *Am. J. Physiol.* 253:F522, 1987.
33. Cserr, H. F., DePasquale, M., and Patlak, C. S. Volume regulatory influx of electrolytes from plasma to brain during acute hyperosmolarity. *Am. J. Physiol.* 253:F530, 1987.
34. DeWitt, L. D., Buonanno, F. S., Kistler, J. P., et al. Central pontine myelinolysis: Demonstration by nuclear magnetic resonance. *Neurology* 34:570, 1984.
35. Dickoff, D. J., Raps, M., and Yahr, M. D. Striatal syndrome following hyponatremia and its rapid correction: A manifestation of extrapontine myelinolysis confirmed by magnetic resonance imaging. *Arch. Neurol.* 45:112, 1988.
36. Dila, C. J., and Pappius, H. M. Cerebral water and electrolytes: An experimental model of inappro-

priate secretion of antidiuretic hormone. *Arch. Neurol.* 26:85, 1972.
37. Endo, Y., Oda, M., and Hara, M. Central pontine myelinolysis: A study of 37 cases in 1,000 consecutive autopsies. *Acta Neuropathol.* 53:145, 1981.
38. Finlayson, M. H., Snider, S., Oliva, L. A., and Gault, M. H. Cerebral and pontine myelinolysis: Two cases with fluid and electrolyte imbalance and hypotension. *J. Neurol. Sci.* 18:399, 1973.
39. Fraser, C. F., and Arieff, A. I. Hepatic encephalopathy: Current concepts. *N. Engl. J. Med.* 313(14):865, 1985.
40. Fraser, C. L., and Arieff, A. I. Water Metabolism and Its Disorders. In R. D. Cohen, K. G. M. M. Alberti, B. Lewis, and A. M. Denman (eds.), *The Metabolic and Molecular Basis of Acquired Disease.* London: Baillière Tindall, 1990.
40a. Fraser, C. L., and Arieff, A. I. Fatal central diabetes mellitus and insipidus resulting from untreated hyponatremia: A new syndrome. *Ann. Intern. Med.* 112:113, 1990.
41. Fraser, C. L., Kucharczyk, J., Arieff, A. I., et al. Sex differences result in increased morbidity from hyponatremia in female rats. *Am. J. Physiol.* 256 (*Regul. Integrative Comp. Physiol.* 25):R880, 1989.
42. Fraser, C. L., Sarnacki, P., and Arieff, A. I. $Na^{+}-K^{+}$ATPase pump function in male rate brain synaptosomes is different from that of females. *Am. J. Physiol.* 257(20):E284, 1989.
43. Gerber, O., Geller, M., Stiller, J., and Yang, W. Central pontine myelinolysis: Resolution shown by computed tomography. *Arch. Neurol.* 40:116, 1983.
44. Ginsberg, M. D. Carbon monoxide intoxication: Clinical features, neuropathology and mechanisms of injury. *Clin. Toxicol.* 23:281, 1985.
45. Ginsberg, M. D., Hedley-Whyte, E. T., and Richardson, E. P., Jr. Hypoxic-ischemic leukoencephalopathy in man. *Arch. Neurol.* 33:5, 1976.
46. Goebel, H. H., and Herman-Ben Zur, P. Central pontine myelinolysis: A clinical and pathological study of 10 cases. *Brain* 95:495, 1972.
47. Gross, S. G., and Bell, R. D. Central pontine myelinolysis and rapid correction of hyponatremia. *Tex. Med.* 78:59, 1982.
48. Haibach, H., Ansbacher, L. E., and Dix, J. D. Central pontine myelinolysis: A complication of hyponatremia or of therapeutic intervention? *J. Forensic Sci.* 32:444, 1987.
49. Hazratji, S. M. A., Kim, R. C., Lee, S. H., and Marasigan, A. V. Evolution of pontine and extrapontine myelinolysis. *J. Comput. Assist. Tomogr.* 7:356, 1983.
50. Illowsky, B. P., and Laureno, R. Encephalopathy and myelinolysis after rapid correction of hyponatremia. *Brain* 110:855, 1987.
51. Kalnins, R. M., Berkovic, S. F., and Bladin, P. F. Central pontine myelinolysis with widespread extrapontine lesions: A report of two cases. *Clin. Exp. Neurol.* 21:189, 1984.
52. Kandt, R. S., Heldrich, F. J., and Moser, H. W. Recovery from probable central pontine myelinolysis associated with Addison's disease. *Arch. Neurol.* 40:118, 1983.
53. Kepes, J. J., Reece, C. A., and Oxley, D. K. Central pontine myelinolysis in a 7 year old boy. *J. Neurol. Neurosurg. Psychiatry* 28:39, 1965.
54. Kleinschmidt-DeMasters, B. K., and Norenberg, M. D. Cerebellar degeneration in the rat following rapid correction of hyponatremia. *Ann. Neurol.* 10:561, 1981.
55. Kleinschmidt-DeMasters, B. K., and Norenberg, M. D. Rapid correction of hyponatremia causes demyelination: Relation to central pontine myelinolysis. *Science* 211:1068, 1981.
56. Kold, A. Hyponatremia: Cerebral symptoms and role in central pontine myelinolysis. *Acta Neurol. Scand.* 73:200, 1986.
57. Krigman, M. R., and Bouldin, T. W. Intoxications and Deficiency Diseases. Oxygen deficiency: Brain hypoxia and ischemia. In S. S. Schochet, Jr. (ed.), *Neuropathology.* The Clinical Neurosciences, Rosenberg, R. N. (series ed.). New York: Churchill Livingstone, 1983. P. 496.
58. Landers, J. W., Chason, J. L., and Samuel, V. N. Central pontine myelinolysis: A pathogenetic hypothesis. *Neurology* 15:968, 1965.
59. Laureno, R. Central pontine myelinolysis following rapid correction of hyponatremia. *Ann. Neurol.* 13:232, 1983.
60. Lipsmeyer, E., and Ackerman, G. L. Irreversible brain damage after water intoxication. *J.A.M.A.* 196:286, 1966.
61. Lopez, R. I., and Collins, G. H. Wernicke's encephalopathy: A complication of chronic hemodialysis. *Arch. Neurol.* 18:248, 1968.
62. Marra, T. R. Hemiparesis apparently due to central pontine myelinolysis following hyponatremia. *Ann. Neurol.* 14:687, 1983.
63. Mathieson, G., and Olszewski, J. Central pontine myelinolysis with other cerebral changes. *Neurology* 10:345, 1960.
64. Matsuoka, T., Miyoshi, K., Saka, K., et al. Central pontine myelinolysis: A report of three cases. *Acta Neuropathol.* 5:117, 1965.
65. McCormick, W. F., and Danneel, C. M. Central pontine myelinolysis. *Arch. Intern. Med.* 119:444, 1967.
66. McKee, A. C., Winkelman, M. D., and Banker, B. Q. Central pontine myelinolysis in severely burned patients: Relationship to serum hyperosmolality. *Neurology* 38:1211, 1988.
67. Messert, B., Orrison, W. W., Hawkins, M. J., and Quaglieri, C. E. Central pontine myelinolysis: Considerations on etiology, diagnosis, and treatment. *Neurology* 29:147, 1979.
68. Norenberg, M. D., Leslie, K. O., and Robertson, A. S. Association between rise in serum sodium

and central pontine myelinolysis. *Ann. Neurol.* 11:128, 1982.

69. Norenberg, M. D., and Papendick, R. E. Chronicity of hypernatremia as a factor in experimental myelinolysis. *Ann. Neurol.* 15:544, 1984.
70. Paguirigan, A., and Lefken, E. B. Central pontine myelinolysis. *Neurology* 19:1007, 1969.
71. Papadakis, M. A., and Arieff, A. I. Hyponatremia and Hypernatremia in Patients with Liver Disease. In M. Epstein (ed.), *The Kidney in Liver Disease* (3rd ed.). Baltimore: Williams & Wilkins, 1988. Pp. 73–88.
72. Pfister, H. W., Einhaupl, K. M., and Brandt, T. Mild central pontine myelinolysis: A frequently undetected syndrome. *Eur. Arch. Psychiatry Neurol. Sci.* 235:134, 1985.
73. Plum, F., Posner, J. B., and Hain R. F. Delayed neurological deterioration after anoxia. *Arch. Intern. Med.* 110:56, 1962.
74. Price, B. H., and Mesulam, M. M. Behavioral manifestations of central pontine myelinolysis. *Arch. Neurol.* 44:671, 1987.
75. Price, D. B., Kramer, J., Hotson, G. C., and Loh, J. P. Central pontine myelinolysis: Report of a case with distinctive appearance on MR imaging. *Am. J. Neuroradiol.* 8:576, 1987.
76. Rodriquez del Castello, A., Battaner, E., Guerra, M., et al. Regional changes of brain Na^+, K^+-transporting adenosine triphosphate related to ovarian function. *Brain Res.* 416:113, 1987.
77. Rosenbloom, S., Buchholz, D., Kumar, A. J., et al. Evolution of central pontine myelinolysis on CT. *Am. J. Neuroradiol.* 5:110, 1984.
78. Rosman, N. P., Kakulas, B. A., and Richardson, E. P. Central pontine myelinolysis in a child with leukemia. *Arch. Neurol.* 14:273, 1966.
79. Rowntree, L. G. Effects on mammals of the administration of excessive quantities of water. *J. Pharmacol. Exp. Ther.* 29:135, 1926.
80. Schneck, S. A. Neuropathological features of human organ transplantation. II. Central pontine myelinolysis and neuroaxonal dystrophy. *J. Neuropathol. Exp. Neurol.* 25:18, 1966.
81. Schroth, G. Clinical and CT confirmed recovery from central pontine myelinolysis. *Neuroradiology* 26:149, 1984.
82. Sherins, R. J., and Verity, M. A. Central pontine myelinolysis associated with acute hemorrhagic pancreatitis. *J. Neurol. Neurosurg. Psychiatry* 31:583, 1968.
83. Shurtliff, L. F., Ajax, E. T., Englert, E., and D'Agostino, A. N. Central pontine myelinolysis and cirrhosis of the liver. *Am. J. Clin. Pathol.* 46:239, 1966.
84. Siebens, A. W. Cellular Volume Control. In D. W. Seldin and G. Giebisch (eds.), *The Kidney: Physiology and Pathophysiology.* New York: Raven, 1985. Pp. 91–115.
85. Skowsky, V. R., Swan, L., and Smith, P. Effects of sex hormones on arginine vasopressin in intact and castrated male and female rats. *Endocrinology* 104:105, 1979.
86. Sterns, R. H. Severe symptomatic hyponatremia: Treatment and outcome. *Ann. Intern. Med.* 107:656, 1987.
87. Sterns, R. H., Riggs, J. E., and Schochet, S. S. Osmotic demyelination syndrome following correction of hyponatremia. *N. Engl. J. Med.* 314:1535, 1986.
88. Sztencel, J., Baleriaux, D., Borenstein, S., et al. Central pontine myelinolysis: Correlation between CT and electrophysiologic data. *Am. J. Neuroradiol.* 4:529, 1983.
89. Telfer, R. B., and Miller, E. M. Central pontine myelinolysis following hyponatremia, demonstrated by computerized tomography. *Ann. Neurol.* 6:455, 1979.
90. Thompson, D. S., Hutton, J. T., Stears, J. C., et al. Computerized tomography in the diagnosis of central and extrapontine myelinolysis. *Arch. Neurol.* 38:243, 1981.
91. Thurston, J. H., and Hauhart, R. E. Brain amino acids decrease in chronic hyponatremia and rapid correction causes brain dehydration: Possible clinical significance. *Life Sci.* 40:2539, 1987.

91a. Tien, R., Arieff, A. I., Kucharczyk, W., et al. Hyponatremic brain damage: Is central pontine myelinolysis common? *Am. J. Med.* 92:(in press), 1992.

92. Tomlinson, B. E., Pierides, A. M., and Bradley, W. G. Central pontine myelinolysis. *Q. J. Med.* 45:373, 1976.
93. Valsamis, M. P., Peress, N. S., and Wright, L. D. Central pontine myelinolysis in childhood. *Arch. Neurol.* 25:307, 1971.
94. Wasterlain, C. G., and Posner, J. B. Cerebral edema in water intoxication: I. Clinical and chemical observations. *Arch. Neurol.* 19:71, 1968.
95. Wolman, L. Ischaemic lesions in the brain-stem associated with raised intracranial pressure. *Brain* 76:364, 1953.
96. Woodbury, D. M. Effect of acute hyponatremia on distribution of water and electrolytes in various tissues of the rat. *Am. J. Physiol.* 185:281, 1956.
97. Worthley, L. I. G., and Thomas, P. D. Treatment of hyponatremic seizures with intravenous 29.2% saline. *Br. Med. J.* 292:168, 1986.
98. Wright, D. G., Laureno, R., and Victor, M. Pontine and extrapontine myelinolysis. *Brain* 102:361, 1979.

15 Neurologic Manifestations of Immunologic Disorders

Daniel W. Giang and Randolph B. Schiffer

The neurologic manifestations of immunologically mediated diseases cover protean symptoms associated with a diverse set of disease entities. Detailed descriptions of such a spectrum of conditions is beyond the scope of a single chapter. Therefore, systemic lupus erythematosus will serve as a model of pathophysiologic mechanisms of collagen vascular disease. Mixed connective tissue disease, progressive systemic sclerosis, Sjögren's syndrome, and rheumatoid arthritis will be discussed more briefly. Isolated angiitis of the nervous system will serve as a model for the effect of vasculitis on the central nervous system, while Cogan's syndrome, polyarteritis nodosa, giant cell arteritis, Wegener's granulomatosis, lymphomatoid granulomatosis, Behçet's disease, and other entities will be discussed more briefly. A number of disorders with immune-mediated etiologies are not considered in this chapter because they are dealt with elsewhere in this volume (e.g., sarcoidosis) or because they are usually covered in standard textbooks of neurology as primary neurologic diseases (e.g., inflammatory myositis and multiple sclerosis).

SYSTEMIC LUPUS ERYTHEMATOSUS

Neuropsychiatric signs and symptoms in systemic lupus erythematosus (SLE) are produced by a variety of processes. Secondary causes of neurologic dysfunction include metabolic derangements (e.g., uremia), iatrogenic effects (e.g., steroid-induced mania), and intercurrent illnesses (e.g., sepsis). One prospective study determined that 60 percent of all central nervous system symptoms in SLE patients were associated with one or more secondary mechanisms [116]. SLE also causes neurologic dysfunction directly. Considerable confusion in the literature has resulted from attempting to attribute all neuropsychiatric symptoms of SLE to a single pathophysiologic mechanism. Although disagreement exists, the broad outlines of three syndromes of neuropsychiatric manifestations of SLE appear to be emerging: (1) antiphospholipid antibodies (strokes, chorea, and some seizures), (2) antineuronal antibodies (nonfocal symptoms such as dementia, psychiatric disorders, and seizures), and (3) vasculitis (intracranial hemorrhages and peripheral nerve disorders). Other symptoms such as headaches, aseptic meningitis, transverse myelitis, and cranial nerve abnormalities may be due to other pathophysiologic mechanisms. Diagnosis, treatment, and prognosis differ according to the mechanism involved, and these will be discussed separately with each syndrome.

Antiphospholipid Antibodies

Antiphospholipid antibodies (APA) refer to a group of circulating antibodies against negatively charged phospholipids including cardiolipin. [93] They are detected in patients with SLE and other systemic diseases as well as in healthy individuals. A group of symptoms including arterial and venous thrombosis, midpregnancy fetal loss, and thrombocytopenia have been recognized to be associated with APA, and the terms *antiphospholipid-antibody syndrome* and *anticardiolipin syndrome* have been widely used [34].

APA can be detected by various methods including prolonged coagulation tests ("lupus anticoagulants"), biologic false-positive tests for syphilis, and anticardiolipin antibody assays by enzyme-linked or radioimmunoassay techniques. These methods may cross react with each other but may occur independently [189]. Thus, all three tests should be performed when suspicion of APA arises.

The term *lupus anticoagulant* misrepresents the pathophysiologic activity of APA. It was originally described in 1952 [44] as an acquired inhibitor of prothrombin conversion that was associated with cerebral hemorrhages in two SLE patients. Subsequently, it has been shown that lupus anticoagulant neither is exclusively associated with SLE nor acts as an anticoagulant in vivo. Rather, it is an IgG or IgM antibody against negatively charged phospholipids that prolongs the activated partial thromboplastin time (aPTT) by interfering with the phospholipid surface upon which the prothrombin activator complex forms in vitro [70]. Its presence is determined by the following laboratory features: (1) prolonged aPTT; (2) failure of a 1:1 mixture of the patient's plasma with normal plasma to correct the aPTT to within 4 seconds of control values; (3) reduced activity of more than one aPTT coagulation factor (VII, IX, XI, XII) by one-stage assay; and (4) increased coagulation-factor activity with dilution of the patient's plasma with normal plasma [86]. Thus, lupus anticoagulant is defined by an abnormality of the aPTT assay. A number of other laboratory coagulation assays are similarly prolonged by the lupus anticoagulant, including Russell viper venom times, kaolin clotting times, and recalcification times [162,166].

False-positive biologic tests for syphilis (VDRL, rapid plasma reagin, and Wasserman tests) constitute one of the 11 American Rheumatological Association criteria used to diagnose SLE [166]. Each of these tests is designed to detect reagin, an antibody associated with syphilis. However, each includes cardiolipin and other phospholipids as substrate. A false-positive biologic test for syphilis represents APA activity against negatively charged phospholipids in the assays themselves [95,132]. False-positive biologic tests for syphilis may not carry the same increased risk for thrombosis as do anticardiolipin antibodies and lupus anticoagulants [94].

Anticardiolipin antibodies are IgG or IgM antibodies directed against cardiolipin and can be detected by using enzyme-linked immunosorbent assays or solid radioimmunoassay. Although titers fluctuate, the persistence of high titers of anticardiolipin antibodies is associated with recurrent thrombosis and other clinical manifestations [92,109,155,160].

Epidemiology

SLE remains the disease most commonly associated with APA. Lupus anticoagulants occur in 34 percent of SLE patients and anticardiolipin antibodies occur in 44 percent [136]. APA has been reported in a wide variety of other diseases including other collagen vascular diseases (Sjögren's syndrome, Behçet's syndrome, rheumatoid arthritis, osteoarthritis, and psoriatic arthritis [70,136]), various immune-mediated neurologic disorders (dermatomyositis, polymyositis, and myasthenia gravis [43]), infectious diseases (acquired immunodeficiency syndrome [25,39], Lyme disease [139], and some bacterial infections [186]) and in patients receiving neuroleptics [32,149], procainamide, quinidine, and phenytoin [189]. In many of these entities, APA are detected at relatively low titers, which may not be predictive of thrombosis [43,136]. Finally, APA are also detected in otherwise healthy individuals with thrombosis or other manifestations of the APA syndrome [16,131]. This has been termed primary APA syndrome. APA have been detected in 11 percent of nonpregnant controls [166] and in up to 22 percent of pregnant women [128]. The frequency at which symptoms occur among such individuals is unclear.

Clinical Features

Clinically significant thromboembolic phenomena occur in 25 percent of patients with APA whether or not SLE is present [73]. Sneddon's syndrome of livedo reticularis and cerebral infarction has been shown to be related to APA [60,113]. Deep venous thrombosis, strokes, myocardial infarctions [90], and other arterial and venous thrombosis have been reported. Thrombocytopenia and Coombs-positive hemolytic anemia occur commonly. Recurrent fetal loss, valvular heart disease, and pulmonary hypertension are also associated with APA [52,121,130].

Cerebral ischemia, transient or fixed, is the neurologic disorder most clearly associated with APA [4,45,52,73,78,131,144,145]. Strokes occur in 2 to 10 percent of SLE patients [144] and multi-infarct dementia can result [18,45]. Cerebral ischemia can also occur in patients with APA who do not have SLE or other immunologic abnormalities [45] and in patients as young as 9 months [171]. Angiography in patients with APA reveals a range of findings from normal to occlusions of various intra- and extracranial vessels [132].

A number of mechanisms have been proposed as explanations of how APA produce thromboembolic phenomena in vivo. APA effects on platelets, various circulating factors of both the intrinsic and extrinsic clotting systems, and components of vessel walls have all been demonstrated. Multiple sites of action appear most likely [132]. Another recently postulated mechanism of antiphospholipid antibody-induced ischemia involves verrucous endocarditis (Libman-Sacks endocarditis), a common postmortem finding in SLE patients. Recent reports note an association between valvular heart disease, cerebral infarctions, and APA, suggesting that emboli from verrucous endocarditis may cause cerebral ischemia [17,54,68,121, 130].

Chorea occurs in 2 percent of patients with SLE. APA have been associated with chorea in patients with and without evidence of SLE. The chorea is of sudden onset, may be unilateral or bilateral, and typically improves gradually although some patients are permanently affected and others experience recurrences [15]. Chorea gravidarum in patients with a history of recurrent fetal loss has also been reported associated with APA [96,132]. Cerebral ischemia often occurs in the same patient as chorea, and it is presumed that chorea is due to basal ganglia ischemia. A direct autoantibody attack upon the basal ganglia is another possible explanation for the association between chorea and APA. Treatment is directed at preventing further strokes and symptomatic control of the chorea [15].

Focal seizures have been associated with APA, perhaps as a result of cerebral infarctions. "Vascular" headaches are frequently reported in patients with SLE, and a possible association with APA has been suggested based on reports of APA found in both SLE and non-lupus migraineurs [132,189]. However, one large series did not detect an association between APA and either seizures or headaches [4].

Treatment

Good therapeutic trials in patients with APA syndrome are not yet available. Anticoagulation with warfarin with or without aspirin appears to prevent further thrombotic complications [92]. Corticosteroids, immunosuppressants, and plasmapheresis have been utilized with mixed results [132].

Our general approach presently is to anticoagulate with heparin (monitored using thromboplastin times) patients with acute thrombosis and evidence of APA. Warfarin anticoagulation is then substituted for heparin. The duration of anticoagulation is based on clinical response and titers of APA.

Antineuronal Antibodies

Subtle changes in concentration, memory, or personality are frequently noted by SLE patients but are often unrecognized by their physicians. When cognitive and behavioral alterations reach levels requiring hospitalization, they are often termed organic brain syndrome or organic psychosis. These terms have limited usefulness, since they also describe metabolically induced delirium secondary to uremia, hypoxia, and so on. Not all patients diagnosed under those terms have primary neuropsychiatric manifestations of SLE, making the actual prevalence of cognitive and psychiatric manifestations in SLE difficult to assess.

Clinical Features

Cognitive abnormalities in the alert patient are common in SLE patients when careful testing is performed. Denburg, Carbotte, and Denburg [51] studied 86 consecutive female SLE patients seen as inpatients and outpatients from two hospitals. Not surprisingly, moderate or severe cognitive impairment was found in 22 of 23 female SLE patients experiencing acute central nervous system symptoms. However, cognitive abnormalities were also noted in 16 of 17 similar patients with history of central nervous system disease but no current symptoms. Furthermore, cognitive abnormalities were more frequently noted among 41 SLE patients without any history of central nervous system disease, as compared to normal controls. Such an increased frequency of cognitive deficits could not be attributed to stroke syndromes, medication, or psychological distress [33]. Cognitive deficits due to primary neuropsychiatric manifestations of SLE appear permanent [51]. Cognitive deficits profound enough to be diagnosed as organic brain syndrome occurred in 6 percent of SLE patients followed prospectively for 6 years [1]. Little is known regarding treatment of these deficits. Such cognitive deficits among SLE patients have been associated with one or more serum IgG antineuronal antibodies [50]. The exact mechanism of action remains unclear.

Depression and anxiety symptoms of moderate severity affect 40 to 50 percent of SLE patients [74]. These symptoms occur more frequently in SLE patients than in comparable rheumatoid arthritis patients [159]. They have been associated with antibodies to ribosomal P protein [175]. These studies suggest that affective symptoms may be attributable to immune-mediated factors and are not solely the result of disability or medications. Affective symptoms in SLE are alleviated by conventional therapies such as antidepressant medications and psychotherapy. Suicide occurred in 4 of 180 SLE patients followed prospectively over 6 years [1].

SLE-induced acute confusional states must be distinguished from metabolic delirium and primary psychiatric disorders, since therapies differ. Psychotic features often occur but are not essential for diagnosis. SLE-induced acute confusional state can be recognized by the occurrence of concurrent neurologic deficits or typical abnormalities in the electroencephalogram, spinal fluid, cerebral blood flow, or serology (rising erythrocyte sedimentation rate or antinuclear antibody). Abel, Gladman, and Urowitz [1] noted 17 episodes of "psychosis" among 180 SLE patients followed prospectively over 6 years. Most SLE-induced acute confusional states resolve with corticosteroid treatment [65,116]. However, corticosteroids can produce mania or psychosis when administered at high doses or can exacerbate underlying conditions [134].

Seizures are another important neuropsychiatric manifestation of SLE. Seizures have been associated with antineuronal antibodies [26] and psychiatric disorders [65]. Seizures occur in roughly 15 to 35 percent of SLE patients [142], but again this represents a mixed group of primary central nervous system events and secondary metabolic, infectious, or treatment complications. In one study, all 10 seizures that occurred in 71 SLE patients could be attributed to such secondary causes [116]. Seizures often occur as an initial symptom of SLE and also as a preterminal event. Although there is reference to "grand mal" and "petit mal" seizures in the literature, it is our impression that the vast majority of seizures in SLE are partial seizures with either secondary generalization or complex features. Electroencephalography is the diagnostic procedure of choice. Seizures are in most cases self-limited and resolve without steroid treatment [65,116]. When SLE is suspected in a patient with a preexisting seizure disorder, consideration should be given to a diagnosis of drug-induced lupus (especially in relation to phenytoin).

Pathophysiology

The etiology of nonfocal cerebral dysfunction remains unclear, but a number of antibodies have been associated with various clinical manifestations. Antilymphocytic antibodies that cross react with neurons have been demonstrated in sera of patients with neuropsychiatric manifestations of SLE [102,188]. Serum antibodies to ribosomal P proteins have been reported in association with acute confusional states and severe affective disorders. The titers of these antibodies fluctuate with clinical manifestations [27,81,175], and rising titers may predict neuropsychiatric symptoms [53]. Elevated titers of antineuronal antibodies have been detected in the cerebrospinal fluid and sera of patients with "organic mental" abnormalities and seizures when compared with patients experiencing focal neurologic symptoms, active nonneurologic SLE disease, and controls [26,36]. Significantly higher antineuronal binding activity is present in sera of patients with neuropsychiatric manifestations of SLE than in SLE patients without neuropsychiatric symptoms, rheumatoid arthritis patients, and normal controls [49]. Finally, serum IgG antineuronal antibodies have been associated with cognitive deficits [50].

Antibodies appear to cross a damaged blood-brain barrier into the cerebrospinal fluid [120]. It is not certain whether cerebrospinal fluid antineuronal antibodies induce cognitive and psychiatric abnormalities or are merely epiphenomena. Neurocytotoxicity has been demonstrated in a chromium release assay, but further evidence for a direct effect of these antibodies on neurons remains to be demonstrated [26].

Vasculitis

Although the neuropsychiatric manifestations of SLE are often referred to as vasculitis, documentation by either angiography or histopathologic examination of actual inflammation of blood vessel walls is infrequent. Only 3 of 24 patients in an autopsy series had evidence of cellular invasion of vessel walls, and in no case was vasculitis prominent [112]. More recent series have uniformly confirmed the rarity of central nervous system vasculitis in SLE [54,58]. Individual cases of proven vasculitis in SLE may involve other predisposing factors such as herpes zoster infection, amphetamine use [174], or pregnancy [184].

Intracranial hemorrhage was noted in 50 percent of SLE patients in older postmortem series usually involving subarachnoid and intraparenchymal hemorrhage [58,112]. A more recent study found only one subarachnoid hemorrhage among 50 cases of SLE [54]. Postmortem series may have a selection bias for hemorrhage due to its high mortality rate. In a prospective study, only 1 of 180 SLE patients had an intracranial hemorrhage over a 6-year period [1]. Cerebral vasculitis (with or without associated infection) is often associated with hemorrhage [58] and probably accounts for cases of intracranial hemorrhages in SLE. Other factors that may contribute to intracranial hemorrhages in SLE include coagulopathies secondary to organ failure and thrombocytopenia in association with antiphospholipid antibodies. Corticosteroids with or without cyclophosphamide would be the treatment of choice for proven cerebral vasculitis (see Isolated Angiitis of the Nervous System).

In contrast to the lack of evidence for central nervous system vasculitis in SLE, the peripheral nervous system is affected by systemic vasculitis. This causes mononeuritis multiplex and may play a role in a distal symmetric polyneuropathy that affects SLE patients. The pathophysiology is similar to that found in polyarteritis nodosa.

Other Neurologic Manifestations of SLE

Headaches are the most frequent neurologic manifestation of SLE, occurring in at least 60 percent of SLE patients. Vascular headaches, both classic and common migraines, account for two-thirds of these, with the remainder being less well characterized [158]. Standard treatments of vascular headaches are often helpful. Although the vast majority of headaches in SLE are benign, they may be the presenting sign of serious complications such as cerebral venous thrombosis [192].

Aseptic meningitis occurs in 5 percent of SLE patients [58], although a number of large series do not mention it [1,54]. It presents with headache, fever, and meningismus. The cerebrospinal fluid shows increased protein concentration and pleocytosis (usually below 300 nucleated cells with lymphocyte predominance). Hypoglycorrhachia is infrequent and should suggest infectious meningitis. Aseptic meningitis usually resolves spontaneously or in response to corticosteroid administration but may recur or become chronic [127]. It is critical to differentiate this entity from infectious meningitis, which tends to occur in the late stages of SLE [31,173]. Whether aseptic meningitis is mediated by antibodies [119] or is actually an as yet unidentified viral meningitis is not clear. A meningitis induced by azathioprine and various nonsteroidal anti-inflammatory drugs occurs more frequently in SLE patients than in the general population [173]. Intrathecal synthesis of IgG has been detected in some of these patients [38].

Transverse myelitis occurs in association with aseptic meningitis [65,173] or alone in scattered cases [141]. Lifetime risk for SLE patients appears to be roughly 2 percent. Spinal fluid findings are similar to those mentioned for aseptic meningitis except that transient hypoglycorrhachia may occur. Ischemic necrosis of the spinal cord is described as a common postmortem finding [14], which may suggest involvement of APA. One case of myelopathy was found to contain vacuoles in the white matter of the posterior and lateral columns similar to those found in subacute combined degeneration [54].

Cranial nerve abnormalities are found in up to 31 percent of retrospectively reviewed SLE inpatients [65] and in 11 out of 180 prospectively followed patients in 6 years [1]. The facial nerve was most frequently involved [65], with third, fifth, and eighth nerve dysfunction also occurring. Multiple cranial neuropathies occur associated with meningitis. Vasculitis may also be a factor in some cases.

Peripheral nerve abnormalities are found in about 10 percent of SLE patients [1] and take varied forms. Two-thirds present as a distal sensorimotor neuropathy, while the remainder suggest mononeuritis multiplex [65]. Carpal tunnel syndrome has been documented in as many as 23 percent of SLE patients [158]. Vasculitis appears to cause mononeuritis multiplex and may also have a role in the symmetric neuropathy.

Diagnosis

Neuropsychiatric manifestations may occur in patients where the diagnosis of SLE is well established. More confusing are situations where the neuropsychiatric symptom is the initial presentation of SLE either alone or as a part of a multisystem illness. No single laboratory test or battery of tests can diagnose a neuropsychiatric manifestation of SLE due to the diversity of pathophysiologic mechanisms noted above. Each laboratory test is useful in certain situations. Diagnostic strategies must be individualized. Few other diseases require the degree of clinical acumen in evaluating neuropsychiatric symptoms.

Serologic Studies

Serologic studies may reveal evidence of systemic disease activity concurrent with the neuropsychiatric symptoms. Elevations of the erythrocyte sedimentation rate or antinuclear antibody titers can suggest that a given neuropsychiatric symptom is being caused by the disease. Interestingly, antibodies to double-stranded DNA are often absent among patients with central nervous system manifestations of SLE [185].

Cerebrospinal Fluid

Some abnormality in the spinal fluid has been found associated with neuropsychiatric SLE in 30 to 40 percent of patients. This usually consists of pleocytosis and elevated protein concentrations. Hypoglycorrhachia suggests an infectious cause, although it may be seen in aseptic meningitis and transverse myelitis [1,14,31,112,142]. Elevated IgG levels and the presence of antibodies to DNA have been found in over 60 percent of SLE patients with neuropsychiatric manifestations [179] and may represent the most specific cerebrospinal fluid parameter.

Neuroimaging

Radionuclide scanning in cases of neuropsychiatric manifestations has yielded mixed results [75]. However, depression of global and regional cerebral blood flow determined by the method of xenon-133 inhalation is correlated with central nervous system symptoms [80]. Positron emission tomography has demonstrated areas of altered metabolism that normalize with clinical improvement and that can predict neurologic symptoms [100], but the utility of this technique is presently limited due to lack of availability.

Computed tomography demonstrates hemorrhages, infarcts, and cerebral atrophy in patients with neuropsychiatric symptoms of SLE. However, atrophy can be mimicked in patients receiving corticosteroids. Furthermore, atrophy induced by SLE probably reflects permanent damage to the cerebrum, and thus computed tomography cannot differentiate active disease and residual cerebral damage [2].

Magnetic resonance imaging has shown gray-white junction abnormalities or transient changes suggestive of cerebral edema in patients with acute neuropsychiatric manifestations of SLE. In some cases, these changes resolve in conjunction with clinical remission, but this is not uniformly noted [3,110]. Magnetic resonance imaging shows focal defects that correlate with clinical abnormalities in nearly all cases of stroke or seizure [143]. Thus, magnetic resonance imaging is the best modality for confirming the presence of an acute focal lesion in SLE.

Angiography demonstrates an abnormality in less than 10 percent of cases of neuropsychiatric SLE patients. It is insensitive to small vessel alterations but can detect large emboli [142]. In view of the rarity of cerebral vasculitis in SLE, cerebral angiography should not be used routinely.

Electroencephalography

Electroencephalography has provided a sensitive marker of neuropsychiatric SLE. The electroencephalogram demonstrated some type of abnormality in 70 to 80 percent of patients with active disease [65,179]. Electroencephalography is sensitive for seizure disorders and can differentiate focal from diffuse disease. Although inexpensive and widely available, electroencephalograms are altered by a host of metabolic encephalopathies and are thus not specific for primary neuropsychiatric manifestations of SLE.

Pathology

On a gross level, infarctions, hemorrhages, and meningitis are abnormalities commonly found on examination of brains of SLE patients with neuropsychiatric symptoms. Microinfarcts (less than 1 cm) are found in the cortex and pons in 35 percent of cases, whereas larger infarcts occurred in only 12 percent [58]. Although the neuropsychiatric effects of SLE are often termed lupus cerebritis, SLE does not cause cerebral inflammation [72]. As noted, vasculitis or evidence of previous vasculitis is rarely encountered in cerebral vessels of SLE patients. Instead, the most common feature is vascular hyalinization with the thickening of the intima of small arterioles. Perivascular inflammation and endothelial proliferation are each noted in approximately 25 percent of cases [54,58,112].

PROGRESSIVE SYSTEMIC SCLEROSIS

Progressive systemic sclerosis (PSS), formerly termed scleroderma, is a systemic inflammatory diseases affecting connective tissue. CREST syndrome and morphea can be considered more limited forms of PSS. The skin is the most frequently involved organ, with joints, heart, lungs, kidneys, and the gastrointestinal tract also commonly affected. In contrast to SLE, central nervous system involvement from the primary disease process is exceedingly rare. In a thoughtful study, Gordon and Silverstein [84] concluded that while 24 of 134 patients with PSS had neurologic symptoms at some point in their illness, none involved a central nervous system process directly attributable to PSS. Malabsorption states secondary to gastrointestinal involvement can cause neurologic dysfunction. No specific neuropathologic correlate with PSS has been found [55].

Trigeminal neuropathy occurs in 4 percent of patients with PSS and can be the presenting complaint. In half the cases, bilateral involvement is noted. It has been associated with high serum titers of antiribonucleoprotein antibodies and with myositis [61]. Other cranial nerves may also be affected in addition to the trigeminal (most commonly the facial nerve). Microangiopathy appears to be the causative mechanism [187].

Peripheral nervous system involvement in PSS is uncommon and usually takes the form of a distal sensorimotor polyneuropathy caused by demyelination secondary to microangiopathy [56]. One patient with marked autonomic dysfunction has been reported. Asymptomatic parasympathetic dysfunction was found in three of six other patients tested [182]. Myopathy also has been described, with half resulting from polymyositis and the other half from a vasculopathy characterized by intimal proliferation [170].

MIXED CONNECTIVE TISSUE DISEASE

Mixed connective tissue disease is an overlap syndrome of SLE, PSS, and polymyositis that is associated with the presence of antibodies against ribonucleoprotein. Neuropsychiatric manifestations occur in 55 percent of patients and generally parallel those found in SLE with the exceptions that aseptic meningitis (25% of patients) and trigeminal neuropathy (10%) appear more common and thromboembolic phenomena are not reported [20].

SJÖGREN'S SYNDROME

Sjögren's syndrome is an autoimmune disease affecting lacrimal and salivary glands, causing symptoms of xerophthalmia and xerostomia (sicca syndrome). It is diagnosed by confirming lacrimal gland dysfunction by either the Schirmer's test (less than 5 mm of fluid migration within 5 minutes on a strip of filter paper placed under an anesthetized lower eyelid) or slit-lamp determination of keratoconjunctivitis sicca plus confirming salivary gland dysfunction by examination of the mouth or biopsy of the salivary glands of the lip. Extraglandular features of the illness are being reported, including a wide range of neurologic disease.

Epidemiology

Prevalence of Sjögren's syndrome has been estimated as high as 5 percent of the population over 55 years. Peak incidence is between ages 40 and 50 years with a female to male ratio of 9 : 1. It also occurs in association with a variety of rheumatologic diseases such as rheumatoid arthritis, PSS, and SLE (secondary Sjögren's syndrome) or alone (primary Sjögren's syndrome) [9]. Seventy percent of patients with primary Sjögren's syndrome are found to have antinuclear antibodies against SS-A (Ro), while 50 percent are found to have antibodies against SS-B (La) [76].

Clinical Features

A significant proportion of patient's with Sjögren's syndrome are stated to have neurologic abnormalities. Approximately 30 percent of patients with primary Sjögren's syndrome have peripheral nervous system dysfunction, and 20 percent have peripheral central system disease. The latter rate is greatly increased if psychopathology is included [140]. Often a single patient is susceptible to both peripheral and central nervous system symptoms [8]. Cutaneous vasculitis is associated with a neurologic morbidity rate of 90 percent. Central nervous system disorders found in Sjögren's syndrome are similar to those in SLE and include stroke (20%), seizure (15%), movement disorder (8%), aseptic meningitis, and encephalopathy. Cognitive abnormalities are demonstrated in 18 percent of patients, consisting of deficits in attention, concentration, and memory. Affective and personality disorders (although not psychosis) may occur with rates as high as 50 percent [140,193]. Migraine-like headaches occur in 46 percent of patients with primary Sjögren's syndrome and appear associated with Raynaud's phenomenon [161].

Alexander and co-workers [8] reported 20 patients with symptomatology mimicking multiple sclerosis who eventually were diagnosed with Sjögren's syndrome. In 13 of the patients, neurologic symptoms antedated the diagnosis of Sjögren's syndrome, but sicca symptoms had begun prior to or concurrent with neurologic symptoms in all patients. Transverse myelitis and optic neuritis were each noted in about half of the patients. Cerebrospinal fluid analysis revealed one or more oligoclonal bands in 16 of 18 patients tested. Sixty percent of these patients have evidence of peripheral neuropathy, vasculitis, or myositis, which distinguishes them from multiple sclerosis patients. Other cases in the series may represent coexistent multiple sclerosis and Sjögren's syndrome. These patients responded to moderate doses of prednisone (40–60 mg/day) with stabilization or improvement. In contrast to the frequency of severe neurologic dysfunction reported by the Baltimore group, other studies have found only rare, relatively minor neurologic morbidity in primary Sjögren's syndrome [24]. Furthermore, no cases of Sjögren's syndrome were found among 192 patients attending a university-based multiple sclerosis clinic [156].

Peripheral nervous system manifestations of Sjögren's syndrome include a distal symmetric pansensory polyneuropathy, which on occasion involves motor neuropathy on the basis of vasculitis of various types including necrotizing vasculitis, lymphocytic, and endarteritis obliterans [167,190]. Mononeuritis multiplex and entrapment neuropathies also occur [13].

Cranial neuropathies on the basis of peripheral entrapment or vasculitis are also found. The most common of these is trigeminal neuropathy, which presents with painless sensory loss over the second and third distributions. Facial nerve palsy (Bell's palsy) also occurs [167]. Inflammatory myopathy has also been associated with Sjögren's syndrome.

Diagnosis

Electroencephalography and cerebrospinal fluid analysis are each abnormal in about two-thirds of patients with active central nervous system manifestations. Magnetic resonance imaging of the head has proved positive in 75 percent of cases with neurologic manifestations of Sjögren's syndrome [7]. Computed tomography and angiography are much less helpful [6].

Pathophysiology

Since vasculitis can play a prominent pathophysiologic role in systemic manifestations of Sjögren's syndrome, one might assume that it is commonly a factor in central nervous system manifestations as well. However, in one report [10], cerebral angiography was normal in 12 out of 13 patients with central nervous system disease, and the remaining patient exhibited stenosis of a distal internal carotid artery. A bland, mononuclear vasculopathy of small vessels is found at postmortem. This is similar to the vasculopathy described in SLE and is unlike the necrotizing angiitis found in peripheral tissues in Sjögren's syndrome [9]. Cases of documented cerebral vasculitis have occurred in complicated clinical settings [66,190] and may represent vasculitis due to another disease process, with Sjögren's syndrome being incidental. However, central nervous system disorders tend to occur in the setting of peripheral vasculitis [140]. Mechanisms similar to those postulated for SLE may account for the pathophysiology of neurologic manifestations of Sjögren's syndrome, but more research in this area is needed.

Treatment

Suggested treatment for central nervous system Sjögren's syndrome or for vasculitis associated with Sjögren's syndrome consists of high-dose steroids with or without cyclophosphamide [9].

RHEUMATOID ARTHRITIS AND SPONDYLARTHROPATHIES

Rheumatoid Arthritis and Juvenile Rheumatoid Arthritis

The rarity of cerebral involvement in rheumatoid arthritis and juvenile rheumatoid arthritis stands in marked contrast to SLE. Twelve cases of cerebral vasculitis producing hemorrhages, infarctions, cognitive impairment, and seizures have been reported in patients with rheumatoid arthritis [178], including cases where vasculitic changes were confined to the cerebrum [195]. Dural nodules may compress the brain or spinal cord in equally rare cases [41]. In all these cases, articular evidence of rheumatoid arthritis was obvious and of long standing.

Cervical myelopathy is the most serious neurologic complication of rheumatoid arthritis. Radiographic changes of subluxation are found in 25 percent of rheumatoid patients, but only a small minority become symptomatic [151,152, 180]. Four types of cervical subluxation have been delineated: (1) C1 moves anteriorly on C2, (2) C1 moves posteriorly on C2, (3) vertical subluxation of odontoid, and (4) "staircase" or multiple lower level subluxations. Types 1 and 4 are the most common [151]. The presentation is of a mild spastic quadriparesis with sensory and sphincter symptoms in a majority [152]. Pontomedullary symptoms caused by transient or permanent vertebrobasilar ischemia are also documented [103,151,180]. Even severe subluxation demonstrated radiographically may remain asymptomatic. In a study of 130 patients with radiographic evidence of subluxation, 46 patients died of other causes, 4 developed myelopathy, and 6 developed vertebrobasilar insufficiency. There was no increased mortality associated with radiographically documented subluxation [180]. Diagnosis can be confirmed with myelography, computed tomography, or magnetic resonance imaging [12]. Conservative treatment may be administered using collars or external traction devices to avoid neck flexion or extension. Aspirin has been used in cases of transient ischemic attacks. Surgical treatment may benefit a selected group of patients [152]. Other portions of the spinal canal may also be affected by articular changes in rheumatoid arthritis [150].

Peripheral nerve disorders are the most common neurologic manifestation of rheumatoid arthritis. Compression neuropathy secondary to arthropathy occurs in 45 percent and involves the median nerve at the wrist (carpel tunnel syndrome), ulnar nerve at the elbow, posterior interosseous nerve, sciatic nerve at the knee (secondary to Baker's cyst rupture), peroneal nerve (or one of its branches), or posterior tibial nerve at the ankle (tarsal tunnel syndrome). A distal sensory neuropathy often accompanied by dysesthesias and mononeuritis multiplex is also noted. Both are secondary to occlusive vascular changes due to arteritis. Sural nerve biopsy is helpful in doubtful cases, and treatment is symptomatic unless an acute necrotizing vasculitis is documented [150].

Seronegative Spondylarthropathies

The seronegative spondylarthropathies include ankylosing spondylitis, psoriatic arthropathy, and Reiter's syndrome and overlap with one another with regard to neurologic symptoms. Neurologic involvement is usually due to compression of the cord or cauda equina by advanced bony disease. Cervical subluxations also occur in these disorders as in rheumatoid arthritis [163]. Reiter's syndrome may be associated with meningoencephalitis and seizures [178].

VASCULITIS

Vasculitis is characterized pathologically by inflammation and necrosis of walls of blood vessels and accurately applies to a relatively small group of conditions. Many factors may trigger vasculitis, but all vasculitides involve invasion of the walls of blood vessels by inflammatory cells that produce necrosis of vessel walls or stenosis of the vessel lumen. Vasculitis usually produces symptoms through ischemia or hemorrhage. Clinical manifestations depend on the nature of the blood vessels affected and the acuteness of the ischemia [147]. Although defined histologically, vasculitis can at times be diagnosed radiologically by angiography [67].

Systematic clinical consideration of the vasculitides is hampered by multiple classification schemata. Division of vasculitides according to the size of the vessels involved is the most widely accepted method of categorization. Large arteries are affected in Takayasu's arteritis and giant cell arteritis. Medium- and small-sized arteries are affected in polyarteritis group, Wegener's granulomatosis, lymphomatoid granulomatosis, and Cogan's syndrome. Small vessels are affected in Henoch-Schönlein purpura, cryoglobulinemia, hypersensitivity vasculitis, and drug-induced vasculitis [133].

Vasculitides can also be grouped by immunologic mechanisms. Polyarteritis nodosa and allergic granulomatosis result from immune complex deposition on vessel walls (Arthus reaction). Granuloma formation is present in Wegener's granulomatosis and isolated angiitis of the nervous system, suggesting cell-mediated immunity involvement in vasculitis. Direct lymphocytic invasion of vessel walls is found in lymphomatoid granulomatosis. Tissue ischemia is the final common pathophysiology of all vasculitides [147].

From the clinician's view, vasculitis affecting the nervous system can best be classified by presentation. Temporal arteritis, Cogan's syndrome, amphetamine-induced angiitis, and isolated angiitis of the nervous system typically present with central nervous system complaints, whereas evidence of generalized vasculitis is usually evident in the other conditions prior to central nervous system involvement [178].

Finally, vasculitis is associated with other conditions such as collagen-vascular diseases, malignancies (especially hairy-cell leukemia) [87], infections (e.g., Lyme disease [191]), drugs, and allergies.

ISOLATED ANGIITIS OF THE NERVOUS SYSTEM

In 1959, Cravioto and Feigin [46] described cases of a vasculitis affecting small arteries and causing symptoms primarily in the central nervous system. Less than 100 similar cases have been reported in the English literature, although the entity is often discussed as a cause of multiple strokes or other obscure neurologic disorders. However, its clinical and laboratory features typify central nervous system vasculitis of all causes. Various terms have been applied to the syndrome such as isolated angiitis of the nervous system, granulomatous angiitis of the nervous system (GANS), and primary angiitis of the central nervous system.

The mean age of onset is 46 years with a range from 3 to 74 years and no clear sex predilection. Histologic examination reveals inflammation of the small arteries and arterioles (200 to 500 microns in diameter) of the leptomeninges and cerebrum. Other blood vessels may also be affected [29]. Lesions are segmental and consist of perivascular lymphocytes and monocytes, granulomata, and multinucleated giant cells [178].

Clinical Features

The hallmarks of isolated angiitis of the central nervous system (or any vasculitis of the central nervous system) are headaches and multifocal neurologic deficits superimposed on delirium [29]. When systemic inflammation or infection is excluded by appropriate tests and either angiography or histologic examination of a biopsy specimen confirms the presence of vascular inflammation, the diagnosis is established [146]. Symptoms may fluctuate or stutter at onset [129,146]. Nonspecific symptoms such as focal or diffuse headache (68%), weakness (56%), and confusion (55%) were the most common presentations. Seizures were part of the presentation in only 23 percent. Physical signs included hemiplegia/monoplegia (56%), abnormalities of cranial nerve examination (36%), aphasias (27%), fever (23%), and hypertension (23%) [178]. Petechiae, intraparenchymal hemorrhage, and rarely subarachnoid hemorrhage are also reported [23,129]. Spinal cord presentations also occur [29].

Laboratory evaluation reveals an elevated erythrocyte sedimentation rate in up to 70 percent of cases. Some abnormality of routine cerebrospinal analysis is present in 94 percent, with increased protein (as high as 800 gm/dl), increased pressure, and pleocytosis (up to 300/hpf) being the most common. Peripheral blood cell counts tended to remain normal, although a leukocytosis can occur [178]. Electroencephalography has been one of the more sensitive diagnostic tools, being abnormal in 81 percent of cases; however, it is nonspecific. Electroencephalography shows diffuse slowing or focal slowing with or without discharges. Computed tomography and magnetic resonance imaging show multiple lesions in both gray and white matter. Normal results of any of the above tests do not exclude isolated angiitis of the central nervous system, but in combination these tests can be suggestive of angiitis and exclude more common explanations for central nervous system symptoms.

Angiographic findings in cerebral arteritis are classically described as intermittent narrowing and dilatation of blood vessels, alteration in blood flow, and at times a mass effect. Such alterations are not entirely specific for vasculitis, as similar findings are seen associated with neoplasms, hemorrhage (vasospasm), atherosclerotic vascular disease, fibromuscular dysplasia, and neurocutaneous syndromes [67,129,146]. In the presence of a high suspicion of vasculitis, a positive angiogram can be accepted as confirming the diagnosis of isolated angiitis of the nervous system [29]. Angiitis confined to small vessels has been found at postmortem in cases with normal angiography [147].

The standard for diagnosis of isolated angiitis of the nervous system remains histopathologic examination. The sensitivity of antemortem examination of biopsy specimens is only 71 percent due to the focal nature of pathologic changes (so-called skip lesions). Sensitivity is improved by biopsy of the extracranial vessels, leptomeninges, and cortex [29]. Biopsy also detects other causes of vascular inflammation [146] and should be performed whenever angiography is not diagnostic and clinical suspicion remains high.

Etiology

No single cause has been found for isolated angiitis of the nervous system. Angiitis restricted to the central nervous system has been regularly reported in the setting of lymphoma and leukemia. Similar angiitis has been associated with hepatitis B, vericella-zoster, and human immunodeficiency virus [196]. This may suggest an infectious agent in an immune-compromised host as an etiology [29]. Finally, sympathomimetic amines can produce vasculitis isolated to the central nervous system.

Treatment

No controlled therapeutic trials have been performed in isolated angiitis of the nervous system; however, it appears that the disease is frequently fatal if untreated (19 out of 20 reported cases). Corticosteroid treatment may reduce mortality (6 out of 13 cases), and a combination of steroids and cytotoxic agents (cyclophosphamide with or without initial induction with nitrogen mustard) may be associated with a further decrease in mortality (1 out of 13) [29,47]. The length of treatment required may be guided by repeat angiography, as vasculitis may persist on angiography even when clinical symptoms have responded to treatment [30,183].

VASCULITIS SECONDARY TO INFECTIOUS AGENTS

A number of infectous diseases cause neurologic dysfunction by means of vasculitis, including syphilis, Lyme disease, tuberculosis, and hepatitis B. A granulomatous angiitis affecting the central nervous system has been reported among patients infected with the human immunodeficiency virus (HIV) without manifestations of the acquired immunodeficiency syndrome (AIDS) or other infections [196].

Delayed Contralateral Hemiplegia Following Herpes Zoster Ophthalmicus

Focal angiitis following cutaneous herpes zoster (shingles) in the region of the ophthalmic branch of the trigeminal nerve is closely related to isolated angiitis of the nervous system. Essentially, the syndrome consists of an ipsilateral middle cerebral artery distribution infarct secondary to vasculitis induced by the herpes zoster. It is postulated that the arteritis is a result of viral invasion of vessel walls following spread from the ophthalmic branch of the trigeminal nerve, which supplies sensation to the proximal intracranial arteries. The mean age of persons affected is 56 years, with a slight male predominance. Hemiplegia contralateral to the herpes zoster ophthalmicus appears an average of 1 month after the skin lesion. More diffuse manifestations of vasculitis such as confusion and headaches are rare. Laboratory tests of blood and cerebrospinal fluid are comparable to those in isolated angiitis of the nervous system except that the erythrocyte sedimentation rate is usually normal. Angiography reveals vasculitic changes affecting the proximal middle cerebral artery, anterior cerebral artery, and occasionally the siphon portion of the internal carotid artery ipsilateral to the skin lesions. Prognosis is similar to that of large hemispheric strokes, with mortality being 22 percent. Corticosteroids, acyclovir, and anticoagulation have been suggested as treatment [178].

SYMPATHOMIMETIC AMINE-INDUCED CENTRAL NERVOUS SYSTEM VASCULITIS

Amphetamine, ephedrine, phenylpropanolamine, and related compounds have been associated with cerebral vasculitis, often with subarachnoid or intracerebral hemorrhage. Arteritis affecting small- to medium-sized vessels without granulomas has been found in pathologic specimens. Inflammation is presumed to be secondary to immune complex deposition in the intima of blood vessels. Clinical presentations are similar to those in isolated angiitis of the nervous system except that hemorrhages appear in 44 percent of reported cases. In diagnosis, care must be taken to differentiate the angiographic appearance of vasculitis from the vasospasm that is often present following subarachnoid hemorrhage. Leptomeningeal and possibly parenchymal biopsy should be performed in cases of doubt. Removal of the offending agent is the suggested treatment. Addition of cyclophosphamide and corticosteroids may be useful based on the experience with other vasculitides [77].

COGAN'S SYNDROME

Cogan's syndrome is thought to represent a systemic vasculitis that often presents with central nervous system symptomatology. The criteria for diagnosis consist of auditory and vestibular dysfunction combined with nonsyphilitic interstitial keratitis. Median age of onset is 25 years, with equal sex distribution in the 78 cases reported in the English language up to 1986. Interstitial keratitis usually manifests as "stromal clouding of the anterior and middle aspects of the cornea, near the limbus." Ocular symptoms include redness, photophobia, and discomfort. Vestibuloauditory symptoms include the sudden onset of hearing loss, tinnitis, and vertigo, which often progresses to bilateral deafness. Systemic symptoms include fever, arthralgias, and lymphadenopathy. Generalized vasculitis and aortic insufficiency occur less frequently [194]. Aseptic meningoencephalitis and cerebral artery occlusions have each been reported in roughly 6 percent of patients [37,194]. Headache occurs in roughly one-third of patients [21].

No proven etiology of Cogan's syndrome exists, and the pathophysiology remains unclear. Biopsies of various blood vessels or muscle have shown evidence of vasculitis in some cases [37]. Lymphocytic infiltration of the cochlea along with demyelination of the proximal eighth nerve was found in one patient [194]. Cell-mediated immune testing in one patient revealed abnormal lymphocyte migration inhibition in response to inner ear extracts [104].

The disease may relapse and remit. Any worsening of interstitial keratitis may predate a relapse of the more devastating vestibuloauditory manifestations [168]. Bilateral deafness eventuates in 44 percent of all patients, whereas only 8 percent of patients become blind [194]. Interstitial keratitis can be treated by topical steroids [104], and systemic corticosteroid therapy appears to improve hearing if initiated early in the course of the disease [97, 194].

GIANT CELL ARTERITIS

Temporal Arteritis and Polymyalgia Rheumatica

Temporal arteritis and polymyalgia rheumatica affect the same population, have similar histopathologies, follow a generally self-limited course, and overlap frequently enough to consider them as a single disease spectrum. The term *giant cell arteritis* is often used to describe the histopathologic similarities.

Temporal arteritis is one of the most prevalent arteritides affecting the central nervous system. A study in Olmsted County, Minnesota [138] found a prevalence rate of 24.1 per 100,000 in individuals over age 50. A review of 831 cases reported in the literature found a mean age of 70.7 years and a female predominance of 5 to 2. Presentation before age 50 is rare [83]. Temporal arteritis may be more prevalent among northern Europeans, but it occurs in blacks and may be overlooked [22,82]. Polymyalgia rheumatica is roughly three times more common than temporal arteritis and affects a similar population [106].

Clinical Features

Temporal arteritis classically presents with headache, jaw claudication, and facial pain secondary to ischemia of the external carotid system. Constitutional symptoms such as malaise, weight loss, anorexia, and depression occur in approximately half of the patients and may represent the presenting complaint. Low-grade fever occurs in roughly one-quarter of patients. Subclavian and axillary artery and visceral organ involvement have also been reported [154], thus blurring the clinical distinction between temporal arteritis and Takayasu's arteritis. Symptoms of polymyalgia rheumatica (see below) occur in 34 percent of temporal arteritis patients. Nodularity and tenderness to palpation over one or more extracranial arteries, usually the temporal artery, are found in 92 percent of patients. Erythrocyte sedimentation rate of greater than 40 mm/hour was found in 97 percent of patients. Erythrocyte sedimentation rate elevation is often greater than 100 mm/hour [83,138]. However, cases with a normal erythrocyte sedimentation rate are reported [88].

Ischemic damage resulting in stroke or blindness may occur within hours of the onset of the symptoms of arteritis or may be delayed for many months. Ischemia of the internal carotid system resulting in strokes affects 10 percent of patients. Visual loss usually results from optic nerve ischemia but occasionally results from central retinal artery occlusion. Visual loss occurs in half of all patients with temporal arteritis and resulted in total blindness in 22 percent of these patients prior to the availability of steroid treatment [83].

Polymyalgia rheumatica presents with pain or morning stiffness of the proximal extremities, neck, or torso. Patients often report such symptoms as "weakness." Constitutional symptoms and laboratory findings similar to those found in temporal arteritis are associated. Actual arthritis or evidence of muscle weakness or atrophy is not found, although the patient is often quite limited in function due to discomfort and stiffness. Electromyography and muscle biopsy yield nonspecific results. Symptoms appear to result from ischemia due to involvement of the aorta by inflammatory changes similar to those of temporal arteritis. Temporal arteritis affects 15 percent of polymyalgia rheumatica patients [106].

Diagnosis

Diagnosis of temporal arteritis may be based on the presence of three of the following five criteria: age greater than 50 years, onset of a new localized headache, temporal artery tenderness or a decreased temporal artery pulse, erythrocyte sedimentation rate of greater than 50 mm/hour, and positive temporal artery biopsy [105]. Temporal arteries are most frequently selected for biopsy because of the relative ease of the procedure and minimal complication rate reported. Even temporal arteries that appear normal clinically (nontender with normal pulse) prove positive on biopsy in 62 percent of patients. However, due to skip lesions and the possibility that giant cell arteritis is affecting arteries other than the temporal artery, a negative biopsy should not exclude the diagnosis in a patient for whom clinical suspicion is strong. The yield of biopsy can be increased by obtaining a larger length of artery

(4–6 cm) and by carefully sectioning the specimen [83,106]. The diagnosis of polymyalgia rheumatica is based on the clinical picture and response to treatment. Muscle biopsy can be performed in perplexing cases.

Pathology

Granuloma-like lesions and cellular infiltration affecting the vasa vasorum and adventitia plus thrombus in the vessel lumen characterize the histopathologic findings in temporal arteritis. Chronic lesions with necrosis reveal giant cells. Lesions may at times be found in other arteries such as the vertebrobasilar system and coronary arteries [83].

Treatment

Treatment of either polymyalgia rheumatica or temporal arteritis consists of corticosteroids usually in the range of 40 to 60 mg of prednisone per day for temporal arteritis and 15 to 30 mg of prednisone for polymyalgia rheumatica [106,126]. Alternate-day therapy has been shown ineffective. Corticosteroids provide dramatic symptomatic relief of pain and prevent cerebral and retinal infarctions. Because irreversible cerebral or retinal damage may occur soon after the onset of symptoms of arteritis, therapy should be initiated as soon as the diagnosis of temporal arteritis is suspected. Biopsy may be delayed for a few days after initiation of therapy, but 1 week of corticosteroid treatment decreases the diagnostic yield of biopsy [11]. After resolution of symptoms of arteritis, prednisone should be gradually tapered to 15 mg/day over a 10-week period. Chronic treatment with doses greater than 10 mg/day has been associated with shortened life span [85]. Treatment is monitored by erythrocyte sedimentation rate and clinical symptoms. Both temporal arteritis and polymyalgia rheumatica remit after variable periods of 6 to 48 months. Steroid therapy must be reinstituted at the first sign of recurrence.

Takayasu's Arteritis

Takayasu's arteritis is a similar giant cell arteritis that affects the aortic arch and its major branches. The disease is most frequently found in Oriental women but has been reported among other groups of patients worldwide. The disease classically presents with arm claudication ("pulseless disease") but can also present with stroke, headache, hypertension, and constitutional symptoms. Physical signs include bruits, diminished pulses, and heart murmurs. The erythrocyte sedimentation rate is elevated, and angiography of the aortic arch or biopsy of an affected artery is diagnostic [89].

As intracerebral vessels are not often affected in Takayasu's arteritis, neurologic manifestations result from thromboembolic phenomena in the carotid and vertebral arteries, which are involved in the disease in about half of patients. Visual disturbances affect one-quarter of patients and stroke syndromes are found in 15 percent. Headache (50%), dizziness (20%), and seizures (6%) also occur [89,176]. Pathology consists of giant cell inflammation of the intima.

Treatment consists of systemic steroids with cyclophosphamide if progression continues with steroid treatment [176]. The prognosis of Takayasu's arteritis has been variously reported but appears relatively good with treatment [89].

POLYARTERITIS NODOSA

Classic polyarteritis nodosa, allergic angiitis, granulomatosis angiitis (Churg-Strauss syndrome), and an overlap syndrome all involve systemic necrotizing vasculitis. All organs of the body are affected, although the lung and spleen are usually spared [147]. Incidence is estimated at 0.2 per 100,000, and males predominate by a 2 : 1 ratio. All age ranges may be affected [150], with peak incidence being between ages 40 and 70 years [71].

Clinical Features

Clinical features include a wide range of symptoms. Constitutional symptoms of fever and weight loss are among the most common, occurring in 70 percent of patients. Skin, joint, and renal involvement are the most frequent non-neurologic findings. Laboratory abnormalities of an elevated sedimentation rate and anemia are almost universal [71].

The nervous system is one of the most frequently affected organs in polyarteritis nodosa. Central nervous system abnormalities occur in 20 to 40 percent of patients usually late in the course. Symptoms include headache, confusion, strokes (infarcts and hemorrhages), seizures, and various cranial neuropathies [69,148]. Thus, fluctuating combinations of focal and diffuse cerebral symptoms and signs typify the central nervous system manifestations of polyarteritis.

Peripheral nervous system abnormalities are the most common neurologic manifestation of polyarteritis. Between 40 and 60 percent of patients will be affected, often presenting with this complaint [71,147]. Mononeuritis multiplex alone affects 30 to 40 percent of all polyarteritis patients. Presentation is one of painful motor and sensory dysfunction of discrete nerves in a sequential pattern. Electrophysiologic studies reveal denervation of muscles supplied by the affected nerves but often further indicate a more widespread pattern of symmetric neuropathy [28,40,148]. Symmetric distal polyneuropathy occurs clinically in approximately 10 percent of patients [69,169].

Myopathy resulting from the necrotizing vasculitis occurs in about half of all polyarteritis patients [172] and is associated with elevation of muscle enzymes and proximal muscle weakness [79].

Diagnosis

Diagnosis of polyarteritis is based on establishing the presence of disseminated necrotizing vasculitis. Serum antineutrophil cytoplasmic autoantibodies (ANCAs) have been associated with necrotizing vasculitis and may participate in vascular injury [111]. Vasculitis may be established by biopsy or angiography. Electromyography and nerve conduction velocity testing may be used to select appropriate sites for biopsy. Biopsy of muscles that have been electromyographically determined to be acutely affected or biopsy of a sural nerve that has had slowed conduction velocities results in yields approaching 100 percent. Skin and other organs may be biopsied when clinically affected. Lack of clinical involvement of a given organ does not necessarily preclude finding angiographic evidence of vasculitis. Highest yields are found in angiography of the hepatic, renal, and mesenteric arteries [40,48,123,172]. In those cases of a primary cerebral event, the evaluation may proceed along the lines suggested for isolated angiitis of the nervous system. Cerebral angiography and biopsy are indicated. Cerebrospinal fluid and electroencephalographic abnormalities also occur in cases of central nervous system involvement. Serum hepatitis B antigens are found in up to 30 percent of patients [147].

A diagnostic problem arises when mononeuritis multiplex presents without other evidence of polyarteritis. Necrotizing vasculitis can be confined to peripheral nerves, thus requiring nerve biopsy for diagnosis [122,123]. Antineutrophil cytoplasmic autoantibodies may be associated in such cases. On the other hand, mononeuritis multiplex is reported to occur without vasculitis in up to half of nondiabetic cases. Interestingly, these patients also responded to treatment with steroids and cyclophosphamide [99].

Pathology

Lesions in polyarteritis involve the entire thickness of the vessel wall. They evolve through four phases, all of which may occur concurrently in a patient in different areas: (1) edema of the media with fibrinoid necrosis, (2) cellular invasion of vessel walls, which is associated with thrombosis of the vessel lumen or hemorrhage, (3) proliferation of fibroblasts in the adventitia, and (4) organization into scar tissue. Granulomas and giant cells are not seen. Central nervous system structures show similar changes most prominently in the meningeal vessels and least evident in the major cerebral vessels. Peripheral nerves show demyelination and axonal degeneration in the middle of nerve fascicles [150].

Treatment

Mortality in untreated patients is as high as 50 percent within 3 months. Combination treatment with corticosteroids (prednisone 60 mg/day) and cyclophosphamide (2 mg/kg/day) is the standard of therapy currently and has been shown to reduce mortality [64].

GRANULOMATOUS ANGIITIS

Wegener's Granulomatosis

Wegener's granulomatosis causes granulomatous lesions in the upper and lower respiratory tract, focal segmental glomerulonephritis, and necrotizing vasculitis. An older term, "lethal midline granuloma," appears to represent a more restricted manifestation of the same disease process. Mean age of onset is 40 years, and there is a slight male predominance [63]. Lymphomatoid granulomatosis represents a related disease (see next section).

Both of the pathologic processes in the disease, granuloma formation and necrotizing vasculitis, lead to neurologic manifestations in up to 50 percent of untreated patients with Wegener's granulomatosis. ANCAs are useful serologic markers for diagnosis and treatment response [42,111]. The central nervous system is affected by granulomas invading the orbit or cranial vault from a contiguous site such as the nasal sinuses. Basilar meningeal involvement also occurs by way of contiguous spread of granulomas and results in cranial neuropathies. Much less frequently, granulomas can present as an isolated mass lesion in the cerebral parenchyma. Necrotizing vasculitis causes hemorrhage (subarachnoid or intracerebral) and thrombosis [57,98]. With modern treatment, the rate of central nervous system complications has been reduced to 12 percent, most of which were cranial neuropathies [63]. Neurologic dysfunction can be caused secondarily by renal failure or hypoxia.

The peripheral nervous system is mostly affected by vasculitis, which causes mononeuritis multiplex and polyneuropathy in 20 percent of Wegener's granulomatosis patients [57]. Mechanisms similar to those in polyarteritis are involved. Inflammatory myopathy has also been reported [63].

Treatment

Treatment consists of corticosteroids (prednisone, 1 mg/kg/day) and cyclophosphamide (2 mg/kg/day). Complete remissions were induced in 93 percent of patients on this regimen [63], although central nervous system disease has also been reported to have progressed on this regimen [125].

Lymphomatoid Granulomatosis

Lymphomatoid granulomatosis is a vasculitis that affects small to medium arteries and that has a predilection for pulmonary involvement. Skin, kidney, and the nervous system are also involved. As the name would suggest, histopathologic examination reveals atypical lymphoreticular cells in and around necrotic vessel walls and poorly formed granulomas [62]. The clinical manifestations of the disease are very similar to Wegener's granulomatosis except that the upper respiratory tract is not involved in lymphomatoid granulomatosis [150]. Lymphomatoid granulomatosis can mimic lymphoproliferative diseases with lymphomic transformation occurring more frequently than in Wegener's granulomatosis [62].

The disease affects young and middle-aged individuals with a male predominance of 2 to 1. Biopsy of affected tissue is crucial in confirming the diagnosis. The disease is almost uniformly fatal within a year of onset if not treated [118].

Clinical Features

Neurologic involvement is noted in approximately one-quarter of patients. Neurologic signs and symptoms may appear years before pulmonary disease is detected. Necrotizing inflammatory parenchymal masses cause focal neurologic deficits. Cranial neuropathies secondary to basilar meningitis, seizures, and confusion also occur in these patients [118,150]. Computed tomography and magnetic resonance imaging may reveal hemorrhagic lesions, which frequently involve the posterior fossa [117]. Cerebral angiography may remain negative [178]. About 7 percent of patients have peripheral nervous system deficits.

Treatment

Neurologic involvement represents an advanced stage of the disease with 3-year mortality approaching 90 percent in neurologically affected patients [118]. Treatment with prednisone and cyclophosphamide induces remission in some patients. However, transformation to lymphoma and neurologic progression can occur despite cytotoxic therapy [62,178].

BEHÇET'S DISEASE

The triad of recurrent oral and genital ulcers and iritis was first described in 1937 by the Turkish dermatologist Hulusi Behçet. Subsequently, erythema nodosum and other diverse skin lesions, arthritis, thrombophlebitis, gastrointestinal symptoms, and epididymitis have been associated with the disease [177]. The disease is most prevelant in the eastern Mediterranean and Japan and has a peak onset in the third decade. Males have a 2 : 1 preponderance [35].

Clinical Features

Neurologic complications are reported in 10 to 50 percent of Behçet's disease patients [35, 114]. Migraine headaches occur frequently [114,175a]. In one large series from Turkey, 5.3 percent of patients with Behçet's syndrome had neurologic involvement beyond headaches. Cerebral mass lesions and cerebral ischemia appear infrequently but may be the presenting sign of Behçet's disease [108,124,135,175a].

Aseptic meningitis occurred in 7 of 25 patients treated at the Mayo Clinic. Cerebrospinal fluid lymphocytic pleocytosis of less than 500 cells, mildly elevated protein, fever, and meningeal signs were found. Transient cranial neuropathies and long tract signs were also noted. Meningitis occurred in the setting of exacerbation of mucocutaneous symptoms [157].

Symptomatic intracranial hypertension occurs secondary to intracranial dural sinus thrombosis in Behçet's disease [91,175a]. Thrombosis in various veins occurs through suspected circulating immune complex mediation [115], and a similar mechanism is probable in the dural sinuses.

Distal symmetric peripheral neuropathy and mononeuritis multiplex have also been reported occasionally [153]. Abnormal nerve conduction velocities that "mimicked" carpal tunnel syndrome were found in 5 of 12 patients screened for participation in a drug study [115].

Diagnosis

The diagnosis of Behçet's disease is based on the presence of recurrent oral ulceration and two of the following: recurrent genital ulceration, eye lesions, skin lesions, and positive pathergy tests [107]. Cerebrospinal fluid analysis shows a varying degree of pleocytosis and an increased IgM index during the acute phases of neurologic symptoms [101]. Magnetic resonence imaging shows high signal lesions involving both gray and white matter of the cerebral hemispheres and brain stem. These show mass effect acutely and may shrink or disappear with time [5].

Pathology

Acute Behçet's disease skin lesions show a neutrophilic vasculitis, whereas autopsy specimens of solid organs including the brain show lymphocytic perivascular inflammation. It is postulated that circulating immune complexes induce a neutrophilic vasculitis, which causes the symptoms observed [115].

Treatment

Although prognosis for Behçet's disease is generally benign, central nervous system complications can prove fatal. Systemic prednisone (1 mg/kg/day) and azathioprine are the mainstays of treatment [114,197].

OTHER VASCULITIDES

Malignant Atrophic Papulosis

Malignant atrophic papulosis (Köhlmeier-Degos disease) is a disseminated occlusive vasculopathy that affects small arteries. It produces distinctive skin lesions (white, round macules surrounded by a telangectatic rim) and bowel perforation [19]. About 20 percent of patients have neurologic involvement, which consists of disseminated infarctions throughout the central nervous system and which may precede or overshadow other manifestations of the disease [164]. Association with antiphospholipid antibodies has been reported in one case [59]. The disease is often fatal, and optimal treatment has not been defined.

Eales's Disease

Eales's disease consists of angiitis restricted to the small veins of the retina and central nervous system. Retinal phlebitis with hemorrhage into the vitreous is the hallmark of the disease. Neurologic involvement occurs infrequently and consists of transverse myelitis or a myelinopathic, relapsing illness similar to multiple sclerosis. Visual loss occurs in 50 percent of patients, but the disease is not usually fatal [150]. Optimal treatment has not been defined.

Uveomeningeal Syndrome

Uveomeningeal syndrome (Vogt-Koyanagi-Harada syndrome) consists of a transient aseptic meningitis followed by ocular (uveitis and iridocyclitis) and cutaneous (alopecia and vitiligo) manifestations. The disease may be more prevalent in Orientals and Native Americans. Neurologic manifestations include tinnitis, hearing loss, and cranial nerve abnormalities as well as encephalopathy more rarely. Loss of visual acuity results from retinal detachments. Corticosteroids and pregnancy may alleviate the retinopathy [137,181].

REFERENCES

1. Abel, T., Gladman, D. D., and Urowitz, M. B. Neuropsychiatric lupus. *J. Rheumatol.* 7:325, 1980.
2. Adelman, D. C., Saltiel, E., and Klinenberg, J. R. The neuropsychiatric manifestations of systemic lupus erythematosus: An overview. *Semin. Arthritis Rheum.* 15:185, 1986.
3. Aisen, A. M., Gabrielsen, T. O., and McCune, W. J. MR imaging of systemic lupus erythematosus involving the brain. *A.J.R.* 144:1027–1031, 1985.
4. Alarcon-Segovia, D., Deleze, M., Oria, C. V., et al. Antiphospholipid antibodies and the antiphospholipid syndrome in systemic lupus erythematosus: A prospective analysis of 500 consecutive patients. *Medicine* 68:353, 1989.
5. Al Kawi, M. Z., Bohlega, S., and Banna, M. MRI findings in neuro-Behçet's disease. *Neurology* 41:405, 1991.
6. Alexander, E. L. Central nervous system (CNS) manifestations of primary Sjögren's syndrome: An overview. *Scand. J. Rheumatol.* [*Suppl.*] 61:161, 1986.
7. Alexander, E. L., Beall, S. S., Gordon, B., et al. Magnetic resonance imaging of cerebral lesions in patients with the Sjögren's syndrome. *Ann. Intern. Med.* 108:815, 1988.
8. Alexander, E. L., Malinow, K., Lejewski, J. E., et al. Primary Sjögren's syndrome with central nervous system disease mimicking multiple sclerosis. *Ann. Intern. Med.* 104:323, 1986.
9. Alexander, E. L., and Provost, T. T. Sjögren's syndrome: Association of cutaneous vasculitis with central nervous system disease. *Arch. Dermatol.* 123:801, 1987.
10. Alexander, E. L., Provost, T. T., Stevens, M. D., and Alexander, G. E. Neurologic complications of primary Sjögren's syndrome. *Medicine* 61:247, 1982.
11. Allison, M. C., and Gallagher, P. J. Temporal artery biopsy and corticosteroid treatment. *Ann. Rheum. Dis.* 43:416, 1984.
12. Anda, S., Nilsen, G., and Røysland, P. Periodontoid changes in rheumatoid arthritis: MRI observations. *Scand. J. Rheumatol.* 17:59, 1988.
13. Andonopoulos, A. P., Lagos, G., Drosos, A. A., and Moutsopoulus, H. M. The spectrum of neurological involvement in Sjögren's syndrome. *Br. J. Rheumatol.* 29:21, 1990.
14. Andrianakos, A. A., Duffy, J., Suzuki, M., and Sharp, J. T. Transverse myelopathy in systemic lupus erythematosus: Report of three cases and review of the literature. *Ann. Intern. Med.* 83:616, 1975.
15. Asherson, R. A., Derksen, R. H. W. M., Harris, E. N., et al. Chorea in systemic lupus erythematosus and "lupus-like" disease: Association with antiphospholipid antibodies. *Semin. Arthritis Rheum.* 16:253, 1987.
16. Asherson, R. A., Khamashta, M. A., Ordi-Ros, J., et al. The "primary" antiphospholipid syndrome: Major clinical and serological features. *Medicine* 68:366, 1989.
17. Asherson, R. A., and Lubbe, W. F. Cerebral and valve lesions in SLE: Association with antiphospholipid antibodies. *J. Rheumatol.* 15:539, 1988.
18. Asherson, R. A., Mercey, D., Phillips, G., et al. Recurrent stroke and multi-infarct dementia in systemic lupus erythematosus: Association with antiphospholipid antibodies. *Ann. Rheum. Dis.* 46:605, 1987.
19. Barlow, R. J., Heyl, T., Simson, I. W., and Schulz,

E. J. Malignant atrophic papulosis (Degos' disease): Diffuse involvement of brain and bowel in an African patient. *Br. J. Dermatol.* 118:117, 1988.

20. Bennett, R. M., Bong, D. M., and Spargo, B. H. Neuropsychiatric problems in mixed connective tissue disease. *Am. J. Med.* 65:955, 1978.
21. Bicknell, J. M., and Holland, J. V. Neurologic manifestations of Cogan syndrome. *Neurology* 28:278, 1978.
22. Bielory, L., Ogunkoya, A., and Frohman, L. P. Temporal arteritis in blacks. *Am. J. Med.* 86:707, 1989.
23. Biller, J., Loftus, C. M., Moore, S. A., et al. Isolated central nervous system angiitis first presenting as spontaneous intracranial hemorrhage. *Neurosurgery* 20:310, 1987.
24. Binder, A., Snaith, M. L., and Isenberg, D. Sjögren's syndrome: A study of its neurological complications. *Br. J. Rheumatol.* 27:278, 1988.
25. Bloom, E. J., Abrams, D. I., and Rodgers, G. Lupus anticoagulant in the acquired immunodeficiency syndrome. *J.A.M.A.* 256:491, 1986.
26. Bluestein, H. G., Williams, G. W., and Steinberg, A. D. Cerebrospinal fluid antibodies to neuronal cells: Association with neuropsychiatric manifestations of systemic lupus erythematosus. *Am. J. Med.* 70:240, 1981.
27. Bonfa, E., Golombek, S. J., Kaufman, L. D., et al. Association between lupus psychosis and antiribosomal P protein antibodies. *N. Engl. J. Med.* 317:265, 1987.
28. Bouche, P., Léger, J. M., Travers, M. A., et al. Peripheral neuropathy in systemic vasculitis: Clinical and electrophysiologic study of 22 patients. *Neurology* 36:1598, 1986.
29. Calabrese, L. H., and Mallek, J. A. Primary angiitis of the central nervous system: Report of 8 new cases, review of the literature, and proposal for diagnostic criteria. *Medicine* 67:20, 1987.
30. Calabrese, L. H., and Mallek, J. A. The treatment of vasculitis of the central nervous system. *J.A.M.A.* 258:778, 1987.
31. Canoso, J. J., and Cohen A. S. Aseptic meningitis in systemic lupus erythematosus: Report of three cases. *Arthritis Rheum.* 18:369, 1975.
32. Canoso, R. T., and Sise, H. S. Chlorpromazine-induced lupus anticoagulant and associated immunologic abnormalities. *Am. J. Hematol.* 13:121, 1982.
33. Carbotte, R. M., Denburg, S. D., and Denburg, J. A. Prevalence of cognitive impairment in systemic lupus erythematosus. *J. Nerv. Ment. Dis.* 174:357, 1986.
34. Case Records of the Massachusetts General Hospital. A 35-year-old woman with recurrent strokes, an intracardiac lesion, anemia, and thrombocytopenia: Case 37-1988. *N. Engl. J. Med.* 319:699, 1988.
35. Chajek, T., and Fainaru, M. Behçet's disease: Report of 41 cases and a review of the literature. *Medicine* 54:179, 1975.
36. Chen, W. Z., Zhang, N. Z., and Jiang M. Antineuronal antibodies and neuropsychiatric systemic lupus erythematosus. *Chung-Hua Nei Ko Tsa Chih* 29:161, 1990.
37. Cheson, B. D., Bluming, A. Z., and Alroy, J. Cogan's syndrome: A systemic vasculitis. *Am. J. Med.* 60:549, 1976.
38. Chez, M., Sila, C. A., Ransohoff, R. M., et al. Ibuprofen-induced meningitis: Detection of intrathecal IgG synthesis and immune complexes. *Neurology* 39:1578, 1989.
39. Cohen, A. J., Philips, T. M., and Kessler, C. M. Circulating coagulation inhibitors in the acquired immunodeficiency syndrome. *Ann. Intern. Med.* 104:175, 1986.
40. Cohen, R. D., Conn, D. L., and Ilstrup, D. M. Clinical features, prognosis, and response to treatment in polyarteritis. *Mayo Clin. Proc.* 55:146, 1980.
41. Cohen, S. B., and Hurd, E. R. Neurological complications of connective tissue and other "collagen-vascular" diseases. *Semin. Arthritis Rheum.* 11:190, 1981.
42. Cohen Tervaert, J. W., Huitema, M. G., Hene, R. J., et al. Prevention of relapses in Wegener's granulomatosis by treatment based on antineutrophil cytoplasmic antibody titre. *Lancet* 336:709, 1990.
43. Colaco, C. B., Scadding, G. K., and Lockhart, S. Anti-cardiolipin antibodies in neurological disorders: Cross reaction with anti-single stranded DNA activity. *Clin. Exp. Immunol.* 68:313, 1987.
44. Conley, C. L., and Hartmann, R. C. A hemorrhagic disorder caused by circulating anticoagulant in patients with disseminated lupus erythematosus. *J. Clin. Invest* 31:621, 1952.
45. Coull, B. M., Bourdette, D. N., Goodnight, Jr., S. H., et al. Multiple cerebral infarctions and dementia associated with anticardiolipin antibodies. *Stroke* 18:1107, 1987.
46. Cravioto, H., and Feigin, I. Noninfectious granulomatous angiitis with a predilection for the nervous system. *Neurology* 9:599, 1959.
47. Cupps, T. R., Moore, P. M., and Fauci, A. S. Isolated angiitis of the central nervous system: Perspective, diagnostic, and therapeutic experience. *Am. J. Med.* 74:97, 1983.
48. Dahlberg, P. J., Lockhart, J. M., and Overholt, E. L. Diagnostic studies for systemic necrotizing vasculitis: Sensitivity, specificity, and predictive value in patients with multisystem disease. *Arch. Intern. Med.* 149:161, 1989.
49. Danon, Y. L., and Garty, B. Z. Autoantibodies to neuroblastoma cell surface antigens in neuropsychiatric lupus. *Neuropediatrics* 17:23, 1986.

50. Denburg, J. A., Carbotte, R. M., and Denburg, S. D. Neuronal antibodies and cognitive function in systemic lupus erythematosus. *Neurology* 37:464, 1987.
51. Denburg, S. D., Carbotte, R. M., and Denburg, J. A. Cognitive impairment in systemic lupus erythematosus: A neuropsychological study of individual and group deficits. *J. Clin. Exp. Neuropsychol.* 9:323, 1987.
52. Derksen, R. H. W. M., Bouma, B. N., and Kater, L. The prevalence and clinical associations of the lupus anticoagulant in systemic lupus erythematosus. *Scand. J. Rheumatol.* 16:185, 1987.
53. Derksen, R. H., van Dam, A. P., Gmelig Meyling, F. H., et al. A prospective study on antiribosomal P proteins in two cases of familial lupus and recurrent psychosis. *Ann. Rheum. Dis.* 49:799, 1990.
54. Devinsky, O., Petito, C. K., and Alonso, D. R. Clinical and neuropathological findings in systemic lupus erythematosus: The role of vasculitis, heart emboli, and thrombotic thrombocytopenic purpura. *Ann. Neurol.* 23:380, 1988.
55. Dierckx, R. A., Aichner, F., Gerstenbrand, F., and Fritstch, P. Progressive systemic sclerosis and nervous system involvement: A review of 14 cases. *Eur. Neurol.* 26:134, 1987.
56. Di Trapani, G., Tulli, A., La Cara, A., et al. Peripheral neuropathy in course of progressive systemic sclerosis: Light and ultrastructural study. *Acta Neuropathol.* 72:103, 1986.
57. Drachman, D. A. Neurological complications of Wegener's granulomatosis. *Arch. Neurol.* 8:145, 1963.
58. Ellis, S. G., and Verity, M. A. Central nervous system involvement in systemic lupus erythematosus: A review of neuropathologic findings in 57 cases, 1955–1977. *Semin. Arthritis Rheum.* 8:212, 1979.
59. Englert, H. J., Hawkes, C. H., Boey, M. L., et al. Degos' disease: Association with anticardiolipin antibodies and the lupus anticoagulant. *Br. Med. J.* 289:576, 1984.
60. Englert, H. J., Loizou, S., Derue, G. G., et al. Clinical and immunologic features of livedo reticularis in lupus: A case-control study. *Am. J. Med.* 87:408, 1989.
61. Farrell, D. A., and Medsger, T. A., Jr. Trigeminal neuropathy in progressive systemic sclerosis. *Am. J. Med.* 73:57, 1982.
62. Fauci, A. S., Haynes, B. F., Costa, J., et al. Lymphomatoid granulomatosis: Prospective clinical and therapeutic experience over 10 years. *N. Engl. J. Med.* 306:68, 1982.
63. Fauci, A. S., Haynes, B. F., Katz, P., and Wolff, S. M. Wegener's granulomatosis: Prospective clinical and therapeutic experience with 85 patients for 21 years. *Ann. Intern. Med.* 98:76, 1983.
64. Fauci, A. S., Katz, P., Haynes, B. F., and Wolff, S. M. Cyclophosphamide therapy of severe systemic necrotizing vasculitis. *N. Engl. J. Med.* 301:235, 1979.
65. Feinglass, E. J., Arnett, F. C., Dorsch, C. A., et al. Neuropsychiatric manifestations of systemic lupus erythematosus: Diagnosis, clinical spectrum, and relationship to other features of the disease. *Medicine* 55:323, 1976.
66. Ferreiro, J. E., Robalino, B. D., and Saldana, M. J. Primary Sjögren's syndrome with diffuse cerebral vasculitis and lymphocytic interstitial pneumonitis. *Am. J. Med.* 82:1227, 1987.
67. Ferris, E. J., and Levine, H. L. Cerebral arteritis: Classification. *Radiology* 109:327, 1973.
68. Ford, P. M., Ford, S. E., and Lillicrap, D. P. Association of lupus anticoagulant with severe valvular heart disease in systemic lupus erythematosus. *J. Rheumatol.* 15:597, 1988.
69. Ford, R. G., and Siekert, R. G. Central nervous system manifestations of periarteritis nodosa. *Neurology* 15:114, 1965.
70. Fort, J. G., Cowchock, F. S., Abruzzo, J. L., and Smith, J. B. Anticardiolipin antibodies in patients with rheumatic diseases. *Arthritis Rheum.* 30:752, 1987.
71. Frohnert, P. P., and Sheps, S. G. Long-term follow-up study of periarteritis nodosa. *Am. J. Med.* 43:8, 1967.
72. Futrell, N., and Millikan, C. The misnomer of "lupus cerebritis." *Ann. Neurol.* 26:158, 1989.
73. Gastineau, D. A., Kazmier, F. J., Nichols, W. L., and Bowie, E. J. W. Lupus anticoagulant: An analysis of the clinical and laboratory features of 219 cases. *Am. J. Hematol.* 19:265, 1985.
74. Giang, D. W. Systemic lupus erythematosus and depression. *Neuropsychiatr. Neuropsychol. Behav. Neurol.* 4:78, 1991.
75. Gibson, T., and Myers, A. R. Nervous system involvement in systemic lupus erythematosus. *Ann. Rheum. Dis.* 35:398, 1975.
76. Gilliland, B. C., and Mannik, M. Rheumatoid Arthritis. In R. G. Petersdorf et al. (eds.), *Harrison's Principles of Internal Medicine* (10th ed.). New York: McGraw-Hill, 1983.
77. Glick, R., Hoying, J., Cerullo, L., and Perlman, S. Phenylpropanolamine: An over-the-counter drug causing central nervous system vasculitis and intracerebral hemorrhage. Case report and review. *Neurosurgery* 20:969, 1987.
78. Glueck, H. I., Kant, K. S., Weiss, M. A., et al. Thrombosis in systemic lupus erythematosus: Relation to the presence of circulating anticoagulants. *Arch. Intern. Med.* 145:1389, 1985.
79. Goetz, C. G. Polyarteritis Nodosa. In P. J. Vinken and G. W. Bruyn (eds.), *Handbook of Clinical Neurology.* Amsterdam: Elsevier/North Holland, 1980. Vol. 39, pp. 295–311.
80. Goldstein, S., Kushner, M. J., Alves, W. M., et al. Regional cerebral blood flow as a laboratory

marker in systemic lupus erythematosus. *Ann. Neurol.* 28:244, 1990.
81. Golombek, S. J., Graus, F., and Elkon, K. B. Autoantibodies in the cerebrospinal fluid of patients with systemic lupus erythematosus. *Arthritis Rheum.* 29:1090, 1986.
82. Gonzalez, E. B., Varner, W. T., Lisse, J. R., et al. Giant-cell arteritis in the southern United States: An 11-year retrospective study from the Texas Gulf Coast. *Arch. Intern. Med.* 149:1561, 1989.
83. Goodwin, J. A. Temporal Arteritis. In P. J. Vinken and G. W. Bruyn (eds.), *Handbook of Clinical Neurology.* Amsterdam: Elsevier/North Holland, 1980. Vol. 39, pp. 313–342.
84. Gordon, R. M., and Silverstein, A. Neurologic manifestations in progressive systemic sclerosis. *Arch. Neurol.* 22:126, 1970.
85. Graham, E., Holland, A., Avery, A., and Russell, R. W. R. Prognosis in giant-cell arteritis. *Br. Med. J.* 282:269, 1981.
86. Green, D., Hougie, C., Kazmier, F. J., et al. Report of the working party on acquired inhibitors of coagulation: Studies of the "lupus anticoagulant." *Thromb. Haemost.* 49:144, 1983.
87. Greer, J. M., Longley, S., Edwards, N. L., et al. Vasculitis associated with malignancy: Experience with 13 patients and literature review. *Medicine* 67:220, 1988.
88. Grodum, E., and Peterson, H. A. Temporal arteritis with normal erythrocyte sedimentation rate. *J. Int. Med.* 227:279, 1990.
89. Hall, S., Barr, W., Lie, J. T., et al. Takayasu arteritis: A study of 32 North American patients. *Medicine* 64:89, 1985.
90. Hamsten, A., Bjorkholm, M., Norberg, R., et al. Antibodies to cardiolipin in young survivors of myocardial infarction: An association with recurrent cardiovascular events. *Lancet* 1:113, 1986.
91. Harper, C. M., O'Neill, B. P., O'Duffy, J. D., and Forbes, G. S. Intracranial hypertension in Behçet's disease: Demonstration of sinus occlusion with use of digital subtraction angiography. *Mayo Clin. Proc.* 60:419, 1985.
92. Harris, E. N., Chan, J. K. H., Asherson, R. A., et al. Thrombosis, recurrent fetal loss, and thrombocytopenia: Predictive value of the anticardiolipin antibody test. *Arch. Intern. Med.* 146: 2153, 1986.
93. Harris, E. N., Gharavi, A. E., and Hughes, G. R. V. Anti-phospholipid antibodies. *Clin. Rheum. Dis.* 11:591, 1985.
94. Harris, E. N., Hughes, G. R. V., and Gharavi, A. E. Thrombosis, fetal loss, and anti-phospholipid antibodies. *Clin. Aspect Autoimmun.* 1:1, 1986.
95. Harris, E. N., Hughes, G. R., and Gharavi, A. E. Antiphospholipid antibodies: An elderly statesman dons new garments. *J. Rheumatol.* 14(Suppl. 13):208, 1987.
96. Hatron, P. Y., Bouchez, B., Wattel, A., et al. Chorea, systemic lupus erythematosus, circulating lupus anticoagulant. *J. Rheumatol.* 13:991, 1986.
97. Haynes, B. F., Pikus, A., Kaiser-Kupfer, M., and Fauci, A. S. Successful treatment of sudden hearing loss in Cogan's syndrome with corticosteroids. *Arthritis Rheum.* 24:501, 1981.
98. Hearne, C. B., and Zawada, E. T., Jr. Survival after intracerebral hemorrhage in Wegener's granulomatosis. *West. J. Med.* 137:431, 1982.
99. Hellmann, D. B., Laing, T. J., Petri, M., et al. Mononeuritis multiplex: The yield of evaluations for occult rheumatic diseases. *Medicine* 67:145, 1988.
100. Hiraiwa, M., Nonaka, C., Abe, T., and Iio M. Positron emission tomography in systemic lupus erythematosus: Relation of cerebral vasculitis to PET findings. *A.J.N.R.* 4:541, 1983.
101. Hirohata, S., Takeuchi, A., and Miyamoto, T. Association of cerebrospinal fluid IgM index with central nervous system involvement in Behçet's disease. *Arthritis Rheum.* 29:793, 1986.
102. How, A., Dent, P. B., Lia, S. K., and Denburg, J. A. Antineuronal antibodies in neuropsychiatric systemic lupus erythematosus. *Arthritis Rheum.* 28:789, 795, 1985.
103. Howell, S. J. L., and Molyneux, A. J. Vertebrobasilar insufficiency in rheumatoid atlantoaxial subluxation: A case report with angiographic demonstration of left vertebral artery occlusion. *J. Neurol.* 235:189, 1988.
104. Hughes, G. B., Kinney, S. E., Barna, B. P., et al. Autoimmune reactivity in Cogan's syndrome: A preliminary report. *Otolaryngol. Head Neck Surg.* 91:24, 1983.
105. Hunder, G. G., Bloch, D. A., Michael, B. A., et al. The American College of Rheumatology 1990 criteria for the classification of giant cell arteritis. *Arthritis Rheum.* 33:1122, 1990.
106. Hunder, G. G., and Michet, C. J. Giant cell arteritis and polymyalgia rheumatica. *Clin. Rheum. Dis.* 11:471, 1985.
107. International Study Group for Behçet's Disease. Criteria for diagnosis of Behçet's disease. *Lancet* 335:1078, 1990.
108. Iragui, V. J., and Marave, E. Behçet syndrome presenting as cerebrovascular disease. *J. Neurol. Neurosurg. Psychiatry* 49:838, 1986.
109. Ishii, Y., Nagasawa, K., Mayumi, T., and Niho, Y. Clinical importance of persistence of anticardiolipin antibodies in systemic lupus erythematosus. *Ann. Rheum. Dis.* 49:387, 1990.
110. Jacobs, L., Kinkel, P. R., Costello, P. B., et al. Central nervous system lupus erythematosus: The value of magnetic resonance imaging. *J. Rheumatol.* 15:601, 1988.

111. Jennette, J. C., and Falk, R. J. Antineutrophil cytoplasmic autoantibodies and associated diseases: A review. *Am. J. Kidney Dis.* 15:517, 1990.
112. Johnson, R. T., and Richardson, E. P. The neurological manifestations of systemic lupus erythematosus: A clinical-pathological study of 24 cases and review of the literature. *Medicine* 47:337, 1968.
113. Jonas, J., Kölbie, K., Völcker, H. E., and Kalden, J. R. Central retinal artery occlusion in Sneddon's disease associated with antiphospholipid antibodies. *Am. J. Ophthalmol.* 102:37, 1986.
114. Jorizzo, J. L. Behçet's disease: An update based on the 1985 International Conference in London. *Arch. Dermatol.* 122:556, 1986.
115. Jorizzo, J. L. Behçet's disease. *Neurol. Clin.* 5:427, 1987.
116. Kaell, A. T., Shetty, M., Lee, B. C. P., and Lockshin, M. D. The diversity of neurologic events in systemic lupus erythematosus: Prospective clinical and computed tomographic classification of 82 events in 71 patients. *Arch. Neurol.* 43:273, 1986.
117. Kapila, A., Gupta, K. L., and Garcia, J. H. CT and MR of lymphomatoid granulomatosis of the CNS: Report of four cases and review of the literature. *A.J.N.R.* 9:1139, 1988.
118. Katzenstein, A. L. A., Carrington, C. B., and Liebow, A. A. Lymphomatoid granulomatosis: A clinicopathologic study of 152 cases. *Cancer* 43:360, 1979.
119. Keeffe, E. B., Bardana, E. J., Harbeck, R. J., et al. Lupus menintigitis: Antibody to deoxyribonucleic acid (DNA) and DNA:anti-DNA complexes in the cerebrospinal fluid. *Ann. Intern. Med.* 80:58, 1974.
120. Kelly, M. C., and Denburg, J. A. Cerebrospinal fluid immunoglobulins and neuronal antibodies in neuropsychiatric systemic lupus erythematosus and related conditions. *J. Rheumatol.* 14:740, 1987.
121. Khamashta, M. A., Cervera, R., Asherson, R. A., et al. Association of antibodies against phospholipids with heart valve disease in systemic lupus erythematosus. *Lancet* 335:1541, 1990.
122. Kissel, J. T., Riethman, J. L., Omerza, J., et al. Peripheral nerve vasculitis: Immune characterization of the vascular lesions. *Ann. Neurol.* 25:291, 1989.
123. Kissel, J. T., Slivka, A. P., Warmolts, J. R., and Mendell, J. R. The clinical spectrum of necrotizing angiopathy of the peripheral nervous system. *Ann. Neurol.* 18:251, 1985.
124. Kozin, F., Haughton, V., and Bernhard, G. C. Neuro-Behçet disease: Two cases and neuroradiologic findings. *Neurology* 27:1148, 1977.
125. Kroneman, O. C., 3d, and Pevzner, M. Failure of cyclophosphamide to prevent cerebritis in Wegener's granulomatosis. *Am. J. Med.* 80:526, 1986.
126. Kyle, V., and Hazleman, B. L. Treatment of polymyalgia rheumatica and giant cell arteritis: I. Steroid regimens in the first two months. *Ann. Rheum. Dis.* 48:658, 1989.
127. Lancman, M. E., Mesropian, H., and Granillo, R. J. Chronic aseptic meningitis in a patient with systemic lupus erythematosus. *Can. J. Neurol. Sci.* 16:354, 1989.
128. Laskin, C. A., and Soloninka, C. A. Anticardiolipin antibodies: Smoking gun or smoke screen. *J. Rheumatol.* 15:7, 1988.
129. Launes, J., Iivanainen, M., Erkinjuntti, T., and Vuorialko, M. Isolated angiitis of the central nervous system. *Acta Neurol. Scand.* 74:108, 1986.
130. Leung, W. H., Wong, K. L., Lau, C. P., et al. Association between antiphospholipid antibodies and cardiac abnormalities in patient with systemic lupus erythematosus. *Am. J. Med.* 89:411, 1990.
131. Levine, S. R., Kim, S., Deegan, M. J., and Welch, K. M. A. Ischemic stroke associated with anticardiolipin antibodies. *Stroke* 18:1101, 1987.
132. Levine, S. R., and Welch, K. M. A. The spectrum of neurologic disease associated with antiphospholipid antibodies: Lupus anticoagulants and anticardiolipin antibodies. *Arch. Neurol.* 44:876, 1987.
133. Lie, J. T. Classification and immunodiagnosis of vasculitis: A new solution or promises undulfilled? *J. Rheumatol.* 15:728, 1988.
134. Ling, M. H. M., Perry, P. J., Tsuang, M. T. Side effects of corticosteroid therapy: Psychiatric aspects. *Arch. Gen. Psychiatry* 38:471, 1981.
135. Litvan, I., Roig, C., Rovira, A., and Ruscalleda, J. Behçet's syndrome masquerading as tumor. *Neuroradiology* 29:103, 1987.
136. Love, P. E., and Santoro, S. A. Antiphospholipid antibodies: Anticardiolipin and the lupus anticoagulant in systemic lupus erythematosus (SLE) and in non-SLE disorders: Prevalence and clinical significance. *Ann. Intern. Med.* 112:682, 1990.
137. Lubin, J. R., Loewenstein, J. I., Frederick, A. R., Jr. Vogt-Koyanagi-Harada syndrome with focal neurologic signs. *Am. J. Ophthalmol.* 91:332, 1981.
138. Machado, E. B. V., Michet, C. J., Ballard, D. J., et al. Trends in incidence and clinical presentation of temporal arteritis in Olmsted County, Minnesota, 1950–1985. *Arthritis Rheum.* 31:745, 1988.
139. Mackworth-Young, C. G., Harris, E. N., Steere, A. C., et al. Anticardiolipin antibodies in Lyme disease. *Arthritis Rheum.* 31:1052, 1988.
140. Malinow, K. L., Molina, R., Gordon, B., et al. Neuropsychiatric dysfunction in primary

Sjögren's syndrome. *Ann. Intern. Med.* 103: 344, 1985.

141. Marabani, M., Zoma, A., Hadley, D., and Sturrock, R. D. Transverse myelitis occurring during pregnancy in a patient with systemic lupus erythematosus. *Ann. Rheum. Dis.* 48:160, 1989.
142. McCune, W. J., and Golbus, J. Neuropsychiatric lupus. *Rheum. Dis. Clin. North Am.* 14:149, 1988.
143. McCune, W. J., MacGuire, A., Aisen, A., and Gebarski S. Identification of brain lesions in neuropsychiatric systemic lupus erythematosus by magnetic resonance scanning. *Arthritis Rheum.* 31:159, 1988.
144. McHugh, N. J., Maymo, J., Skinner, R. P., et al. Anticardiolipin antibodies, livedo reticularis, and major cerebrovascular and renal disease in systemic lupus erythematosus. *Ann. Rheum. Dis.* 47:110, 1988.
145. Meyer, O., Piette, J. C., Bourgeois, P., et al. Antiphospholipid antibodies: A disease marker in 25 patients with antinuclear antibody negative systemic lupus erythematosus (SLE). Comparison with a group of 91 patients with antinuclear antibody positive SLE. *J. Rheumatol.* 14:502, 1987.
146. Moore, P. M. Diagnosis and management of isolated angiitis of the central nervous system. *Neurology* 39:167, 1989.
147. Moore, P. M., and Cupps, T. R. Neurological complications of vasculitis. *Ann. Neurol.* 14:155, 1983.
148. Moore, P. M., and Fauci, A. S. Neurologic manifestations of systemic vasculitis: A retrospective and prospective study of the clinicopathologic features and responses to therapy in 25 patients. *Am. J. Med.* 71:517, 1981.
149. Mueh, J. R., Herbst, K. D., and Rapaport, S. I. Thrombosis in patients with the lupus anticoagulant. *Ann. Intern. Med.* 92:156, 1980.
150. Nadeau, S. E., and Watson, R. T. Neurologic Manifestations of Vasculitis and Collagen Vascular Syndromes. In A. B. Baker and R. J. Joynt (eds.), *Clinical Neurology.* Philadelphia: Harper & Row, 1983.
151. Nakano, K. K. Neurologic complications of rheumatoid arthritis. *Orthop. Clin. North Am.* 6:861, 1975.
152. Nakano, K. K., Schoene, W. C., Baker, R. A., and Dawson, D. M. The cervical myelopathy associated with rheumatoid arthritis: Analysis of 32 patients, with 2 postmortem cases. *Ann. Neurol.* 3:144, 1978.
153. Namer, I. J., Karabudak, R., Zileli, T., et al. Peripheral nervous system involvement in Behçet's disease: Case report and review of the literature. *Eur. Neurol.* 26:235, 1987.
154. Ninet, J. P., Bachet, P., Dumontet, C. M., et al. Subclavian and axillary involvement in temporal arteritis and polymyalgia rheumatica. *Am. J. Med.* 88:13, 1990.
155. Norberg, R., Nived, O., Sturfelt, G., et al. Anticardiolipin and complement activation: Relation to clinical symptoms. *J. Rheumatol.* 14(Suppl. 13):149, 1987.
156. Noseworthy, J. H., Bass, B. H., Vandervoort, M. K., et al. The prevalence of primary Sjögrens's syndrome in a multiple sclerosis population. *Ann. Neurol.* 25:95, 1989.
157. O'Duffy, J. D., and Goldstein, N. P. Neurological involvement in seven patients with Behçet's disease. *Am. J. Med.* 61:170, 1976.
158. Omdal, R., Mellgren, S. I., and Husby, G. Clinical neuropsychiatric and neuromuscular manifestations in systemic lupus erythematosus. *Scand. J. Rheumatol.* 17:113, 1988.
159. O'Neil, M. L., Giang, D. W., Como, P., and Schiffer, R. B. Anxiety and depression as neuropsychiatric symptoms of systemic lupus erythematosus. *Ann. Neurol.* 28:255, 1990.
160. Out, H. J., de Groot, P. B., Hasselaar, P., et al. Fluctuations of anticardiolipin antibody levels in patients with systemic lupus erythematosus: A prospective study. *Ann. Rheum. Dis.* 48:1023, 1989.
161. Pal, B., Gibson, C., Passmore, J., et al. A study of headaches and migraine in Sjögren's syndrome and other rheumatic disorders. *Ann. Rheum. Dis.* 48:312, 1989.
162. Pauzner, R., Rosner, E., and Many, A. Circulating anticoagulant in systemic lupus erythematosus: Clinical manifestations. *Acta Haematol.* 76:90, 1986.
163. Pease, C. T., and Pozo, J. L. Atlantoaxial subluxation and spinal compression in psoriatic arthropathy. *Ann. Rheum. Dis.* 46:717, 1987.
164. Petit, W. A., Jr., Soso, M. J., and Higman, H. Degos disease: Neurologic complications and cerebral angiography. *Neurology* 32:1305, 1982.
165. Petri, M., Golbus, M., Anderson, R., et al. Antinuclear antibody, lupus anticoagulant and anticardiolipin antibody in women with idiopathic habitual abortion. *Arthritis Rheum.* 30:601, 1987.
166. Petri, M., Rheinschmidt, M., Whiting-O'Keefe, Q., et al. The frequency of lupus anticoagulant in systemic lupus erythematosus: A study of sixty consecutive patients by activated partial thromboplastin time, Russell viper venom time, and anticardiolipin level. *Ann. Intern. Med.* 106:524, 1987.
167. Pittsley, R. A., and Talal, N. Neuromuscular Complications of Sjögren's Syndrome. In P. J. Vinken and G. W. Bruyn (eds.), *Handbook of Clinical Neurology.* Amsterdam: Elsevier/North Holland, 1980. Vol. 39, pp. 419–433.
168. Rabinovitch, J., Donnenfeld, E. D., and Laibson,

P. R. Management of Cogan's syndrome. *Am. J. Ophthalmol.* 101:494, 1986.
169. Reeves, A., and Bresnihan, B. Clinical features, treatment and outcome of polyarteritis nodosa. *Irish J. Med. Sci.* 156:90, 1987.
170. Ringel, R. A., Brick, J. E., Brick, J. F., et al. Muscle involvement in the scleroderma syndromes. *Arch. Intern. Med.* 150:2550, 1990.
171. Roddy, S. R., and Giang, D. W. Antiphospholipid antibodies and stroke in an infant. *Pediatrics* 48:312, 1991.
172. Sack, M., Cassidy, J. T., and Bole, G. G. Prognostic factors in polyarteritis. *J. Rheumatol.* 2:411, 1975.
173. Sands, M. L., Ryczak, M., and Brown, R. B. Recurrent aseptic meningitis followed by transverse myelitis as a presentation of systemic lupus erythematosus. *J. Rheumatol.* 15:862, 1988.
174. Scharre, D., Petri, M., Engman, E., and DeArmond, S. Large intracranial arteritis with giant cells in systemic lupus erythematosus. *Ann. Intern. Med.* 104:661, 1986.
175. Schneebaum, A. B., Singleton, J. D., West, S. G., et al. Association of psychiatric manifestations with antibodies to ribosomal P proteins in systemic lupus erythematosus. *Am. J. Med.* 90:54, 1991.
175a. Serdaroğlu, P., Yazici, H., Özdemer, C., et al. Neurologic involvement in Behçet's syndrome: A prospective study. *Arch. Neurol.* 46:265, 1989.
176. Shelhamer, J. H., Volkman, D. J., Parrillo, J. E., et al. Takayasu's arteritis and its therapy. *Ann. Intern. Med.* 103:121, 1985.
177. Shimizu, T., Ehrlich, G. E., Inaba, G., and Hayashi, K. Behçet's disease (Behçet's syndrome). *Semin. Arthritis Rheum.* 8:223, 1979.
178. Sigal, L. H. The neurologic presentation of vasculitic and rheumatologic syndromes: A review. *Medicine* 66:157, 1987.
179. Small, P., Mass, M. F., Kohler, P. F., et al. Central nervous system involvement in SLE: Diagnostic profile and clinical features. *Arthritis Rheum.* 20:869, 1977.
180. Smith, P. H., Benn, R. T., and Sharp, J. Natural history of rheumatoid cervical luxations. *Ann. Rheum. Dis.* 31:431, 1972.
181. Snyder, D. A., and Tessler, H. H. Vogt-Koyanagi-Harada syndrome. *Am. J. Ophthalmol.* 90:69, 1980.
182. Sonnex, C., Paice, E., and White, A. G. Autonomic neuropathy in systemic sclerosis: A case report and evaluation of six patients. *Ann. Rheum. Dis.* 45:957, 1986.
183. Stein, R. L., Martino, C. R., Weinert, D. M., et al. Cerebral angiography as a guide for therapy in isolated central nervous system vasculitis. *J.A.M.A.* 257:2193, 1987.
184. Suzuki, Y., Kitagawa, Y., Matsuoka, Y., et al. Severe cerebral and systemic necrotizing vasculitis developing during pregnancy in a case of systemic lupus erythematosus. *J. Rheumatol.* 17:1408, 1990.
185. Swaak, A. J., Huysen, V., Nossent, J. C., and Smeenk, R. J. Antinuclear antibody profiles in relation to specific disease manifestations of systemic lupus erythematosus. *Clin. Rheumatol.* 9(Suppl. 1):82, 1990.
186. Syrjanen, J., Vaarala, O., Iivanainen, M., et al. Anticardiolipin response and its association with infections in young and middle-aged patients with cerebral infarction. *Acta Neurol. Scand.* 78:381, 1988.
187. Teasdall, R. D., Frayha, R. A., and Shulman, L. E. Cranial nerve involvement in systemic sclerosis (scleroderma): A report of 10 cases. *Medicine* 59:149, 1980.
188. Temesvari, P., Denburg, J., Denburg, S., et al. Serum lymphocytotoxic antibodies in neuropsychiatric lupus: A serial study. *Clin. Immunol. Immunopathol.* 28:243, 1983.
189. Triplett, D. A., Brandt, J. T., Musgrave, K. A., and Orr, C. A. The relationship between lupus anticoagulants and antibodies to phospholipid. *J.A.M.A.* 259:550, 1988.
190. Tsokos, M., Lazarou, S. A., and Moutsopoulos, H. M. Vasculitis in primary Sjögren's syndrome: Histologic classification and clinical presentation. *Am. J. Clin. Pathol.* 88:26, 1987.
191. Veenendall-Hilbers, J. A., Perquin, W. V. M., Hoogland, P. H., and Doornbos, L. Basal meningo-vasculitis and occlusion of the basilar artery in two cases of *Borrelia burgdorferi* infection. *Neurology* 38:1317, 1988.
192. Vidailhet, M., Piette, J. C., Wechsler, B., et al. Cerebral venous thrombosis in systemic lupus erythematosus. *Stroke* 21:1226, 1990.
193. Vitali, C., Tavoni, A., Neri, R., et al. Fibromyalgia features in patients with primary Sjögren's syndrome: Evidence of a relationship with psychological depression. *Scand. J. Rheumatol.* 18:21, 1989.
194. Vollertsen, R. S., McDonald, T. J., Younge, B. R., et al. Cogan's syndrome: 18 cases and a review of the literature. *Mayo Clin. Proc.* 61:344, 1986.
195. Watson, P., Fekete, J., and Deck, J. Central nervous system vasculitis in rheumatoid arthritis. *Can. J. Neurol. Sci.* 4:269, 1977.
196. Yankner, B. A., Skolnik, P. R., Shoukimas, G. M., et al. Cerebral granulomatous angiitis associated with isolation of human T-lymphotropic virus type III from the central nervous system. *Ann. Neurol.* 20:362, 1986.
197. Yazici, H., Pazarli, H., Barnes, C. G., et al. A controlled trial of azathioprine in Behçet's syndrome. *N. Engl. J. Med.* 322:281, 1990.

16 Neurosarcoidosis

Barney J. Stern and Steven A. Schonfeld

Sir Jonathan Hutchinson described the first two patients with cutaneous sarcoidosis 100 years ago. His now classic report of the cutaneous lesions of "Mortimer's Malady" marked the beginning of the early investigative era of descriptive sarcoidology [74]. In the late nineteenth century, many of the cutaneous manifestations were attributed to syphilis and tuberculosis, common diseases of the times. At the turn of the century, Caesar Boeck [11] described sarcoidosis of the lymph nodes and skin as resembling sarcoma or "multiple benign sarkoid," from which was derived the term *sarcoidosis.* In 1936, Schaumann [161] put forward the concept of a single disease entity that he called "lymphogranuloma benignum," which was characterized by epithelioid granulomas in multiple organs. Common symptom complexes were identified by Heerfordt (uveoparotid fever with parotid gland enlargement, cranial nerve palsies, and uveitis) and Lofgren (bilateral hilar lymphadenopathy, erythema nodosum, and fever) in the early twentieth century. It is now well recognized that sarcoidosis can involve any body tissue (Table 16-1).

The first internationally accepted definition of sarcoidosis was proposed at the Seventh International Conference on Sarcoidosis and Other Granulomatous Disorders in 1975 as "a multisystem granulomatous disorder of unknown etiology . . . . Immunologic features are *depression* of late-type hypersensitivity suggesting impaired cell mediated immunity and raised or abnormal immunoglobulins" [170]. This view of sarcoidosis as functionally a depression of immunologic mechanisms was first challenged by Kataria, Lo Buglio, and Bromberg [86] in 1976 who suggested that "the immune apparatus of patients with sarcoidosis may be hyperactive" based on in vitro studies of macrophage function. This landmark observation heralded the

This work was supported, in part, by the Lloyd M. Gerber Memorial Neurology Fund.

Table 16-1. Percentage frequency of organ involvement in sarcoidosis

Manifestation	*Frequency [79,130,171]*
Intrathoracic	87
Hilar nodes	72
Lung parenchyma	46
Upper respiratory tract	6
Dermatologic	
Skin	18
Erythema nodosum	15
Ocular	15
Lacrimal	3
Parotid	6
Splenomegaly	10
Peripheral lymphadenopathy	28
Bone	3
Cardiac	3
Hepatomegaly	10
Hypercalcemia	13
Neurologic	5
Hematologic, endocrinologic, gastrointestinal, & genitourinary	Rare

beginning of what might be called the second era of sarcoidosis investigation, that of the immunopathogenesis. Kataria's concept was formalized in statements at the Ninth (1981) and Tenth (1984) International Conferences that modified the earlier definition of sarcoidosis to characterize it as a "multi-system granulomatous disorder of unknown cause, characterized by *enhanced* cellular immune processes at sites of involvement" [25,81].

Sarcoidosis occurs in all age groups, with a peak incidence in the third and fourth decades. Although some studies have reported a female predilection, worldwide there does not appear to be any sex predominance. Sarcoidosis occurs in all races and has been reported on all continents. An unexplained but well-documented observation is a 10- to 17-fold increased incidence of sarcoidosis in blacks in the United States compared to whites. There is also a tendency for more severe disease to occur in black Americans. The observed worldwide distribution of the disease is largely a reflection of the available diagnostic tools, the use of screening radiographs, and the local prevalence of tuberculosis. In underdeveloped countries where tuberculosis is prevalent, it is very difficult to distinguish sarcoidosis from tuberculosis on the basis of the chest film alone. However, where mass radiographic surveys have been performed, such as in Sweden, prevalence rates as high as 64 per 100,000 have been determined. Limited autopsy surveys in Sweden have suggested that this, too, may grossly underestimate the actual prevalence, which may be as high as 600 per 100,000 [60]. Sarcoidosis does occur in families, but there is very low penetrance, and HLA typing has revealed no significant correlations. In spite of the vast epidemiologic efforts over the past century, no significant positive insights have been made as to the etiology of the disease.

Neurologic disease occurs in 5 percent of patients with sarcoidosis [179]. Nervous system dysfunction is the presenting feature of sarcoidosis in one-half or more of the patients with neurosarcoidosis [23,134,137,143,179]. Some 50 to 75 percent of sarcoid patients who are destined to develop neurologic disease do so within the first 2 years of their systemic illness [137,179].

Neurosarcoidosis is a diagnostic consideration in patients with sarcoidosis who develop neurologic signs or symptoms and in patients without known sarcoidosis who develop an illness consistent with neurosarcoidosis. Sarcoidosis presents with a variety of neurologic problems, as outlined in Table 16-2.

PATHOPHYSIOLOGY

Overview

Although the etiology of sarcoidosis remains unknown, the pathology of the disease is well described and an unraveling of the underlying immunologic aberrations is underway. The key pathologic finding in sarcoidosis is the noncaseating granuloma [50]. Formation of the granuloma begins with blood-derived mono-

Table 16-2. Neurosarcoidosis

Clinical manifestation	*Approximate frequency (%)*
Cranial neuropathy (facial palsy)	50–75 (25–50)
Aseptic meningitis	10–20
Hydrocephalus	10
Parenchymal disease	
Endocrinopathy	10–15
Mass lesion(s)	5–10
Encephalopathy/ vasculopathy	5–10
Seizures	5–10
Neuropathy	5–10
Myopathy	10

cytes being transformed into epithelioid cells. A granuloma forms as an aggregation of epithelioid cells, lymphocytes, and monocytes. Multinucleated giant cells appear. Surrounding the granuloma is a fine reticulin network as well as fibroblasts, collagen, lymphocytes, capillaries, and lymphatic channels. Granulomas often regress, but they may be replaced by fibrosis. Freiman [50] describes the granuloma as an "organized chronic inflammatory response to persistent irritation." Recently, increasing attention has been given to the microangiopathy associated with sarcoidosis: endothelial cell proliferation and basal lamina thickening and layering occur at multiple sites and probably contribute to symptomatology [95].

Thomas and Hunninghake [184] have provided an overview of the pathogenesis of sarcoidosis. The lymphocytes involved in early granuloma formation are predominantly of the CD4 (helper/inducer) type. As the lesion matures, CD8 (suppressor/cytotoxic) cells become prominent, especially surrounding the granuloma [116,120,191]. B cells and plasma cells are also present and are stimulated to produce immunoglobulins. It seems that much of the antibody synthesis is nonspecific, although some immunoglobulin may be involved in granuloma formation by producing insoluble immune complexes.

Monocyte/macrophage secretion of the lymphokine, interleukin-1, accounts, in part, for the movement of T-lymphocytes to sites of disease activity. The activated monocytes secrete monocyte activating and inhibitory factors, which may augment granuloma formation [6,7]. Lymphokine secretion also increases local T-cell proliferation. Activated T cells in turn secrete monocyte chemotactic factor, which draws more monocytes to the area [31]. Movement of T cells from the blood leads to a peripheral lymphopenia and low CD4/CD8 ratio with an excess of CD4 cells at sites of active inflammation where the CD4/CD8 ratio may be as high as 5 to 20 : 1 [58,116,120,165,191]. Inactive disease, on the other hand, is characterized by a relative decrease in the CD4/CD8 ratio [73]. The helper CD4 lymphocytes release interleukin-2, T-cell growth factor, and thereby reinforce the local inflammation and disease compartmentalization [159]. The activation of the interleukin-2 gene occurs only at sites of disease activity and may require local stimuli to remain active [123]. Interleukin-2 receptors are present on lymphocytes obtained by bronchoalveolar lavage from patients with active sarcoidosis [164], and there are elevated concentrations of soluble interleukin-2 receptors in the serum and bronchoalveolar lavage fluid of patients with active disease [96].

Fibroblast activity, and subsequent fibrosis, is modulated in part by interleukin-1, interferon (produced by T cells), and fibronectin. Prostaglandin E_2 (PGE_2) secretion by macrophages is decreased in sarcoidosis; PGE_2 diminishes granuloma formation and fibroblast proliferation and affects collagen production.

Neuropathology

Noncaseating granulomas and an accompanying diffuse mononuclear cell infiltrate can be found in any part of the neuraxis and in peripheral nerve and muscle. The most common site of inflammation is the meninges, especially the basal areas [35,196]. The granulomas can be distributed widely or be particularly concentrated in one or more areas to form a mass. Sarcoidosis is not usually considered to be a primary vasculitis [122], but arteriolar and venous infiltration does occur and can lead to infarction [19,35,39,110,115,190]. The granulomatous inflammation can be clinically silent or correlate with signs and symptoms [107,196].

Central nervous system (CNS) involvement can be *conceptualized* as an inflammatory process primarily affecting the leptomeninges (Fig. 16-1). Inflammation may spread along the Virchow-Robin perivascular spaces to invade the brain or spinal cord or remain more localized to involve the cranial nerves [115,188,196]. Presumably the active inflammation is reversible, although irreversible damage may occur due to ischemia. Ultimately fibrosis can develop and lead to a static neurologic insult.

Granulomas are apparent in the epineurium and perineurium of peripheral nerve in symptomatic patients. The endoneurium may contain a mononuclear cell infiltrate. Perivascular and vascular inflammation can be seen in the epineurial and perineurial vessels. All nerve fiber sizes can be affected. There seems to be a predominantly axonal neuropathy with only a minor component of segmental demyelination. Nerve damage may result from an arteriolar insult or direct compression from granulomas [51].

Asymptomatic noncaseating granulomas have been found in up to one-half of sarcoid patients having a muscle biopsy [180]. Muscle biopsy of symptomatic patients reveals noncaseating granulomas, and there may be a more diffuse inflammation as well as muscle fiber degeneration and regeneration and fibrosis [4,68].

Neuroimmunology

Detailed study of the immunologic features of CNS sarcoidosis has been limited to analysis of the cerebrospinal fluid (CSF). An excess of CSF CD4 lymphocytes has been demonstrated in some patients [83,177]. This finding may be dependent on the intensity of the CNS inflammation, the anatomic areas involved and their contiguity to the CSF, the temporal course of the illness, and concurrent therapy [177].

There seems to be an abnormally permeable blood-brain barrier in CNS sarcoidosis [118], and this may account for the occasional finding of an apparent increase in intrathecal IgG levels [92,118]. Oligoclonal bands can be seen in the CSF [55,92] but are rare [118,177]. The IgG index can also be elevated [92,134], although this too is somewhat unusual [118,177] unless there is intense inflammation. The immunoglobulin profiles can vary with clinical course and treatment [92]. The finding of abnormal immunoglobulin profiles in the CSF of patients with CNS sarcoidosis is not unexpected given the B-cell infiltration associated with the granulomas. Furthermore, continuing inflammation

Fig. 16-1. CNS sarcoidosis: a clinopathologic construct.

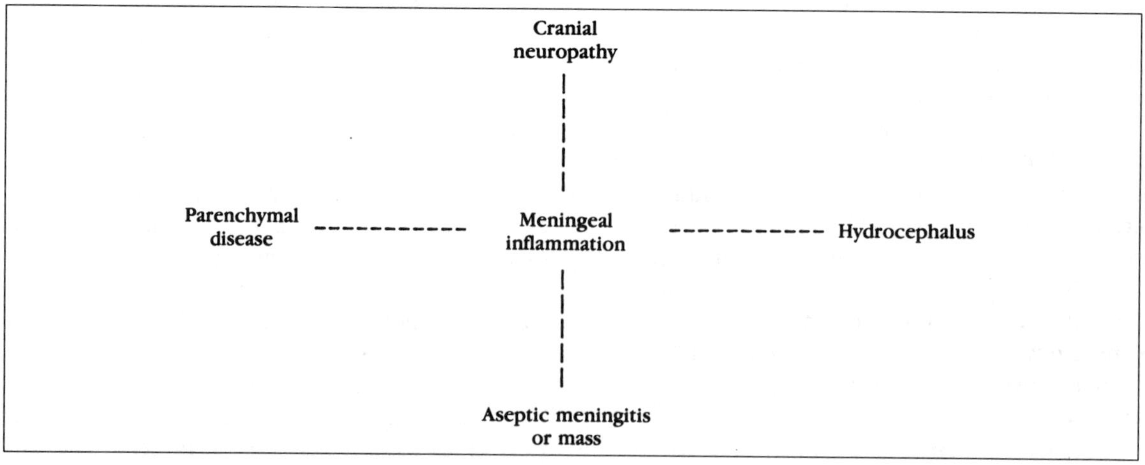

may predispose to the formation of a few dominant immunocyte clones [131] and thereby allow oligoclonal bands to develop.

CLINICAL MANIFESTATIONS

The frequency of neurologic manifestations of sarcoidosis is outlined in Table 16-2. Approximately one-third of patients have more than one neurologic lesion [134,179].

Cranial Neuropathy

The most frequent neurologic complication of sarcoidosis is cranial neuropathy [179]. This occurs in approximately three-quarters of patients with neurosarcoidosis, and over one-half have multiple cranial nerve lesions [179].

Olfactory nerve dysfunction can occur secondary to meningeal sarcoidosis involving the subfrontal region [37]. Anosmia also results from local nasal granulomatous inflammation, and therefore an otolaryngological evaluation with nasal biopsy is necessary before attributing impaired olfaction to CNS disease.

Optic nerve sarcoidosis can present as papilledema, papillitis, optic disc edema, retrobulbar neuritis, or optic atrophy [19,55,59,61,158]. A chiasmal syndrome can develop [52]. Patients can present with an acute or subacute painful or chronic painless visual loss [55]. These manifestations result from either diffuse optic nerve inflammation, compression from a granulomatous mass, or meningeal inflammation.

Disorders of ocular motility may follow involvement of the third, fourth, or sixth cranial nerves in the granulomatous process [179]. Typically, the nerves are damaged in their extra-axial course in the subarachnoid space and as they traverse the meninges. However, these nerves may be involved in orbital disease, and rarely the cell bodies or intra-axial pathways can be affected by brain stem inflammation [93]. Occasionally, pupillary dysfunction is apparent [28,65,93,146]. Disordered motility rarely is due to inflammation of the extraocular muscles [132].

Trigeminal nerve disease may present as facial numbness or, rarely, trigeminal neuralgia [179]. Involvement of the muscles of mastication is unusual.

Peripheral facial nerve palsy is the single most common neurologic manifestation of neurosarcoidosis [134,172,179,197]. Fifty percent of the neurologic complications of sarcoidosis are due to this problem. The facial weakness can be unilateral or bilateral; it may be recurrent. Rarely is the facial palsy caused by parotid inflammation. Oksanen [134,139] has suggested that facial paresis can be due to intra-axial inflammation involving the facial nerve. Because of its relatively high prevalence, facial weakness is accompanied by other neurologic problems in over one-half of patients affected.

Eighth nerve disease can involve the auditory or vestibular components of the nerve [134,179]. Hearing loss can be sudden or insidious and may fluctuate over time [75,78,85]. Bilateral disease may occur, and bilateral seventh and eighth nerve dysfunction is highly suggestive of neurosarcoidosis [134,179,197].

Glossopharyngeal and vagus nerve involvement by sarcoidosis causes dysphagia and dysphonia. Hoarseness is more commonly due to laryngeal nerve dysfunction from intrathoracic disease than CNS inflammation involving the vagus nerve [42,187].

Eleventh and twelfth cranial nerve disease seems to be quite rare.

Meningeal Disease

Aseptic meningitis can be a manifestation of sarcoidosis, but it is rarely the presenting feature [179]. The patient typically has headache and meningismus, and a predominantly mononuclear cell pleocytosis is found in the sterile CSF. Hypoglycorrhachia occasionally occurs, and there is often a CSF protein elevation. An aseptic meningitis may be recurrent or become chronic [145]. A patient presenting as though she had benign intracranial hypertension developed aseptic meningitis and ultimately was thought to have sarcoidosis [151].

Occasionally granulomas can coalesce on the meninges to form a mass. The collection can present as a space-occupying lesion and may resemble a meningioma [76,140,166].

Hydrocephalus

Hydrocephalus can be of the communicating or noncommunicating type. Inflammation or fibrosis impairing CSF flow can involve the ependymal surfaces, cerebral aqueduct, foramina of Lushka or Magendie, or subarachnoid space [104,162]. A granulomatous mass can compress the cerebral aqueduct or fourth ventricle, causing ventricular enlargement.

CNS Parenchymal Disease

Neuroendocrinologic dysfunction is due to either a hypothalamic or pituitary granulomatous mass or a more diffuse "local" encephalopathy [18,22,76,117,182]. Given the predilection of the granulomatous inflammation for the basal meninges, the relative frequency of endocrinologic disturbances is not surprising [14]. A disorder of thirst is the most common abnormality and may be due to a change in the hypothalamic "osmostat" [183]. Occasionally diabetes insipidus [183] or the syndrome of inappropriate secretion of antidiuretic hormone can occur [94]. Hormonal disruptions have been documented to involve any of the other neuroendocrinologic systems [182]. Disorders of appetite, libido, temperature control, and weight regulation have been found [14,64,101]. An empty sella syndrome has been associated with CNS sarcoidosis [24].

Solitary or multiple granulomatous masses can involve any area of the brain or spinal cord. These lesions can present as a space-occupying mass and cause signs and symptoms appropriate to their location [16,26,147]. Spinal cord involvement can manifest as an intramedullary or extramedullary lesion and even as a radiculopathy, cauda equina syndrome, an atrophic spinal cord, or arachnoiditis [17,45,69,108,127,192]. The development of a postinflammatory syrinx has been related to sarcoidosis [148]. Granulomatous infiltration of the pineal gland is reported [194].

A diffuse encephalopathy/vasculopathy can involve the cerebral hemispheres or basilar regions. Patients may present with a delirium, personality change, or isolated memory disturbance [29,70,185]. Rarely is large-vessel disease evident on angiography. The development of transient ischemic attacks or ischemic stroke has been reported [13,19,30,166]. The presence of a retinal phlebitis has been associated with diffuse encephalopathy and angiopathy [19]. Dural sinus obstruction causing intracranial hypertension has been related to inflammation from sarcoidosis [15,22].

Seizures have been associated with mass lesions or a diffuse encephalopathy/vasculopathy. Convulsions often imply active inflammation but can be associated with a static lesion such as a small infarct. The presence of seizures has been related to a poor prognosis [36] and is likely related to the intensity of the inflammatory process. Seizure control, per se, is usually not difficult if the underlying inflammatory state can be successfully treated.

Neuropathy

The peripheral nervous system disease can occur as a diffuse sensorimotor polyneuropathy, generalized sensory or motor neuropathy, or mononeuritis multiplex [21,51,53,142]. Rarely an isolated peripheral nerve palsy may occur. Electrodiagnostic testing has suggested the occurrence of an asymptomatic mononeuropathy multiplex in over one-half of patients with sarcoidosis [21].

Myopathy

Muscle involvement in sarcoidosis can take the form of incidentally discovered granulomas, acute or chronic myositis, focal mass lesions, muscle atrophy, pseudohypertrophy, or contractures [4].

DIAGNOSIS OF SARCOIDOSIS

General Considerations

Given the spectrum of clinical disease in sarcoidosis, a low threshold for considering this diagnosis in the proper clinical setting must be maintained. At one end of the spectrum is the patient with asymptomatic bilateral hilar lymphadenopathy requiring little more than observation, while at the other extreme is the patient with life-threatening disease for which rapid diagnosis and treatment is critical.

In virtually every situation, the diagnosis of sarcoidosis rests on securing a biopsy demonstrating noncaseating granulomata without evidence of fungal or mycobacterial organisms. Biopsy should be from the most accessible site. For this reason, a detailed examination of the skin and mucous membranes is advised, as these sites are readily biopsied with virtually no morbidity. Biopsy of palpable lymph nodes is also a high-yield approach, although specificity becomes an issue, since granulomas may be present in lymph nodes associated with regions harboring a carcinoma and other nonsarcoid disease. In the absence of superficially accessible tissue, and with the high prevalence of pulmonary disease, transbronchial biopsy through the fiberoptic bronchoscope in patients with roentgenographs demonstrating bilateral hilar lymphadenopathy or parenchymal lung disease has a diagnostic yield of 60 to 90 percent. This procedure has a low morbidity and virtually no mortality. In general, the presence of granulomas in a biopsy specimen is not, in itself, pathognomonic for sarcoidosis; the total clinical presentation needs to be considered [80]. On the other hand, some clinical presentations are highly characteristic of sarcoidosis and pathologic confirmation is not necessary; for instance, the patient with symmetric bilateral hilar lymphadenopathy and erythema nodosum almost certainly has sarcoidosis.

The Kveim-Siltzbach test is not widely available but offers yet another means for diagnosing sarcoidosis. Kveim-Siltzbach reagent is a suspension derived from the spleen of a patient with sarcoidosis. This suspension is injected intracutaneously and when positive will produce a cutaneous nodule that on biopsy will reveal noncaseating granulomata. While this represents a very specific and sensitive test, it does require a waiting period of 4 to 6 weeks before biopsy can be performed, making this a poor test for patients with acute manifestations requiring early corticosteroid treatment.

Over 90 percent of patients with sarcoidosis have evidence of pulmonary involvement [79]. Suspicion of sarcoidosis is most often raised by an abnormal chest roentgenogram. However, the chest x-ray is not considered diagnostic but only suggestive and supportive of the diagnosis. Pulmonary function testing is considered mandatory as part of the evaluation of patients with sarcoidosis, as the vast majority do manifest pulmonary disease.

Though many blood studies may be abnormal, there is no specific diagnostic test yet available. Patients may demonstrate anemia, leukopenia, thrombocytopenia, hypergammaglobulinemia, hypercalcemia, hypercalciuria, and hepatic or renal dysfunction. Lieberman [99] demonstrated that active sarcoidosis may cause an elevation in serum angiotensin converting enzyme (SACE), which can then serve as a possible marker for the disease. SACE is thought to be produced by alveolar macrophages and epithelioid giant cells and, in effect, reflects the "granulomatous load" of the patient. SACE, however, may only be elevated in 50 to 60 percent of active sarcoidosis patients and is elevated in patients with other conditions such as liver disease, diabetes mellitus, and hyperthyroidism. Nevertheless, although controversy still exists as to the proper role of the SACE assay [8], many investigators have shown it to be a useful marker for disease activity that can be followed during therapy [38].

Gallium-67 scanning has been touted as another method of disease detection [22] but has limited utility for clinical longitudinal follow-up because of its expense and radiation exposure [189]. Detection of inflammation in the lacrimal and parotid glands is especially suggestive of sarcoidosis [160].

A thorough ocular examination, especially in patients with possible neurosarcoidosis, is indicated to search for uveitis, periphlebitis, or superficial lesions for conjunctival biopsy.

In summary, the diagnosis of sarcoidosis is best made on the basis of the finding of granulomata in multiple nonreticuloendothelial organs. Clinically, the diagnosis will usually be secure with a compatible biopsy in the presence of typical signs and symptoms of this disease. Many recent excellent monographs on sarcoidosis are available and review in considerable detail the various organ system manifestations, pathophysiology, epidemiology, and present avenues of research investigation [48,100,167].

Neurodiagnosis

Although evidence for multisystem disease may not be evident at the time of neurologic presentation, other systemic manifestations of sarcoidosis develop in 80 to 90 percent of patients [134,179]. If there is no definite evidence of multisystem inflammation, the diagnosis of sarcoidosis should remain suspect unless there is pathologic examination of tissue from an area of neurologic disease [22]. Although CNS tissue is not readily available for examination, unique opportunities for pathologic review do occur. For instance, a ventriculoperitoneal shunt revision has provided enough material to help solidify the diagnosis of CNS sarcoidosis in one patient (Fig. 16-2). Other systemic features of sarcoidosis can develop over time [134], although corticosteroid therapy may mask this.

Neurodiagnostic testing must be tailored to the presenting problems. For instance, nerve conduction studies and electromyography are appropriate for the patient with a suspected myopathy or neuropathy, and electroencephalography is indicated for the patient with seizures or encephalopathy.

CSF analysis of patients with CNS sarcoidosis can reveal an elevated pressure, a high protein level, hypoglycorrhachia, and a predominantly mononuclear pleocytosis of up to several hundred cells. Over 50 percent of patients will have some CSF abnormality [134,179]. As discussed, most patients do not have oligoclonal bands in the CSF or an elevated IgG index, although these abnormalities can be present especially in patients with intense inflammation.

Newer CSF assays may permit more refined assessment of CNS sarcoidosis. CSF angiotensin converting enzyme (ACE) activity tends to be

Fig. 16-2. The patient is a 35-year-old woman with bilateral hilar adenopathy and noncaseating granulomas demonstrated on biopsy of the nasal mucosa. A midbrain mass developed, which caused hydrocephalus and required the insertion of a ventriculoperitoneal shunt. The CT scan abnormalities developed while the patient was taking prednisone, 8 mg daily. A. Computed cranial tomography with contrast administration demonstrating multiple nodules and enhancement of the ependymal surfaces. A ventricular shunt is present. B. At the time of a shunt revision, examination of adherent tissue revealed choroid plexus with an adherent noncaseating epithelioid granuloma. (Hematoxylin and eosin × 600.) C. An adjacent microscopic field demonstrates a noncaseating granuloma. No foreign material was identified. (Hematoxylin and eosin × 600.)

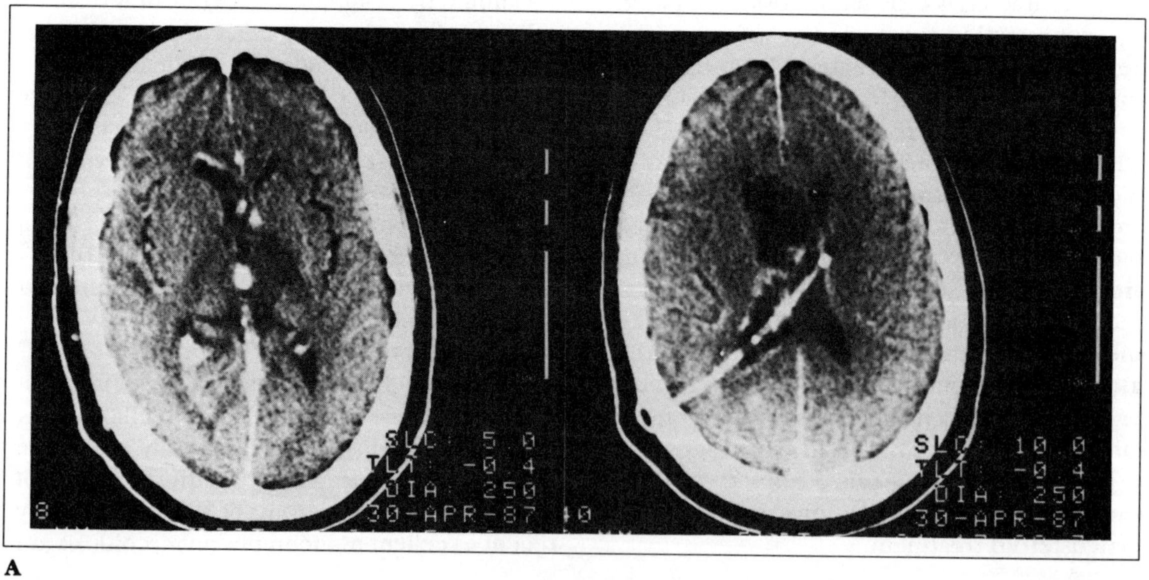

A

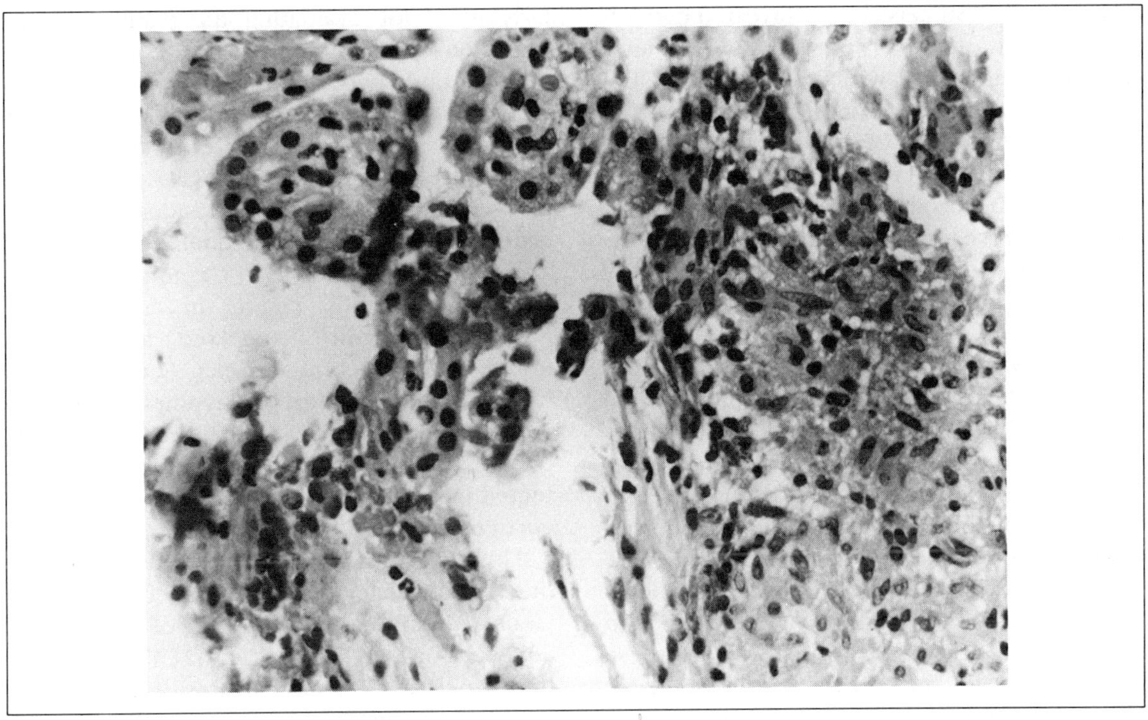

B

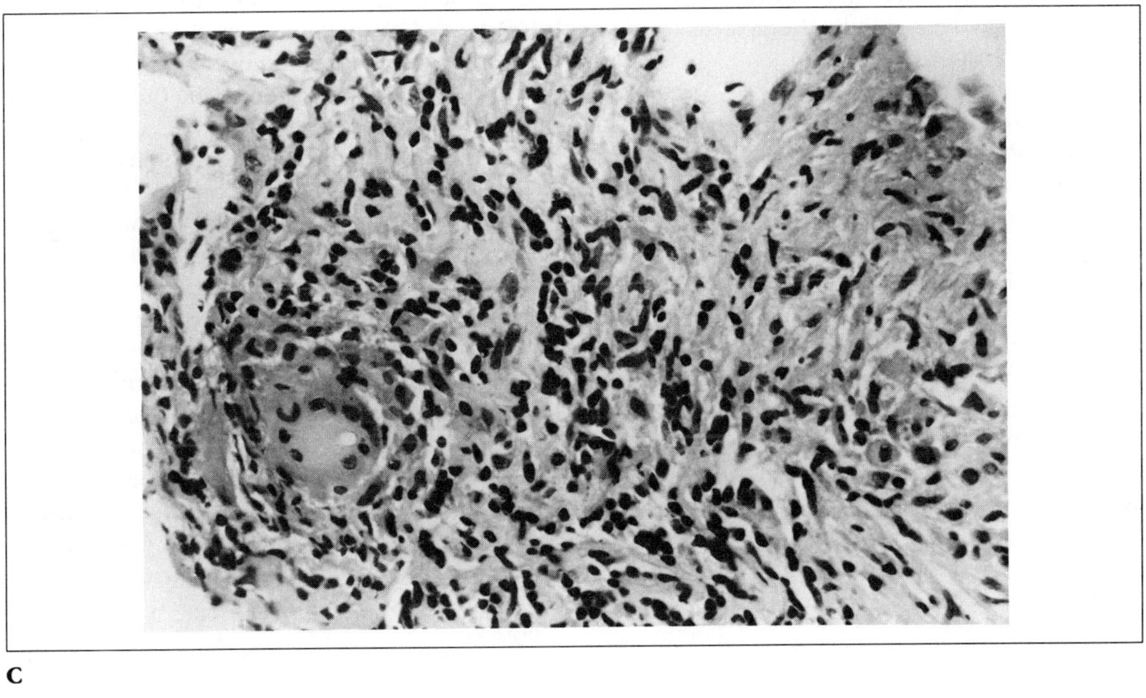

C

raised in some 50 percent of untreated patients with CNS sarcoidosis [136]. The CSF ACE level can still be abnormal with steroid therapy but less consistently than in untreated patients. The degree of elevation of CSF ACE seems to parallel the clinical course [135,136,163]. CSF ACE is thought to be produced by CNS granulomas, especially those on or near the meninges, and its presence in the CSF is unlikely to be a result of leakage through a diseased blood-brain barrier [136].

As previously mentioned, an excess of helper lymphocytes is found in the CSF of some patients with CNS sarcoidosis [83,177]. The utility of this analysis remains to be determined. Lysozyme and beta-2 microglobulin are elevated in the serum of some patients with systemic sarcoidosis. These proteins are elevated in the CSF of 75 and 53 percent, respectively, of patients with CNS sarcoidosis and do not correlate with serum levels [138]. The CSF levels of these proteins may fluctuate with neurologic status [138].

None of the aforementioned CSF analyses are in and of themselves pathognomonic of CNS sarcoidosis but taken together may be highly suggestive of the diagnosis. The utility of these tests in potentially differentiating CNS sarcoidosis from other diseases requires close scrutiny. Furthermore, the potential that these new techniques may have for guiding therapy makes further study particularly exciting.

A brain computed tomography (CT) scan can detect discrete meningeal or brain mass lesions, multiple nodules, hydrocephalus, diffuse inflammation (usually extending from the leptomeninges), and areas of periventricular white matter hypodensity [90,98]. Orbital disease including optic nerve and muscle can also be assessed with CT scan [41,46,176]. The typical granulomatous mass is isodense or slightly hyperdense on a nonenhanced scan and enhances relatively uniformly with the administration of contrast dye. CT scanning is helpful in monitoring disease activity as judged by the size of a mass lesion or the degree of enhancement of diffuse inflammation [88].

Magnetic resonance imaging (MRI) is very sensitive in detecting CNS lesions and is particularly good for evaluating the parasellar area [193], posterior fossa, and spinal cord. MRI has demonstrated hypothalamic lesions not seen on CT scan and has revealed clinically unsuspected disease involving white matter in the periventricular regions [62,91,114] (Fig. 16-3). The periventricular white matter lesions may represent the clinically silent sequelae of a sarcoid angiopathy [39,62,66,91]. Granulomatous inflammation usually results in an increased MRI signal intensity (compared) to the signal intensity of cerebral cortex). Some patients however, will demonstrate hypointense or isointense lesions on T1- or T2-weighted images [62]. A granulomatous lesion may fail to be detected in patients being treated with high-dose corticosteroids [62].

Although both CT scan and MRI easily demonstrate hydrocephalus, MRI may better define an obstructing lesion at the level of the cerebral aqueduct or fourth ventricle [62]. Furthermore, MRI can assess CSF flow at sites of possible obstruction by the CSF flow void sign (flowing CSF often has a low signal intensity at areas of narrowing within the ventricular system) [168]. There is some evidence that MRI can also demonstrate disease regression [152].

MRI with gadopenetate-dimeglumine-enhanced T1-weighted images is the preferred technique for evaluating CNS sarcoidosis (Fig. 16-4) [169,198]. Enhanced images frequently reveal diffuse or focal leptomeningeal disease and can demonstrate inflammation of the dura; pituitary and infundibulum; optic nerves, chiasm, and tract; gray and white matter regions; periventricular areas; and spinal cord. A normal enhanced MRI scan does not exclude the diagnosis of sarcoidosis, especially if the only clinical manifestation is that of a cranial neuropathy. Furthermore, enhancement can resolve with corticosteroid treatment.

Angiography usually has little to contribute in the evaluation of CNS sarcoidosis [12,13]. Granulomatous masses are typically avascular and cause vessel shifts appropriate to their size and location [88]. Rarely, angiographic abnormalities are found: a smooth narrowing of the caudal internal carotid artery [88], a tapering occlusion of the anterior cerebral artery [30], or multiple

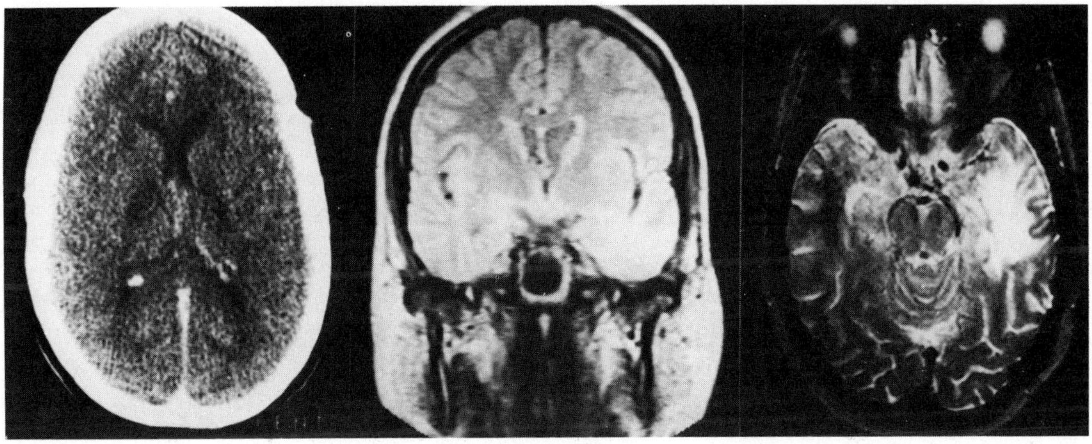

Fig. 16-3. A 27-year-old woman developed complex partial seizures and was found to have an area of enhancement in the left temporal lobe. Exploration demonstrated noncaseating granulomas within cerebral tissue surrounded by chronic inflammatory cells. Left: Computed cranial tomography with contrast administration reveals an area of subtle enhancement in the left posterior medial temporal lobe. Center: A coronal 0.5 Tesla T2-weighted magnetic resonance scan of the same patient reveals subtle increased signal in the left temporal lobe, hypothalamus, and periventricular area. Right: A transverse 1.5 Tesla T2-weighted magnetic resonance scan done 6 months later demonstrates dramatic increased signal in the white matter of the left temporal lobe and subtle increased signal in the right temporal lobe.

small-vessel segmental narrowings suggesting an arteritis [97]. Patients with a diffuse encephalopathy or stroke-like episodes are most likely to demonstrate clinically relevant angiographic findings [134].

Traditional spinal cord imaging involves myelography, and it can demonstrate changes suggesting an intramedullary or extramedullary lesion as well as arachnoiditis or cauda equina disease [88,127]. MRI is the imaging technique of choice, for defining intramedullary spinal cord disease. Sarcoidosis can cause enhancing lesions that are well demarcated or relatively diffuse [129]. Cystic structures have been visualized [27].

Gallium radionuclide imaging has demonstrated increased uptake in the meninges and a brain mass due to sarcoidosis [5].

Visual evoked potentials (VER) can reveal abnormalities of the anterior visual pathways. Brain stem auditory evoked responses (BAER) can evaluate the integrity of the eighth cranial nerve and pontomesencephalic auditory circuits. VERs are often abnormal in patients with symptomatic optic nerve disease and may be abnormal in some patients with CNS sarcoidosis but no clinical evidence of optic nerve dysfunction [139,179,181]. Occasional patients with sarcoidosis, including ocular sarcoidosis, but no known neurologic disease can have abnormal VERs [181], although this finding is not certain [179]. BAERs are often abnormal in CNS sarcoid patients with brain stem or eighth nerve symptoms and can be abnormal in neurologically ill patients without overt disease in these areas [139]. Extensive evidence for abnormal BAERs in patients without CNS sarcoidosis is lacking. Interestingly, the degree of abnormality of an evoked potential can fluctuate depending on disease activity, and an abnormal pattern can even normalize [139]. Somatosensory evoked responses remain to be comprehensively evaluated for their role in the assessment of patients with a sarcoid myelopathy as well as in patients with extraspinal CNS disease or no overt neurosarcoidosis.

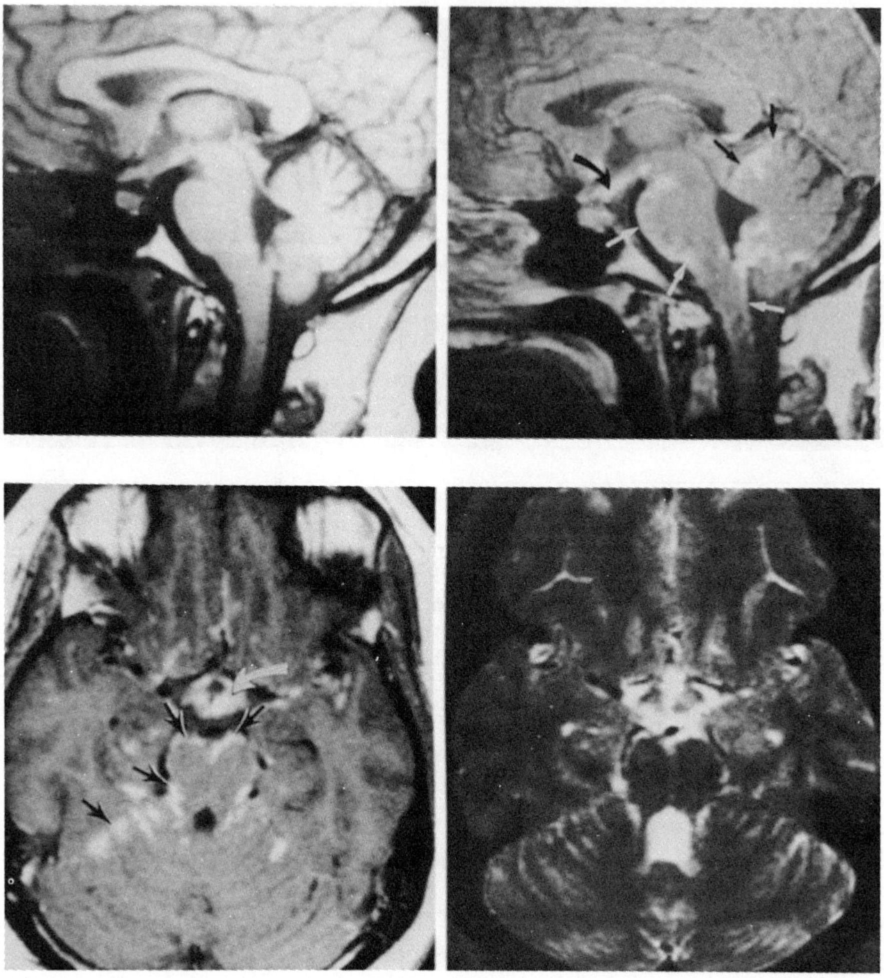

Fig. 16-4. A 34-year-old woman with CNS leptomeningeal sarcoid. Top left: Normal unenhanced T1-weighted midsagittal image. Top right: Contrast-enhanced T1-weighted midsagittal image shows diffuse leptomeningeal enhancement. Note enhancement of chiasm (*curved arrow*), cerebellum, tectum, and margin of brain stem (*straight arrows*). Bottom left: Enhanced T1-weighted axial image. Enhancement around midbrain and cerebellar hemisphere (*straight arrows*) indicates breakdown of blood-CSF barrier. Optic chiasm involvement (*curved arrow*). Bottom right: T2-weighted image at same level shows no evidence of abnormal signal in brain stem. CSF-brain barrier is probably intact. (From J. L. Sherman and B. J. Stern, Sarcoidosis of the CNS: Comparison of unenhanced and enhanced MR images. *A.J.N.R.* 11:915, 1990. Copyright by American Society of Neuroradiology.)

Nerve conduction studies in patients with sarcoid neuropathy usually reveal changes compatible with an axonal neuropathy, though slowing can be more pronounced and suggestive of demyelinating disease [21,51]. Electromyography can demonstrate a denervation pattern in patients with a neuropathy and myopathic changes in patients with a symptomatic myopathy [4]. MRI may reveal a characteristic "star-shaped" pattern for muscle nodules [141].

A neuroendocrine assessment should include inquiry of the patient's thirst sensation, fluid intake, and urinary habits. Libido, potency, and menstrual pattern should be discussed as appropriate. Sleep and eating patterns need to be documented. Screening tests for hypothalamic-pituitary integrity include determination of serum sodium and osmolality, urinary osmolality, thyroid function tests, serum prolactin [105,128] and cortisol, and, as appropriate, testosterone or estradiol levels.

Other Diagnostic Considerations

Given the diverse manifestations of neurosarcoidosis, sarcoidosis is a diagnostic consideration in many clinical settings. Conversely, if sarcoidosis is thought to be the primary diagnosis, many other conditions warrant attention in the differential diagnosis. Table 16-3 lists selected diagnostic points pertinent to neurosarcoidosis. This table is not meant to be inclusive, and other references should be consulted for a broader discussion of differential diagnosis.

Several rare diseases that have protean neurologic sequelae can pose diagnostic challenges. This is especially true of processes that affect younger patients and are associated with granulomatous vasculitis: Wegener's granulomatosis, lymphomatoid granulomatosis, and granulomatous angiitis (isolated CNS vasculitis) [122,126]. These entities can cause cranial nerve, meningeal, and CNS parenchymal disease, and therefore the distinction among these conditions and CNS sarcoidosis can be difficult. The distinction between the degree of vascular, meningeal, and parenchymal inflammation in the CNS and the pattern of systemic involvement seems to be critical in defining the diagnosis.

Multiple sclerosis is associated with a remitting-relapsing neurologic illness with a well-described CSF profile and MRI picture. Similar findings can occur in isolated CNS sarcoidosis. However, except for optic nerve disease, extra-axial cranial neuropathies are unusual, and this fact is important in distinguishing the two entities. Moreover, leptomeningeal enhancement with MRI seems to be quite common in CNS sarcoidosis. Sjögren's syndrome can imitate multiple sclerosis, but peripheral neuropathy or myopathy can also occur [2,72,106,121]. Patients with Sjögren's syndrome can therefore present diagnostic difficulty. The presence of the sicca complex and appropriate biopsy findings can help sort out the potential confusion, but it is important to remember that sarcoidosis can cause dry eyes [40].

Several complications of neurosarcoidosis have been identified, and these are enumerated in Table 16-4. Again, these conditions are representative of the problem and are not meant to be a comprehensive analysis.

PROGNOSIS AND THERAPY

Most patients with neurosarcoidosis do well [22]. Two-thirds of patients seem to have a monophasic illness with minimal neurologic residual deficit [102,134,143]. These patients typically have one or more cranial nerve lesions. Approximately one-third of patients have a remitting-relapsing or chronically progressive illness that is associated with considerable morbidity and potential mortality. These patients often have CNS mass lesions, hydrocephalus, or a diffuse encephalopathy/vasculopathy [102,134,143]. Patients with recurrent aseptic meningitis, cranial polyneuropathies, myopathy, or neuropathy can have a protracted course but tend not to succumb to their illness [4,22,102]. It is not possible to identify with confidence which patients will have a relapsing course, but those patients that do have recurrent disease tend to develop similar neurologic manifestations over time [102].

There have been no rigorous treatment trials for neurosarcoidosis [22,102]. There is a consensus, however, that patients with neurosarcoidosis deserve corticosteroid treatment to decrease the inflammatory reaction and treat symptoms and perhaps prevent the development of irreversible fibrosis [125,179]. Corticosteroids normalize the elevated CD4/CD8 lymphocyte ratio found in the active alveolitis of pulmonary sarcoidosis [20], decrease interleukin-2 production [54,144], and inhibit collagen synthesis [133]. Prior to beginning immunosuppressive treatment, the absence of intercurrent infection, especially tuberculosis, should be established.

The intensity of treatment should be appropriate to the neurologic problem and what is known of its natural history [22,178]. For in-

Table 16-3. Other diagnostic considerations in patients with suspected neurosarcoidosis

Neurosarcoidosis feature	*Selected diagnostic considerations*
Cranial neuropathy	
Optic neuropathy	Multiple sclerosis
	Giant cell arteritis
	Wegener's granulomatosis
	Polyarteritis nodosa
	Meningioma
Cranial nerve 3,4,6	Horner's syndrome (due to mediastinal and cervical adenopathy)
	Graves' ophthalmopathy
	Wegener's granulomatosis
Trigeminal neuropathy	Sjögren's syndrome
Peripheral facial palsy	Bell's palsy
	Borrelia burgdorferi infection (Lyme disease) [199]
	Parotitis
	Wegener's granulomatosis
Eighth nerve dysfunction	Cogan's syndrome
	Vogt-Koyanagi-Harada syndrome
Recurrent laryngeal nerve palsy	Mediastinal adenopathy
Meningeal disease	
Aseptic meningitis	Cryptococcosis
	HIV infection
	Tuberculosis
	Borrelia burgdorferi infection
	Behçet's syndrome
	Vogt-Koyanagi-Harada syndrome
	Mollaret's meningitis
	Wegener's granulomatosis
	Brucellosis
	Meningeal carcinomatosis
Meningeal mass	Meningioma
	Fibrosclerosis
Parenchymal disease	
Mass lesion	Lymphoma [174]
	Glioma [147]
	Metastases
	Tuberculoma
	Wegener's granulomatosis
	Lymphomatoid granulomatosis
	Dysgerminoma
	Pinealoma
	Reticulum cell sarcoma
Spinal cord dysfunction	Multiple sclerosis
	Intramedullary tumor
Encephalopathy and vasculopathy	Fungal, bacterial, tuberculous infection
	Granulomatous angiitis
	HIV infection
	Sjögren's syndrome
	Systemic lupus erythematosus
	Multiple sclerosis
	Polyarteritis nodosa
	Wegener's granulomatosis
	Lymphomatoid granulomatosis
	Cerebral emboli due to:
	Left atrial myxoma
	Sarcoid cardiomyopathy
	Borrelia burgdorferi infection [112]
	Whipple's disease [1]
	Behçet's disease
	Vogt-Koyanagi-Harada syndrome

(*Continued*)

Neurosarcoidosis feature	*Selected diagnostic considerations*
Peripheral neuropathy	Guillain-Barré syndrome
	Polyarteritis nodosa
	Sjögren's syndrome
	Wegener's granulomatosis
	Lymphomatoid granulomatosis
	Borrelia burgdorferi infection
Myopathy	Polymyositis
	Dermatomyositis
	Granulomatous myopathy
CSF analysis	
Hypoglycorrhachia	Carcinomatous and tuberculous meningitis
Elevated IgG index	Multiple sclerosis
	Sjögren's syndrome
	Progressive multifocal leukoencephalopathy
	HIV infection
Oligoclonal bands	Multiple sclerosis
	Sjögren's syndrome
	HIV infection
Elevated angiotensin converting enzyme	CNS infections
	CNS malignancy
	Behçet's disease
Increased CD4/CD8 ratio	?Multiple sclerosis [95]
	?Aseptic meningoencephalitis [95]
Increased beta-2 microglobulin	Infection
	Malignancy (especially lymphoma)
	Syphilis
	AIDS dementia complex
Eosinophilia	Lymphoma
	Tuberculosis
	Syphilis
	Parasites
	Foreign body reaction
CT scan	
Basilar enhancement	Tuberculous, fungal, and bacterial meningitis
	Meningeal carcinomatosis
Convexity mass(es)	Meningioma
Parenchymal mass(es)	Metastasis
	Glioma
	Toxoplasmosis
	Lymphoma
Orbital disease	Optic neuritis
	Malignancy
	Graves' ophthalmopathy
	Orbital pseudotumor
MRI	
Periventricular white matter lesions	Multiple sclerosis
	Sjögren's syndrome
	Progressive multifocal leukoencephalopathy
	Borrelia burgdorferi infection
Angiography	
Arteritis	Granulomatous angiitis [190]
	Drug abuse (sympathomimetics)
	Granulomatous angiitis associated with HIV infection [200]
Evoked potentials	
Abnormal VERs	Multiple sclerosis
	Sjögren's syndrome
Abnormal BAERs	Multiple sclerosis
	Sjögren's syndrome

Table 16-4. Some neurologic complications associated with sarcoidosis and its therapy

Cryptococcal meningitis
Tuberculous meningitis [71]
Progressive multifocal leukoencephalopathy [157]
Herpes simplex encephalitis [119]
Steroid myopathy
Inclusion body myositis [33]

stance, the patient with a solitary peripheral facial nerve palsy attributed to sarcoidosis might be treated with a 2-week course of prednisone. Generally, prednisone, 40 mg/day for 1 week and a second week of tapering dose, is sufficient therapy. Similarly, a bout of aseptic meningitis often responds to a limited course of prednisone.

Patients with a neuropathy or myopathy need more extended therapy, over weeks or months, to control disease activity. Corticosteroid doses should be decreased gradually, for instance at 5-mg decrements of prednisone every other week. A return to higher doses is indicated if there is an exacerbation.

Hydrocephalus can be associated with active CNS inflammation or be the result of an end-stage fibrotic process. Evidence for acute inflammation includes basilar enhancement on CT or MRI scans, a CSF pleocytosis, hypoglycorrhachia, and a CNS mass obstructing the CSF pathways. An enhanced MRI scan is particularly effective for demonstrating a lesion blocking CSF flow in the area of the cerebral aqueduct or fourth ventricle. If active inflammation is present and the patient is asymptomatic or only mildly symptomatic, a course of corticosteroids can lead to resolution or stabilization of the hydrocephalus [49]. Even if no inflammation can be demonstrated, a 1- or 2-week trial of prednisone, 40 mg/day, may be worthwhile to try to quell a subclinical process. Life-threatening elevated intracranial pressure should be treated as an emergency with a ventricular shunt [49]. Patients with chronic hydrocephalus may require shunt revisions and are at risk for infectious complications.

Patients with a CNS mass lesion or encephalopathy/vasculopathy often require protracted corticosteroid therapy [102]. Although a dose of prednisone, 40 mg daily may be sufficient to control the disease process, occasionally much higher corticosteroid doses are needed. The dose should be decreased slowly, for instance, 5-mg decrements every 2 to 4 weeks, and the clinical status monitored. Often the corticosteroid dose will have to be repeatedly raised to minimize recurrent neurologic deficits. Our practice has been initially to double the patient's current dose at the time of relapse to try to obtain a clinical response. A maintenance dose of prednisone, usually in the range of 10 mg daily, is often required to keep the inflammation quiescent.

Rarely is surgery indicated to treat a mass lesion [63]. The patient with known sarcoidosis who develops a CNS mass that is typical of granulomatous disease can often be given a trial of corticosteroid therapy to assess the therapeutic effect. If the lesion does not respond to corticosteroids, biopsy of the lesion is indicated to ensure that an alternative diagnosis is not missed. If noncaseating granulomas are found on biopsy of a CNS mass in a patient without known sarcoidosis, resection of the mass is generally not indicated; enough tissue for pathologic and microbiologic evaluation should be obtained. After a search for other organ involvement with sarcoidosis, a trial of corticosteroids is appropriate. Resection of a sarcoid mass lesion should be reserved for life-threatening disease.

Occasional patients with neurosarcoidosis will not respond to moderately high corticosteroid doses. Six to eight treatments of weekly pulse therapy with up to 30 mg/kg of methylprednisolone, coupled with 0.25 mg/kg/day maintenance prednisone, can be tried to treat severe disease [3,195]. We have successfully used high-dose dexamethasone, 100 mg daily for 3 days, followed by decremental dexamethasone dosing over 2 weeks and ultimate conversion to prednisone, 40 to 60 mg/day, in several patients.

The patient with chronic active inflammation or recurrent disease is at risk not only for the development of neurologic disability associated with sarcoidosis, but also to develop complications from therapeutic interventions. The long-term sequelae of corticosteroid therapy are well known. Recurrent disease should be treated with the lowest corticosteroid dose possible to control inflammation. By judicious adjustment of medication over time, this goal can be achieved. However, a maintenance dose of prednisone, usually in the range of 10 mg daily, may be necessary to control the inflammatory reaction on a long-term basis [102].

New Therapeutic Strategies

Because rare patients with neurosarcoidosis can have life-endangering disease, other therapeutic maneuvers besides corticosteroid treatment and surgery have been suggested [22]. Radiation therapy [9,57], methotrexate [175], and azathioprine [43,52] have been used to treat refractory neurosarcoidosis. Cyclosporine has received increasing attention as an immunosuppressive agent to treat neurologic conditions such as myasthenia gravis and multiple sclerosis and may have a role in the therapy of refractory neurosarcoidosis [82,124,186].

Cyclosporine is an attractive therapeutic agent because of its relatively specific effect on T-lymphocyte function while sparing other host defense mechanisms [89]. Cyclosporine inhibits CD4 (helper) cell performance by inhibiting the generation of interleukin-2 and other lymphokines [67,84], although this effect may not be evident clinically in sarcoid patients [109]. Furthermore, the ability of precursor cytotoxic effector lymphocytes to respond to interleukin-2 is impaired by cyclosporine, perhaps by inhibition of interleukin-2 receptor formation [67]. Also, PGE_2 concentrations are increased by cyclosporine [47,84]. There is a reduction of the (blood) CD4/CD8 ratio in some renal transplantation patients treated with cyclosporine, and this is associated with a good outcome [84]. Cyclosporine has been used successfully to treat pulmonary sarcoidosis [44,149,150], sarcoid uveitis [56], and CNS sarcoidosis [10,22,23,32,87]. A formal protocol to evaluate the safety and efficacy of cyclosporine for refractory neurosarcoidosis has recently been completed (Stern, personal communication).

Other Therapeutic Considerations

Because sarcoid patients can be on chronic corticosteroid therapy, their corticosteroid response to stress is potentially inadequate. Therefore, during intercurrent stress, supplemental corticosteroid therapy is indicated.

Corticosteroid-treated sarcoid patients frequently develop osteoporosis [155], as do patients who are hypogonadal [77,111]. Sarcoidosis is associated with hypercalcemia and hypercalciuria, and corticosteroid therapy itself can cause hypercalciuria [173]. On the other hand, corticosteroid therapy will normalize sarcoid-associated hypercalcemia by inhibiting macrophage synthesis of 1,25-dihydroxyvitamin D and secondarily decreasing bone resorption [173]. Therefore, attention to calcium and bone metabolism is important in the chronic care of sarcoidosis patients, especially if there is concurrent hypogonadism.

Optimal prevention and therapy of osteoporosis are still being investigated [103]. Using as little corticosteroid medication as possible, maintaining physical activity and nutrition, restricting sodium intake to 2 to 3 gm daily, and replacing estrogen and testosterone, as appropriate, are general management guidelines [103]. If hypercalciuria is present, a thiazide diuretic and a potassium-sparing diuretic can be given [103]. 25-Hydroxyvitamin D levels should be maintained in the normal range with supplements, as appropriate. Serum calcium and urinary calcium excretion should be monitored if diuretics or vitamin D is prescribed. Calcitonin administration can reduce the risk of osteoporosis in corticosteroid-treated sarcoid patients [154,156]. Etidronate may also be effective in preventing and treating osteoporosis, but further studies are needed in the treatment of corticosteroid-induced osteoporosis. Deflazacort is a corticosteroid that has few adverse effects on bone and calcium metabolism and is effective in treating sarcoidosis [153].

Needless to say, other endocrine deficiencies are treated as indicated. Patients with disordered thirst are counseled about the dangers of electrolyte derangements; the association of hyponatremia and seizures is stressed. Propranolol may help normalize thirst in patients with hypothalamic disorders [94].

Care of the patient with neurosarcoidosis is a challenge. The diagnosis is often difficult, and although most patients do well, a small number experience considerable morbidity and even death. Optimal management involves a team approach to utilize the expertise of the neurologist, neurosurgeon, pulmonologist, and ophthalmologist as well as potentially many other physicians. With an increasing understanding of the basic processes leading to granulomatous disease, sarcoidosis will remain a fertile area of study.

REFERENCES

1. Adams, M., Rhyner, P. A., Day, J., et al. Whipple's disease confined to the central nervous system. *Ann. Neurol.* 21:104, 1987.
2. Alexander, E. L., Malinow, K., Lejewski, J. E., et al. Primary Sjögren's syndrome with central nervous system disease mimicking multiple sclerosis. *Ann. Intern. Med.* 104:323, 1986.
3. Allen, R. K. A., and Merory, J. Intravenous pulse methylprednisolone in the successful treatment of severe sarcoid polyneuropathy with pulmonary involvement. *Aust. N.Z. J. Med.* 15:45, 1985.
4. Ando, D. G., Lynch, J. P., III, and Fantone, J. C., III. Sarcoid myopathy with elevated creatine phosphokinase. *Am. Rev. Respir. Dis.* 131:298, 1985.
5. Ayres, J. G., Hicks, B. H., and Maisey, M. N. Gallium-67 uptake in meningeal sarcoidosis. *Clin. Nucl. Med.* 11:507, 1986.
6. Baba, T., Ochiya, T., Yamaguchi, K., et al. Monocyte activating factor in sarcoidosis: I. Existence of the factor in sarcoidosis sera. *Clin. Immunol. Immunopathol.* 39:24, 1986.
7. Baba, T., Yamaguchi, K., Ochiya, T., et al. Monocyte activating factor in sarcoidosis: II. Secretion of the factor from monocytes. *Clin. Immunol. Immunopathol.* 39:37, 1986.
8. Baughman, R. P., Ploysongsang, Y., Roberts, R. D., et al. Effects of sarcoid and steroids on angiotensin-converting enzyme. *Am. Rev. Respir. Dis.* 128:631, 1983.
9. Bejar, J. M., Kerby, G. R., Ziegler, D. K., et al. Treatment of central nervous system sarcoidosis with radiotherapy. *Ann Neurol.* 18:258, 1985.
10. Bielory, L., Holland, C., Gascon, P., et al. Uveitis, cutaneous and neurosarcoid: Treatment with low-dose cyclosporine A. *Transplant. Proc.* 20:144, 1988.
11. Boeck, C. Multiple benign sarkoid of skin. *J. Cutan. Genito-urin. Dis.* 17:543, 1899.
12. Brooks, B. S., Gammal, T. E., Hungerford, G. D., et al. Radiologic evaluation of neurosarcoidosis: Role of computed tomography. *A.J.N.R.* 3:513, 1982.
13. Brown, M. M., Thompson, A. J., Wedzicha, J. A., et al. Sarcoidosis presenting with stroke. *Stroke* 20:400, 1989.
14. Brust, J. C. M., Rhee, R. S., Plank, C. R., et al. Sarcoidosis, galactorrhea, and amenorrhea: 2 autopsy cases, 1 with Chiari-Frommel syndrome. *Ann. Neurol.* 2:130, 1977.
15. Byrne, J. V., and Lawton, C. A. Meningeal sarcoidosis causing intracranial hypertension secondary to dural sinus thrombosis. *Br. J. Radiol.* 56:755, 1983.
16. Cahill, D. W., Botero, E., and Robinson, W. L. Neurosarcoidosis presenting as an intracranial mass. *J. Fla. Med. Assoc.* 73:35, 1986.
17. Campbell, J. N., Black, P., and Ostrow, P. T. Sarcoid of the cauda equina. *J. Neurosurg.* 47:109, 1977.
18. Capellan, J. I. L., Olmedo, L. C., Martin, J. M. et al. Intrasellar mass with hypopituitarism as a manifestation of sarcoidosis. *J. Neurosurg.* 73:283, 1990.
19. Caplan, L., Corbett, J., Goodwin, J., et al. Neuro-ophthalmologic signs in the angiitic form of neurosarcoidosis. *Neurology* 33:1130, 1983.
20. Ceuppens, J. L., Lacquet, L. M., Marien, G., et al. Alveolar T-cell subsets in pulmonary sarcoidosis. *Am. Rev. Respir. Dis.* 129:563, 1984.
21. Challenor, Y. B., Felton, C. P., and Brust, J. C. M. Peripheral nerve involvement in sarcoidosis: An electrodiagnostic study. *J. Neurol. Neurosurg. Psychiatry* 47:1219, 1984.
22. Chapelon, C., Ziza, J. M., Piette, J. C., et al. Neurosarcoidosis: Signs, course and treatment in 35 confirmed cases. *Medicine* 69:261, 1990.
23. Chen, R. C. Y., McLeod, J. G. Neurologic complications of sarcoidosis. *Clin. Exp. Neurol.* 26:99, 1989.
24. Chiang, R., Marshall, M. C., Rosman, P. M., et al. Empty sella turcica in intracranial sarcoidosis. *Arch. Neurol.* 41:662, 1984.
25. Chretien, J., Marsar, J., Saitiel, J. C. (eds.). *Ninth International Conference on Sarcoidosis and Other Granulomatous Disorders.* Paris: Pergamm, 1981.
26. Clark, W. C., Acker, J. D., Dohan, F. C., Jr., et al. Presentation of central nervous system sarcoidosis as intracranial tumors. *J. Neurosurg.* 63:851, 1985.
27. Clifton, A. G., Stevens, J. M., Kapoor, R., et al. Spinal cord sarcoidosis with intramedullary cyst formation. *Br. J. Radiol.* 63:805, 1990.
28. Cohen, D. M., and Reinhardt, R. A. Systemic sarcoidosis presenting with Horner's syn-

drome and mandibular paresthesia. *Oral Surg.* 53:577, 1982.
29. Cordingley, G., Navarro, C., Brust, J. C. M., et al. Sarcoidosis presenting as senile dementia. *Neurology* 31:1148, 1981.
30. Corse, A. M., and Stern, B. J. Neurosarcoidosis and stroke. *Stroke* 21:152, 1990.
31. Costabel, U., Bross, K. J., Ruhle, K. H., et al. Ia-like antigens on T-cells and their subpopulations in pulmonary sarcoidosis and in hypersensitivity pneumonitis. *Am. Rev. Respir. Dis.* 131:337, 1985.
32. Cunnah, D., Chew, S., and Wass, J. Cyclosporin for central nervous system sarcoidosis. *Am. J. Med.* 85:580, 1988.
33. Danon, M. J., Perurena, O. H., Ronan, S., et al. Inclusion body myositis associated with systemic sarcoidosis. *Can. J. Neurol. Sci.* 13:334, 1986.
34. Day, A. L., and Sypert, G. W. Spinal cord sarcoidosis. *Ann. Neurol.* 1:79, 1977.
35. Delaney, P. Neurologic manifestations in sarcoidosis. *Ann. Intern. Med.* 87:336, 1977.
36. Delaney, P. Seizures in sarcoidosis: A poor prognosis. *Ann. Neurol.* 7:494, 1980.
37. Delaney, P., Henkin, R. I., Manz, H., et al. Olfactory sarcoidosis. *Arch. Otolaryngol.* 103:717, 1977.
38. DeRemee, R. A., and Rohrbach, M. S. Serum angiotensin-converting enzyme activity in evaluating the clinical course of sarcoidosis. *Ann. Intern. Med.* 92:361, 1980.
39. Douglas, A. C., and Maloney, A. F. J. Sarcoidosis of the central nervous system. *J. Neurol. Neurosurg. Psychiatry* 36:1024, 1973.
40. Drosos, A. A., Constantopoulos, S. H., Psychos, D., et al. The forgotten cause of sicca complex: Sarcoidosis. *J. Rheumatol.* 16:1548, 1989.
41. Dubois, P. J., Beardsley, T., Klintworth, G., et al. Computed tomography of sarcoidosis of the optic nerve. *Neuroradiology* 24:179, 1983.
42. El-Kassimi, F. A., Ashour, M., Vijayaraghavan, R. Sarcoidosis presenting as recurrent left laryngeal nerve palsy. *Thorax* 45:565, 1990.
43. Elkin, R., and Willcox, P. A. Neurosarcoidosis. *S. Afr. Med. J.* 67:943, 1985.
44. Endres, P., and de Wall, N. Ciclosporin A: Experiences with two patients with refractory active sarcoidosis in need of treatment. *Prax. Klin. Pneumol.* 40:96, 1986.
45. Espinosa, G. A., Michael, A., Wilbur, A., et al. Spinal cord sarcoidosis. *Milit. Med.* 150:309, 1985.
46. Ey, E. H., Wall, M., Numaguchi, Y., et al. Neurosarcoidosis involving optic nerves and leptomeninges: Computed tomography findings. *J. Comput. Tomogr.* 10:129, 1986.
47. Fan, T. D., Cox, J. H., and Chisholm, P. M. Mechanism of action of cyclosporine in preventing cardiac allograft rejection: II. Graft tissue levels of prostacyclin and thromboxane. *Transplantation* 43:343, 1987.
48. Fanburg, B. L. (ed). Sarcoidosis and Other Granulomatous Diseases of the Lung. In *Lung Biology in Health and Disease.* New York: Marcel Dekker, 1983. Vol. 20.
49. Foley, K. T., Howell, J. D., and Junck, L. Progression of hydrocephalus during corticosteroid therapy for neurosarcoidosis. *Postgrad. Med. J.* 65:481, 1989.
50. Freiman, D. G. The pathology of sarcoidosis. *Semin. Roentgenol.* 20:327, 1985.
51. Galassi, G., Gibertoni, M., Mancini, A., et al. Sarcoidosis of the peripheral nerve: Clinical, electrophysiological and histological study of two cases. *Eur. Neurol.* 23:459, 1984.
52. Gelwan, M. J., Kellen, R. I., Burde, R. M., et al. Sarcoidosis of the anterior visual pathway: Successes and failures. *J. Neurol. Neurosurg. Psychiatry* 51:1473, 1988.
53. Godwin, J. E., and Sahn, S. A. Sarcoidosis presenting as progressive ascending lower extremity weakness and asymptomatic meningitis with hypoglycorrhachia. *Chest* 97:1263, 1990.
54. Goodwin, J. S., Atluru, D., Sierakowski, S., et al. Mechanism of action of glucocorticosteroids. *J. Clin. Invest.* 77:1244, 1986.
55. Graham, E. M., Ellis, C. J. K., Sanders, M. D., et al. Optic neuropathy in sarcoidosis. *J. Neurol Neurosurg. Psychiatry* 49:756, 1986.
56. Graham, E. M., Sanders, M. D., James, D. G., et al. Cyclosporin A in the treatment of posterior uveitis. *Trans. Ophthalmol. Soc. U.K* 104:146, 1985.
57. Grizzanti, J. N., Knapp, A. B., Schecter, A. J., et al. Treatment of sarcoid meningitis with radiotherapy. *Am. J. Med.* 73:605, 1982.
58. Groman, G. S., Castele, R. J., Altose, M. D., et al. Lymphocyte subpopulations in sarcoid pleural effusion. *Ann. Intern. Med.* 100:75, 1984.
59. Gudeman, S. K., Selhorst, J. B., Susac, J. O., et al. Sarcoid optic neuropathy. *Neurology* 32:597, 1982.
60. Hagerstrand, I., and Lineli, F. The prevalence of sarcoidosis in the autopsy material from a Swedish town. *Med. Scand.* 425:171, 1963.
61. Hart, W. M., Jr., and Burde, R. M. Optic disk edema in sarcoidosis. *Am. J. Ophthalmol.* 88:769, 1979.
62. Hayes, W. S., Sherman, J. L., Stern, B. J., et al. MR and CT in the evaluation of intracranial sarcoidosis. *A.J.N.R.* 8:841, 1987.
63. Healton, E. B., Zito, G., Chauhan, P., et al. Intracranial subdural sarcoid granuloma. *J. Neurosurg.* 56:728, 1982.
64. Hefferman, A., Cullen, M., Towers, R., et al. Sarcoidosis of the hypothalamus. *Hormones* 2:1, 1971.

65. Henkind, P., and Gottlieb, M. B. Bilateral internal ophthalmoplegia in a patient with sarcoidosis. *Br. J. Ophthalmol.* 57:792, 1973.
66. Herring, A. B., and Urich, H. Sarcoidosis of the central nervous system. *J. Neurol. Sci.* 9:405, 1969.
67. Hess, A. D., Colombani, P. M., and Esa, A. H. Cyclosporine and the immune response: Basic aspects. *C.R.C. Crit. Rev. Immunol.* 6:123, 1986.
68. Hewlett, R. H., and Brownell, B. Granulomatous myopathy: Its relationship to sarcoidosis and polymyositis. *J. Neurol. Neurosurg. Psychiatry* 38:1090, 1975.
69. Hitchon, P. W., Haque, A. U., Olson, J. J., et al. Sarcoidosis presenting as an intramedullary spinal cord mass. *Neurosurgery* 15:86, 1984.
70. Ho, S. U., Berenberg, R. A., Kim, K. S., et al. Sarcoid encephalopathy with diffuse inflammation and focal hydrocephalus shown by sequential CT. *Neurology* 29:1161, 1979.
71. Hopkins, A. Tuberculous meningitis as a complication of sarcoidosis. *J. Neurol. Neurosurg. Psychiatry* 37:644, 1974.
72. Hull, R. G., Morgan, S. H., Harding, A. E., et al. Sjögren's syndrome presenting as a severe sensory neuropathy including involvement of the trigeminal nerve. *Br. J. Rheumatol.* 23:301, 1984.
73. Hunninghake, G. W., and Crystal, R. G. Pulmonary sarcoidosis: A disorder mediated by excess helper T-lymphocyte activity at sites of disease activity. *N. Engl. J. Med.* 305:429, 1981.
74. Hutchinson, J. Cases of Mortimer's malady (lupus vulgaris multiplex non-ulcerous and non-serpiginous). *Arch. Surg.* 9:307, 1898.
75. Hybels, R. L., and Rice, D. H. Neuro-otologic manifestations of sarcoidosis. *Laryngoscope* 86:1873, 1976.
76. Ismail, F., Miller, J. L., Kahn, S. E., et al. Hypothalamic-pituitary sarcoidosis. *S. Afr. Med. J.* 67:139, 1985.
77. Jackson, J. A., and Kleerekoper, M. Osteoporosis in men: Diagnosis, pathophysiology, and prevention. *Medicine* 69:137, 1990.
78. Jahrsdoerfer, R. A., Thompson, E. G., Johns, M. M. E., et al. Sarcoidosis and fluctuating hearing loss. *Ann. Otol. Rhinol. Laryngol.* 90:161, 1981.
79. James, D. G., and Williams, W. J. Multisystem Clinical Features. In *Sarcoidosis and Other Granulomatous Disorders.* Philadelphia: Saunders, 1985.
80. James, D. G., and Williams, W. J. Report of the commission on granulomatous diseases. *Ann. N.Y. Acad. Sci.* 465:304, 1986.
81. Johns, C. J. (ed). Tenth International Conference on sarcoidosis and Other Granulomatous Disorders. *Ann. N.Y. Acad. Sci.* 465:1, 1986.
82. Johnson, K. P., and Belendiuk, G. Use of cyclosporine in neurological autoimmune disease? *Arch. Neurol.* 42:1043, 1985.
83. Juozevicius, J. L., and Rynes, R. I. Increased helper/suppressor T-lymphocyte ratio in the cerebrospinal fluid of a patient with neurosarcoidosis. *Ann. Intern. Med.* 104:807, 1986.
84. Kahan, B. D. Individualization of cyclosporine therapy using pharmacokinetic and pharmacodynamic parameters. *Transplantation* 40:457, 1985.
85. Kane, K. Deafness in sarcoidosis. *J. Laryngol. Otol.* 90:531, 1976.
86. Kataria, Y. P., LoBuglio, A. F., and Bromberg, P. A. Sarcoid lymphocytes: Spontaneous transformation and release of macrophage migration inhibition activity. *Am. Rev. Respir. Dis.* 113:315, 1976.
87. Kavanaugh, A. F., Andrew, S. L., Cooper, B., et al. Cyclosporine therapy of central nervous system sarcoidosis. *Am. J. Med.* 82:387, 1987.
88. Kendall, B. E., and Tatler, G. L. V. Radiological findings in neurosarcoidosis. *Br. J. Radiol.* 51:81, 1978.
89. Keown, P. A., Stiller, C. R., Carruthers, G., et al. Cyclosporine: Mechanism of action, measurement and clinical use. *Br. J. Clin. Pract.* 40:149, 1986.
90. Ketonen, L., Oksanen, V., Kuuliala, I., et al. Hypodense white matter lesions in computed tomography of neurosarcoidosis. *J. Comput. Assist. Tomogr.* 10:181, 1986.
91. Ketonen, L., Oksanen, V., and Kuuliala, I. Preliminary experience of magnetic resonance imaging in neurosarcoidosis. *Neuroradiology* 29:127, 1987.
92. Kinnman, J., and Link, H. Intrathecal production of oligoclonal IgM and IgG in CNS sarcoidosis. *Acta Neurol. Scand.* 69:97, 1984.
93. Kirkham, T. H., and Kline, L. B. Monocular elevator paresis, Argyll Robertson pupils and sarcoidosis. *Can. J. Ophthalmol.* 11:330, 1976.
94. Kirkland, J. L., Pearson, D. J., Goddard, C., et al. Polyuria and inappropriate secretion of arginine vasopressin in hypothalamic sarcoidosis. *J. Clin. Endocrinol. Metab.* 56:269, 1983.
95. Kuroda, Y., and Shibasaki, H. CSF mononuclear cell subsets in active MS: Lack of disease-specific alteration. *Neurology* 37:497, 1987.
96. Lawrence, E. C., Brousseau, K. P., Berger, M. B, et al. Elevated concentrations of soluble interleukin-2 receptors in serum samples and bronchoalveolar lavage fluids in active sarcoidosis. *Am. Rev. Respir. Dis.* 137:759, 1988.
97. Lawrence, W. P., Gammal, T. E., Pool, W. H., Jr., et al. Radiological manifestations of neurosarcoidosis: Report of three cases and review of literature. *Clin. Radiol.* 25:343, 1974.
98. Leeas, N. E., Zimmerman, R. D., Elkin, C. M., et al. Neurosarcoidosis of the brain and meninges. *Semin. Roentgenol.* 20:387, 1985.

99. Lieberman, J. Elevation of serum angiotensin-converting enzyme (ACE) level in sarcoidosis. *Am. J. Med.* 59:365, 1975.
100. Lieberman, J. (ed). *Sarcoidosis.* Orlando, FL: Grune & Stratton, 1985.
101. Lipton, J. M., Kirkpatrick, J., and Rosenberg, R. N. Hypothermia and persisting capacity to develop fever. *Arch. Neurol.* 34:498, 1977.
102. Luke, R. A., Stern, B. J., Krumholz, A., et al. Neurosarcoidosis: The long-term clinical course. *Neurology* 37:461, 1987.
103. Lukert, B. P., and Raisz, L. G. Glucocorticoid-induced osteoporosis: Pathogenesis and management. *Ann. Intern. Med.* 112:352, 1990.
104. Lukin, R. R., Chambers, A. A., and Soleimanpour, M. Outlet obstruction of the fourth ventricle in sarcoidosis. *Neuroradiology* 10:65, 1975.
105. Malarkey, W. B., and Kataria, Y. P. Sarcoidosis and hyperprolactinemia. *Ann. Intern. Med.* 81:116, 1974.
106. Malinow, K. L., Molina, R., Gordon, B., et al. Neuropsychiatric dysfunction in primary Sjögren's syndrome. *Ann. Intern. Med.* 103: 344, 1985.
107. Manz, H. J. Pathobiology of neurosarcoidosis and clinicopathologic correlation. *Can. J. Neurol. Sci.* 10:50, 1983.
108. Martin, C. A., Murali, R., and Trasi, S. S. Spinal cord sarcoidosis. *J. Neurosurg.* 61:981, 1984.
109. Martinet, Y., Pinkston, P., Saltini, C., et al. Evaluation of the in vitro and in vivo effects of cyclosporine on the lung T-lymphocyte alveolitis of active pulmonary sarcoidosis. *Am. Rev. Respir. Dis.* 138:1242, 1988.
110. Matthews, W. B. Neurosarcoidosis. In P. J. Vinken and G. W. Bruyn (ed.), *Handbook of Clinical Neurology.* New York: Elsevier/North-Holland, 1979. Vol. 38, pp. 521–542.
111. Melton, L. J., Eddy, D. M., Johnston, Jr., C. C. Screening for osteoporosis. *Ann. Intern. Med.* 112:516, 1990.
112. Midgard, R., and Hofstad, H. Unusual manifestations of nervous system *Borrelia burgdorferi* infection. *Arch. Neurol.* 44:781, 1987.
113. Mikami, R., Sekiguchi, M., Ryuzin, Y., et al. Changes in the peripheral vasculature of various organs in patients with sarcoidosis: Possible role of microangiopathy. *Heart Vessels* 2:129, 1986.
114. Miller, D. H., Kendall, B. E., Barter, S., et al. Magnetic resonance imaging in central nervous system sarcoidosis. *Neurology* 38:378, 1988.
115. Mirfakhraee, M., Crofford, M. J., Guinto, F. C., Jr., et al. Virchow-Robin space: A path of spread in neurosarcoidosis. *Radiology* 158:715, 1986.
116. Mirshra, B. B., Poulter, L. W., Janossy, G., et al. The distribution of lymphoid and macrophage like cell subsets of sarcoid and Kveim granulomata: Possible mechanism of negative PPD reaction in sarcoidosis. *Clin. Exp. Immunol.* 54:705, 1983.
117. Missler, U., Mack, M., Nowack, G., et al. Pituitary sarcoidosis. *Klin. Wochenschr.* 68:342, 1990.
118. Mitchell, J. D., Yap, P. L., Milne, L. A., et al. Immunological studies on the cerebrospinal fluid in neurological sarcoidosis. *J. Neuroimmunol.* 7:249, 1985.
119. Modi, C. M., and Valaitis, J. Herpesvirus encephalitis and pulmonary sarcoidosis. *Neurology* 24:1096, 1974.
120. Modlin, R. L., Gottlieb, B., Hofman, F. M., et al. Demonstration in situ of subsets of T-lymphocytes in sarcoidosis. *Am. J. Dermatopathol.* 6:423, 1984.
121. Molina, R., Provost, T. T., and Alexander, E. L. Peripheral inflammatory vascular disease in Sjögren's syndrome. *Arthritis Rheum.* 28:1341, 1985.
122. Moore, P. M., and Cupps, T. R. Neurological complications of vasculitis. *Ann. Neurol.* 14:155, 1983.
123. Muller-Quernheim, J., Saltini, C., Sondermeyer, P., et al. Compartmentalized activation of the interleukin 2 gene by lung T lymphocytes in active pulmonary sarcoidosis. *J. Immunol.* 137:3475, 1986.
124. The Multiple Sclerosis Study Group. Efficacy and toxicity of cyclosporine in chronic progressive multiple sclerosis: A randomized, double-blinded, placebo-controlled clinical trial. *Ann. Neurol.* 27:591, 1990.
125. Muthiah, M. M., and MacFarlane, J. T. Current concepts in the management of sarcoidosis. *Drugs* 40:231, 1990.
126. Nadeau, S. E. Collagen vascular disease: Vasculitis, systemic lupus erythematosus, and rheumatoid arthritis. *Semin. Neurol.* 5:324, 1985.
127. Nagai, H., Ohtsubo, K., and Shimada, H. Sarcoidosis of the spinal cord. *Acta Pathol. Jpn.* 35:1007, 1985.
128. Nakao, K., Noma, K., Sato, B., et al. Serum prolactin levels in eighty patients with sarcoidosis. *Eur. J. Clin. Invest.* 8:37, 1978.
129. Nesbit, G. M., Miller, G. M., Baker, Jr., H. L., et al. Spinal cord sarcoidosis: A new finding at MR imaging with Gd-DTPA enhancement. *Radiology* 173:839, 1989.
130. Neville, E., Walker, A. N., James, D. G. Prognostic factors predicting the outcome of sarcoidosis: An analysis of 818 patients. *Q. J. Med.* 208:525, 1983.
131. Nossal, G. J. V. The basic concepts of the immune system. *N. Engl. J. Med.* 316:1320, 1987.
132. Obenauf, C. D., Shaw, H. E., Sydnor, C. F., et al. Sarcoidosis and its ophthalmic manifestations. *Am. J. Ophthalmol.* 86:648, 1978.

133. Oikarinen, A. I., Uitto, J., Oikarinen, J. Glucocorticoid action on connective tissue: From molecular mechanisms to clinical practice. *Med. Biol.* 64:221, 1986.
134. Oksanen, V. Neurosarcoidosis: Clinical presentations and course in 50 patients. *Acta Neurol. Scand.* 73:283, 1986.
135. Oksanen, V., Fyhrquist, F., Gronhagen-Riska, C., et al. CSF angiotensin-converting enzyme in neurosarcoidosis. *Lancet* 1:1050, 1985.
136. Oksanen, V., Fyhrquist, F., Somer, H., et al. Angiotensin converting enzyme in cerebrospinal fluid: A new assay. *Neurology* 35:1220, 1985.
137. Oksanen, V., Gronhagen-Riska, C., Fyhrquist, F., et al. Systemic manifestations and enzyme studies in sarcoidosis with neurologic involvement. *Acta Med. Scand.* 218:123, 1985.
138. Oksanen, V., Gronhagen-Riska, C., Tikanoja, S., et al. Cerebrospinal fluid lysozyme and B_2-microglobulin in neurosarcoidosis. *J. Neurol. Sci.* 73:79, 1986.
139. Oksanen, V., and Salmi, T. Visual and auditory evoked potentials in the early diagnosis and follow-up of neurosarcoidosis. *Acta Neurol. Scand.* 74:38, 1986.
140. Osenbach, R. K., Blumenkopf, B., Ramirez, H., Jr., et al. Meningeal neurosarcoidosis mimicking convexity en-plaque meningioma. *Surg. Neurol.* 26:387, 1986.
141. Otake, O., Banno, T., Ohba, S., et al. Muscular Sarcoidosis: Findings at MR imaging. *Radiology* 176:145, 1990.
142. Payne, C. R., Tait, D., and Batten, J. C. Sarcoidosis and chronic sensory neuropathy. *Postgrad. Med. J.* 56:781, 1980.
143. Pentland, B., Mitchell, J. D., Cull, R. E., et al. Central nervous system sarcoidosis. *Q. J. Med.* 56:457, 1985.
144. Pinkston, P., Saltini, C., Müller-Quernheim, J., et al. Corticosteroid therapy suppresses spontaneous interleukin 2 release and spontaneous proliferation of lung T lymphocytes of patients with active pulmonary sarcoidosis. *J. Immunol.* 139:755, 1987.
145. Plotkin, G. R., and Patel, B. R. Neurosarcoidosis presenting as chronic lymphocytic meningitis. *Pa. Med.* 89:36, 1986.
146. Poole, C. J. M. Argyll Robertson pupils due to neurosarcoidosis: Evidence for site of lesion. *Br. Med. J.* 289:356, 1984.
147. Powers, W. J., and Miller, E. M. Sarcoidosis mimicking glioma: Case report and review of intracranial sarcoid mass lesions. *Neurology* 31:907, 1981.
148. Rawlings, C. E., III, Saris, S. C., Muraki, A., et al. Syringomyelia in a man with sarcoidosis. *Neurosurgery* 18:805, 1986.
149. Rebuck, A. S., Sanders, B. R., MacFadden, D. K., et al. Cyclosporin in pulmonary sarcoidosis. *Lancet* 1:1486, 1987.
150. Rebuck, A. S., Stiller, C. R., Braude, A. C., et al. Cyclosporin for pulmonary sarcoidosis. *Lancet* 1:1174, 1984.
151. Redwood, M. D., Winer, J. B., and Rosser, M. Neurosarcoidosis presenting as benign intracranial hypertension. *Eur. Neurol.* 30:282, 1990.
152. Reed, L. D., Abbas, S., Markivee, C. R., et al. Neurosarcoidosis responding to steroids. *A.J.R.* 146:819, 1986.
153. Rizzato, G., and Fraioli, P. Natural and corticosteroid-induced osteoporosis in sarcoidosis: Prevention, treatment, follow up and reversibility. *Sarcoidosis* 7:89, 1990.
154. Rizzato, G., Schiraldi, G., Tosi, G., et al. Administration of salmon calcitonin nasal spray for long-term treatment of corticosteroid-induced osteoporosis: A preliminary report. *Curr. Ther. Res.* 45:761, 1989.
155. Rizzato, G., Tosi, G., Mella, C., et al. Researching osteoporosis in prednisone treated sarcoid patients. *Sarcoidosis* 4:45, 1987.
156. Rizzato, G., Tosi, G., Schiraldi, G., et al. Bone protection with salmon calcitonin (SCT) in the long-term steroid therapy of chronic sarcoidosis. *Sarcoidosis* 5:99, 1988.
157. Rosenbloom, M. A., and Uphoff, D. The association of progressive multifocal leukoencephalopathy and sarcoidosis. *Chest* 83:572, 1983.
158. Rush, J. A. Retrobulbar optic neuropathy in sarcoidosis. *Ann. Ophthalmol.* 12:390, 1980.
159. Saltini, C., Spurzem, J. R., Lee, J. J., et al. Spontaneous release of interleukin 2 by lung T lymphocytes in active pulmonary sarcoidosis is primarily from the Leu3+Dr+ T cell subset. *J. Clin. Invest.* 77:1962, 1986.
160. Savolaine, E. R., and Schlembach, P. J. Gallium scan diagnosis of sarcoidosis in the presence of equivocal radiographic and CT findings: Value of lacrimal gland biopsy. *Clin. Nucl. Med.* 15:198, 1990.
161. Schaumann, J. Lupus Pernio: Zambaco Prize Essay. Stockholm: PA Norstedt & Soner, 1936.
162. Schlitt, M., Duvall, E. R, Bonnin, J., et al. Neurosarcoidosis causing ventricular loculation, hydrocephalus, and death. *Surg. Neurol.* 26:67, 1986.
163. Seem, C. P. C., Norfolk, G., and Spokes, E. G. CSF angiotensin-converting enzyme in neurosarcoidosis. *Lancet* 1:456, 1985.
164. Semenzato, G., Agostini, C., Trentin, L., et al. Evidence of cells bearing interleukin-2 receptor at sites of disease activity in sarcoid patients. *Clin. Exp. Immunol.* 57:331, 1984.
165. Semenzato, G., Pezzutto, A., Pizzolo, G., et al. Immunohistological study in sarcoidism: Eval-

uation at different sites of disease activity. *Clin. Immunol. Immunopathol.* 30:29, 1984.
166. Sethi, K. D., Gammal, T. E., Patel, B. R., et al. Dural sarcoidosis presenting with transient neurologic symptoms. *Arch. Neurol.* 43:595, 1986.
167. Sharma, O. P. *Sarcoidosis: Clinical Management.* London: Butterworth, 1984.
168. Sherman, J. L., Citrin, C. M., Bowen, B. J., et al. MR demonstration of altered cerebrospinal fluid flow by obstructive lesions. *A.J.N.R.* 7:571, 1986.
169. Sherman, J. L., and Stern, B. J. Sarcoidosis of the CNS: Comparison of unenhanced and enhanced MR images. *A.J.N.R.* 11:915, 1990.
170. Siltzbach, L. E. (ed). Seventh international conference on sarcoidosis and other granulomatous disorders. *Ann. N.Y. Acad. Sci.* 278:1, 1976.
171. Siltzbach, L. E., James, D. G., Neville, E., et al. Course and prognosis of sarcoidosis around the world. *Am. J. Med.* 57:847, 1974.
172. Silverstein, A., Feuer, M. M., and Siltzbach, L. E. Neurologic sarcoidosis. *Arch. Neurol.* 12:1, 1965.
173. Singer, F. R., and Adams, J. S. Abnormal calcium homeostasis in sarcoidosis. *N. Engl. J. Med.* 315:755, 1986.
174. Singh, A., Strobos, R. J., Singh, B. M., et al. Steroid-induced remissions in CNS lymphoma. *Neurology* 32:1267, 1982.
175. Soriano, F. G., Caramelli, P., Nitrini, R., et al. Neurosarcoidosis: Therapeutic success with methotrexate. *Postgrad. Med. J.* 66:142, 1990.
176. Stannard, K., and Spalton, D. J. Sarcoidosis with infiltration of the external ocular muscles. *Br. J. Ophthalmol.* 69:562, 1985.
177. Stern, B. J., Griffin, D. E., Luke, R. A., et al. Neurosarcoidosis: Cerebrospinal fluid lymphocyte subpopulations. *Neurology* 37:878, 1987.
178. Stern, B. J., and Krumholz, A. Neurosarcoidosis. In R. T. Johnson (ed.), *Current Therapy in Neurologic Disease-2.* Toronto: Decker, 1987. Pp. 135–137.
179. Stern, B. J., Krumholz, A., Johns, C., et al. Sarcoidosis and its neurological manifestations. *Arch. Neurol.* 42:909, 1985.
180. Stjernberg, N., Cajander, S., Truedsson, H., et al. Muscle involvement in sarcoidosis. *Acta Med. Scand.* 209:213, 1981.
181. Streletz, L. J., Chambers, R. A., Bae, S. H., et al. Visual evoked potentials in sarcoidosis. *Neurology* 31:1545, 1981.
182. Stuart, C. A., Neelon, F. A., and Lebovitz, H. E. Hypothalamic insufficiency: The cause of hypopituitarism in sarcoidosis. *Ann. Intern. Med.* 88:589, 1978.
183. Stuart, C. A., Neelon, F. A., and Lebovitz, H. E. Disordered control of thirst in hypothalamic-pituitary sarcoidosis. *N. Engl. J. Med.* 303:1078, 1980.
184. Thomas, P. D., and Hunninghake, G. W. Current concepts of the pathogenesis of sarcoidosis. *Am. Rev. Respir. Dis.* 135:747, 1987.
185. Thompson, C., and Checkley, S. Short term memory deficit in a patient with cerebral sarcoidosis. *Br. J. Psychiatry* 139:160, 1981.
186. Tindall, R. S. A., Rollins, J. A., Phillips, J. T., et al. Preliminary results of a double-blind, randomized placebo-controlled trial of cyclosporine in myasthenia gravis. *N. Engl. J. Med.* 316:719, 1987.
187. Tobias, J. K., Santiago, S. M., and Williams, A. J. Sarcoidosis as a cause of left recurrent laryngeal nerve palsy. *Arch. Otolaryngol. Head Neck Surg.* 116:971, 1990.
188. Trombley, I. K., Mirra, S. S., and Miles, M. L. An electron microscopic study of central nervous system sarcoidosis. *Ultrastruct. Pathol.* 2:257, 1981.
189. Turner-Warwick, M., Haslem, P. L., McAllister, W., et al. Do measurements of bronchoalveolar lymphocytes and neutrophils, serum angiotensin-converting enzyme and gallium uptake help the clinician to treat patients with sarcoidosis? In C. J. Johns (ed.), The Tenth International Conference on Sarcoidosis and Other Granulomatous Diseases. *Ann. N.Y. Acad. Sci.* 465:387, 1986.
190. Urich, H. Neurosarcoidosis or granulomatous angiitis: A problem of definition. *Mt. Sinai J. Med.* 44:718, 1977.
191. Viale, G., Codecasa, L., Bulgheroni, P., et al. T-cell subsets in sarcoidosis: An immunocytochemical investigation of blood, bronchoalveolar lavage fluid, and prescalenic lymph nodes from eight patients. *Hum. Pathol.* 17:476, 1986.
192. Vighetto, A., Fischer, G., Collet, P., et al. Intramedullary sarcoidosis of the cervical spinal cord. *J. Neurol. Neurosurg. Psychiatry* 48:477, 1985.
193. Walker, F. O., McLean, Jr., W. T., Elster, A., et al. Chiasmal sarcoidosis: *A.J.N.R.* 11:1205, 1990.
194. Wall, M. J., Peyster, R. G., Finkelstein, S. D., et al. A unique case of neurosarcoidosis with pineal and suprasellar involvement: CT and pathological demonstration. *J. Comput. Assist. Tomogr.* 9:381, 1985.
195. Wallaert, B., Ramon, P., Fournier, E. C., et al. High-dose methylprednisolone pulse therapy in sarcoidosis. *Eur. J. Respir. Dis.* 68:256, 1986.
196. Waxman, J. S., and Sher, J. H. The spectrum of central nervous system sarcoidosis: A clinical and pathologic study. *Mt. Sinai J. Med.* 46:309, 1979.

197. Wiederholt, W. C., and Siekert, R. G. Neurological manifestations of sarcoidosis. *Neurology* 15:1147, 1965.
198. Williams, D. W., Elster, A. D., and Kramer, S. I. Neurosarcoidosis: Gadolinium-enhanced MR imaging. *J. Comput. Assist. Tomogr.* 14:704, 1990.
199. Wokke, J. H. J., van Gijn, J., Elderson, A., et al. Chronic forms of *Borrelia burgdorferi* infection of the nervous system. *Neurology* 37:1031, 1987.
200. Yankner, B. A., Skolnik, P. R., Shoukimas, G. M., et al. Cerebral granulomatous angiitis associated with isolation of human T-lymphotrophic virus type III from the central nervous system. *Ann. Neurol.* 20:362, 1986.

17 Neurologic Manifestations of the Acquired Immunodeficiency Syndrome

Robert M. Wachter

As experience with the clinical spectrum of the acquired immunodeficiency syndrome (AIDS) has grown, an increasing number of neurologic manifestations have been recognized. During the early years of the epidemic, opportunistic infections and malignancies of the central nervous system (CNS) accounted for most of reported clinical manifestations of neurologic disease in patients with AIDS [100]. The last few years have brought an increasing awareness of the varied disorders of the CNS caused by human immunodeficiency virus (HIV) itself. Studies of these CNS infections by the neurotropic HIV are yielding new insights into the biologic properties of both the virus and the CNS. The frequency of neurologic complications in AIDS patients is approximately 35 percent [61,100]. This frequency, coupled with predictions of more than 250,000 AIDS cases in the United States by 1991 [85], have fueled the search for greater understanding of and treatments for the neurologic sequelae of AIDS.

SPECTRUM OF NEUROLOGIC MANIFESTATIONS OF AIDS

Three large series [61,66,100] have reviewed the spectrum of neurologic disorders seen in patients with AIDS (Table 17-1). Because these series generally report patients referred for neurologic consultation, they may underestimate the frequency or overestimate the severity of these neurologic disorders. In general, the disorders can be divided into six groups:

1. Manifestations of primary CNS infection with HIV
2. Other CNS viral infections
3. Nonviral CNS opportunistic infections
4. CNS malignancies
5. Disorders of the spinal cord and peripheral nervous system
6. Other manifestations

Invasion of the CNS by HIV itself carries importance beyond its clinical sequelae. For antivi-

Table 17-1. The spectrum of neurologic complications in patients with AIDS

Complications	*Snider et al. [100]*	*Levy et al. [61]*	*McArthur [66]*	*Total (%)*
CNS HIV infections				
Aseptic meningitis	17	4	13	34 (10)
AIDS dementia complex	35	18	30	83 (24)
Other CNS viral infections				
CMV encephalitis	2	0	3	5 (1)
CMV retinitis	NA	1	9	10 (3)
Herpes encephalitis	8	0	0	8 (2)
PML	2	2	1	5 (1)
Nonviral CNS infections				
CNS Toxoplasmosis	18	5	15	38 (11)
Cryptococcal meningitis	16	2	11	29 (8)
Neurosyphilis	1	0	1	2 (1)
Atypical mycobacteria	1	3	0	4 (1)
Mycobacterium tuberculosis	0	0	0	0 (0)
Candida albicans	2	1	0	3 (1)
Aspergillus fumigatus	0	0	0	0 (0)
Coccidiomycosis	1	0	0	1 (0)
Bacteria	0	0	0	0 (0)
Neoplasms				
CNS lymphoma	9	3	7	19 (6)
Systemic lymphoma with CNS involvement	2	4	1	7 (2)
Kaposi's sarcoma	2	0	0	2 (1)
Spinal cord and peripheral nervous system				
Vacuolar myelopathy	0	0	12	12 (3)
IDP	17	8	11	36 (10)
Sensory neuropathy	5	0	26	31 (9)
Myopathy	0	1	0	1 (0)
Others				
Cerebrovascular events	2	6	1	9 (3)
Metabolic encephalopathy	NA	NA	5	5 (1)
Total complications	140	58	146	344

* Percentages are given as percent of total number of complications (344). CMV = cytomegalovirus, PML = progressive multifocal leukoencephalopathy, IDP = inflammatory demyelinating polyneuropathy, NA = not available.

ral agents or modulators of the immune response to be effective, they will have to penetrate the blood-brain barrier to eradicate the virus in the CNS and destroy a potentially persistent reservoir of replication and infection [5].

INFECTIONS OF THE CNS BY HIV

Biologic Properties of HIV

The HIV is a retrovirus, a diverse family of enveloped RNA viruses. Each retrovirus contains an RNA-dependent DNA polymerase (reverse transcriptase), which produces an intermediate DNA (provirus). This provirus is incorporated into the host genome and is utilized in the infected cell for the transcription of virus RNA [11,43].

The HIV has been called a "lentivirus," or "slow virus," because of its ability to evade host defenses and cause persistent infection. Like other lentiviruses, the HIV has a long incubation period and manifests many of its biologic effects as a result of its cellular tropism. In the case of HIV, this tropism is directed primarily at the T4 (helper/inducer) lymphocyte and leads to destruction of the cells and persistent immunosuppression [103]. Recent evidence suggests that HIV is not only lymphotropic but neurotropic as well [44].

HIV-Related Meningitis

Infection of the CNS by the HIV itself is common [49,83,93] and may occur with or without symptoms. In a cohort of 11 HIV infected but asymptomatic homosexual men, 2 had mononuclear pleocytosis and 4 had HIV isolated from the cerebrospinal fluid (CSF) [67]. Other reports have documented that the meningitis that occurs at the time of HIV seroconversion may be clinically silent [10,89]. However, a number of patients will manifest an aseptic meningitis at the time of primary HIV infection, usually weeks after exposure to the virus [13,45,93]. This aseptic meningitis usually occurs as part of a mononucleosis-like illness and may be manifested by headache, fever, meningismus, and cranial neuropathies [45,49,61,100].

Thirteen patients with HIV-related meningitis were studied by McArthur [66]. Seven had AIDS-related complex (ARC), and 6 were asymptomatic at the time of meningitis; none had frank AIDS. Symptoms were as described above; although the most common symptoms were headache and fever, these were seen in only 5 (38%) and 3 (23%) of the patients, respectively. All had a mononuclear CSF pleocytosis, with a mean white blood cell count of 41 WBC/mm^3 (range, 5–176). Total protein was elevated in 6 of these 13 patients (46%), with a mean value of 65 mg/dl (range, 20–186). HIV was isolated from the CSF in 4 of 8 patients in whom it was attempted. The aseptic meningitis in these 13 patients was usually self-limited, with symptoms resolving within 1 to 4 weeks without specific therapy. None of the patients developed recurrent meningitis or AIDS dementia complex in 8 months of follow-up, although 3 patients had persistent CSF pleocytosis.

AIDS Dementia Complex

Although early reports highlighted the frequency of cognitive dysfunction in patients with AIDS [100], these deficits were often attributed to depression or delirium. However, over the past few years, it has become increasingly clear that many AIDS patients suffer cognitive and behavioral changes as a consequence of their infection [30,53,61,72,84]. Although the term *HIV encephalopathy* has been used by the Centers for Disease Control [9] to describe the varied manifestations of HIV on cognition and behavior, most investigators refer to this entity as AIDS-related dementia [66] or AIDS dementia complex (ADC) [72, 84]. Price, Sidtis, and Rosenblum [84] prefer the term *ADC* to HIV encephalopathy in light of the absence of brain inflammation in many affected patients and the fact that the evidence that HIV *causes* ADC, although convincing, remains somewhat circumstantial. Navia and Price [74] have outlined some of the clinical and laboratory findings that are suggestive of ADC; no single finding is pathognomonic (Table 17-2).

The clinical manifestations of ADC range from subtle memory loss and behavioral change to severe, disabling dementia. Some patients

Table 17-2. Findings that suggest the diagnosis of AIDS dementia complex

Clinical presentation
Dementia
Motor dysfunction (slowed movements, tremor, ataxia, paraparesis)
Behavioral disturbance (social withdrawal, organic psychosis)
Neurodiagnostic studies
Computed tomographic or magnetic resonance imaging: brain atrophy, white matter changes
Epidemiologic background
Risk group: male homosexual, intravenous drug abuser, transfusion recipient, offspring or heterosexual partner of HIV-infected person
Systemic conditions
Full-blown AIDS
AIDS-related complex
Systemically asymptomatic
Immunology
Reduced T4/T8 peripheral lymphocyte ratio; other indexes of impaired T-cell function
Serology
Serum antibodies against HIV
Viral culture
Isolation of HIV from blood, cerebrospinal fluid, or brain
Neuropathology (biopsy or autopsy)
White matter changes; multinucleated cells and macrophage infiltrates

Source: Navia and Price [74].

with early ADC will be free of constitutional symptoms; their dementia may be the only clinical manifestation of HIV infection [74]. These patients frequently score normally on the Mini-Mental Status examination [32], although more detailed testing often demonstrates subtle abnormalities of memory, attention, or concentration. Since about 40 percent of these patients with early ADC demonstrate normal neurologic examinations (and in many of the others, diffuse hyperreflexia is the only abnormality) [66], their dementia is frequently confused with mild depression.

In contrast to these patients with early ADC, some patients present with severe cognitive deficits and are incapable of independent living. Also, unlike patients with early ADC, these patients generally have known AIDS or ARC and suffer from other constitutional symptoms [66,72]. The Mini-Mental Status examination is usually abnormal in these patients, as is the neurologic examination, which may demonstrate hyperreflexia, hypertonia, or frontal release signs. Approximately 40 percent of these patients have an accompanying myelopathy with signs of spastic paraparesis [66]. The mean survival of patients with ADC ranges from about 3 to 9 months [66,74].

Common laboratory abnormalities in ADC include elevated CSF protein and immunoglobulin (IgG) fraction [66,72,100]. Pleocytosis is found in about one-fifth of patients [66]. Although HIV can be isolated from the CSF in 40 to 60 percent of patients with ADC [44,49,66], it can also be isolated in up to 30 percent of neurologically normal HIV-seropositive subjects [67]; it is therefore neither sensitive nor specific for the diagnosis of ADC. Radiologic studies demonstrate diffuse cerebral atrophy in about two-thirds of patients; magnetic resonance imaging (MRI) does not appear to be more sensitive than computed tomography (CT) in demonstrating this finding. MRI does appear to be more sensitive than CT in demonstrating subtle abnormalities of white matter, usually as increased signal intensity on T2-weighted images [19,57,72].

Pathologically, patients with ADC are generally found to have cerebral atrophy. Pathologic examination also often demonstrates multiple inflammatory nodules composed of lymphocytes, macrophages, and microglia distributed in both gray and white matter. Other common findings in patients with ADC include multinucleated giant cells, focal demyelination, and vacuolar (spongiform) myelopathy [7,17,71,75,78,90,96]. Despite the wide variety of pathologic findings, Navia and co-workers [71] were struck by the "remarkable blandness" of histologic findings in approximately one-third of their patients dying with severe dementia.

The expression of ADC in children born with HIV infection can be more striking than that seen in adults. These children may suffer any or all of the following: encephalopathy, acquired microcephaly, movement disorders, visual loss, or seizures. Pathologic examination of the brains of these children demonstrates gross atrophy, multinucleated giant cells in the white matter, microglial nodules, and vascular calcifications [28,97]. Although half the children followed by Belman and colleagues [4] succumbed to their illness within 2 years of diagnosis, the others entered a static phase with delayed attainment of developmental milestones.

Contradictory evidence has accumulated as to the efficacy of azidothymidine (AZT) in the treatment of ADC. AZT is capable of penetrating the blood-brain barrier [115]. One small study demonstrated temporary clinical improvement in 4 of 7 patients with mild dementia [114]. However, a larger study involving 32 patients failed to demonstrate a benefit in neuropsychiatric testing, although there was a significant decrease in mortality and the frequency of opportunistic infections [31,39]. If AZT or other antiviral agents prove to be effective in the therapy of ADC, then this condition will need to be added to the list of treatable dementias. As in all patients with dementia, other therapeutic interventions include the avoidance of unnecessary psychoactive medications and judicious use of neuroleptics for patients with agitation or hallucinosis [58]. Psychological and emotional support for patient, family, and loved ones is essential, as is practical assistance to help patients manage daily living activities. One practical matter, that of the ascertainment of the patient's wishes regarding life-sustaining treatments, should be attended to early in the patient's course [104]. Some but not all states now allow the patient to designate a durable power of attorney for health care decisions should he or she later lose competence [101,102].

In the first few years of the AIDS epidemic, cytomegalovirus (CMV) was generally felt to be responsible for ADC [100]. However, over the past half-decade, convincing evidence has accumulated implicating HIV in the pathogenesis of ADC. This evidence includes failure to isolate other pathogens (including CMV) in most cases of ADC, frequent isolation of HIV from brain or CSF in patients with ADC, and localization of HIV within macrophages and multinucleated giant cells of inflammatory nodules in the brains of patients with ADC [17,35,40,44,60,83,84,86,98,112]. However, a number of scientific issues surrounding ADC remain unresolved, including the mechanism by which AIDS gains access to the CNS and that by which the neuropathogenicity of HIV is expressed. This may involve actual genetic changes in human immunodeficiency virus type 1 (HIV-1) [83]. Elucidation of these mechanisms may lead to improvements in our understanding of the pathogenicity of viral infections, the structure and function of the blood-brain barrier, and the biochemical basis of cognitive function.

Recent evidence suggests a possible mechanism of action of the AIDS virus on the CNS [22]. It has been demonstrated in rat retinal ganglion cells that a coat protein, gp120 from HIV-1, may increase intracellular calcium in nerve cells in the hippocampus. Under experimental conditions, calcium channel blockers prevented the gp120 protein from causing neurologic injury and from increasing intracellular calcium in neurons (rat retinal ganglion cells) [22]. Although by no means definitive, these findings provide strong evidence that an increase of intracellular calcium may be important in the neurotoxicity of HIV-1. In the particular case of HIV-1 infection of the retina, recent studies of a total of 12 patients who had AIDS document that the retina is indeed often infected with the AIDS virus [8, 80].

OTHER VIRAL INFECTIONS OF THE CNS

Cytomegalovirus Encephalitis

As noted earlier, many cases of encephalitis previously attributed to CMV are now attributed to infection with HIV [109]. Because of the high prevalence of HIV infection of the CNS and the coexistence of other opportunistic pathogens in many cases of encephalitis with histologic changes characteristic of CMV, it is difficult to define a true CMV encephalitis adequately. Post and associates [81] described six patients with AIDS, progressive confusion, and fever. At autopsy, all six patients had evidence of disseminated CMV infection outside the CSF, intranuclear inclusions typical of CMV in the brain, and no evidence of other opportunistic infections of the CSF. There were no distinguishing clinical, radiologic, or laboratory features that would have permitted a secure antemortum diagnosis of CMV encephalitis in these patients. At the present time, no therapy has proved effective for CMV encephalitis [51].

Cytomegalovirus Retinitis

CMV retinitis is the most common ocular infection in patients with AIDS [34]. Fluffy white exudates are seen at ophthalmoscopy, often with associated hemorrhage that follows a vascular pattern of distribution [12,23,24,76] (Fig. 17-1). Pathologically, the lesion is one of retinal necrosis with intranuclear and intracytoplasmic inclusions [47]. In situ hybridization studies have demonstrated that CMV is a major pathogen in these cases of retinitis [54], but HIV-1 may actually facilitate retinal infection by CMV. Treatment with zidovudine of some patients with retinitis associated with AIDS has been demonstrated to improve CMV retinitis, even though zidovudine has little activity against CMV. Thus, retinitis associated with AIDS is probably a com-

Fig. 17-1. Cytomegalovirus retinitis in a patient with known disseminated cytomegalovirus infection. (From W. R. Freeman et al., A prospective study of the ophthalmologic findings in the acquired immune deficiency syndrome. *Am. J. Ophthalmol.* 97:133, 1984. Published with permission from *The American Journal of Ophthalmology.* Copyright by The Ophthalmic Publishing Company.)

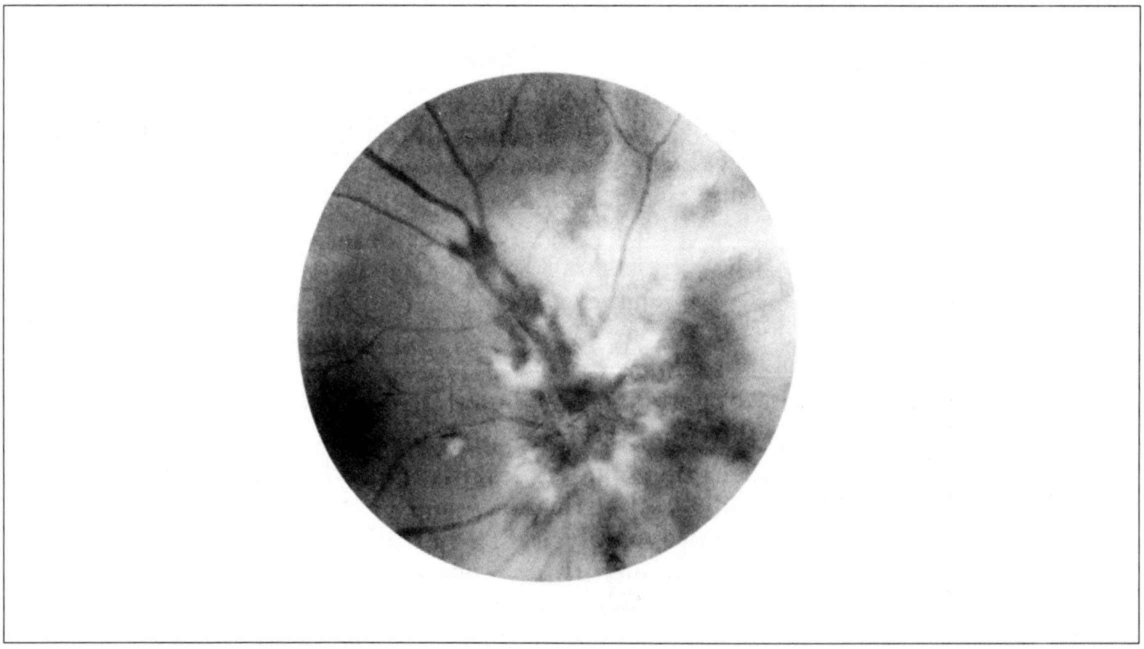

bination of infection with HIV-1 and CMV [8,80].

Retinitis associated with AIDS is generally painless. Patients usually present with blurred vision, decreased visual acuity, or visual field defects. The visual loss tends to progress with time and, if untreated, leads to blindness [51]. When blindness occurs suddenly, retinal detachment (resulting from a scar in a thinned portion of the retina) should be suspected [48]. Although the majority of patients who develop AIDS associated retinitis already have a known AIDS diagnosis, CMV retinitis represents the index diagnosis of AIDS in about 1 in 10 patients at San Francisco General Hosptial [51]. Although the diagnosis of CMV retinitis may be confirmed by isolation of CMV from other body sites such as urine or blood, therapy should be initiated based on symptoms and funduscopic appearance; this will often be before culture results are available.

Ganciclovir (formerly known as DHPG) is effective in the treatment of CMV retinitis. A number of studies [12,48,59,65] have confirmed the efficacy of intravenous ganciclovir, given for 10 or 20 days, in inducing remission of CMV retinitis. Most patients developed clinical and virologic relapse on cessation of induction therapy. Therefore, trials of maintenance therapy have been initiated. Early evidence has demonstrated the value of intravenous maintenance therapy in sustaining remission [51]. Because lifelong maintenance therapy appears to be required, future studies will concentrate on the efficacy of other routes of administration of ganciclovir, including oral and intravitreal [51].

The major toxicity of ganciclovir is neutropenia, which may be severe but is almost always reversible within a few days of discontinuing the drug. Less common side effects include thrombocytopenia, disorientation, hepatitis, nausea, rash, and pain at the injection site.

Herpes Encephalitis

Both herpes simplex and herpes zoster encephalitis have been reported in patients with AIDS [21,61,72,94]. The clinical presentation of herpes encephalitis, with fever and focal neurologic deficits, is similar in AIDS patients to that seen in patients without AIDS. As in non-AIDS patients, the treatment of choice is intravenous acyclovir [18].

Progressive Multifocal Leukoencephalopathy

Progressive multifocal leukoencephalopathy (PML), characterized by altered mentation or focal neurologic signs, including aphasia, ataxia, or hemiparesis, was previously reported in patients with lymphoma or leukemia or patients on immunosuppressive therapy. In the last few years, AIDS has become the most common predisposing disorder leading to PML [2,6]. PML is caused by the reactivation of CNS infection by a papovavirus (slow virus), which results in the destruction of oligodendroglia. The CT appearance shows single or multiple areas of low density in the white matter without evidence of mass effect or contrast enhancement [26,62]. Biopsy may be necessary to distinguish the lesions of PML from those of lymphoma or toxoplasmosis. At present, there is no effective therapy.

NONVIRAL CNS OPPORTUNISTIC INFECTION

Cerebral Toxoplasmosis

Infection with the protozoan *Toxoplasma gondii* is common; 10 to 50 percent of the general population of the United States is infected by the age of 12 [68]. Despite the frequency of infection, clinically apparent infection was unusual before the AIDS epidemic. In AIDS patients, however, cerebral toxoplasmosis is a relatively common syndrome, occurring in about 10 percent of all patients [29].

Infection of the CNS is by far the most common manifestation of toxoplasmosis in patients with AIDS. Most patients have signs of a focal CNS process, with motor deficits ranging from mild hand weakness to hemiparesis or aphasia. Focal seizures are also a relatively common finding. This focality can be attributed to the lesions of *T. gondii,* which are multifocal necrotic and inflammatory abscesses. Headache, fever, and altered mentation are seen only in a minority of patients [64,66,73].

The lumbar puncture is not helpful in making the diagnosis of toxoplasmosis; the usual finding is a nonspecific lymphocytic pleocytosis. It is useful in excluding other pathogens, however. Imaging of the brain with CT is the most useful diagnostic test for toxoplasmosis. CT will generally reveal single or multiple abscesses with enhancement (frequently in a ring pattern) after the injection of intravenous contrast (Fig. 17-2). These abscesses show a moderate predilection for the basal ganglia [26,66,73,82,111]. MRI appears to be somewhat more sensitive than CT for demonstrating the lesions of cerebral toxoplasmosis [61,62]. Serologic testing for IgG antibodies to *T. gondii* is often positive in patients with or without cerebral toxoplasmosis; therefore, such testing may support the diagnosis but cannot be diagnostic [68]. A negative IgG serology does help exclude the diagnosis, although exceptions to this general rule have been reported [66]. CSF serologic testing is not helpful.

Brain biopsy remains the only definitive procedure for confirming the diagnosis of toxoplasmosis. Its role in the evaluation of suspected cerebral toxoplasmosis remains controversial, however. Many authorities would make a presumptive diagnosis of cerebral toxoplasmosis in a patient with risk factors for AIDS, a positive HIV serology, positive IgG or IgM antibodies to *T. gondii,* ring-enhancing lesions on CT scan, and no evidence of other CNS infections or tumors. Biopsy should probably be reserved for patients who fail to improve with therapy or in whom diagnostic confusion exists (e.g., a patient with a negative IgG antibody to *Toxoplasma* or with a single or non-contrast-enhancing lesion on CT [66, 68]. Whether open or sterotactic needle biopsy is chosen, tissue should be stained with immunoperoxidase for *T. gondii* antigens, a technique with a much higher yield than routine hematoxylin-eosin staining [64,70].

The treatment of choice for cerebral toxoplasmosis is the combination of pyrimethamine with a sulfonamide. After 2 to 3 weeks of therapy with 25 mg/day of pyrimethamine and 100 mg/

Fig. 17-2. CT scan (A) and MRI (T2-weighted image) (B) of a patient with cerebral toxoplasmosis. Studies were done at the same time on the same patient, demonstrating the increased sensitivity of MRI. (From McArthur [66].)

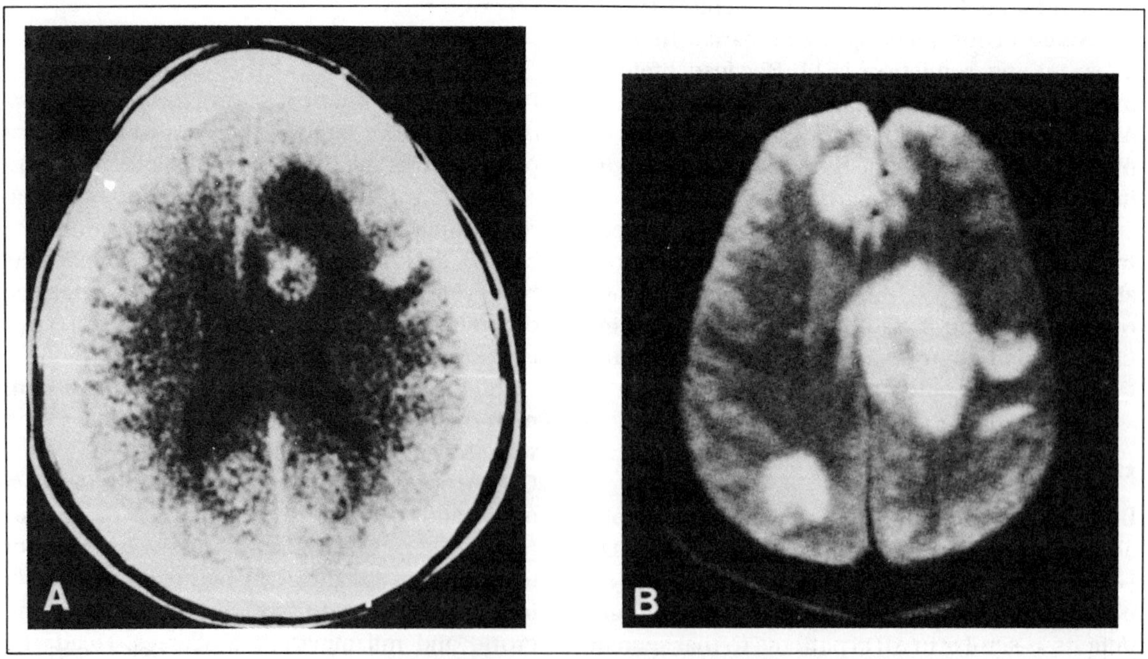

kg/day of sulfadiazine in divided doses, most patients experience a clinical and radiologic improvement [66,107]. Unfortunately, virtually all patients relapse quickly upon cessation of the drugs. Therefore, lifetime maintenance therapy is necessary but often poorly tolerated because of leukopenia, thrombocytopenia, or rash. These toxicities have fueled the search for other agents, and trials with trimetrexate and clindamycin are ongoing [18]. The adjunctive use of corticosteroids, although popular, is of unproven benefit [68,107]. Many authorities reserve steroids for patients with definite signs of increased intracranial pressure or early herniation.

Cryptococcal Meningitis

Although the yeast *Cryptococcus neoformans* can infect normal hosts, it tends to show a predilection toward patients with depressed cell-mediated immunity. With the development of the AIDS epidemic, the frequency of cryptococcal infection has grown. Between 6 and 13 percent of AIDS patients suffer cryptococcal infection at some time during the course of their disease [27,61,117].

The large majority of AIDS patients with cryptococcal infection present with signs and symptoms of CNS infection. The most common symptoms are fever and headache, each found in more than 80 percent of patients [56,117]. The most common presenting syndrome is meningitis; however in Zuger's series [117], fewer than one-third of patients showed signs of meningeal irritation in the form of stiff neck or photophobia. In contrast to toxoplasmosis, seizures and focal neurologic deficits are uncommon, although they may be present in the rare patient with a cryptococcoma of the brain. Approximately one-third of patients with CNS cryptococcosis also have infection outside the nervous system; the lung, blood, and skin are the most common sites [56,117].

Examination of the CSF demonstrates a surprisingly benign formula in cryptococcal infection. In Kovac's series [56], the CSF white blood cell count was less than 6 WBC/mm^3 in 65 percent of patients, the protein was less than 45 mg/110 ml in 31 percent, and the glucose was greater than 40 mg/ml in 69 percent. Three of the 17 patients with proven cryptococcal meningitis had normal values for CSF protein, glucose, and leukocytes [56]. CSF cryptococcal antigen is almost invariably positive in patients with cryptococcal meningitis, with titers ranging from 1:2 to 1:20,000 (mean 1:200). Patients with CNS cryptococcoma without meningitis may have negative cryptococcal antigens. CSF culture is positive in almost all patients with cryptococcal meningitis, as is serum cryptococcal antigen. The India ink preparation of the CSF is somewhat less sensitive than serum or CSF cryptococcal antigen and CSF culture; it was positive in about 75 percent of patients with cryptococcal meningitis in two large series [56,117]. In patients with crytpococcal meningitis, CNS imaging studies (CT or MRI) are usually normal. The finding of mass lesions should suggest alternative diagnoses, such as toxoplasmosis, lymphoma, or cryptococcoma [61].

The two standard regimens for treating cryptococcal meningitis are amphotericin B alone (0.4–0.6 mg/kg/day) or a combination of oral flucytosine (150 mg/kg/day) and amphotericin B (0.3–0.6 mg/kg/day). Although some 60 percent of patients enjoy an initial response to one of these regimens, few patients achieve a complete and sustained remission [56,117]. Therefore, after completion of an initial 6-week course of one of the standard regimens, lifetime maintenance therapy (in the form of once or twice weekly intravenous amphotericin B given through an indwelling Hickman catheter) is generally recommended [117]. Successful therapy is accompanied by a resolution of clinical symptoms and signs and a fall in CSF and serum cryptococcal antigen titers by at least four dilutions.

Available therapies for cryptococcal meningitis are highly toxic. Common toxicities of amphotericin B include renal impairment, chills, and fever. Flucytosine causes leukopenia, thrombocytopenia, and abnormal liver and renal function. Intraventricular amphotericin (given through an indwelling Ommaya reservoir) has been tried both electively and in patients refractory to standard therapy. No obvious increase in efficacy has been demonstrated by this technique, which carries a high risk of chemical arachnoiditis [117].

AIDS patients with cryptococcal meningitis have a poor prognosis. Kovacs and associates [56] reported that 14 of 26 patients (54%) treated for cryptococcosis failed therapy by virtue of death or persistance of positive cultures despite therapy. In 8 of the 14 patients who failed therapy (57%), death could be attributed directly to cryptococcal disease. The mean survival after the diagnosis of cryptococcal meningitis is 9 months. Clearly, the search for the optimal treatment regimen has not ended.

Neurosyphilis

In 1987, Johns, Tierney, and Felsenstein [52] reported the cases of four AIDS patients with CNS syphilis; two had meningovascular syphilis, one had acute syphilitic meningitis, and one had asymptomatic neurosyphilis. In two patients, neurosyphilis developed despite previous adequate therapy for early syphilis with benzathine penicillin. It appears that the course of *Treponema pallidum* infection is more virulent in patients with AIDS and that the usual serologic response to the treponeme may be modified [52,108]. It is recommended that high-dose penicillin (2–4 million units/day given intravenously for 10 days) be the minimum antibiotic regimen used for the treatment of AIDS patients with neurosyphilis. Although this regimen ensures that adequate treponemicidal levels are reached in the CSF, Johns, Tierney, and Felsenstein [52] suggest that maintenance therapy (as is required for toxoplasmosis and cryptococcus in AIDS) may prove necessary to control the course of neurosyphilis in some HIV-infected patients.

Other CNS Opportunistic Infections

Although toxoplasmosis and cryptococcosis are by far the most frequent CNS opportunistic infections seen in patients with AIDS, a wide variety of other pathogens have been reported to cause infection. These pathogens, which include mycobacteria (both typical and atypical), *Candida albicans, Aspergillus fumigatus,* and *Coccidioides immitis,* are indistinguishable from other opportunistic pathogens and each other on clinical grounds [61]. Therefore, a bacteriologic diagnosis is often needed to tailor appropriate therapy. AIDS patients may have multiple infections or the coexistence of infection and lymphoma [61]. However, they rarely suffer from routine bacterial infections [61,100].

TUMORS OF THE CNS

CNS Lymphoma

Primary malignant lymphoma of the CNS is a rare entity, representing less than 2 percent of all primary brain tumors and about 1 percent of all newly diagnosed lymphomas in America [41]. In the last few years, AIDS has replaced congenital and iatrogenic immunodeficiency states as the most common predisposing cause of CNS lymphoma.

The most common presenting symptom of AIDS-associated CNS lymphoma is altered mentation, which may be subtle and thus simulate ADC. The onset of encephalopathy is generally less acute than that seen with toxoplasmosis, and headache, focal neurologic deficits, and seizures are less common than with toxoplasmosis [66]. CT scanning usually demonstrates single or multiple hypodense areas with homogenous contrast enhancement (Fig. 17-3), although in a minority of patients the scan is normal [61, 66]. These hypodense lesions are in contrast to the isodense or hypodense lesions reported in primary CNS lymphoma without underlying immunodeficiency [37]. Rapid growth of the mass may be seen in AIDS-associated CNS lymphoma and thus does not help differentiate this entity from opportunistic infection [26]. Unfortunately, neither the clinical presentation, location, multicentricity, nor the pattern of contrast enhancement reliably distinguishes toxoplasmosis from lymphoma in the work-up of a CNS mass lesion in a patient with known or suspected AIDS. Since therapy for toxoplasmosis usually leads to an initial shrinking of toxoplasma lesions and therapy for CNS lymphoma is unrewarding, many would treat empirically for *T. gondii* when diagnostic confusion exists and reserve biopsy for lesions that fail to regress.

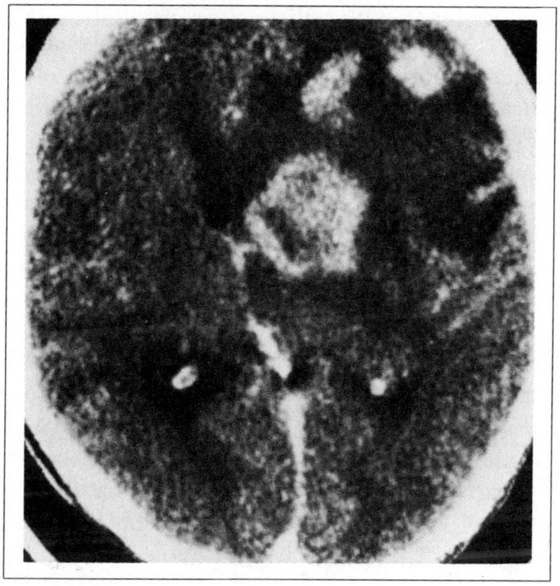

Fig. 17-3. Contrast-enhanced CT scan of a patient with biopsy proven CNS lymphoma. Note the multicentricity, contrast enhancement, and extensive edema. (From Gill et al. [37].)

Pathologically, CNS lymphomas in AIDS are usually high-grade small-cell noncleaved or large-cell immunoblastic lymphomas [37,66, 92]. Although some initial response to radiation therapy and steroids may be seen, the prognosis is dismal. Of seven patients treated by McArthur [66], none survived longer than 4 months. However, one patient who had a complete response to radiation and chemotherapy and remained well after 28 months of follow-up has been reported [37].

Other CNS Tumors

Systemic lymphoma may invade the CNS in patients with AIDS. The presentation is as commonly one of carcinomatous meningitis as one that suggests a mass lesion. Therefore, common presenting complications include cranial neuropathy and epidural cord compression. Most of these lymphomas are extranodal diffuse high-grade B-cell lymphomas [20,116]. Transient response to therapy is common, but most patients die within 1 year of diagnosis [61].

Involvement of the CNS by Kaposi's sarcoma is extremely rare. When it does metastasize to the brain, it usually causes hemorrhagic lesions [61]. Kaposi's sarcoma can also infiltrate peripheral nerves and lead to peripheral neuropathy or plexopathy [61, 66].

DISORDERS OF THE SPINAL CORD AND PERIPHERAL NERVOUS SYSTEM

Vacuolar Myelopathy

Vacuolar myelopathy, which is characterized pathologically by vacuolar degeneration of the spinal cord white matter, appears to be the most common myelopathy associated with HIV infection [79]. The vacuolation is generally found of the lateral and posterior columns of the thoracic spinal cord. Consistent with this pathology, the most common clinical manifestation is spastic paraparesis and sensory ataxia. Sixty to 75 percent of patients also have accompanying ADC [66,79], and most have known AIDS. However, McArthur [66] reported an HIV seropositive patient who presented with a mild spastic paraparesis without dementia or other AIDS manifestations. Therefore, vacuolar myelopathy can be seen as a first clinical manifestation of acquired immunodeficiency.

The pathogenesis of vacuolar myelopathy is still uncertain. The primary role of HIV infection of the spinal cord has been supported by the occurrence of a similar vacuolation of the spinal cord in mice infected with certain murine retroviruses [36]. The isolation of HIV from the CSF (antemortem) and spinal cord (postmortem) of an AIDS patient who developed incontinence and paraplegia and the pathologic finding of vacuolar changes in the patient's spinal cord provide further evidence for the primary role of HIV [44]. Petito and colleagues [79] found no evidence of spinal cord infection with CMV, adenovirus, herpes simplex virus, herpes zoster virus, or *T. gondii* on detailed histochemical and pathological examination of the spinal cords of seven patients dying with vacuolar myelopathy. It thus appears that strong but circumstantial evidence implicates HIV in the pathogenesis of this entity, for which no effective treatment has been identified.

Other Myelopathies in AIDS

Other clinical syndromes associated with myelopathy have been described in patients with AIDS. Rance and co-workers [87] reported four patients with AIDS who had severe acral paresthesiae, suggestive of a sensory neuronopathy. All four patients also suffered from ADC. Degeneration of the fasciculus gracilis was found on pathologic examination, although direct evidence of HIV infection was not. The authors speculated that the pathogenesis of the myelopathy may have been direct infection of lumbar dorsal root ganglia.

Other viral pathogens may cause myelopathy in immunocompromised patients. For example, CMV appears to be pathogenic in some patients with demyelination of the posterior column [69]. Herpes simplex type I and II and herpes zoster have also been implicated as causes of myelitis, although not in known HIV-infected patients [42,46,55]. In herpes simplex infections, the pathogenesis involves retrograde viral spread from sacral nerves to the spinal cord [42,55].

Inflammatory Demyelinating Polyneuropathy

The clinical manifestations of inflammatory demyelinating polyneuropathy can take on two forms. In some patients, the presentation is that of an acute demyelinating neuropathy (Guillain-Barré syndrome), while others will demonstrate a more chronic course with a predominance of motor weakness [15,66]. Examination of the CSF in patients with these disorders reveals pleocytosis, elevated protein, reversal of the normal T-cell helper-suppressor ratios, and an abnormal immunoglobulin index (ratio of CSF to serum immunoglobulins divided by the ratio of CSF to serum albumin) [15, 61, 66]. Nerve biopsies have revealed typical changes of inflammatory demyelinating polyneuropathy with mononuclear-macrophage infiltration and demyelination with no evidence of vasculitis [15,61], while nerve conduction studies have shown the characteristic pattern of demyelination [15].

Although many of the patients with inflammatory polyneuropathy improve spontaneously, Cornblath and associates [15] suggest that patients should be treated with plasmapheresis. Corticosteroids have also been tried, with mixed results [15,61].

Interestingly, unlike most of the neurologic manifestations of AIDS, inflammatory demyelinating polyneuropathy is frequently a very early manifestation of HIV infection, usually occurring before the onset of frank AIDS. This suggests that infection with HIV may, during its early phase, disrupt the immune system in a way that manifests itself as an autoimmune attack on neuronal myelin [66]. This autoimmune phenomenon often resolves spontaneously, thereby distinguishing itself from most other manifestations of direct HIV infection, and may not portend a rapid progression to full-blown AIDS [50]. The frequent occurrence of inflammatory polyneuropathy before other clinical manifestations of AIDS dictates that serologic tests for HIV should be checked in patients presenting with this syndrome [15].

Although most reported patients with demyelinating peripheral nerve disorders have had a symmetric polyneuropathy, Lipkin and coworkers [63] described nine patients with generalized lymphadenopathy and mononeuropathy, often presenting as mononeuritis multiplex. McArthur [66] also reported two patients with multiple mononeuropathies. Nerve biopsies in these patients revealed vasculitic changes and centrofascicular necrosis, suggestive of an immune complex pathogenesis. In Lipkin's series [63], trials of corticosteroids were ineffective, but two patients went into prolonged spontaneous remissions.

Sensory Neuropathy

Unlike the syndrome of inflammatory demyelinating polyneuropathy, which often presents early in the course of HIV infection, a painful sensory neuropathy has been described in patients with known AIDS or ARC. Cornblath and McArthur [14] described 26 patients with sensory neuropathy; 20 had AIDS and 6 had ARC. The most common presenting complaints were pains in the soles and paresthesia of the feet. On examination, most had diminished or absent ankle jerks, while nearly half had increased patellar reflexes. Nerve conduction studies revealed a neuropathy affecting both sensory and motor fibers, while sural nerve biopsies demonstrated vasculitis and axonal loss. The investigators were unable to culture HIV from sural nerve specimens. Therefore, the etiology of sensory neuropathy in AIDS remains uncertain, although McArthur [66] suggests that HIV infection of dorsal root ganglion neurons, immune complex vasculitis, and nutritional and toxic factors might all play a role.

At the present time, treatment of sensory neuropathy is limited to the use of drugs with efficacy against neuropathic pain, like carbamazepine or amitriptyline [14]. Although the use of AZT lead to clinical and electrophysiologic improvement in one patient [33], many more patients show no improvement [14,66].

Myopathy

Fewer than 15 patients have been reported with myositis and HIV infection [1,16,99]. The presentations were classic for myositis, that is, myalgias, proximal muscle weakness, and elevated serum creatine phosphokinase. Muscle biopsies have revealed the presence of HIV in some cases, along with muscle necrosis and inflammatory cells. The course has been variable, although some patients have demonstrated clinical improvement (usually transient) with corticosteroid therapy [16,99].

Radiculitis

The most common cause of nerve root infection (radiculitis) in patients with AIDS is herpes zoster [61]. Up to 10 percent of AIDS patients develop dermatomal shingles at some time in their course, and about one-quarter of these develop disseminated zoster. Pain control and local care are probably all that are necessary for dermatomal shingles involving thoracic nerve roots. However, the incidence of severe myeloradiculitis and motor deficts appears to increase markedly with involvement of cervical and lumbar dermatomes. The use of high-dose (30 mg/kg/day) intravenous acyclovir has been recommended in these patients [66]. In patients who develop post-herpetic neuralgia, agents like amitriptyline may be necessary to control pain. Because of the dangers of further immunosuppression, no studies have evaluated the use of corticosteroids (in an attempt to prevent post-herpetic neuralgia) in patients with AIDS and dermatomal zoster.

A small number of cases of progressive radiculopathy involving sacral and lumbar roots have been reported and attributed to infection with CMV [3,25,77]. In some of these patients, cytomegalic inclusions, demyelination, and inflammatory infiltrates have been demonstrated in nerve roots, and CMV has been identified in cells [25]. The efficacy of anticytomegaloviral agents like ganciclovir in the treatment of CMV radiculitis is unknown [51].

OTHER NEUROLOGIC MANIFESTATIONS OF AIDS

Cerebrovascular Complications

The incidence of cerebrovascular complications in AIDS patients has ranged from 0.5 to 7.0 percent in two large series [61,66]. These complications have been almost evenly divided between bland infarction and hemorrhage. In the case of infarction, the most common predisposing cause appears to be nonbacterial thrombotic endocarditis, although vasculitis has rarely been implicated [61,113]. The major risk factors for CNS hemorrhage are thrombocytopenia and CNS tumors, especially when the tumors are biopsied [61].

Metabolic Encephalopathy

As in any seriously ill patient with multi-organ system disease, metabolic derangements can both cause altered mentation and exacerbate an underlying CNS process [66]. Any of the pulmonary infections in AIDS patients may cause hypoxemia and thus encephalopathy. Electrolyte disorders such as hyponatremia may be caused by an AIDS-related infection (e.g., CMV adrenalitis) or may be side effect of therapy (e.g., secondary to hypotonic fluids given with intravenous trimethoprim-sulfamethoxazole). Hyponatremia may be present in a majority of hospitalized patients with AIDS [117,110] and a substantial percent of those with ARC. Most patients with hyponatremia and AIDS have inappropriately elevated plasma vasopressin levels [110]. A substantial number will have adrenal insufficiency, often secondary to adrenal damage associated with the AIDS virus [38,106]. In the near future, AIDS will probably be a major cause of hyponatremia in hospitalized subjects [38,110]. Renal failure has been reported in AIDS [38] and may lead to uremic encephalopathy [33,88]. A number of the therapeutic agents used in AIDS patients, such as AZT and ganciclovir, can cause reversible somnolence or delirium [12,91], and pentamidine isethionate can cause hypoglycemia [95]. Of course, patients with ADC may be particularly prone to develop altered sensorium with the use of psychoactive medications.

AREAS FOR FUTURE RESEARCH

The frequency and severity of the neurologic manifestations of HIV infection present a number of difficult problems and challenges for future research. First, we still do not know exactly when HIV enters the CNS, although recent evidence points to early invasion near the time of seroconversion. Second, we remain uncertain about the elapsed time between CNS infection and neurologic manifestations. Accumulating evidence points to a long latency period in some patients. Even if effective systemic therapies for HIV or opportunistic infections were available, this long latency period raises the specter of late neurologic relapses if the therapies were unable to destroy the reservoir of HIV in the CNS. Third, we do not know where or how HIV induces neurologic deterioration. Delineating the site of infection may prove to be of vital importance, since systemically administered drugs may eradicate infection in CNS vascular endothelium but not in glial cells. Similarly, determining the mode of pathogenesis of HIV will also impact on strategies to design effective therapies. Many observers have been struck by the paucity of histologic findings and the small numbers of infected cells in patients with clinically (and often radiologically) severe CNS disease. It may be that HIV exerts its neuropathogenicity through indirect mechanisms, which will need to be understood and overcome before effective treatments can be designed.

Finally, the possibility exists that effective therapy for many of the neurologic manifestations of AIDS will not be forthcoming in the near future. Although discovery of a vaccine would prevent further HIV infection, it would not deter the progression of disease in the millions of people in the United States who are already infected. The provision of compassionate supportive care to these individuals will prove to be a complex and perhaps overwhelming challenge to our medical, economic, and political institutions.

REFERENCES

1. Bailey, R. O., Turok, D. I., Jaufmann, B. P., and Singh, J. K. Myositis and acquired immunodeficiency syndrome. *Hum. Pathol.* 18:749, 1987.
2. Bedri, J., Weistein, W., and DeGregorio, P. Progressive multifocal leukoencephalopathy in acquired immunodeficiency syndrome. *N. Engl. J. Med.* 309:492, 1983.
3. Behar, R., Wiley, C., and McCutchan, J. A. Cytomegalovirus polyradiculopathy in acquired immune deficiency syndrome. *Neurology* 37:557, 1987.
4. Belman, A. L., Ultmann, M. H., Horoupian, D., et al. Neurological complication in infants and children with acquired immunodeficiency syndrome. *Ann. Neurol.* 18:560, 1985.
5. Black P. HIV, AIDS, and the brain. *N. Engl. J. Med.* 313:1538, 1985.
6. Blum, L. W., Chambers, R. A., Schwartzman, R. J., and Streletz, L. J. Progressive multifocal leukoencephalopathy in acquired immune deficiency syndrome. *Arch. Neurol.* 42:137, 1985.
7. Budka, H. Multinucleated giant cells in brain: A hallmark of the acquired immune deficiency syndrome (AIDS). *Acta Neuropathol. (Berl.)* 69:253, 1986.
8. Cantrill, H. L., Henry, K., Sannerud, K., et al. HIV infection of the retina (correspondence). *N. Engl. J. Med.* 318:1539, 1988.
9. Centers for Disease Control. Revision of CDC surveillance case definition for acquired

immunodeficiency syndrome. *M.M.W.R.* 36 (Suppl. 1s):3, 1987.

10. Chiodi, F., Asjo, B., Fenyo, E.-M., et al. Isolation of human immunodeficiency virus from cerebrospinal fluid of antibody-positive virus carrier without neurological symptoms. *Lancet* 2:1276, 1986.
11. Clements, J. E. Hypothesis on the molecular basis of nononcogenic retroviral diseases. *Rev. Infect. Dis.* 7:68, 1985.
12. Collaborative DHPG Treatment Study Group. Treatment of serious cytomegalovirus infections with 9-(1,3 dihydroxy-2-propoxymethyl) guanine in patients with AIDS and other immunodeficiencies. *N. Engl. J. Med.* 314:801, 1986.
13. Cooper, D. A., Gold, J., Maclean, P., et al. Acute AIDS retrovirus infection: Definition of a clinical illness associated with seroconversion. *Lancet* 1:537, 1985.
14. Cornblath, D. R., and McArthur, J. C. Predominantly sensory neuropathy in patients with AIDS and AIDS-related complex. *Neurology* 38:794, 1988.
15. Cornblath, D. R., McArthur, J. C., Kennedy, P. G. E., et al. Inflammatory demyelinating peripheral neuropathies associated with human T-cell lymphotropic virus type III infection. *Ann. Neurol.* 21:32, 1987.
16. Dalakas, M. C., Pezeshkpour, G. H., Gravell, M., and Sever, J. L. Polymyositis associated with AIDS retrovirus. *J.A.M.A.* 256:2381, 1986.
17. de la Monte, S. M., Ho, D. D., Schooley, R. T., et al. Subacute encephalomyelitis of AIDS and its relation to HTLV-III infection. *Neurology* 37:562, 1987.
18. Devita, V. T., Jr., Broder, S., Fauci, A. S., et al. Developmental therapeutics and the acquired immunodeficiency syndrome. *Ann. Intern. Med.* 106:568, 1987.
19. DeWitt, L. D., Buonanno, F. S., Kistler, J. P., et al. Central pontine myelinolysis: Demonstration by nuclear magnetic resonance. *Neurology* 34:570, 1984.
20. DiCarlo, E. F., Amberson, J. B., Metroka, C. A., et al. Malignant lymphomas and the acquired immunodeficiency syndrome. *Arch. Pathol. Lab. Med.* 110:1012, 1986.
21. Dix, R. D., Waitzman, D. M., Follansbee, S., et al. Herpes simplex virus type 2 encephalitis in two homosexual men with persistent lymphadenopathy. *Ann. Neurol.* 17:203, 1985.
22. Dreyer, E. B., Kaiser, P. K., Offermann, J. T., et al. HIV-1 coat protein neurotoxicity prevented by calcium channel antagonists. *Science* 248:364, 1990.
23. Egbert, P. R., Pollard, R. B., Gallagher, J. G., and Merigan, T. C. Cytomegalovirus retinitis in immunosuppressed hosts: I. Natural history and effects of treatment with adenine arabinoside. *Ann. Intern. Med.* 93:655, 1980.
24. Egbert, P. R., Pollard, R. B., Gallagher, J. G., and Merigan, T. C. Cytomegalovirus retinitis in immunosuppressed hosts: II. Ocular manifestations. *Ann. Intern. Med.* 93:664, 1980.
25. Eidelberg, D., Sotrel, A., Vogel, H., et al. Progressive polyradiculopathy in acquired immune deficiency syndrome. *Neurology* 36:912, 1986.
26. Elkin, C. M., Leon, E., Grenell, S. L., and Leeds, N. E. Intracranial lesions in the acquired immunodeficiency syndrome. *J.A.M.A.* 253:393, 1985.
27. Eng, R. H. K., Bishburg, E., Smith, S. M., and Kapila, R. Cryptococcal infections in patients with the acquired immune deficiency syndrome. *Am. J. Med.* 81:19, 1986.
28. Epstein, L. G., Sharer, L. R., Joshi, V. V., et al. Progressive encephalopathy in children with acquired immunodeficiency syndrome. *Ann. Neurol.* 17:488, 1985.
29. Fauci, A. S., Masur, H., Gelmann, E. P., et al. The acquired immunodeficiency syndrome: An update. *Ann. Intern. Med.* 102:800, 1985.
30. Fischer, P.-A., and Enzensberger, W. Neurological complications in AIDS. *J. Neurol.* 234:269, 1987.
31. Fischl, M. A., Richman, D. D., Grieco, M. H., et al. The efficacy of azidothymidine (AZT) in the treatment of patients with AIDS and AIDS-related complex. *N. Engl. J. Med.* 317:185, 1987.
32. Folstein, M. F., Folstein, S. E., and McHugh, P. R. Mini-Mental State: A practical method for grading the cognitive state of patients for the clinician. *J. Psychiatr. Res.* 12:189, 1975.
33. Fraser, C. L., and Arieff, A. I. Nervous system complications in uremia. *Ann. Intern. Med.* 109:143, 1988.
34. Freeman, W. R., Lerner, C. W., Mines, J. A., et al. A prospective study of the ophthalmologic findings in the acquired immune deficiency syndrome. *Am. J. Ophthalmol.* 97:133, 1984.
35. Gabuzda, D. H., Ho, D. D., de la Monte, S. M., Hirsch, M. S., et al. Immunohistochemical identification of HTLV-III antigen in brains of patients with AIDS. *Ann. Neurol.* 20:289, 1986.
36. Gardner, M. B. Retroviral spongiform polioencephalomyelopathy. *Rev. Infect. Dis.* 7:99, 1985.
37. Gill, P. S., Levine, A. M., Meyer, P. R., et al. Primary central nervous system lymphoma in homosexual men: Clinical, immunologic and pathological features. *Am. J. Med.* 78:742, 1985.
38. Glassock, R. J., Cohen, A. H., Danovitch, G., and Parsa, K. P. Human immunodeficiency virus (HIV) infection and the kidney. *Ann. Intern. Med.* 112:35, 1990.

39. Grant, I., Atkinson, J. H., Kennedy, C., et al. Neuropsychological findings in HIV infection: Relation to seropositivity and treatment with azidothymidine. *J. Clin. Exp. Neuropsychol.* 9:261, 1987.
40. Gyorkey, F., Melnick, J. L., and Gyorkey, P. Human immunodeficiency virus in brain biopsies of patients with AIDS and progressive encephalopathy. *J. Infect. Dis.* 155:870, 1987.
41. Henry, J. M., Heffner, R. R., Jr., Dillard, S. H., et al. Primary malignant lymphomas of the central nervous system. *Cancer* 34:1293, 1974.
42. Hinthorn, D. R., Baker, L. H., Romig, D. A., and Lui, C. Recurrent conjugal neuralgia caused by herpesvirus hominis type 2. *J.A.M.A.* 236:587, 1976.
43. Ho, D. D., Pomerantz, R. J., and Kaplan, J. C. Pathogenesis of infection with human immunodeficiency virus. *N. Engl. J. Med.* 317:278, 1987.
44. Ho, D. D., Rota, T. R., Schooley, R. T., et al. Isolation of HTLV-III from cerebrospinal fluid and neural tissues of patients with neurologic syndromes related to the acquired immunodeficiency syndrome. *N. Engl. J. Med.* 313:1493, 1985.
45. Ho, D. D., Sarngadharan, M. G., Resnick, L., et al. Primary human T-lymphotropic virus type III infection. *Ann. Intern. Med.* 103:880, 1985.
46. Hogan, E. L., and Krigman, M. R. Herpes zoster myelitis: Evidence for viral invasion of the spinal cord. *Arch. Neurol.* 29:253, 1973.
47. Holland, G. N., Pepose, J. S., Pettit, T. H., et al. Acquired immune deficiency syndrome: Ocular manifestations. *Ophthalmology* 90:859, 1983.
48. Holland, G. N., Sakamoto, M. J., Hardy, D., et al. Treatment of cytomegalovirus retinopathy in patients with acquired immunodeficiency syndrome. *Arch. Ophthalmol.* 104:1794, 1986.
49. Hollander, H., and Levy, J. A. Neurologic abnormalities and recovery of human immunodeficiency virus from cerebrospinal fluid. *Ann. Intern. Med.* 106:692, 1987.
50. Holzman, R. S., Walsch, C. M., and Karpatkin, S. Risk of the acquired immunodeficiency syndrome among thrombocytopenic and nonthrombocytopenic homosexual men seropositive for the human immunodeficiency virus. *Ann. Intern. Med.* 106:383, 1987.
51. Jacobson, M. A., and Mills, J. Serious cytomegalovirus disease in the acquired immunodeficiency syndrome (AIDS). *Ann. Intern. Med.* 108:585, 1988.
52. Johns, D. R., Tierney, M., and Felsenstein, D. Alteration in the natural history of neurosyphilis by concurrent infection with the human immunodeficiency virus. *N. Engl. J. Med.* 316:1569, 1987.
53. Jordan, B. D., Navia, B. A., Petito, C., et al. Neurological syndromes complicating AIDS. *Front. Radiat. Ther. Oncol.* 19:82, 1985.
54. Kennedy, P. G., Newsome, D. A., Hess, J., et al. Cytomegalovirus but not human T lymphotropic virus type III/lymphadenopathy associated virus detected by in situ hybridization in retinal lesions in patients with the acquired immune deficiency syndrome. *Br. Med. J.* [*Clin. Res.*] 293:162, 1986.
55. Klastersky, J., Cappel, R., Snoeck, J. M., et al. Ascending myelitis in association with herpes simplex virus. *N. Engl. J. Med.* 287:182, 1972.
56. Kovacs, J. A., Kovacs, A. A., Polis, M., et al. Cryptococcosis in the acquired immunodeficiency syndrome. *Ann. Intern. Med.* 103:533, 1985.
57. Kucharczyk, W., Brant-Zawadzki, M., and Norman, D. Magnetic resonance imaging of the central nervous system: An update. *West. J. Med.* 142:54, 1985.
58. Larson, E. B., Lo, B., and Williams, M. E. Evaluation and care of elderly patients with dementia. *J. Gen. Intern. Med.* 1:116, 1986.
59. Laskin, O. L., Stahl-Bayliss, C. M., Kalman, C. M., and Rosecan, L. R. Use of ganciclovir to treat serious cytomegalovirus infections in patients with AIDS. *J. Infect. Dis.* 155:323, 1987.
60. Levy, J. A., Shimabukuro, J., Hollander, H., et al. Isolation of AIDS-associated retrovirus from cerebrospinal fluid and brain of patients with neurological symptoms. *Lancet* 2:586, 1985.
61. Levy, R. M., Bredesen, D. E., and Rosenblum, M. L. Neurological manifestations of the acquired immunodeficiency syndrome (AIDS): Experience of UCSF and review of the literature. *J. Neurosurg.* 62:475, 1985.
62. Levy, R. M., Rosenbloom, S., and Perrett, L. V. Neuroradiologic findings in AIDS: A review of 200 cases. *A.J.R.* 147:977, 1986.
63. Lipkin, W. I., Parry, G., Kiprov, D., and Abrams, D. Inflammatory neuropathy in homosexual men with lymphadenopathy. *Neurology* 35:1479, 1985.
64. Luft, B. J., Brooks, R. G., Conley, F. K., et al. Toxoplasmic encephalitis in patients with acquired immunodeficiency syndrome. *J.A.M.A.* 252:913, 1984.
65. Masur, H., Lane, H. C., Palestine, A., et al. Effect of 9-(1,3-dihydroxy-2-propoxymethyl) guanine on serious cytomegalovirus disease in eight immunosuppressed homosexual men. *Ann. Intern. Med.* 104:41, 1986.
66. McArthur, J. C. Neurologic manifestations of AIDS. *Medicine* (Baltimore) 66:407, 1987.
67. McArthur, J. C., Cohen, B. A., Farzedegan, H., et al. Cerebrospinal fluid abnormalities in homosexual men with and without neuropsychiatric findings. *Ann. Neurol.* 23(Suppl.):S34, 1988.

68. Mills, J. *Pneumocystis carinii* and *Toxoplasma gondii* infections in patients with AIDS. *Rev. Infect. Dis.* 8:1001, 1986.
69. Moskowitz, L. B., Gregorios, J. B., Hensley, G. T., and Berger, J. R. Cytomegalovirus: Induced demyelination associated with acquired immune deficiency syndrome. *Arch. Pathol. Lab. Med.* 108:873, 1984.
70. Moskowitz, L. B., Hensley, G. T., Chan, J. C., et al. Brain biopsies in patients with acquired immunodeficiency syndrome. *Arch. Pathol. Lab. Med.* 108:368, 1984.
71. Navia, B. A., Cho, E.-S., Petito, C. K., and Price, R. W. The AIDS dementia complex: II. Neuropathology. *Ann. Neurol.* 19:525, 1986.
72. Navia, B. A., Jordan, B. D., and Price, R. W. The AIDS dementia complex: I. Clinical features. *Ann. Neurol.* 19:517, 1986.
73. Navia, B. A., Petito, C. K., Gold, J. W. M., et al. Cerebral toxoplasmosis complicating the acquired immune deficiency syndrome: Clinical and neuropathological findings in 27 patients. *Ann. Neurol.* 19:224, 1986.
74. Navia, B. A., and Price, R. W. The acquired immunodeficiency syndrome dementia complex as the presenting or sole manifestation of human immunodeficiency virus infection. *Arch. Neurol.* 44:65, 1987.
75. Nielsen, S. L., Petito, C. K., Urmacher, C. D., and Posner, J. B. Subacute encephalitis in acquired immune deficiency syndrome: A postmortem study. *Am. J. Clin. Pathol.* 82:678, 1984.
76. Palestine, A. G., Stevens, G., Jr., Lane, H. C., et al. Treatment of cytomegalovirus retinitis with dihydroxy propoxymethyl guanine. *Am. J. Ophthalmol.* 101:95, 1986.
77. Parry, G. J. Peripheral neuropathies associated with human immunodeficiency virus infection. *Ann. Neurol.* 23(Suppl.):S49, 1988.
78. Petito, C. K. Review of central nervous system pathology in human immunodeficiency virus infection. *Ann. Neurol.* 23(Suppl.):S54, 1988.
79. Petito, C. K., Navia, B. A., Cho, E.-S., et al. Vacuolar myelopathy pathologically resembling subacute combined degeneration in patients with the acquired immunodeficiency syndrome. *N. Engl. J. Med.* 312:874, 1985.
80. Pomerantz, R. J., Kuritzkes, D. R., de la Monte, S. M., et al. Infection of the retina by human immunodeficiency virus type I. *N. Engl. J. Med.* 317:1643, 1987.
81. Post, M. J., Hensley, G. T., Moskowitz, L. B., and Fischl, M. Cytomegalic inclusion virus encephalitis in patients with AIDS: CT, clinical and pathologic correlation. *A.J.R.* 146:1229, 1986.
82. Post, M. J., Sheldon, J. J., Hensley, G. T., et al. Central nervous system disease in acquired immunodeficiency syndrome: Prospective correlation using CT, MR imaging, and pathologic studies. *Radiology* 158:141, 1986.
83. Price, R. W., Brew, B., Sidtis, J., et al. The brain in AIDS: Central nervous system HIV-1 infection and AIDS dementia complex. *Science* 239:586, 1988.
84. Price, R. W., Sidtis, J., and Rosenblum, M. The AIDS dementia complex: Some current questions. *Ann. Neurol.* 23(Suppl.):S27, 1988.
85. Public Health Service. Coolfont report: A PHS plan for prevention and control of AIDS and the AIDS virus. *Public Health Rep.* 101:341, 1986.
86. Pumarola-Sune, T., Navia, B. A., Cordon-Cardo, C., et al. HIV antigen in the brains of patients with the AIDS dementia complex. *Ann. Neurol.* 21:490, 1987.
87. Rance, N. E., McArthur, J. C., Cornblath, D. R., et al. Gracile tract degeneration in patients with sensory neuropathy and AIDS. *Neurology* 38:265, 1988.
88. Rao, T. K. S., Friedman, E. A., and Nicastri, A. D. The types of renal disease in the acquired immunodeficiency syndrome. *N. Engl. J. Med.* 316:1062, 1987.
89. Resnick, L., Berger, J. R., Shapshak, P., and Tourtellotte, W. W. Early penetration of the blood-brain-barrier by HIV. *Neurology* 38:8, 1988.
90. Rhodes, R. H. Histopathology of the central nervous system in the acquired immunodeficiency syndrome. *Hum. Pathol.* 18:636, 1987.
91. Richman, D. D., Fischl, M. A., Grieco, M. H., et al. The toxicity of azidothymidine (AZT) in the treatment of patients with AIDS and AIDS-related complex. *N. Engl. J. Med.* 317:192, 1987.
92. Rosenblum, M. L., Levy, R. M., Bredesen, D. E., et al. Primary central nervous system lymphomas in patients with AIDS. *Ann. Neurol.* 23(Suppl.):S13, 1988.
93. Royal, W., III, and McArthur, J. C. HIV-associated neurologic disorders: Part 1. Noninfectious problems. *J. Crit. Illness* 4(7):24, 1989.
94. Ryder, J. W., Croen, K., Kleinschmidt-DeMasters, B. K., et al. Progressive encephalitis three months after resolution of cutaneous zoster in a patient with AIDS. *Ann. Neurol.* 19:182, 1986.
95. Sands, M., Kron, M. A., and Brown, R. B. Pentamidine: A review. *Rev. Infect. Dis.* 7:625, 1985.
96. Sharer, L. R., Cho, E.-S., and Epstein, L. G. Multinucleated giant cells and HTLV-III in AIDS encephalopathy. *Hum. Pathol.* 16:760, 1985.
97. Sharer, L. R., Epstein, L. G., Cho, E.-S., et al. Pathology of AIDS encephalopathy in children: Evidence for LAV/HTLV-III infection in brain. *Hum. Pathol.* 17:271, 1986.

98. Shaw, G. M., Harper, M. E., Hahn, B. H., et al. HTLV-III infection in brains of children and adults with AIDS encephalopathy. *Science* 227:177, 1985.
99. Simpson, D. M., and Bender, A. N. HTLV-III-associated myopathy. *Neurology* 37(Suppl.):319, 1987.
100. Snider, W. D., Simpson, D. M., Nielson, G., et al. Neurological complication of acquired immune deficiency syndrome: Analysis of 50 patients. *Ann. Neurol.* 14:403, 1983.
101. Snyder, L. Life, death, and the American College of Physicians: The Cruzan case. *Ann. Intern. Med.* 112:802, 1990.
102. Steinbrook, R., and Lo, B. Decision making for incompetent patients by designated proxy: California's new law. *N. Engl. J. Med.* 310:1598, 1984.
103. Stoler, M. H., Eskin, T. A., Benn, S., et al. Human T-cell lymphotropic virus type III infection of the central nervous system. *J.A.M.A.* 256:2360, 1986.
104. Steinbrook, R., Lo, B., Tirpack, J., et al. Ethical dilemmas in caring for patients with the acquired immunodeficiency syndrome. *Ann. Intern. Med.* 103:787, 1985.
105. Tang, W. W., Feinstein, E. I., and Massry, S. G. Hyponatremia in patients with AIDS and the AIDS related complex. *Kidney Int.* 33:211, 1988.
106. Tapper, M. L., Rotterdam, H. Z., Lerner, C. W., et al. Adrenal necrosis in the acquired immune deficiency syndrome. *Ann. Intern. Med.* 100:357, 1984.
107. The TE Study Group. Assessment of therapy for toxoplasma encephalitis. *Am. J. Med.* 82:907, 1987.
108. Tramont, E. C. Syphilis in the AIDS era. *N. Engl. J. Med.* 316:1600, 1987.
109. Vazeux, R., Brousse, N., Jarry, A., et al. AIDS subacute encephalitis: Identification of HIV-infected cells. *Am. J. Pathol.* 126:403, 1987.
110. Vitting, K. E., Gardenswartz, M. H., Zabetakis, P. M., et al. Frequency of hyponatremia and nonosmolar vasopressin release in the acquired immunodeficiency syndrome. *J.A.M.A.* 263:973, 1990.
111. Wanke, C., Tuazon, C. U., Kovacs, A., et al. Toxoplasma encephalitis in patients with the acquired immune deficiency syndrome: Diagnosis and response to therapy. *Am. J. Trop. Med. Hyg.* 36:509, 1987.
112. Wiley, C. A., Schrier, R. D., Nelson, J. A., et al. Cellular localization of human immunodeficiency virus infection within the brains of acquired immunodeficiency syndrome patients. *Proc. Natl. Acad. Sci.* 83:7089, 1986.
113. Yanker, B. A., Skolnik, P. R., Shoukimas, G. M., et al. Cerebral granulomatous angiitis associated with isolation of human T-lymphotropic virus type III from central nervous system. *Ann. Neurol.* 20:362, 1986.
114. Yarchoan, R., Berg, G., Brouwers, P., et al. Response of human immunodeficiency-virus-associated neurological disease to 3′-azido-3′-deoxythymidine. *Lancet* 1:132, 1987.
115. Yarchoan, R., and Broder, S. Development of antiretroviral therapy for the acquired immunodeficiency syndrome and related disorders. *N. Engl. J. Med.* 316:557, 1987.
116. Ziegler, J. L., Beckstead, J. A., Volberding, P. A., et al. Non-Hodgkin's lymphoma in 90 homosexual men: Relation to generalized lymphadenopathy and the acquired immunodeficiency syndrome. *N. Engl. J. Med.* 311:565, 1984.
117. Zuger, A., Louie, E., Holzman, R. S., et al. Cryptococcal disease in patients with the AIDS: Diagnostic features and outcome of treatment. *Ann. Intern. Med.* 104:234, 1986.

18 Recent Advances in Bacterial Meningitis

Keith R. Powell

In 1913 Flexner [8] published the results of a study demonstrating that antiserum therapy could reduce the mortality of meningococcal meningitis from about 70 to 30 percent. Antiserum therapy was perceived as an improvement in outcome but not as the solution. Investigators continued attempts to develop vaccines to prevent bacterial infections as well as seeking to improve the treatment of infections once they had begun. As early as the 1930s an effective pneumococcal vaccine was licensed for use in the United States. However, when antimicrobial agents became readily available, there was little interest in preventing infections that could be treated so easily. The pneumococcal vaccine was a commercial failure, and research necessary to develop vaccines to prevent infections with bacteria that cause meningitis was largely abandoned until the 1960s.

With time it became apparent that antimicrobial agents do not change the morbidity and mortality associated with bacterial meningitis as dramatically as hoped for. In fact, the overall mortality due to bacterial meningitis has remained at about 14 percent since 1950. Because the success of antimicrobial therapy was incomplete, investigations in all aspects of bacterial meningitis have begun anew. Selected recent advances in our knowledge about bacterial meningitis will be reviewed.

PATHOGENESIS

Species of Bacteria that Cause Meningitis

It is striking that only a few species of bacteria cause an overwhelming majority of cases of bacterial meningitis. For normal hosts who are no longer neonates, meningitis is caused by *Haemophilus influenzae* type b (Hib), *Streptococcus pneumoniae,* and *Neisseria meningitidis.* Meningitis in neonates is caused primarily by *Escherichia coli, Streptococcus agalactia* (group B streptococci), and *Lysteria monocytogenes.* Although *H. influenzae* type b causes the greatest number of cases of bacterial meningitis overall, disease caused by this bacteria occurs mainly in the first 5 years of life.

Serotypes of Species of Bacteria that Cause Meningitis

The bacteria that cause meningitis are almost always encapsulated, as are most organisms that cause bacteremia. However, the bacteria that usually cause bacteremia are not the same species that cause meningitis. Thus, while encapsulation seems to be an important virulence factor in the pathogenesis of bacteremia, the role of the capsule in the pathogenesis of meningitis is not as clear. Encapsulated bacteria of the same species are subclassified as serotypes based on differences in capsular polysaccharides.

Although the number of species of bacteria that cause meningitis is limited, more than one serotype of most species is associated with meningitis (Table 18-1). However, there are apparently some capsular polysaccharides that facilitate entry into the cerebrospinal fluid (CSF) more readily than others. *E. coli* of the K1 capsular serotype is responsible for 84 percent of cases of neonatal meningitis caused by *E. coli,* despite the fact that there are over 100 capsular serotypes of *E. coli.* Furthermore, the K1 capsular polysaccharide is almost identical to the capsular polysaccharides of *N. meningitidis* group B and group B streptococcus type III. Thus the majority of cases of neonatal meningitis can be attributed to bacteria with similar capsular polysaccharides.

Some role for the type of capsular polysaccharide in pathogenesis is also supported by the limited number of serotypes of other species that cause meningitis. Of the 84 serotypes of *S. pneumoniae,* 15 are responsible for 80 percent of serious streptococcal infections in the United States. There are at least six capsular types of *H. influenzae* (types a–f), yet meningitis is caused almost exclusively by type b. Likewise, there are 12 serotypes of *N. meningitidis,* yet groups A, B, and C are responsible for most cases of meningitis.

Exactly what it is about these relatively few serotypes of encapsulated bacteria that allows them to invade the central nervous system is not known. It might be that these selected organisms are truly neurotrophic by virtue of enhanced attachment to or penetration of the blood-brain barrier, or it may simply be that particular capsular structures allow for more successful evasion of host defenses that normally clear bacteria from the bloodstream.

Aquisition of Bacteria that Cause Meningitis

It is fairly clear that the minimal requirements for acquiring bacterial meningitis are for a person without specific antibodies to become colonized with one of these pathogens. Young infants are generally protected from disease caused by *H. influenzae* type b, *S. pneumoniae,* and *N. meningitidis* by maternal immunoglobulin G (IgG) antibodies, which they receive transplacentally. Antibody against *E. coli* K1 capsular polysaccharide tends to be of the IgM class, which does not cross the placenta. Since *E. coli* and group B streptococci are normally found in stool and colonizing the birth canal, infants are likely to be heavily exposed to these bacteria

Table 18-1. Serotypes of bacterial species associated with bacterial meningitis

Bacteria	*Number of serotypes*	*Serotypes responsible for most meningitis*
Escherichia coli	> 100	K1
Streptococcus agalactia	5	Group III
Haemophilus influenzae type b	6	Type b
Streptococcus pneumoniae	84	≈15 serotypes
Neisseria meningitidis	12	Groups A, B, C

during passage through the birth canal. Thus, infants are likely to be heavily exposed to *E. coli* and group B streptococci at a time when they are unlikely to have protective antibodies.

The bacteria responsible for the majority of meningitis outside of the neonatal period are part of the "normal respiratory" flora. For example, a prospective study done by Murphy and co-workers [21] showed that 71 percent of toddlers and 48 percent of preschool children attending a day care center were colonized with *H. influenzae* type b at some time over a period of 18 months. During this time no *H. influenzae* type b disease occurred in the day care center. On the other hand, passive protection from transplacentally acquired maternal antibodies is generally gone by 3 months of age. By 5 years of age most children will have protective levels of anticapsular antibody against *H. influenzae* type b. Thus, *H. influenzae* type b resides on the respiratory mucosa of most children at a time when they are susceptible to invasive disease, yet only about 1 in 1000 will have *H. influenzae* type b meningitis.

It is not known why some children get meningitis and others do not. There is evidence, however, for a genetically determined factor or factors being important. For example, the incidence of *H. influenzae* type b meningitis in Navajo Indians is 1.7 per 1000 per year and in Alaskan Eskimos 4.1 per 1000 per year [12]. Equally as striking is the near absence of *H. influenzae* type b disease among some Asian populations like the Japanese. Bacterial genetics also play a role in human disease. In studies involving over 2000 strains of *H. influenzae* type b from all over the world, Musser and colleagues [22] have identified electropherotypes that are more likely to result in asymptomatic carriage as well as types that are more likely to result in invasive disease. Despite these interesting clues, the final relationship between host and bacterial genetics that results in bacterial meningitis is yet to be determined.

Bacteremia

The relative role of inoculum size versus some other virulence factor is not known. In an infant rat model of *H. influenzae* type b meningitis, it takes an intranasal inoculum of at least 100,000 virulent bacteria to consistently cause bacteremia and meningitis [20]. Using the infant rat model of *H. influenzae* type b meningitis, Moxon and Murphy [19] showed that *H. influenzae* type b meningitis could result from the survival of a single bacterium in the bloodstream. Within a few hours of inoculating the nares of infant rats with a mixture of streptomycin-susceptible and streptomycin-resistant *H. influenzae* type b mutants, blood isolates were seldom a mixture of susceptible and resistant organisms. Also, animals with meningitis had *H. influenzae* type b with the same susceptibilities in blood and CSF isolates except in two instances [19]. Thus, although it takes an inoculum of at least 100,000 bacteria to cause bacteremia in this model, the survival of a single bacterium in the blood can result in meningitis.

The role of inoculum size in human disease is not known. However, it would seem that as few as a single bacterium that finds its way into the bloodstream and is able to evade host defenses could result in bacterial meningitis.

Penetration of the Blood-Brain Barrier

Once encapsulated bacteria have invaded the respiratory mucosa, reached the intravascular space, and evaded opsonization, phagocytosis, and clearance, they must then penetrate the blood-brain barrier. The arachnoid membrane, the epithelium of the choroid plexus, and the endothelium of cerebral capillaries are the major sites of the blood-brain barrier. Quagliarello, Long, and Scheld [28] have studied the effects of microorganisms on the blood-brain barrier using an in vitro preparation of cerebral microvessels as well as a rat model of lethal meningitis. Based on these models, it has been shown that the earliest host response at the level of the capillary endothelium is pinocytotic vesicle formation followed by the separation of intercellular tight junctional complexes. These morphologic changes in the endothelium result in increased permeability to albumin and probably to other macromolecules as well. All of the different types of bacteria tested resulted in alterations in the morphology and function of cerebral capillaries. Unencapsulated *H. influenzae* also resulted in increased pinocytotic vesicle formation and increased permeability to albumin, but separation of tight junctions did not occur and animals infected intracisternally did not go on to become bacteremic. The comparisons between encapsulated and unencapsulated *H. influenzae* suggest that encapsulation is not necessary to give rise to morphologic and functional changes in the blood-brain barrier, but encapsulation might result in the progression of the pathologic events by allowing the bacteria to evade host defense mechanisms [28].

The Inflammatory Response

Just as the blood-brain barrier can be injured by nonencapsulated bacteria, it is becoming apparent that whole bacteria are not necessary to stimulate the inflammatory response that follows invasion of the subarachnoid space by bacterial pathogens.

Using a rabbit model of meningitis, Tuomanen and colleagues [37] showed that although infection with encapsulated *S. pneumoniae* was associated with a higher and more sustained CSF bacterial density, encapsulation did not account for changes in CSF chemistry. In fact, CSF leukocytosis and increases in protein and lactic acid concentrations were associated with bacterial densities of 10^5 per milliliter regardless of encapsulation. Glucose concentration began to decrease when the density of *S. pneumoniae* reached 10^6 per milliliter. The authors went on to show that a partially purified cell wall preparation from *S. pneumoniae* induced an inflammatory response when injected into the CSF, while capsular polysaccharides at equivalent concentrations evoked little response [37]. Further experiments with the same model showed that both peptidoglycan and teichoic acid could contribute to inflammation, but the greatest specific activity on a weight basis was induced by teichoic acid [36]. These studies suggest that although the inflammatory response may result in a slowing of bacterial growth, bacterial lysis and the release of cell wall components may in fact result in further inflammation and host injury.

Teichoic acid is a major component of the cell wall of many gram-positive bacteria but is generally not found in gram-negative bacteria. Lipopolysaccharides are a major component of the cell wall of gram-negative bacteria and are made of lipid A, core, and O-side chains. The O-side chains are polysaccharides and are responsible for differences between species and serotypes of bacteria. When the O-side chains are short, the complex is referred to as lipo-oligosaccharide. Experiments with lipo-oligosaccharides similar to the experiments described for teichoic acid showed that when lipo-oligosaccharide derived from the outer membrane of *H. influenzae* type b is injected into rabbits intracisternally, there is a dose-dependent increase in CSF protein concentration as well as CSF pleocytosis [34]. Polymyxin B binds to the lipid A region of endotoxin. When lipo-oligosaccharide is preincubated with polymyxin B before intracisternal injection, the inflammatory response is greatly reduced [34].

The role of polymorphonuclear neutrophils in the inflammatory response has been studied by making rabbits neutropenic by the administration of nitrogen mustard prior to infecting them with *S. pneumoniae* [6]. Somewhat surprisingly, the increase in the number of bacteria was the same in neutropenic and non-neutropenic rabbits. Increases in CSF protein and lactate concentrations were similar in neutropenic and non-neutropenic animals, as were decreases in CSF glucose concentrations [6].

MANAGEMENT OF PATIENTS WITH MENINGITIS

Antimicrobial Therapy

The most important therapeutic intervention in the management of bacterial meningitis is still to administer bactericidal antimicrobial agents that enter the CSF well, as early in the course of disease as possible. Bactericidal antimicrobial agents are preferred in the treatment of meningitis because the subarachnoid space, particularly early in the course of infection, is immunodeficient. Uninfected CSF contains no polymorphonuclear leukocytes and virtually no antibody or complement. Thus bacteria proliferate rapidly and are cleared slowly. Because bacterial cell wall components like teichoic acid, peptidoglycan, and lipo-oligosaccharide are released when cells lyse, Tuomanen and colleagues [36] have proposed that the ideal antimicrobial agent would kill the bacteria without causing cell lysis. This hypothesis has yet to be tested in the treatment of bacterial meningitis in humans.

Selection of Antimicrobial Agents

With the recent proliferation of antimicrobial agents, the choices for initial therapy of suspected bacterial meningitis include several possibilities in each age group. Differences in recommendations between a consensus report on the treatment of bacterial meningitis in infants and children [18] and a "white paper" on bacterial meningitis [38] indicate that experts of equal stature have different opinions on which of several possible antimicrobial agents should be recommended as "state of the art."

Because the bacteria that cause meningitis vary with age, the selection of antimicrobial agents must also be age dependent. The major divisions in age are neonates (birth to 1 month of age), infants (1–2 months of age), infants and children (3 months–6 years of age), and children and adults (older than 6 years of age). Table 18-2 lists the bacterial pathogens of greatest concern by age and choices of antimicrobial agents. The major change in antimicrobial therapy is the availability of third-generation cephalosporins that achieve therapeutic concentrations in the cerebrospinal fluid.

As shown in Table 18-3, the specific activity (inhibitory quotient) of some third-generation cephalosporins against the bacterial pathogens that often cause meningitis is usually 100- to more than 1000-fold that which can be achieved with more traditional antimicrobial agents [38]. Major advantages of the newer cephalosporins include single-agent antimicrobial therapy; avoidance of the potential toxicities of chloramphenicol or aminoglycosides because of predictable pharmacokinetics and low toxicity; and, with ceftriaxone, once-a-day intramuscular administration for the patient who is stable.

A major concern regarding the use of the cephalosporins is the relative lack of experience compared to penicillin (ampicillin) and chloramphenicol. As evidence accumulates that selected third-generation cephalosporins are equivalent to ampicillin and chloramphenicol in terms of early outcome, clinicians still argue that long-term sequelae have not been sufficiently evaluated to recommend changes. There is also evidence that cefuroxime (a second-generation cephalosporin) does not sterilize the

Table 18-2. Antimicrobial therapy for bacterial meningitis by age and pathogen

Age	*Major bacterial pathogens*	*Antimicrobial therapy*
Birth–1 month	*Escherichia coli* Group B streptococci *Listeria monocytogenes*	Ceftriaxone* (or cefotaxime) plus ampicillin or ampicillin plus an aminoglycoside (amikacin or gentamicin)
1–2 months	*Escherichia coli* Group B streptococci *Listeria monocytogenes* *Haemophilus influenzae* type b *Streptococcus pneumoniae* *Neisseria meningitidis*	Ceftriaxone plus ampicillin or ampicillin plus an aminoglycoside plus chloramphenicol
3 months–6 years	*Haemophilus influenzae* type b *Streptococcus pneumoniae* *Neisseria meningitidis*	Ceftriaxone or ampicillin (penicillin) plus chloramphenicol
> 6 years–adult	*Streptococcus pneumoniae* *Neisseria meningitidis*	Penicillin (or ceftriaxone)

* With hyperbilirubinemia, use cefotaxime.

Table 18-3. Inhibitory quotients[a] for selected antimicrobial agents and bacteria

Bacteria	*Ampicillin (3.1–27.3 μg/ml)*[b]	*Chloramphenicol (4.2–16.6 μg/ml)*[b]	*Gentamicin (0.3–3.7 μg/ml)*[b]	*Cefotaxime (0.8–27.2 μg/ml)*[b]	*Ceftriaxone 2.2–13.5 μg/ml)*[b]
Haemophilus influenzae	8–68	5–21	≤1	32–1088	88–540
Neisseria meningitidis	155–1365	5–21	<1	110–3400	550–3375
Streptococcus pneumoniae	62–546	1–5	<1	2–68	22–1350
Escherichia coli	1–9	<1–3	≤1	2–54	9–54
Group B streptococcus	16–137	3–17	<1	8–272	22–1350
Listeria monocytogenes	8–68	<1	<1	0	0

[a] Inhibitory quotient = $\frac{\text{CSF concentration}}{\text{minimum inhibitory concentration}}$

[b] μg/ml of antimicrobial agent in CSF.

Source: Modified from R. Yogev, Advances in diagnosis and treatment of childhood meningitis. *Pediatr. Infect. Dis.* 4:321, 1985. Copyright by Williams & Wilkins.

CSF as rapidly as ceftriaxone [14]. Since delayed sterilization of the CSF is associated with adverse outcomes [15], the use of cefuroxime is not recommended for the treatment of bacterial meningitis.

Because of ceftriaxone's tremendous activity in the CSF against bacterial pathogens (Table 18-3), it is currently the antimicrobial agent preferred for the treatment of bacterial meningitis. Ceftriaxone should be used alone or with ampicillin, depending on the age of the patient and the clinical setting (see Table 18-2). Since the goal is rapid sterilization of the CSF, it is reasonable to give an initial loading dose of 100 mg/kg (not to exceed 2 gm) intravenously, followed by 80 mg/kg (not to exceed 2 gm) once a day. Ampicillin should be included in the treatment of neonates and young infants to cover *Listeria monocytogenes* and enterococci, and its use should also be considered in immunocompromised patients.

Length of Treatment

Recommendations regarding the length of antimicrobic therapy for bacterial meningitis are also changing [29]. There is consensus that it is not necessary to treat uncomplicated *N. meningitidis* meningitis any longer than 7 days. Investigators in Spain treated 50 patients with penicillin for 4 days and saw no relapse or recurrence [7]. Two studies on bacterial meningitis in infants and children suggest that, in uncomplicated cases, 7 days of antimicrobial therapy results in a successful clinical outcome without relapse or recurrence [10,17].

Perhaps of more import, with the current emphasis on the reduction of health care costs, is the completion of therapy for bacterial meningitis in an ambulatory setting. Bradley, Ching, and Phillips [4] completed treatment for bacterial meningitis in 54 infants and children in an ambulatory setting. All patients received ceftriaxone intravenously, 18 on an every 12-hour dosing schedule and 36 dosed once daily. All children who completed therapy at home were afebrile at the time of discharge as well as meeting other criteria. The mean duration of outpatient therapy for these patients was 4.6 days. Relapse or recurrence did not occur. Ceftriaxone therapy was complicated by diarrhea in 13 percent of the meningitis patients [4]. We have treated a number of infants and children with bacterial meningitis as outpatients with once daily intramuscular ceftriaxone [25]. Patients are followed daily and ceftriaxone is administered intramuscularly either at the local doctor's office or at home by a visiting nurse. To date we have observed neither relapse nor recurrence, and both physicians and families prefer outpatient treatment.

Antimicrobial agents remain the most important part of treatment for bacterial meningitis. However, with the availability of new antimicrobial agents that are extremely active against the usual bacterial pathogens and attain good concentrations in the CSF, it is possible to consider shortening therapy and administering antibiotics in an ambulatory setting for selected patients.

Steroids in the Treatment of Bacterial Meningitis

The concept of using steroids early in the course of bacterial meningitis to minimize deleterious effects that might result from the inflammatory process itself is not new. Two prospective placebo-controlled studies were published a few months apart in 1969 [3,5]. DeLemos and Haggerty [5] studied 117 patients and found that the only measurable benefit to the 54 patients who received 40 mg of methylprednisolone every 6 hours for 12 doses was a more rapid lysis of fever. The patients who received methylprednisolone also had a more severe illness at the time of hospitalization.

Likewise, Belsey, Hoffpauir, and Smith [3] showed that there were fewer complications in the patients who received dexamethasone (8 of 41) compared with those who received placebo (18 of 42). Dexamethasone-treated patients also had fewer subdural effusions, became afebrile sooner, and had a more rapid normalization of the CSF glucose concentration [3]. The authors minimized these differences because children in the placebo group were ill for a longer time before being hospitalized.

Recent work in animal models as well as a placebo-controlled clinical trial again suggest a role for dexamethasone in the early management of bacterial meningitis. Using a rabbit model, Scheld, Dacey, and Winn [32] studied the CSF outflow resistance during experimental meningitis. After the induction of acute *S. pneumoniae* meningitis, CSF outflow resistance increased to over 20 times that of controls. When rabbits were treated beginning 12 hours after inoculation, their CSF was uniformly sterile within 8 hours of an 8-hour infusion of penicillin. Nonetheless outflow pressures were remarkably elevated 5 and 10 days after infection. In contrast, the peak outflow pressure in infected rabbits that received methylprednisolone was only twice normal. These studies suggest that elevated CSF outflow pressures due to increased resistance to CSF outflow can be reduced almost 10-fold with methylprednisolone treatment.

Another series of experiments using the rabbit meningitis model looked at the effects of ampicillin, methylprednisolone, and dexamethasone on brain water content, CSF pressure, and CSF lactate concentrations [35]. Both methylprednisolone and dexamethasone reversed the development of brain edema, but only dexamethasone reduced the CSF lactate concentration and reduced the CSF pressure [35]. Clinical studies showed that fewer dexamethasone-treated patients (0.6 mg/kg/day in four doses for 4 days) had hearing impairment than placebo recipients [13] and that steroid-treated children with bad prognostic scores at the time of diagnosis had better neurologic outcomes than similar children who did not receive steroids [9]. At present the American Academy of Pediatrics Committee on Infectious Diseases states that dexamethasone probably reduces the likelihood of deafness after *H. influenzae* meningitis. However, the committee has deferred making unqualified recommendations until further data are available [1].

Fluid Therapy in Bacterial Meningitis

It has long been known that fluid and electrolyte imbalances can occur during acute bacterial meningitis. Nyhan and Cook [23] described four children with bacterial meningitis who developed excessive restlessness, extreme irritability, or convulsions associated with serum sodium concentrations that ranged from 112 to 125 mEq/liter. The authors suggested that the patients demonstrated a limited capacity to excrete water because of an excessive release of antidiuretic hormone (ADH). The authors also advised "careful limitations of water intake" in the management of patients with meningitis. Since the measurement of ADH has been and remains a research tool rather than a readily available clinical test, other laboratory and clinical criteria have been used to diagnose the "inappropriate secretion" of ADH. Over time it became standard practice to restrict fluids to two-thirds to three-fourths of calculated maintenance requirements to prevent the syndrome of inappropriate ADH secretion (SIADH).

The practice of fluid restriction was supported by the finding that plasma AVP concentrations are elevated in children with bacterial meningitis compared to selected controls [11]. These authors recommended that every child with meningitis be carefully evaluated and "if retention of fluid in excess of solute is suspected or documented, fluid administration should be restricted to 800–1000 ml/M^2/day" (about two-thirds maintenance) [11]. Regardless of the authors' intent, SIADH is "suspected" in most cases of bacterial meningitis and fluid restriction is begun at the time of diagnosis.

Not everyone has been in agreement with recommendations to restrict fluids in patients with bacterial meningitis. Prince and Neu [27] reviewed fluid management in 50 children with *H. influenzae* type b meningitis. Of the 50 patients, 33 were clinically well hydrated at the time of hospitalization. The serum sodium concentration was between 125 and 135 mEq/liter in 18 of the 33. One of 20 patients who were managed with fluid restriction developed SIADH, while none of the 13 patients who received unrestricted fluids developed the syndrome. These authors did not recommend fluid restriction unless SIADH developed [27].

Since ADH secretion can be stimulated by a number of factors, inappropriate secretion has to be compared to something. To review briefly, arginine vasopressin (ADH) is a heptapeptide hormone that is synthesized along with its carrier protein, neurophysin, in the supraoptic and paraventricular nuclei of the hypothalamus. After production, it is transported in neurosecretory granules via axoplasmic streaming to the posterior pituitary, where it is stored and released under the control of the hypothalamic nuclei. ADH is released in response to a number of perturbations, the strongest of which is thought to be a change in body fluid osmolality, which stimulates osmoreceptors located in the area of the supraoptic nuclei. Aortic and carotid artery baroreceptors and left atrial volume receptors relay impulses to the hypothalamus via the vagus nerve to regulate ADH. In addition to changes in osmolality and volume, hypoxia, hypercapnia, hyperthermia, hypertension, and pain also affect ADH secretion. Once released, ADH causes increased permeability of the distal renal tubule to water, resulting in water retention and a concentrated urine.

Since Kaplan and Feigin [11] clearly showed that ADH concentrations were higher in patients with meningitis than in control patients, we wondered whether this might represent an "appropriate" response to a regulator other than osmolality. To test this hypothesis, patients with meningitis were randomized to receive maintenance fluids (maintenance requirements plus replacement of any estimated deficit) or two-thirds of their calculated maintenance requirements [26]. Plasma ADH concentrations and serum osmolality were measured before beginning fluid therapy and again 24 hours later. Children in the maintenance plus replacement fluid therapy group received a mean of 1.42 times their calculated maintenance requirements and a mean of 6.3 mEq/kg/24 hours of sodium. The fluid restriction group received a mean of 0.65 times their maintenance fluid requirements and a mean of 2.0 mEq/kg/24 hours of sodium. Plasma ADH concentrations and serum osmolality were comparable in the two groups before fluid therapy was begun. After 24 hours of fluid therapy, ADH concentrations returned to normal in children who received maintenance plus replacement fluids (Fig. 18-1), while ADH concentrations remained elevated in children who were fluid restricted (Fig. 18-2). These differences are sta-

Fig. 18-1. Maintenance fluid therapy. Clear symbols represent relationship between plasma arginine vasopressin (AVP) concentration and serum osmolality at time of hospitalization for individual patients and are connected by rule to dark symbols, which represent this relationship after 24 hours of maintenance plus replacement fluid therapy. Adm = admission. (From Powell et al. [26].)

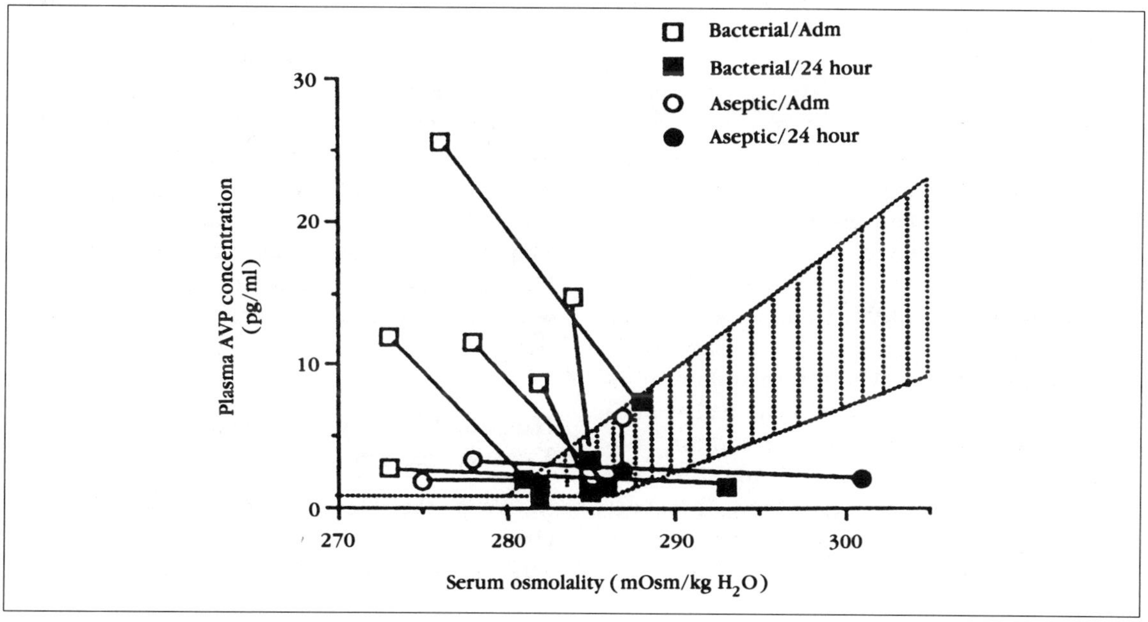

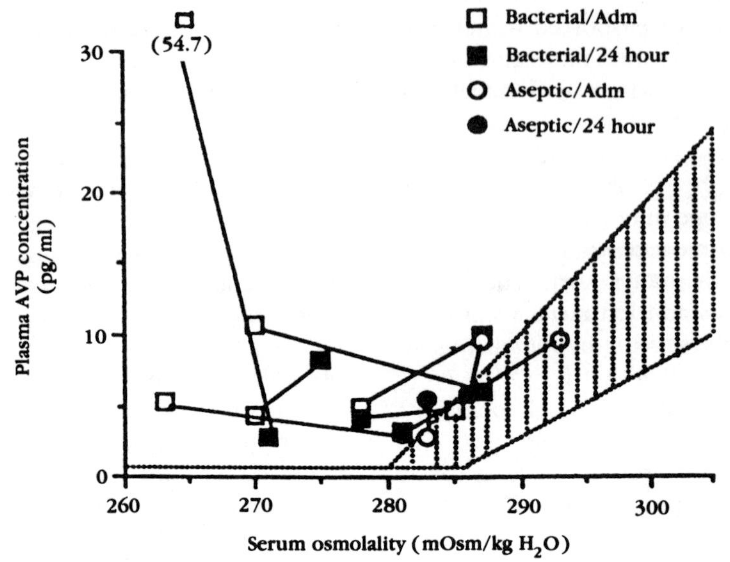

Fig. 18-2. Fluid restriction. Clear symbols represent relationship between plasma AVP concentration and serum osmolality at time of hospitalization for individual patients and are connected by rule to dark symbols, which represent this relationship after 24 hours of fluid restriction. Adm = admission. (From Powell et al. [26].)

tistically significant, and the change in ADH correlated to the amount of sodium given ($p < .02$) [26].

Our study suggests that ADH concentrations are appropriately elevated in children with meningitis because the children are volume depleted. With the administration of sodium the proximal renal tubule reabsorbs water. This explains why there was no difference in serum sodium concentrations between the two groups after 24 hours of therapy despite the maintenance plus replacement group receiving three times as much sodium [26].

Based on these data, it is recommended that meningitis patients be given maintenance fluids plus any replacement deemed necessary based on clinical evaluation. The serum sodium concentration should be checked daily until it becomes normal. If the serum sodium concentration falls to less than 125 mEq/liter, the test should be repeated immediately. If this degree of hyponatremia persists, fluid restriction should be begun.

PREVENTION OF BACTERIAL MENINGITIS

Vaccines

As presented earlier, most cases of bacterial meningitis are caused by a limited repertoire of bacteria. As can be seen from Table 18-4, almost half of the cases of meningitis in the United States are caused by *H. influenzae* type b, and over 85 percent of cases are accounted for if *N. meningitidis, S. pneumoniae*, group B streptococcus, and *E. coli* are included [33]. Thus a vaccine efficacious in the prevention of *H. influenzae* type b meningitis alone would result in nearly a 50 percent reduction in cases of bacterial meningitis.

Haemophilus influenzae Type b Vaccines

In 1985 the first purified capsular polysaccharide vaccine against *H. influenzae* type b was licensed for use in the United States. The

Table 18-4. Total number of bacterial meningitis cases and fatality rates from 27 participating states*

Organism	*Cases reported*	*% of total*	*Case fatality rate (%)*
Haemophilus influenzae	6756	48.3	6.0
Neisseria meningitidis	2742	19.6	10.3
Streptococcus pneumoniae	1865	13.3	26.3
Group B streptococcus	476	3.4	22.5
Listeria monocytogenes	265	1.9	28.5
Escherichia coli	115	0.8	—

* In the National Bacterial Meningitis Surveillance System, 1978 through 1981.
Source: Modified from W. F. Schlech et al., National bacterial meningitis surveillance system 1978–1981. *J.A.M.A.* 253:1749, 1985. Copyright 1985, American Medical Association.

vaccine had been shown to be efficacious in Finnish children who were older than 20 months of age when vaccinated [24]. Based on the results of the Finnish trial and the age distribution of patients with *H. influenzae* type b meningitis, immunization of all children 24 to 60 months of age was expected to result in a 25 to 40 percent reduction in *H. influenzae* type b meningitis. Because the majority of cases of *H. influenzae* type b meningitis occur in infants less than 2 years of age, it has always been clear that a vaccine that could confer protection to young infants is necessary.

Bacterial polysaccharides in general are poor immunogens in infants less than 2 years of age, while protein antigens are perfectly good immunogens. The strategy that has been pursued in recent years is the development of vaccines in which the capsular polysaccharide of *H. influenzae* type b is coupled with a carrier protein. The infant recognizes the protein as foreign, processes the antigen, and makes antibodies against the capsular polysaccharide as well as the protein carrier. Currently two conjugate vaccines for the prevention of *H. influenzae* type b disease have been licensed for use in infants 2 months of age and older [30]. Recommendations of the Immunization Practices Advisory Committee (ACIP) of the Centers for Disease Control are detailed in reference 30.

As conjugate vaccines become extensively used in young infants in the United States, the incidence of *H. influenzae* type b bacterial meningitis should fall dramatically. Nonetheless, there will probably be a period of vulnerability between when vaccine administration begins and when children are immune. Recent observations suggest that this period of vulnerability could also be eliminated by the passive administration of bacterial polysaccharide immune globulin to newborns or by the active immunization of pregnant women near term.

Passive Immunization

Santosham and associates [31] prepared hyperimmune serum globulin from adult donors who were immunized with bacterial polysaccharide vaccines. Infants received either immune globulin or saline intramuscularly in a double-blind fashion. No *H. influenzae* type b or *S. pneumoniae* infections were detected in the 90 days following administration of the bacterial polysaccharide immune globulin, while seven *H. influenzae* type b and four *S. pneumoniae* infections occurred in the placebo group [31]. Further studies showed that the passive administration of antibody does not interfere with active immunization [16]. Thus, a scenario of passive-active immunization whereby *H. influenzae* type b disease could be eradicated is possible. There are obviously practical problems that make eradication unlikely in the foreseeable future.

Neisseria meningitidis Vaccines

Purified capsular polysaccharide vaccines against groups A and C *N. meningitidis* have been shown to be safe and efficacious. Vaccines containing capsular polysaccharides of groups Y and W-135 have been shown to be safe and immunogenic, but efficacy is not known because of the low incidence of disease caused by groups Y and W-135. The major drawback to the prevention of *N. meningitidis* disease is the fact that in some areas over 50 percent of *N. meningitidis* disease is caused by group B bacteria, for which there is currently no effective vaccine.

Like *H. influenzae* type b capsular polysaccharides, *N. meningitidis* capsular polysaccharides are poor immunogens in children less than 2 years of age. Presumably conjugate vaccines could be made, but the lack of a group B immunogen has discouraged this work. In my opinion, the prevention of any cases of meningococcal disease is desirable and the currently available four-component vaccine (A,C,Y,W-135) should be administered to persons over 2 years of age and conjugates should be developed for use in infants. A reduction of *N. meningitidis* disease of even 40 to 50 percent would be more than worth the effort.

Streptococcus pneumoniae Vaccines

Although there are at least 84 different serotypes of *S. pneumoniae,* about 15 serotypes are associated with over 80 percent of the cases of meningitis. Most of the serotypes associated with meningitis are included in the multivalent capsular polysaccharide vaccine that is presently available for use. Unlike *H. influenzae* type b and *N. meningitidis,* which have their highest attack rates during infancy and childhood, *S. pneumoniae* continues to cause meningitis throughout life. The incidence of pneumococcal meningitis is so low, however, that it is unlikely that a study to demonstrate efficacy in the prevention of meningitis will be undertaken.

The vaccine currently marketed in the United States contains capsular polysaccharides from 23 serotypes of *S. pneumoniae* responsible for close to 90 percent of pneumococcal disease in the United States. Like other capsular polysaccharide vaccines, pneumococcal vaccine is poorly immunogenic in children less than 2 years of age. Because the total polysaccharide content is so large, the vaccine is more reactogenic than other capsular polysaccharide vaccines. Reduction in the amount of each type of polysaccharide from 50 to 25 μg per dose has decreased this problem, but there is still concern about Arthus reactions, particularly following second injections. To make a vaccine that would protect young infants would require making conjugates using the most prevalent capsular types. For all of these reasons, it seems unlikely that pneumococcal vaccines will be widely used in attempts to prevent meningitis in the near future.

Escherichia coli and Group B Streptococci Vaccines

Because *E. coli* and group B streptococci cause meningitis almost exclusively in the neonatal period, prevention of disease by immunization would have to involve the vaccination of women of childbearing age. Such vaccines would need to stimulate high enough IgG antibody titers in the mother so that protective concentrations could be achieved transplacentally in the neonate. Since protective antibodies against *E. coli* K1 are largely of the IgM class, even this strategy will not work because IgM does not cross the placenta. Prospects are better for the prevention of group B streptococcal infections. Barker and co-workers [2] vaccinated 40 women during the third trimester of pregnancy with purified capsular polysaccharide from type III group B streptococci. The overall response rate to this vaccine was only 63 percent [2]. However, the study suggests that a more immunogenic vaccine has the potential for reducing neonatal group B streptococcal disease.

Ongoing research continues to increase our understanding of the pathogenesis of bacterial meningitis, which in turn suggests improvement in therapeutic interventions. The future, however, lies in prevention, and new vaccine technologies are bringing us closer to this goal.

REFERENCES

1. American Academy of Pediatrics, Committee on Infectious Diseases 1989–90. Dexamethasone therapy for bacterial meningitis in infants and children. *Pediatrics* 86:130, 1990.

2. Baker, C. J., Rench, M., Edwards, M. S., et al. Immunization of pregnant women with a polysaccharide vaccine of group B streptococcus. *N. Engl. J. Med.* 319:1180, 1988.
3. Belsey, M. A., Hoffpauir, C. W., and Smith, M. H. Dexamethasone in the treatment of acute bacterial meningitis: The effect of study design on the interpretation of results. *Pediatrics* 44:503, 1969.
4. Bradley, J. S., Ching, D. K., and Phillips, S. E. Outpatient therapy of serious pediatric infections with ceftriaxone. *Pediatr. Infect. Dis. J.* 7:160, 1988.
5. De Lemos, R. A., and Haggerty, R. J. Corticosteroids as an adjunct to treatment in bacterial meningitis: A controlled clinical trial. *Pediatrics* 44:30, 1969.
6. Ernst, J. D., Decazes, J. M., and Sande, M. A. Experimental pneumococcal meningitis: Role of leukocytes in pathogenesis. *Infect. Immun.* 41:275, 1983.
7. Fernandez-Villadvich, P., Pallares, R., Ariza, J., et al. Four days of intravenous penicillin for the treatment of meningococcal meningitis [abstract 878]. Presented at 25th Interscience Conference on Antimicrobial Agents and Chemotherapy, September 29–October 2, 1985, Minneapolis, MN.
8. Flexner, S. The results of serum treatment in thirteen hundred cases of epidemic meningitis. *J. Exp. Med.* 5:553, 1913.
9. Gary, N., Powers, N., and Todd, J. K. Clinical identification and comparative prognosis of high-risk patients with *Haemophilus influenzae* meningitis. *Am. J. Dis. Child.* 143:307, 1989.
10. Jadavji, T., Biggar, W. D., Gold, R., and Prober, C. G. Sequelae of acute bacterial meningitis in children treated for seven days. *Pediatrics* 78:21, 1986.
11. Kaplan, S. L., and Feigin, R. D. The syndrome of inappropriate secretion of antidiuretic hormone in children with bacterial meningitis. *J. Pediatr.* 92:758, 1978.
12. Klein, J. O., Feigin, R. D., and McCracken, G. H., Jr. Report of the task force on diagnosis and management of meningitis. *Pediatrics* 78 (Suppl.):958, 1986.
13. Lebel, M. H., Freij, B. J., Syrogianopoulos, G. A., et al. Dexamethasone therapy for bacterial meningitis: Results of two double-blind, placebo-controlled trials. *N. Engl. J. Med.* 319:964, 1988.
14. Lebel, M. H., Hoyt, M. J., and McCracken, G. H., Jr. Comparative efficacy of ceftriaxone and cefuroxime for treatment of bacterial meningitis. *J. Pediatr.* 114:1049, 1989.
15. Lebel, M. H., and McCracken, G. H., Jr. Delayed cerebrospinal fluid sterilization and adverse outcome of bacterial meningitis in infants and children. *Pediatrics* 83:161, 1989.
16. Letson, G. W., Santosham, M., Reid R et al. Comparison of active and combined passive/active immunization of Navajo children against *Haemophilus influenzae* type b. *Pediatr. Infect. Dis. J.* 7:747, 1988.
17. Lin, T. Y., Chrane, D. F., Nelson, J. D., and McCracken, G. H., Jr. Seven days of ceftriaxone therapy is as effective as ten days' treatment for bacterial meningitis. *J.A.M.A.* 253:3559, 1985.
18. McCracken, G. H., Jr., Nelson, J. D., Kaplan, S. L., et al. Consensus report: Antimicrobial therapy for bacterial meningitis in infants and children. *Pediatr. Infect. Dis. J.* 6:501, 1987.
19. Moxon, E. R., and Murphy, P. A. *Haemophilus influenzae* bacteremia and meningitis resulting from survival of a single organism. *Proc. Natl. Acad. Sci. U.S.A.* 75:1534, 1978.
20. Moxon, E. R., Smith, A. L., Averill, D. R., and Smith, D. H. *Hemophilus influenzae* meningitis in infant rats after intranasal inoculation. *J. Infect. Dis.* 129:154, 1974.
21. Murphy, T. V., Granoff, D., Chrane, D. F., et al. Pharyngeal colonization with *Haemophilus influenzae* type b in children in a day care center without invasive disease. *J. Pediatr.* 106:712, 1985.
22. Musser, J. M., Kroll, J. S., Granoff, D. M., et al. Global genetic structure and molecular epidemiology of encapsulated *Haemophilus influenzae. Rev. Infect. Dis.* 12:75, 1990.
23. Nyhan, W. L., and Cooke, R. E. Symptomatic hyponatremia in acute infections of the central nervous system. *Pediatrics* 18:604, 1956.
24. Peltola, H., Käyhty, H., Virtanen, M., and Mäkelä P. H. Prevention of *Haemophilus influenzae* type b bacteremic infections with capsular polysaccharide vaccine. *N. Engl. J. Med.* 310: 1561, 1984.
25. Powell, K. R., and Mawhorter, S. D. Outpatient treatment of serious infections in infants and children with ceftriaxone. *J. Pediatr.* 110:898, 1987.
26. Powell, K. R., Sugarman, L. I., Eskenazi, A. E., et al. Normalization of plasma arginine vasopressin concentrations when children with meningitis are given maintenance plus replacement fluid therapy. *J. Pediatr.* 117:515, 1990.
27. Prince, A. S., and Neu, H. C. Fluid management in *Haemophilus influenzae* meningitis. *Infection* 8:5, 1980.
28. Quagliarello, V. J., Long, W. J., and Scheld, W. M. Morphologic alterations of the blood-brain barrier with experimental meningitis in the rat. *J. Clin. Invest.* 77:1084, 1986.
29. Radetsky, M. Duration of treatment in bacterial meningitis: A historical inquiry. *Pediatr. Infect. Dis. J.* 9:2, 1990.
30. Recommendations and reports: *Haemophilus* b conjugate vaccines for prevention of *Haemophilus influenzae* type b disease among in-

fants and children two months of age and older. *M.M.W.R.* 40:RR1-7, 1991.

31. Santosham, M., Reid, R., Ambrosino, D. M., et al. Prevention of *Haemophilus influenzae* type b infections in high-risk infants treated with bacterial polysaccharide immune globulin. *N. Engl. J. Med.* 317:923, 1987.
32. Scheld, W. M., Dacey, R. G., and Winn, R. H. Cerebrospinal fluid outflow resistance in rabbits with experimental meningitis: Alterations with penicillin and methylprednisolone. *J. Clin. Invest.* 66:243, 1980.
33. Schlech, W. F., III, Ward, J. I., Band, J. D., et al. Bacterial meningitis in the United States, 1978–1981: The National Bacterial Meningitis Surveillance Study. *J.A.M.A.* 253:1749, 1985.
34. Syrogiannopoulos, G. A., Hansen, E. J., Erwin, A. L., et al. *Haemophilus influenzae* type b lipooligosaccharide induces meningeal inflammation. *J. Infect. Dis.* 157:237, 1988.
35. Täuber, M. G., Khayam-Bashi, H., and Sande, M. A. Effects of ampicillin and corticosteroids on brain water content, cerebrospinal fluid pressure, and cerebrospinal fluid lactate levels in experimental pneumococcal meningitis. *J. Infect. Dis.* 151:528, 1985.
36. Tuomanen, E., Hengstler, B., Zak, O., and Tomaz, A. The induction of meningeal inflammation by components of the pneumococcal cell wall. *J. Infect. Dis.* 151:859, 1985.
37. Tuomanen, E., Tomaz, A., Hengstler, B., and Zak, O. The relative role of bacterial cell wall and capsule in the induction of inflammation in pneumococcal meningitis. *J. Infect. Dis.* 151: 535, 1985.
38. Yogev, R. Advances in diagnosis and treatment of childhood meningitis. *Pediatr. Infect. Dis. J.* 4:321, 1985.

19 Viral Infections of the Central Nervous System

John E. Greenlee

Invasion of the central nervous system by viral agents may result in acute meningitis or encephalitis, latent infection, or slow infections in which neurologic signs and symptoms develop months or years after initial exposure to the causative agent. Viruses may also cause neurologic injury indirectly, by immune, vascular, or metabolic mechanisms. In some instances, such as the progressive encephalopathy caused by human immunodeficiency virus, the mechanisms of neurologic injury are not yet understood. This chapter will review current concepts of viral pathogenesis as related to central nervous system infections and will then discuss acute viral meningitis and encephalitis, slow viral infections, and the neurologic complications of infection with the human T-lymphotrophic retroviruses.

This work was supported by the United States Department of Veterans Affairs.

PATHOGENESIS OF VIRAL INFECTIONS

Virus-Host Interactions

A variety of DNA and RNA viruses may infect the central nervous system (Table 19-1). Each of these viruses, to cause neurologic disease, must penetrate the cutaneous or mucosal surfaces of the host, breach the barrier systems separating brain and cerebrospinal fluid (CSF) from blood, and attach to susceptible cells within brain, spinal cord, or meninges. Polio, Coxsackie, and echoviruses enter their human hosts across the intestinal mucosa. Measles, mumps, and influenza viruses are acquired by the respiratory route. The arthropod-borne viruses and rabies virus are carried through the skin by the bite of an insect vector or infected animal. Human immunodeficiency virus (HIV) is transmitted across mucosal surfaces during sexual intercourse or may be inoculated directly into veins by use of illicit drugs or by blood transfusion.

The majority of viruses causing central nervous system infection reach the central nervous

Table 19-1. Viruses associated with central nervous system infections in humans

Family and genus	*Agents*	*Genome*	*Infections*
Adenoviridae	Adenoviruses	DSDNA[a]	Encephalitis
Herpetoviridae			
Alpha herpesvirus	Herpes simplex virus type 1	DSDNA	Encephalitis Meningitis, encephalitis
	Herpes simplex virus type 2		Radiculitis, encephalomyelitis, vasculitis
	Herpes zoster virus		
Beta herpesvirus	Cytomegalovirus		Encephalitis, postinfectious syndromes
Gamma herpesvirus	Epstein-Barr virus		Postinfectious syndromes
Papovaviridae	JC virus SV40 virus	DSDNA	Progressive multifocal leukoencephalopathy
Arenaviridae	Lymphocytic choriomeningitis virus	SS(−)RNA[b]	Meningitis Encephalitis
Orthomyxoviridae	Influenza viruses	SS(−)RNA	Postinfectious syndromes Reye's syndrome
Paramyxoviridae			
Paramyxovirus	Mumps virus	SS(−)RNA	
Morbillivirus	Measles virus		Postinfectious encephalomyelitis Progressive encephalitis (immunosuppressed patients) Subacute sclerosing panencephalitis
Picornaviridae			
Enterovirus	Poliovirus	SS(+)RNA[c]	Meningitis, poliomyelitis
	Coxsackie virus		Meningitis, encephalitis (poliomyelitis)
	Echovirus		Meningitis, encephalitis (poliomyelitis)

[a] DSDNA: double-stranded DNA.
[b] SS(−)RNA: negative-sense RNA. Virus contains RNA-dependent RNA polymerase for production of messenger RNA from viral RNA genome. Viral RNA alone is not infectious.
[c] SS(+)RNA: positive-sense RNA. Viral RNA acts as messenger RNA and is itself infectious.
[d] Retroviruses contain diploid, SS(+)RNA molecules.

system by hematogenous spread following systemic infection. Entry may be across the choroid plexus or through parenchymal capillaries [71]. Infection with polio, Coxsackie, and echoviruses begins in Peyer's patches and intestinal lymphatics [10,71]. Mumps virus replicates in epithelial tissues including parotid glands, pancreas, and testes. Measles virus infects epithelial and vascular endothelial cells, as well as macrophages and T-lymphocytes. HIV infection outside the central nervous system is restricted to $CD4^+$ T-lymphocytes [76]. The arthropod-borne viruses initially infect subcutaneous tissues and may subsequently replicate in vascular endothelial cells [70].

A minority of viral agents reach the central nervous system by neurotropic rather than hematogenous spread. Rabies virus enters peripheral nerves within muscle at the site of inoculation and is carried centrally by retrograde axoplasmic transport to reach dorsal root and spinal neurons. Replication of virus at these sites is followed by ascending transneuronal spread of infection within spinal cord and brain [96,97,119]. Herpes simplex, herpes zoster, and simian B viruses are also capable of neurotropic spread following initial cutaneous or mucosal infection [71,79]. Poliovirus may disseminate within the brain by neurotropic spread once central nervous system invasion has occurred [10,25].

(*Continued*)

Family and genus	*Agents*	*Genome*	*Infections*
Bunyaviridae	California encephalitis virus	SS(−)RNA	Encephalitis
Reoviridae			
Orbivirus	Colorado tick fever virus	DSRNA[d]	Encephalitis
Togaviridae			
Alphavirus	Eastern equine encephalitis virus Western equine encephalitis virus Venezuelan equine encephalitis virus	SS(+)RNA	Encephalitis
Flavivirus	St. Louis encephalitis virus Japanese encephalitis virus		Encephalitis
Rubivirus	Rubella virus		Congenital encephalitis Progressive rubella encephalitis
Rhabdoviridae			
Lyssavirus	Rabies virus	SS(−)RNA	Furious, dumb, or ascending rabies
Retroviridae			
Lentivirus	HIV-1	Diploid SS(+)RNA[d]	AIDS meningitis AIDS-related encephalopathy Vacuolar myelopathy
	HIV-2		Probably same as HIV-1
Oncornavirus	HTLV-1		Tropical spastic paraparesis(?)

Virus-Cell Interactions

Viral infection at a cellular level begins with attachment of the virus to specific receptors on the cell surface. Only a few of these receptors have been identified. Rabies virus appears to bind at or near the peripheral acetylcholine receptors and may also interact with acetylcholine receptors centrally [119,135]. HIV attaches to CD4 receptors on the surfaces of T-lymphocytes and could conceivably interact with similar receptors on cells within brain [76,86].

Mechanisms of viral replication vary with the DNA or RNA virus involved (Table 19-1) [71]. DNA viruses transcribe messenger RNA directly from the viral genome. Small DNA viruses such as the papovaviruses transcribe only limited numbers of proteins and are almost completely dependent on cellular enzyme systems. Herpesviruses also depend on host cellular systems, but in addition code for a virus-specific thymidine kinase. This enzyme is of clinical importance, since it is involved in the phosphorylation of the antiviral drug acyclovir to active form within infected cells [36]. Single-stranded RNA (SSRNA) viruses may have positive- or negative-sense polarity. Positive-sense single-stranded RNA (SS(+)RNA) viruses such as the picornaviruses, coronaviruses, and togaviruses function directly as messenger RNA and hence are themselves infectious. Single-stranded RNA (SS(−)RNA) viruses include paramyxoviruses, orthomyxoviruses, and rhabdoviruses. These agents contain an RNA-dependent RNA polymerase that enables synthesis of messenger RNA from the viral genome. The RNAs of these agents are not infectious in the absence of this viral enzyme. Retroviruses, such as HIV, employ a virus-coded reverse transcriptase to develop a double-stranded DNA proviral copy of the viral genome. During viral replication, proviral DNA integrates into the genome of the host cell. In this integrated state, infectious viral genetic material can persist in a form not recognized by host immune response and can be transmitted to daughter cells during cell mitosis. The ability of retroviruses to persist as integrated DNA presents a major problem in developing effective treatment for HIV infections.

Adenoviruses, papovaviruses, and enteroviruses are released by rupture of the infected cell. Cell rupture may be the consequence of virus-induced shutoff of cellular metabolic activities, virus-induced disruption of lysosomes, or, in the case of adenoviruses, toxicity of virus-coded proteins [71]. Enveloped viruses, including herpesviruses, measles and mumps viruses, rabies virus, and retroviruses, are released by budding across the cell membrane. In this process the protein coat of the immature virus acquires a lipid envelope as it passes through the host cell membrane.

Host Response to Viral Infections

Initial host response to viral infection involves nonspecific phagocytosis of virus by reticuloendothelial cells within blood, lymph nodes, skin, spleen, and liver. Early, nonspecific host defenses also include interferon production and destruction of infected cells' natural killer lymphocytes [71]. B-cell-mediated immune response begins within days after the onset of infection and results in production of antiviral IgM followed by IgG antibody. Antibody facilitates reticuloendothelial clearance of extracellular virus, prevents virus attachment to susceptible cells, and mediates destruction of infected cells by fixing complement or by antibody-mediated cellular cytotoxicity [71]. Development of T-cell-mediated antiviral immunity develops more slowly. T-lymphocytes have important modulating effects on production of specific antibody and provide a mechanism of dealing with intracellular virus in cells expressing viral antigens on their surfaces [133]. Although B-cell- and T-cell-mediated immune responses are often considered separately, the two are mutually interdependent, and compromise of T-cell-mediated immune response, as in AIDS, may be accompanied by blunting of humoral immune response as well [12].

Impairment of host immune response may result in central nervous system infection by unusual agents or lead to prolonged or atypical infection by more common viruses. Infants with congenital agammaglobulinemia may develop widespread encephalitis with poliovirus or echovirus [27,139,147]. Children receiving chemotherapy for acute lymphocytic leukemia may develop a progressive measles encephalitis [98]. Suppression of T-cell response in adult cancer or transplant patients is almost always present in the opportunistic infection by papovavirus JC, progressive multifocal leukoencephalopathy (PML). Defective T-cell-mediated immune response in adults has also been associated with atypical, prolonged herpes simplex virus encephalitis and with encephalitis caused by varicella-zoster virus, cytomegalovirus, adenovirus, and measles virus [19,35,92,110,150]. Central nervous system infections during acquired immunodeficiency syndrome (AIDS) are discussed later in the chapter.

Mechanisms of Injury in Viral Central Nervous System Infections

Most viral encephalitides produce diffuse infection involving multiple cell types [71]. A few agents produce infection confined to specific cell populations or anatomic regions. Rabies virus replicates predominantly in neurons [68]. Poliovirus infects motor neurons in spinal cord and brain [10]. JC virus produces lytic infection of oligodendrocytes [154]. Herpes simplex virus infects multiple cell types. The pathologic changes of herpes simplex encephalitis, however, are largely confined to orbitofrontal cortex, temporal lobes, and cingulate cortex [4].

Neurologic injury in viral infections may also occur by indirect mechanisms. Host immune response directed against viral antigens expressed on surfaces of infected cells may cause cellular destruction. Virus-induced perturbations of host immune response may also result in immune-mediated injury of normal components of the nervous system. Acute disseminated encephalomyelitis, with multifocal demyelination of brain, spinal cord, and optic nerves, has been classically associated with measles virus infection and may occur without actual viral invasion of brain [45]. Acute hemorrhagic leukoencephalitis, with immunologic injury of small vessels within brain, may accompany acute disseminated encephalomyelitis or may occur independently [56,71]. Landry-Guillain-Barré syndrome, with segmental demyelination of cranial, peripheral, and autonomic nerves, may follow infection with cytomegalovirus, Epstein-Barr virus, or, less frequently, mumps, measles, hepatitis viruses, or HIV [71]. None of these three syndromes—acute disseminated encephalomyelitis, acute hemorrhagic leukoencephalitis, and Landry-Guillain-Barré syndrome—is specific to any agent or group of agents, and identical clinical and pathologic findings may follow viral, bacterial, and *Mycoplasma pneumoniae* infections, as well as immunizations.

Viral infection may also produce neurologic injury by causing ischemic infarction or by producing metabolic derangement. Hepatitis B infection is occasionally associated with a necrotizing vasculitis that is believed to be immune-mediated [37,126]. Ophthalmic herpes zoster may be followed by spread of infection to carotid or other vessels, with vascular occlusion and ipsilateral cerebral infarction [58,117]. More extensive vasculitis may complicate herpes zoster infection in immunosuppressed patients [85]. Virus-induced ischemic injury, as discussed later, may also be a key element in the pathogenesis of progressive rubella panencephalitis.

Reye's syndrome of severe hepatic dysfunction accompanied by cerebral edema is often preceded by viral infection. The relationship between infection and the subsequent encephalopathy is unclear. However, experimental work by Davis [26] employing influenza virus in a mouse model indicates that development of Reye's syndrome in these animals following influenza B virus infection is accompanied by nonproductive viral infection of livers and brain capillary endothelial cells.

Rabies virus infection has long represented an enigma, since this most lethal of all neurotropic viruses usually causes surprisingly little inflammation or cellular destruction [68]. Work by Tsiang [135] has demonstrated that binding of acetylcholine to muscarinic receptors within brains diminishes progressively during acute rabies. These data suggest that rabies may possibly produce fatal disease by interfering with neurotransmitter function [135].

ACUTE VIRAL INFECTIONS

Acute viral infection of the central nervous system results in a meningoencephalitis in which either meningitis or encephalitic symptoms may predominate. The clinical consequences of this meningoencephalitis may vary from trivial or asymptomatic infection to overwhelming, rapidly fatal illness.

Viral Agents Associated with Meningitis and Encephalitis

Viruses commonly associated with meningitis in the United States are shown in Table 19-2. Coxsackie and echoviruses account for 80 to 90 percent of cases of viral meningitis in which an etiologic agent is identified [116]. Arthropod-borne viruses, herpes simplex type 2 virus, Epstein-Barr virus, and lymphocytic choriomeningitis virus account for a minority of cases. Mumps virus, once a common cause of viral meningoencephalitis, has become unusual with the widespread use of mumps vaccine [116]. Although poliovirus is no longer an important cause of meningitis in North America or Europe, it remains a frequent cause of viral meningitis in underdeveloped countries.

The majority of cases of acute viral encephalitis are caused by arthropod-borne viruses (Table 19-3) [49,61]. St. Louis encephalitis virus and California encephalitis virus are the most common agents of acute, epidemic encephalitis in the United States [49,61,71]. Western equine encephalitis virus and Eastern equine encephalitis virus account for a minority of cases. Encephalitis caused by Colorado tick fever virus or Powassan virus is rare. Despite their frequent occurrence as agents of viral meningitis, enteroviruses account for only 2 percent of cases of viral encephalitis. Cytomegalovirus encephalitis, although frequent in congenitally infected infants and in patients with AIDS, is unusual in immunologically normal children and adults.

Many of the agents that cause viral encephalitis are agents indigenous to wild animals or

Table 19-2. Viruses associated with acute meningitis

Group	*Agent*	*Seasonal distribution*
Picornaviridae	Echovirus Coxsackie virus (Polio virus)	Late summer–early fall
Paramyxoviridae	Mumps virus	Late winter
Arenaviridae	Lymphocytic choriomeningitis virus	Fall–spring
Herpetoviridae	Herpes simplex virus type 2	Sporadic
Togaviridae	St. Louis encephalitis virus Western equine encephalitis virus	Late summer–early fall
Bunyaviridae	California virus	Late summer–early fall
Reoviridae	Colorado tick fever virus	Late spring–early summer

birds, and human infection is almost always the inadvertent consequence of contact with infected animal hosts or their invertebrate vectors [71]. Rabies is predominantly a sylvatic infection, involving skunks, raccoons, and bats in the United States. Lymphocytic choriomeningitis virus is an agent of mice. Point-source epidemics of lymphocytic choriomeningitis infection have also been traced to infected hamsters purchased from pet stores [31]. The arthropod-borne viruses are agents of birds and small mammals [71].

Several viruses associated with meningitis and encephalitis have predictable seasonal occurrences (see Table 19-2) [49,61,71]. Enterovirus infections are most common in the late summer and early fall but may occur at other times during the year [109]. The arthropod-borne viruses, with the exception of Colorado tick fever, also occur in late summer and early fall. The peak incidence of infections with these agents is similar to that of the enteroviruses. Colorado tick fever is most common in late spring and early summer, coinciding in seasonal incidence with Rocky Mountain spotted fever. Lymphocytic choriomeningitis virus is identified most frequently during the late fall and winter [1]. Mumps virus infections are more frequent in the late winter and early spring but may occur throughout the year [61,71].

Clinical Features of Viral Meningitis

The clinical presentation of viral meningitis is similar to but usually milder than that of bacterial meningitis [116]. Symptoms may begin abruptly or gradually over several days. Systemic complaints of fever, chills, and malaise may precede or accompany the onset of meningitis. Patients may complain of headache, photophobia, and neck or back stiffness. Nausea and vomiting occur in some but not all patients [116]. The presence of focal neurologic signs in addition to those of meningeal irritation should suggest bacterial or viral infection of brain parenchyma, with secondary meningeal irritation.

Clinical Features of Viral Encephalitis

Viral encephalitis, like viral meningitis, may be abrupt or insidious in onset. Although meningeal signs are often present, these are overshadowed by involvement of brain parenchyma, with confusion, stupor, or coma. Examination reveals global attenuation of higher intellectual function, with or without corticospinal tract findings. Focal neurologic signs, although most frequently associated with herpes simplex encephalitis, may occur during encephalitis by other viral agents as well. Focal or generalized seizures may occur at any point during the course of viral encephalitis and may be the presenting symptom. Rabies virus infection may present with agitated behavior and psychosis (furious rabies), as a more typical encephalitis with depressed mental function and stupor (dumb rabies), or as an ascending, paralytic infection similar to Guillain-Barré syndrome [7].

Diagnosis of Acute Viral Meningitis and Encephalitis

Viral meningitis is diagnosed by lumbar puncture. Spinal fluid usually shows normal pressure, lymphocytic pleocytosis in the range of 10 to 1000 cells/mm^3, mild elevation of protein, and normal glucose [116]. During the first 24 to 36 hours of infection, the CSF may contain polymorphonuclear leukocytes as well as lymphocytes, raising the possibility of bacterial rather than viral infection [116]. In these cases, the presence of a normal CSF glucose—unusual in bacterial meningitis—suggests a viral infection, and repeat lumbar puncture within 24 to 36 hours reveals a lymphocytic pleocytosis. Low CSF glucose has been reported in meningoencephalitis caused by herpes zoster, mumps, and lymphocytic choriomeningitis viruses and may occasionally be seen in herpes simplex meningitis and encephalitis [49,142]. Empiric antibiotic therapy should be instituted presumptively where suspicion of bacterial meningitis is high.

CSF findings in viral encephalitis are similar to those in viral meningitis, although cell counts may be higher and greater numbers of polymorphonuclear leukocytes may be present where encephalitis is severe [49,61]. The electroencephalogram [EEG] in viral encephalitis characteristically shows diffuse slowing, occasionally with focal predominance of slow waves or with focal electrographic evidence of seizure activity [49,61,74]. Magnetic resonance imaging (MRI) is the most sensitive means of localizing focal infection. Computed tomography (CT) and radionuclide scans are less sensitive.

Specific identification of the etiologic agent in viral meningitis or encephalitis has classically involved isolation of virus or documentation of a rise in titers of specific antiviral antibody. Echovirus, Coxsackie virus, mumps virus, and lymphocytic choriomeningitis virus may be recovered from CSF. Herpes simplex virus may be recovered from CSF in cases of viral meningitis but is only rarely recovered from CSF in cases of encephalitis [116,144]. Attempts to isolate the arthropod-borne viruses or herpes zoster virus are not usually successful. Because virus isolation may not be successful in all cases, serum drawn at the time of presentation should be held for comparison of antibody titers with serum obtained 3 to 4 weeks into the patient's course. The recent development of the polymerase chain reaction (PCR), which is capable of amplifying extremely small amounts of selected sequences of viral or other nucleic acids, has provided an extremely powerful tool for viral diagnosis, whose applications are only beginning to be explored [40]. The use of PCR in herpes simplex virus infections is discussed later.

A number of infections by nonviral agents may mimic viral meningitis or encephalitis (Table 19-4). Partially treated bacterial meningitis may mimic viral meningitis in severity and in CSF findings, as may brain abscess, especially if the abscess is located in an area of brain not likely to produce focal neurologic signs. Infections by *Toxoplasma gondii* and *Cryptococcus neoformans* may resemble viral encephalitis and are common infections in AIDS. Lyme disease, caused by *Borrelia burgdorferi,* may produce lymphocytic meningitis or encephalitis. Rocky Mountain spotted fever may produce an acute encephalopathy and may occasionally do so in the absence of a rash. *Listeria monocytogenes* may produce focal or diffuse encephalitis, at times with normal CSF cell count, protein, and glucose [32]. A number of conditions of unknown etiology, such as sarcoidosis, Behçet's syndrome, and Mollaret's meningitis, may also cause lymphocytic meningitis, as may leakage of dermoid or epidermoid cysts [71].

Herpes Simplex Encephalitis

Pathogenesis

Herpes simplex viruses are ubiquitous human agents. Herpes simplex virus type 1 is acquired as a symptomatic or asymptomatic gingivostomatitis during childhood. Herpes simplex virus type 2 is usually acquired as a venereal infection during or after adolescence. Both viruses are capable of producing latent infection of neurons within sensory ganglia [4,71]. Herpes simplex virus type 1 is most frequently recovered from trigeminal and superior cervical ganglia [4]. Latent infection by herpes simplex virus type 2 is more common in sacral ganglia [4].

The sequence of events by which herpes sim-

Table 19-3. Viral agents associated with acute encephalitis

Group	*Agent*	*Frequency*[a]	*Seasonal incidence*	*Reservoir*	*Vector*	*Age group affected*	*Mortality*
Togaviridae	St. Louis encephalitis virus	29%	Late summer–early fall	Birds, small rodents	Mosquitoes	All ages but more severe in the elderly	2–20%
	Western equine encephalitis virus	9%	Late summer–early fall	Birds, small mammals	Mosquitoes	Children > adults	2–3%
	Eastern equine encephalitis virus	Rare	Late summer–early fall	Birds	Mosquitoes	Children > adults	80%
	Venezuelan equine encephalitis virus	Rare	Late summer–early fall	Rodents	Mosquitoes	Children > adults	1%
	Rubella virus	Rare				Children > adults	Rare
	Powassan virus	Rare		Small mammals	Ticks	Children > adults	
Bunyaviridae	California encephalitis virus	14%	Late summer–early fall	Small rodents	Mosquitoes	Children > adults	2%
Reoviridae	Colorado tick fever virus	Rare	Late spring–early summer	Small rodents	Ticks	Children > adults	Rare
Paramyxoviridae	Mumps virus	3%	Late winter			Children > adults	< 3%
	Measles virus	Rare				Children > adults	15%

Picornaviridae[b]	Echovirus	2%	Late summer–early fall		Children > adults	Rare
	Coxsackie virus	1%	Late summer–early fall		Children > adults	Rare
	Poliovirus	Rare	Late summer–early fall		Children > adults	
Herpetoviridae	Herpes simplex virus	14%			Adults, children (neonates)	70%[c]
	Herpes zoster virus	3%			Adults (neonates)	50%
	Epstein-Barr virus	1%			Children, adolescents, young adults	Rare
	Cytomegalovirus	Rare			Adults (neonates)	
Arenaviridae	Lymphocytic chorio-meningitis	Rare	Fall–spring	Mice (hamsters)	All ages especially young adults	Rare
Rhabdoviridae	Rabies virus	Rare		Wild animals (raccoons, skunks)	All ages	100%
Adenoviridae		Rare			Children, adults	Rare

[a] Frequency is expressed as percentage of cases of encephalitis in which an agent was identified by virus isolation or serology. Based on case reports to the Centers for Disease Control for 1977.
[b] Picornavirus cases are probably underrepresented because of the mild nature of many cases and difficulties in serologic diagnosis.
[c] Mortality from herpes simplex encephalitis based on data from Whitley et al. [142,143].
Source: Adapted from J. E. Stein, et al. (eds.), *Internal Medicine* (2nd ed.). Boston: Little, Brown, 1986.

Table 19-4. Nonviral causes of encephalitis

Rickettsiae
Rickettsia rickettsii (Rocky Mountain spotted fever)
Rickettsia prowazekii (epidemic typhus)
?Other rickettsial species
Mycoplasma pneumoniae
Bacteria
Mycobacterium tuberculosis
Brucella species
Borrelia species (relapsing fever; Lyme disease)
Leptospira species
Treponema pallidum
Fungi
Cryptococcus neoformans
Histoplasma capsulatum
Candida albicans
Protozoa
Toxoplasma gondii
Trypanosoma species
Plasmodium falciparum
Naegleria species
Trichinella spiralis
Disease of unknown origin
Behçet's disease
Whipple's disease
Sarcoidosis
Vogt-Koyanagi-Harada syndrome

Source: Stein, J. E., et al. (eds.). *Internal Medicine* (2nd ed.). Boston: Little, Brown, 1986.

plex virus causes severe encephalitis is not understood. Over 95 percent of cases are caused by herpes simplex virus type 1 [7,32,154]. Spread from infected trigeminal ganglia to meninges covering temporal lobes has been suggested but not proved, as has infection by the olfactory route [28]. A growing body of experimental data suggests that individual strains of herpes simplex virus may vary considerably in neurovirulence, so that certain strains of herpes simplex virus may be particularly likely to cause encephalitis [34]. Approximately 70 percent of patients with herpes simplex encephalitis have antiviral antibody at the time of presentation [99]. It is not clear, however, whether encephalitis in these patients results from reactivation of infection within sensory ganglia or brain or whether it follows reinfection with a more virulent strain of virus.

Clinical Features

Herpes simplex encephalitis has a bimodal age distribution, with the majority of cases occurring in patients less than 19 or over 40 years of age [142,144]. There is no seasonal distribution of infection. Patients typically develop clinical signs of temporal lobe injury, often with accompanying evidence of diffuse cerebral dysfunction. Symptoms may develop abruptly or over several days. Seizures are present in 67 percent of patients and may be indicative of temporal lobe localization [4,144]. Superior quadrantanopic visual field defects may be detected on examination but are rarely reported by the patient. Receptive or conductive aphasia may be seen where dominant temporal lobe is involved. A minority of cases present with loss of recent memory, suggesting bilateral hippocampal injury, or with psychosis. Occasional patients may present with clinical signs of brain stem involvement [30].

Diagnosis

Diagnosis of herpes simplex virus encephalitis is a matter of urgency, since antiviral therapy must be instituted promptly in order to be effective. Localization of clinical signs to temporal lobes suggests the diagnosis [144]. CSF characteristically shows a lymphocytic pleocytosis, with mild to moderate elevation of protein and normal glucose [99]. Large numbers of polymorphonuclear leukocytes may be seen in overwhelming infection, however, and glucose levels may occasionally be depressed [99,144, 154]. Because herpes simplex virus typically produces a hemorrhagic encephalitis, much has been made of the presence of red blood cells in the CSF of affected patients. Numbers of red blood cells may be extremely low, however, and the presence of red blood cells, even with careful comparison of serial tubes of CSF, is usually not helpful [99,144]. Documentation of temporal lobe involvement may be obtained by EEG, radionuclide brain scan, CT scan, or MRI [124, 144,154]. The role of each of these modalities in the diagnosis of herpes simplex virus encephalitis is changing. The EEG has been felt to be the most consistently useful diagnostic modality early in the course of infection [142,144]. Radionuclide and CT scans should be used together, since either test may be initially normal [142–144]. The diagnostic accuracy of MRI as compared to radionuclide and CT methods has not yet been established. MRI, however, with its much greater clarity of morphologic detail, has been shown to provide elegant localizing information in herpes simplex encephalitis [124] and, in particular with gadolinium enhancement, should provide earlier, more precise localization of temporal lobe injury than can be achieved using CT.

Specific diagnosis of herpes simplex encephalitis during the acute phase of illness has traditionally required brain biopsy. Comparison of serum versus CSF titers of anti-herpesvirus antibodies has been proposed as a diagnostic test, but the test, which is dependent on intrathecal antibody synthesis, is only rarely of value at the time of presentation [78,80,99]. Brain biopsy has a complication rate of 1 percent of patients [141–143]. Since acyclovir has become available for treatment of herpes simplex encephalitis, however, many physicians have felt that localization of the pathologic process to one or both temporal lobes provides sufficient evidence of herpetic infection that biopsy is not needed [43,54]. In deciding whether to biopsy a given patient, it is important to note that a variety of other pathologic processes may produce similar electroencephalographic or radiologic findings of temporal lobe involvement [9,140–144]. These conditions include treatable disorders such as brain abscess, tuberculosis, toxoplasmosis, and cryptococcal infection [140,142,144]. Initiation of antiviral therapy for herpes simplex virus encephalitis based on temporal localization of a lesion alone may thus occasionally result in serious neurologic injury or patient death from other conditions for which definitive treatment exists. Biopsy should thus be strongly considered at initial presentation in all patients in whom herpes simplex encephalitis is suspected. The need for biopsy should also be reconsidered in any patient in whom disease progression occurs despite presumptive antiviral therapy. Proper handling of biopsy material should be ensured prior to surgery by discussion with the various laboratories involved in handling the specimen.

Within the past 2 years, development of PCR, with its ability to amplify minute amounts of specific viral nucleic acids, has provided the first potential means of achieving a specific diagnosis of herpes simplex encephalitis by CSF examination rather than brain biopsy. Rowley and associates [118], using PCR, detected herpes simplex virus nucleic acid sequences in CSF from 4 of 4 patients with proven herpes simplex virus encephalitis but in none of 6 controls. Puchhammer and co-workers [113] detected herpes simplex virus type I nucleic acid sequences in 7 of 8 CSF samples obtained between the second and eighth day of encephalitis; herpesvirus DNA was not detected in any of 42 controls with other central nervous system conditions. Aurelius and colleagues [3] detected viral DNA in the CSF of 42 out of 43 patients with virologically or serologically proven herpes simplex virus encephalitis, the negative patient having been treated with acyclovir from 20 hours after the onset of symptoms. In this study, 87 control samples from patients with other inflammatory neurologic disorders initially thought to be herpes simplex virus encephalitis were negative.

Therapy

The nucleoside analogue adenine arabinoside (Vidarabine) was the first drug shown in controlled trials to reduce mortality in herpes simplex encephalitis [142]. In subsequent trials, a second agent, acyclovir, was found to be superior to adenine arabinoside [141]. Acyclovir is readily phosphorylated to active form by virus-coded thymidine kinase but is poorly phosphorylated by cellular thymidine kinase, resulting in a 200-fold amplification of active drug in virus-infected cells. Use of acyclovir, at a dosage of 30 mg/kg/day for 10 days, has been shown to reduce mortality from 70 to 28 percent, as compared to 54 percent for patients treated with vidarabine [141]. Mortality in patients treated with acyclovir (or with adenine arabinoside) is heavily influenced by level of consciousness at the time of presentation and is higher in patients over 30 years of age

[141,142]. Relapse of encephalitis following cessation of therapy has been reported with both agents but is less common with acyclovir [29,33,137].

Other Neurologic Conditions due to Herpes Simplex Virus Infection

Herpes simplex virus type 2 is associated with systemic infection with encephalitis in neonates and lymphocytic meningitis in adults. In occasional adult patients, herpes simplex virus type 2 has been associated with myelitis, myeloradiculitis, or encephalitis [4,94,120]. Rare cases of acute and recurrent meningitis, myelitis, and radiculitis have been associated with herpes simplex virus type 1 [94,101,131].

Neurologic Complications of Epstein-Barr Virus Infections

Neurologic conditions associated with Epstein-Barr virus infection have included aseptic meningitis, encephalitis, transverse myelitis, Guillain-Barré syndrome, brachial and lumbar plexopathies, cranial and peripheral neuropathies, and optic neuritis [129]. In some of these cases, the association of the neurologic syndrome with Epstein-Barr virus infection is tenuous. Nonetheless, convincing serologic evidence does exist in a number of instances [51,114,129]. The mechanism of injury in Epstein-Barr virus infections has not been clearly established. Epstein-Barr virus has been isolated from CSF lymphocytes in one instance but not from brain or spinal fluid per se [123]. It is most probable that the constellation of neurologic syndromes associated with Epstein-Barr virus infection, like measles encephalomyelitis, results from host immune response rather than viral invasion of the nervous system. Rarely, Epstein-Barr virus–induced thrombocytopenia may result in cerebral hemorrhage [129].

Prognosis in Acute Meningitis and Encephalitis

Prognosis for recovery from viral meningitis in children and adults is excellent. Studies by Sells, Carpenter, and Ray [125] and by Wilfert and associates [148], however, suggest that enteroviral meningitis in patients less than 1 year of age may adversely affect intellectual development. Prognosis for recovery in viral encephalitis, although dependant on the infectious agent, is less favorable. Mortality from Eastern equine encephalitis is in the range of 70 percent. Mortality from the other arthropod-borne encephalitides in the United States is far lower (see Table 19-2). Mumps meningoencephalitis may be followed by injury to cranial nerve VIII with transient or permanent deafness [42]. In rare cases, mumps may be followed by aqueductal stenosis [134]. Rabies virus infection is almost universally fatal; only three surviving cases have been reported, all in patients who received postexposure immunization [7]. Survivors from herpes simplex encephalitis may be left with dementia and a variety of temporal lobe deficits including temporal lobe seizures, receptive aphasia, and loss of the ability to store and recall new information [141–143,154]. Recovery in viral encephalitis may be prolonged over months, as may persistence of CSF abnormalities.

SLOW VIRUS INFECTIONS

Slow infections are characterized by a prolonged asymptomatic period between initial infection and the onset of illness and a progressive course to death or serious neurologic deficit once symptoms begin [71]. Six slow infections have been described in humans. Three of these, subacute sclerosing panencephalitis, progressive rubella encephalitis, and progressive multifocal leukoencephalopathy, are caused by conventional viruses. Kuru, Creutzfeldt-Jakob disease, and Gerstmann-Straussler syndrome are caused by as yet uncharacterized agents whose properties are unlike those of other infectious agents. Central nervous system infections by HIV-1 in AIDS and human T-lymphotrophic virus 1-(HTLV-1) in tropical spastic paraparesis behave in large measure as slow infections and are discussed separately.

Slow Virus Infections Due to Conventional Agents

Subacute Sclerosing Panencephalitis

Subacute sclerosing panencephalitis (SSPE) is caused by measles virus. The disorder is characterized pathologically by meningeal and perivascular lymphocytic infiltrates, astrocytic hypertrophy, proliferation of microglial cells, and the presence of intranuclear inclusions in neurons, astrocytes, and oligodendrocytes. Demyelination may be present in more slowly progressive cases [48]. Symptoms usually begin in childhood after the age of 6. Although most cases occur before adolescence, rare cases have been reported in adults. The affected child is initially noticed to have become withdrawn or to have developed a change in personality, usually with deterioration in school performance [48]. Nightmares and hallucinations may be present. Myoclonic jerking develops and is often thought initially to be clumsiness or restlessness. Visual difficulties occur in as many as 50 percent of patients and may represent either retinal or occipital lobe infection [48]. These early symptoms are followed by intellectual deterioration, development of spasticity, dementia, and eventually deterioration to a persistent vegetative state. In 80 percent of cases, death occurs within 3 years of onset of symptoms. In 10 percent of patients, illness is fulminant, and death occurs over weeks rather than months. In a few cases, the disease may be protracted over 4 to 8 years, with periods of clinical remission and at times improvement. Rare cases of apparent recovery have been described, usually with severe neurologic deficits. Even prior to the advent of measles vaccine, SSPE was a rare disease, with an incidence of one case of SSPE per million cases of measles. SSPE has essentially vanished from this country since the advent of compulsory measles immunization.

SSPE, despite its rarity, should be considered in any child developing progressive deterioration in intellectual function, in particular if there is a history of measles infection or exposure to measles virus infection in early childhood prior to measles vaccination or in children born in Third World countries. General physical examination is unremarkable, except for retinitis in occasional patients. Neurologic examination reveals attenuation of mental status and, in more advanced cases, myoclonus, corticospinal and extrapyramidal signs. Visual field defects may be due either to retinitis or to injury to central visual pathways. The EEG characteristically shows paroxysmal bursts of high-voltage sharp waves or spikes, which may coincide with myoclonic jerks [87]. These initially appear with fairly normal background and may antedate the appearance of clinical signs. Subsequently, a suppression burst pattern emerges in which high-voltage sharp waves and spikes alternate with periods of attenuated background activity [46]. Spinal fluid cell count, protein, and glucose are usually normal. CSF IgG content is greatly increased and may constitute as much as 60 percent of total CSF protein. Oligoclonal bands are present. High titers of antibody to measles virus are present in CSF, and serum anti-measles antibody titers are usually higher than those seen during convalescence from acute infection. Treatment with isoprinosine has produced improvement in SSPE in some but not all controlled studies [39,52,73]. Intraventricular instillation of human leukocyte interferon has been followed by clinical remission in three cases [103].

A disproportionately large number of patients with SSPE have a history of measles infection before the age of 2 years [48,53]. In some cases, no history of clinically evident measles is obtained, suggesting that measles virus infection during infancy may have been masked by passively transferred maternal antibody. Work from several laboratories has demonstrated that measles isolates from cases of SSPE are defective in their ability to code for M protein, a virus-coded protein that is necessary for the adherence of the developing measles virion to the inner surface of the cell membrane [84]. Deficiency of this protein is believed to prevent virus release from infected cells, so that development of infection in SSPE may occur by the much slower process of cell-to-cell spread. More recent work indicates that SSPE strains of measles virus may be deficient in their ability to code for other proteins as well [16]. The connection between acquisition of measles infection at an early age and persistence of defective strains of virus within the central nervous system is not understood.

Progressive Rubella Encephalitis

Slow infection following rubella is a rare condition. Ten cases of progressive rubella encephalitis (PRP) have been identified [149]. All have been males. Seven of the 10 had stigmata of congenital rubella. Onset of symptoms was between 8 and 19 years of age. Initial symptoms of global mental deterioration are similar to SSPE, although the progression of the disease is usually slower, and myoclonus is less frequently seen. The EEG usually shows only generalized slowing; the suppression burst pattern of SSPE has been reported but is unusual. Spinal fluid frequently manifests a lymphocytic pleocytosis of up to 40 cells/mm^3. Large amounts of IgG are present, with oligoclonal bands. High titers of anti-rubella antibodies are present in both sera and CSF. The major neuropathologic finding in PRP is extensive destruction of cerebral and cerebellar white matter. Loss of myelin and axons is prominent, as are gliosis, perivascular inflammation, and deposition of amorphous material in vessel walls [149].

Despite the clinical similarity of PRP to SSPE, the mechanisms of neurologic injury in the two conditions appear to be quite different. Although rubella virus has been isolated from the brain of one patient, attempts to identify infected cells by histology, electron microscopy, or immunofluorescence methods have been unsuccessful [21,149]. The pathologic changes of PRP are unlike those of SSPE and are most suggestive of immune-mediated vasculitis with microvascular ischemia.

Progressive Multifocal Leukoencephalopathy

PML is associated with central nervous system invasion by a papovavirus, JC virus. In five cases, a papovavirus similar to the simian agent SV40 virus has been reported [50]. Brains of PML patients show lytic infection of oligodendrocytes, with resultant multifocal foci of demyelination, which may become confluent to produce larger lesions [50]. JC virus also causes nonproductive infection of astrocytes, causing these cells to develop morphologic features suggestive of cell transformation. PML occurs almost without exception in patients with impaired cell-mediated immunity [50]. Prior to 1985, PML occurred predominantly in patients with chronic lymphocytic and other leukemias and lymphomas. Smaller numbers of cases were associated with immunosuppressive or cytotoxic therapy. Occasional cases have occurred in patients with sarcoidosis, tuberculosis, or nontropical sprue. In the past few years, PML has been increasingly associated with AIDS, occurring in 2 to 4 percent of AIDS patients [5].

PML is characterized clinically by the development of multifocal neurological signs involving the cerebrum, cerebellum, and brain stem. In most cases, cerebral symptoms predominate [50]. These may consist of confusion, dementia, expressive or receptive aphasia, and disturbances of parietal lobe function with apraxias or neglect. Visual field abnormalities are ultimately present in approximately 50 percent of cases. Brain stem or cerebellar findings may be present and may occasionally be the most prominent symptoms of the disease [50]. Most patients with PML die within 12 months, but survival of up to 10 years has been reported [75]. Therapy with adenine arabinoside and acyclovir is ineffective [50]. Therapy with cytosine arabinoside has been reported in nine patients, two of whom had AIDS. Stabilization or clinical improvement was reported in four patients, but five patients succumbed, including both AIDS patients [50]. In rare instances, including in AIDS-PML, the disorder may undergo spontaneous remission [5,6,50].

The sequence of host-virus interactions that leads to PML is not understood. Over 70 percent of persons have antibody to JC virus by late adult life [50]. Asymptomatic urinary excretion of the virus occurs in both immunosuppressed states and during pregnancy. The virus has been detected in extraneural tissues of both normal and PML patients [50,66]. Houff and colleagues [66] have detected JC virus DNA in bone marrow and splenic B-lymphocytes of patients developing PML in the setting of AIDS and have postulated that entry of infected B-lymphocytes into the central nervous system may initiate the disease.

It is not known, however, whether similar infection of B-lymphocytes occurs in non-AIDS patients as well. Additional studies will be required before it is known whether PML invariably represents a complication of ongoing systemic JC virus infection in immunosuppressed patients or whether it may also result from reactivation of latent infection within the central nervous system. The origin of PML-associated SV40 virus, if such actually exists, is unknown.

Transmissible Spongiform Encephalopathies

The transmissible spongiform encephalopathies include four diseases of animals—scrapie of sheep, spongiform encephalopathy of domestic cattle ("mad cow disease"), transmissible mink encephalopathy, and transmissible encephalopathy of mule deer—and three diseases of humans—kuru, Creutzfeldt-Jakob disease, and Gerstmann-Straussler syndrome. The infectious nature of these diseases has been repeatedly demonstrated by their transmission to laboratory animals and, in the case of kuru and Creutzfeldt-Jakob disease, by transmission from human to human [8,14,38,44,115]. The neuropathologic changes characteristic of these disorders are more typical of degenerative than infectious conditions and include neuronal loss, astrocytic glial response, development of amyloid plaques, and spongiform change within surviving neurons. Inflammation, viral inclusions, and other hallmarks of viral infection are absent.

Kuru

Kuru was the first of the human spongiform encephalopathies to be transmitted to laboratory animals [44]. The condition was confined to the highlands of the Fore Peninsula of New Guinea and was characterized by progressive cerebellar ataxia and dysarthria, ending in death. Spread of infection from human to human is believed to have occurred through cutaneous and mucosal inoculation with infected brain material during cannibalistic mourning rituals. At the time the disease was first discovered, kuru had an incidence of 1 percent and accounted for up to 50 percent of deaths in some villages. The incidence of the disease has diminished steadily since suppression of cannibalism [44].

Creutzfeldt-Jakob Disease

Creutzfeldt-Jakob disease is a subacute dementia, characteristically accompanied by stimulus-sensitive myoclonus and by development of high-voltage periodic complexes on the EEG. Although the most common of the subacute spongiform encephalopathies, the incidence of Creutzfeldt-Jakob disease is only 0.9 to 1.2 cases per million [89]. Areas of increased incidence have been reported among Lybian Jews and within Czechoslovakia [89]. The disorder is predominantly a condition of middle age, with a mean age of onset of 52 years, but cases have been reported in persons as young as 17 years and as old as 78 years. A familial history of progressive dementia is obtained in approximately 15 percent of cases. Conjugal cases of the disease are rare, however, suggesting that the familial occurrence of Creutzfeldt-Jakob disease reflects genetically determined susceptibility rather than common exposure [89]. The means by which the disease is transmitted in nature is not known. Creutzfeldt-Jakob disease has occurred following transplantation of a cornea from an infected donor, use of contaminated electrodes for cerebral cortical depth recordings, and use of contaminated dura mater grafts in neurosurgical procedures [8,38,44,115]. Several cases have occurred in patients receiving human growth hormone prepared from pooled human pituitary glands obtained at autopsy [14].

The onset of Creutzfeldt-Jakob disease is usually subacute, with impairment of memory, alteration in personality, and blunting of intellect [15]. Patients may note changes in visual perception. As the disease progresses, myoclonus appears, which may be elicited by auditory stimuli. The disease may produce symptoms referable to virtually any part of the central nervous system, with pyramidal and extrapyramidal symptoms, cerebellar ataxia, and evidence of brain stem injury. Involvement of the occipital lobes may produce hemianopsias or, in a minority of patients, Haidenhain's syndrome, in which the predominant initial feature of the disease is cortical blindness. Involvement of spinal motor neurons may produce fasciculations and depression of reflexes suggestive of amyotrophic lateral sclerosis. As the disease progresses, the patient enters a persistent vegetative state, with decorticate or decerebrate posturing. Death usually occurs within 9 months of onset of symptoms. The disease may occasionally run a more rapid course, however, and instances of clinical survival of 5 years or more have been reported [15]. There is no known therapy.

Creutzfeldt-Jakob disease is an important differential condition in any adult patient developing rapidly progressive dementia. Routine studies of blood, urine, and CSF are nondiagnostic. CT and MRI are unhelpful. The EEG may initially be normal or show only generalized slowing. Over time, triphasic high-voltage waves appear, superimposed on generalized slowing [18]. During the terminal stages of the disease, high-voltage activity may disappear, leaving only profound slowing. In rare cases, the EEG may remain normal late into the course of disease. In some cases, presumptive diagnosis may be made on the basis of the typical history, neurologic examination, and EEG findings. In many patients, however, the diagnosis becomes clear only as the patient is followed over weeks or months. Definitive diagnosis by brain biopsy may be required in atypical cases but requires specific measures of decontamination as discussed below.

Gerstmann-Straussler Syndrome

In 1981, Masters, Gajdusek, and Gibbs [88] described four patients whose clinical course was characterized by prominent cerebellar ataxia accompanying dementia and corticospinal tract signs. Median survival in these patients was 59 months, significantly longer than that seen in Creutzfeldt-Jakob disease. Neuropathologic examination revealed prominent amyloid plaques. A familial history of similar illness was present in one case. The clinical and neuropathologic findings in these cases were strongly reminiscent of Gerstmann-Straussler syndrome, a familial degenerative condition of unknown etiology. Inoculation of brain material from these patients into laboratory primates, however, produced spongiform changes identical to those seen in experimental Creutzfeldt-Jakob disease. The relationship of transmissible Gerstmann-Straussler syndrome to Creutzfeldt-Jakob disease and the reasons for the atypical features of this syndrome are not understood.

Etiology and Pathogenesis of the Transmissible Spongiform Encephalopathies

Extensive efforts to identify virus particles, antigens, or nucleic acids in scrapie, kuru, or Creutzfeldt-Jakob material have been unsuccessful, and work from multiple laboratories has demonstrated that the causative agents of these disorders possess unique properties including extreme resistance to heat, ionizing radiation, agents known to destroy nucleic acids, and most materials normally used to decontaminate infectious material. A major conceptual advance in understanding the pathogenesis of these disorders has come through the work of Prusiner and associates [67,112], who identified a unique 27-30 kd glycoprotein, termed PrP 27-30, which was absent from controls and which copurified with the scrapie agent. Subsequent investigations have demonstrated similar proteins in brains of humans dying of Creutzfeldt-Jakob disease and of Gerstmann-Straussler syndrome [112]. PrP 27-30 forms the core of a 33-35 kd protein, which is encoded by a host chomosomal gene and not by nucleic acid from some extrinsic agent. The PrP gene has been localized to the short arm of human chromosome 20 and to the homologous region of chromosome 2 in the mouse. PrP 33-35 is present in both normal and infected brains but exists in two isoforms, each consisting of 253 amino acids in mice or hamsters and 254 amino acids in humans [112]. PrP 33-35 isolated from scrapie-infected brains, PrP^{sc}, is degraded by proteinase K to PrP 27-30. In contrast, PrP 33-35 obtained from uninfected material, PrP^{c}, is completely degraded by proteinase K, without formation of PrP 27-30. Formation of PrP^{sc} appears does not appear to be a due to abnormalities in the host mRNA encoding the protein but rather appears to result from posttranslational modification of the normal protein. PrP^{sc} is found in aggregates, rods, tubules, and detergent-lipid-protein aggregates obtained from brains of mice or hamsters with scrapie and of patients with Creutzfeldt-Jakob disease or

Gerstmann-Straussler syndrome [18,89,100]. PrP^{sc} is also found in amyloid within infected brains but not in amyloid deposits associated with other conditions. Recently, Hsaio and co-workers [67] have created transgenic mice by microinjecting into fertilized mouse oocytes the human PrP gene and have demonstrated that these animals develop a spontaneous disease histopathologically similar to scrapie. Further work with transgenic mice carrying the hamster PrP^{sc} gene show that PrP^{sc} influences other aspects of scrapie as well, including species specificity, length of incubation time, and synthesis of the pathologic PrP protein [67,112]. The mechanisms by which this pathologic protein might cause transmissible, progressive central nervous system pathology, however, is not yet known.

Containment of the Infectious Agent in Transmissible Virus Dementias

The agents of Creutzfeldt-Jakob disease and Gerstmann-Straussler syndrome, like those of scrapie and kuru, are resistant to autoclaving at conventional temperatures and to routine chemical methods of decontamination including alcohols, formaldehyde, glutaraldehyde, and iodine. Methods of decontamination must thus be altered when treating materials potentially contaminated with these agents [20]. This necessity is obvious where the issue involves fresh brain biopsy or autopsy of suspected or confirmed cases. Equally stringent precautions should be considered in patients with rapidly progressive dementia undergoing lumbar puncture, neurosurgical or ophthalmologic procedures of any sort, or procedures more routine in the elderly, such as transurethral prostatic resection or hip replacement. The resistance of the agent of Creutzfeldt-Jakob disease to formalin suggests that precautions should also be taken in situations involving handling of fixed tissues [93]. Disposable materials such as needles, syringes, or lumbar puncture supplies should be incinerated. Material that can be autoclaved should be heated at 132°C for 1 hour. Nonautoclavable material should be treated with 1N sodium hydroxide for 1 hour. Sodium hypochlorite (household bleach), previously recommended as a method of decontamination, is only partially effective.

RETROVIRUS INFECTIONS OF THE CENTRAL NERVOUS SYSTEM: ACQUIRED IMMUNODEFICIENCY SYNDROME

Within the past several years, several retroviruses have been associated with human disease. These agents were initially termed human T-lymphotrophic viruses 1–4 (HTLV-1, 2, 3, and 4), based on their ability to infect T-lymphocytes. Subsequently, HTLV-3 was renamed human immunodeficiency virus (HIV-1) to emphasize its association with acquired human immunodeficiency. HTLV-1 and 2 produce transformation of T-lymphocytes. HTLV-1 is associated with adult T-cell leukemia and non-Hodgkin T-cell lymphoma [121,122]. HTLV-2 has been isolated from cases of hairy-cell leukemia [121,122]. HIV-1 produces lytic rather than transforming infection of T-lymphocytes and is the agent most frequently associated with AIDS. HIV-2, a closely related virus, has recently been recovered from AIDS cases in Africa and from 12 patients, largely of African origin, in this country [2]. Lytic infection of T-lymphocytes by HIV-1 and HIV-2 is confined to those cells bearing the CD4 marker (Helper-inducer T-lymphocytes) [76]. Destruction of these cells results in profound impairment of cell-mediated immunity, with attenuation of T-cell-associated B-cell-mediated immune function as well [133]. Commonly seen immunologic findings include cutaneous anergy, depressed response in lymphocyte transformation assays, impaired natural killer cell activity, and failure to mount an antibody response to ongoing opportunistic infections.

The central nervous system is symptomatically involved in over 30 percent of patients with AIDS, and AIDS patients frequently present with neurologic complaints (Table 19-5). [11,13,55,82,90, 107,130]. Infection may be caused by HIV itself or by a variety of opportunistic agents. Neurologic symptoms may also be produced by hemorrhage, embolic events from marantic endocarditis, or spontaneous tumors,

Table 19-5. Neurologic syndromes associated with HIV infection

Lymphocytic (aseptic) meningitis
AIDS-related encephalopathy
Vacuolar myelopathy
Demyelinating neuropathy
Polymyositis
Vasculitis

usually primary central nervous system non-Hodgkin lymphomas.

Neurologic Syndromes Associated Directly with HIV Infection of the Central Nervous System

AIDS Meningitis

Lymphocytic meningitis occurs in approximately 13 percent of AIDS patients developing central nervous system signs or symptoms and is particularly common at the time of seroconversion [64,90]. Less frequently, meningitis may occur after seroconversion or in the setting of AIDS-related encephalopathy. Onset may be abrupt, with typical meningeal symptoms; chronic, with mild headache; or asymptomatic. Cranial nerve palsies, in particular of cranial nerves V, VII, and VIII, may be present, as may long tract signs. Spinal fluid shows a lymphocytic pleocytosis [13,64,82,90]. Protein may be normal or mildly elevated. Glucose is normal. HIV can be detected in the CSF of some but not all patients [90]. The meningitis may occur as a single, self-limited episode or may be chronic or recurrent [64,90].

AIDS-Related Encephalopathy (AIDS-Related Dementia, AIDS Encephalopathy, AIDS Dementia Complex)

AIDS-related encephalopathy may accompany systemic manifestations of AIDS or may be the initial feature of the disorder. Early symptoms consist of personality change, loss of usual interests, blunting of intellect, withdrawal, and apathy. Psychological testing in such patients reveals findings consistent with a subcortical dementia, with psychomotor slowing, diminished spontaneity, impaired problem-solving, and loss of fine motor control [11,13,67,82,90, 107,111,130]. Progression of the disorder over weeks to months may lead to profound dementia with urinary and fecal incontinence. Focal neurologic signs are present in a minority of patients [111]. Occasional patients may develop seizures [111]. Gross examination of brains from affected patients reveals deep and superficial cerebral atrophy [82,106,107,111]. Early histologic findings include pallor of cerebral white matter, gemistocytic astrocytosis, and sparse infiltrates of lipid-laden macrophages, lymphocytes, and microglia. More advanced cases exhibit multinucleated giant cells. Neuronal loss and astrocytosis are frequently present within caudate, putamen, and other subcortical structures. Clinical improvement has been reported following therapy with 3′-azido-2′3′-deoxythymidine (zidovudine [azidothymidine, AZT]), a drug that is believed to inhibit virus-coded reverse transcriptase [60,152,153]. The long-term efficacy of AZT in AIDS-related encephalopathy is still under investigation.

Vacuolar Myelopathy

Vacuolar myelopathy occurs in approximately 30 percent of patients with AIDS but does not produce symptoms in all patients [108,127]. The disorder may accompany or occur independently of the AIDS-related encephalopathy. Lateral and posterior columns of the thoracic cord are most severely affected. Clinical symptoms include progressive spastic mono- or paraparesis. Ataxia is frequently present and may be out of keeping with the apparent degree of proprioceptive involvement. Pathologic findings are similar to those of subacute combined degeneration, with vacuolation of myelin lamellae within posterior and lateral fiber tracts.

Other Neurologic Conditions Associated with HIV Infection

Disorders of peripheral nerve or muscle occur in approximately 15 percent of patients with AIDS. Peripheral nervous system involvement may be asymptomatic or may result in acute Guillain-Barré syndrome, chronic progressive demyelinating polyneuropathies, axonal neuropathies, mononeuritis multiplex, or a cauda equina syndrome [22,104]. Improvement in AIDS-related neuropathies has been reported with the use of AZT [24]. Typical polymyositis with proximal muscle weakness has been reported in AIDS [22,23], as has a syndrome of proximal muscle weakness with atrophy of type II fibers [22,23,104]. A single case of upper and lower motor neuron degeneration indistinguishable from amyotrophic lateral sclerosis has been described in a 26-year-old man in whom seroconversion to HIV and isolation of HIV from peripheral blood were documented [63]. Pathologic confirmation of motor neuron disease was not obtained, however, and the association between the patient's neuromuscular disease and his HIV infection is not clear. Vasculitis with multifocal cerebral infarcts not associated with herpes zoster virus infection has also been reported [151].

Mechanisms of Neurologic Injury by HIV

The pathogenesis of the neurologic disorders associated with HIV infection is poorly understood. AIDS meningitis, encephalopathy, and vacuolar myelopathy appear to be directly related to viral infection. CSF abnormalities are frequent in asymptomatic HIV-positive individuals, suggesting that central nervous system invasion by HIV may occur very early in the course of infection [91]. HIV-1 has been identified in brains of both adults and children with AIDS encephalopathy [62,81,128]. HIV virions have been detected in multinucleated giant cells within AIDS brains. HIV genomic material has been identified by in situ nucleic acid hybridization methods in multinucleated giant cells and, in a few reports, in neurons and astrocytes [77,132,146]. It is not known whether neurologic injury is initiated by infected macrophages or by infection of other cell types, nor is it known whether the neuropathologic syndromes seen in AIDS result from virus-induced disturbances in metabolic function or secretion of neurotoxins by HIV-infected mononuclear phagocytes [47,105]. HIV has not been identified within lesions of the vacuolar myelopathy, and the pathogenesis of this disorder is unknown. Some of the conditions, such as Guillain-Barré syndrome, are probably of autoimmune origin.

Opportunistic Central Nervous System Infections in AIDS

The impairment of T-cell- and antibody-mediated immune response characteristic of AIDS permits central nervous system infection by a variety of opportunistic bacterial, fungal, protozoal, and viral agents (Table 19-6) [11,13,55,82,90,107,130]. Of these agents, the protozoan organism *Toxoplasma gondii* is the most common, followed by *Cryptococcus neoformans*. Opportunistic viral infections are also common. Cytomegalovirus (CMV) has been associated with encephalitis in the setting of AIDS [57,90,145]. The frequency of CMV encephalitis is not known with certainty, however, since some of the early cases attributed to CMV may in fact have been cases of AIDS-related encephalopathy. Diagnosis of CMV encephalitis in the

Table 19-6. Agents of opportunistic central nervous system infection in patients with acquired immunodeficiency syndrome

Bacteria
Mycobacterium tuberculosis
(*Mycobacterium avium intracellulare*)*
(*Listeria monocytogenes*)
(*Nocardia asteroides*)
Spirochetes
Treponema pallidum
Fungi
Cryptococcus neoformans
(*Candida albicans*)
(*Aspergillus fumigatus*)
(*Coccidioides immitis*)
(*Rhizopus* species)
Protozoa
Toxoplasma gondii
Viruses
Cytomegalovirus
Herpes simplex virus type 1
Herpes simplex virus type 2
Herpes zoster virus
Papovavirus JC
(Adenovirus type 2)

* Parentheses indicate infrequently reported agents as causes of central nervous system infections in AIDS.

setting of AIDS may be difficult; extraneural infection with CMV may accompany central nervous system infections by other agents. Because CMV is not usually recovered from CSF, definitive diagnosis of CMV encephalitis during life may require brain biopsy, although further work with the polymerase chain reaction may permit definitive diagnosis from CSF alone. CMV may cause progressive retinitis in AIDS patients and has also been associated with demyelination of the posterior columns of the spinal cord and ascending myelitis [90,95]. The acyclovir analogue 9-(1,3-dihydroxy-2-propoxymethyl) guanine (DHPG) is under investigation in CMV retinitis and may offer a therapy for CMV encephalitis.

Progressive multifocal leukoencephalopathy, as mentioned above, is seen in 2 to 4 percent of patients with AIDS. Herpes simplex virus has been associated with myelitis, encephalitis, and ventriculitis in AIDS patients. Cutaneous infection with varicella-zoster virus occurs in 5 to 10 percent of AIDS patients. Herpes zoster virus may produce a multifocal, demyelinating encephalomyelitis similar to that seen in other immunosuppressed conditions [65] and also a vasculitis with cerebral infarction.

Neurologic Complications of HIV Infection in Children

The neurologic complications of AIDS in children differ to some extent from those seen in adults. Progressive encephalopathy is present in 30 to 50 percent of infected children [41]. The clinical symptoms of AIDS-related encephalopathy in children may be intermittent, with periods of apparent stabilization. Pathologic findings include prominent demyelination, at times with severe atrophy of the deep white matter, corpus callosum, and descending corticospinal tracts. Perivascular inflammation is more prominent in children than is usual in adults and may be accompanied by vessel calcification [72,106]. In children, as opposed to adults, neurologic involvement by opportunistic infections is relatively uncommon. Vacuolar myelopathy has not been reported in children.

ASSOCIATION OF HUMAN RETROVIRUSES WITH OTHER NEUROLOGIC DISEASES

HTLV-1 has recently been suggested as the causative agent of two syndromes of chronic progressive myelopathy: tropical spastic paraparesis (TSP) and HTLV-1-associated myelopathy (HAM) [72,102,138]. TSP occurs predominantly in Caribbean and South American countries but has also been reported in the southeastern United States [72,138]. HAM is a similar condition described in Japan [102]. Both disorders are characterized clinically by progressive lower extremity spasticity and weakness. Pathologic findings include chronic inflammation of spinal cord gray and white matter and demyelination of the lateral columns. Antibodies to HTLV-1 have been detected in sera and CSF of patients with disorders, with evidence of intrathecal antibody synthesis [17,102,138]. Retrovirus-like particles have been detected in the spinal cord of a patient with TSP [83]. Isolation of HTLV-1 has been achieved from CSF in both TSP and HAM [59,69]. The mechanism by which HIV-1 might cause TSP or HAM is not yet known. Studies of patients from Japan suggest that immunogenetic factors may determine whether HTLV-1 virus infection results in acute T-cell leukemia as opposed to HAM [136].

REFERENCES

1. Addair, C. V., Gauld, R. L., and Smadel, J. E. Aseptic meningitis, a disease of diverse etiology: Clinical and etiologic studies on 854 cases. *Ann. Intern. Med.* 39:675, 1953.
2. Centers for Disease Control. Update: HIV-2 infection. *M.M.W.R.* 38:572, 1989.
3. Aurelius, E., Johansson, B., Skoldenberg, B., et al. Rapid diagnosis of herpes simplex encephalitis by nested polymerase chain reaction assay of cerebrospinal fluid. *Lancet* 337(8735):189, 1990.
4. Baringer, J. R. Herpes Simplex Virus Infections of the Nervous System. In P. J. Vinken and G. W. Bruyn (eds.), *Handbook of Clinical Neurology.* Amsterdam: North-Holland, 1978. Vol. 34, pp. 145–159.
5. Berger, J. R., Kaszovitz, B., Post, J. D., and Dick-

erson, G. Progressive multifocal leukoencephalopathy associated with human virus infection. *Ann. Intern. Med.* 107:78, 1987.
6. Berger, J. R., and Mucke, L. Prolonged survival and partial recovery in AIDS-associated progressive multifocal leukoencephalopathy. *Neurology* 38:1060, 1988.
7. Bernard, K. W., and Hattwick, M. A. W. Rabies Virus. In G. L. Mandell, R. G. Douglas, Jr., and J. E. Bennett (eds.), *Principles and Practice of Infectious Diseases* (3rd ed.). New York: Wiley, 1985. Pp. 897–909.
8. Bernoulli, C., Siegried, J., Baumgartner, G., et al. Danger of accidental person-to-person transmission of Creutzfeldt-Jakob disease by surgery. *Lancet* 1:478, 1977.
9. Bia, F. J., Thornton, G. F., Main, A. J., et al. Western equine encephalitis mimicking herpes simplex encephalitis. *J.A.M.A.* 244: 367, 1980.
10. Bodian, D., and Horstmann, D. M. Polioviruses. In F. L. Horsfall and I. Tamm (eds.), *Viral and Rickettsial Infections of Man* (4th ed.). Philadelphia: Lippincott, 1965. Pp. 430–473.
11. Booss, J., and Harris, S. A. Neurology of AIDS virus infection: A clinical classification. *Yale J. Biol. Med.* 60:537, 1987.
12. Bowen, D. L., Lane, H. C., and Fauci, A. S. Immunopathogenesis of the acquired immunodeficiency syndrome. *Ann. Intern. Med.* 103:704, 1985.
13. Britton, C. B., and Mills, J. R. Neurological complications in acquired immunodeficiency syndrome (AIDS). *Neurol. Clin.* 2:315, 1984.
14. Brown, P. The decline and fall of Creutzfeldt-Jakob disease associated with human growth hormone therapy. *Neurology* 38:1135, 1988.
15. Brown, P., Cathala, F., Castaigne, P., and Gajdusek, D. C. Creutzfeldt-Jakob disease: Clinical analysis of a consecutive series of 230 neuropathologically verified cases. *Ann. Neurol.* 20:597, 1986.
16. Cattaneo, R., Schmid, A., Billeter, M. A., et al. Multiple viral mutations rather than host factors cause defective measles virus gene expression in a subacute sclerosing panencephalitis cell line. *J. Virol.* 62:1388, 1988.
17. Ceroni, M., Piccardo, P., Rodgers-Johnson, P., et al. Intrathecal synthesis of IgG antibodies to HTLV-I supports an etiological role for HTLV-I in tropical spastic paraparesis. *Ann. Neurol.* 23(Suppl.):S188, 1988.
18. Chiofalo, N., Fuentes, A., and Galvez, S. Serial EEG findings in 27 cases of Creutzfeldt-Jakob disease. *Arch. Neurol.* 37:143, 1980.
19. Chou, S. M., Ross, R., Burrell, R., et al. Subacute focal adenovirus encephalitis. *J. Neuropathol. Exp. Neurol.* 323:34, 1973.
20. Committee on Health Care Issues, American Neurological Association. Precautions in handling tissues, fluids, and other contaminated materials from patients with documented or suspected Creutzfeldt-Jakob disease. *Ann. Neurol.* 19:75, 1986.
21. Cremer, N. E., Oshiro, L. S., Weil, M. L., et al. Isolation of rubella virus from brain in chronic progressive panencephalitis. *J. Gen. Virol.* 29:143, 1975.
22. Dalakas, M. C., and Pezeshkpour, G. H. Neuromuscular diseases associated with human immunodeficiency virus infection. *Ann. Neurol.* 32(Suppl.):S38, 1987.
23. Dalakas, M. C., Pezeshkpour, G. H., Gravell, M., and Sever, J. L. Polymyositis associated with AIDS retrovirus. *J.A.M.A.* 256:2381, 1986.
24. Dalakas, M. C., Yarchoan, R., Spitzer, R., et al. Treatment of human immunodeficiency virus-related polyneuropathy with 3′-azido-2′3′-deoxythymidine *Ann. Neurol.* 32(Suppl.):S92, 1987.
25. Dal Canto, M. C., Barbano, R. L., and Jubelt, B. Ultrastructural immunohistochemical localization of poliovirus during virulent infection of mice. *J. Neuropathol. Exp. Neurol.* 45:613, 1986.
26. Davis, L. E. Influenza B virus model of Reye's syndrome: Evidence for a nonpermissive infection of liver and brain. *Lab. Invest.* 56:32, 1987.
27. Davis, L. E., Bodian, D., Price, D., et al. Chronic progressive poliomyelitis secondary to vaccination of an immunosuppressed child. *N. Engl. J. Med.* 297:241, 1977.
28. Davis, L. E., and Johnson, R. T. An explanation for the localization of herpes simplex encephalitis? *Ann. Neurol.* 5:2, 1979.
29. Davis, L. E., and McLaren, L. C. Relapsing herpes simplex encephalitis following antiviral therapy. *Ann. Neurol.* 13:192, 1983.
30. Dayan, A. D., Gooddy, W., Harrison, M. J. G., and Rudge, P. Brain stem encephalitis caused by herpesvirus hominis. *Br. Med. J.* 4:405, 1972.
31. Deibel, R., Woodall, J. P., Decher, W. J., and Schryver, G. D. Lymphocytic choriomeningitis virus in man: Serological evidence of association with pet hamsters. *J.A.M.A.* 232:501, 1975.
32. Delacour, J. L., Floriot, C., Ritz, A., et al. Rhombencephalites listeriennes sans atteinte meningee. *Presse Med.* 16:735, 1987.
33. Dix, R. D., Baringer, J. R., Panitch, H. S., et al. Recurrent herpes simplex encephalitis: Recovery of the virus after Ara-A treatment. *Ann. Neurol.* 13:196, 1983.
34. Dix, R. D., McKendall, R. R., and Baringer, J. R. Comparative neurovirulence of herpes simplex virus type 1 strains after peripheral or intracerebral inoculation of BALB/c mice. *Infect. Immun.* 40:103, 1983.

35. Dorfman, L. J. Cytomegalovirus encephalitis in adults. *Neurology* 23:136, 1973.
36. Dorsky, D. I., and Crumpacker, C. S. Drugs five years later: Acyclovir. *Ann. Intern. Med.* 107:859, 1987.
37. Duffy, J., Lidsky, M. D., Sharp, J. T., et al. Polyarthritis, polyarteritis, and hepatitis B. *Medicine* 55:19, 1976.
38. Duffy, P., Wolf, J., Collins, G., et al. Possible person-to-person transmission of Creutzfeldt-Jakob disease. *N. Engl. J. Med.* 290:692, 1974.
39. Dyken, P. R., Swift, A., and DuRant, R. H. Long-term follow-up of patients with subacute sclerosing panencephalitis treated with inosiplex. *Ann. Neurol.* 11:359, 1982.
40. Eisenstein, B. I. The polymerase chain reaction a new method of using molecular genetics for medical diagnosis. *N. Engl. J. Med.* 322:178, 1990.
41. Epstein, L. G., Sharer, L. R., and Goudsmit, J. Neurological and neuropathological features of human immunodeficiency virus infection in children. *Ann. Neurol.* 23(Suppl.):S19, 1988.
42. Everberg, G. Deafness following mumps. *Acta Otolaryngol.* 48:397, 1957.
43. Fishman, R. A. No, brain biopsy need not be done in every patient suspected of having herpes simplex encephalitis. *Arch. Neurol.* 44:1291, 1987.
44. Gajdusek, D. C. Unconventional viruses and the origin and disappearance of kuru. *Science* 197:943, 1977.
45. Gendelman, H. E., Wolinsky, J. S., Johnson, R. T., et al. Measles encephalomyelitis: Lack of evidence of viral invasion of the central nervous system and quantitative study of the nature of demyelination. *Ann. Neurol.* 15:353, 1984.
46. Gimenez-Roldan, S., Martin, M., Mateo, D., and Lopez-Fraile, I. P. Preclinical EEG abnormalities in subacute sclerosing panencephalitis. *Neurology* 31:763, 1981.
47. Giulian, D., Vaca, K., and Noonan, C. A. Secretion of neurotoxins by mononuclear phagocytes infected with HIV1. *Science* 250:1593, 1990.
48. Graves, M. C. Subacute sclerosing panencephalitis. *Neurol. Clin.* 2:267, 1984.
49. Greenlee, J. E. Encephalitis. In J. H. Stein, (ed.), *Internal Medicine* (2nd ed.). Boston: Little, Brown, 1987. Pp. 2224–2228.
50. Greenlee, J. E. Progressive multifocal leukoencephalopathy. *Curr. Clin. Topics Infect. Dis.* 10:141, 1989.
51. Grose, C., Henle, W., Henle, G., and Feorino, P. M. Primary Epstein-Barr-virus infections in acute neurologic diseases. *N. Engl. J. Med.* 292:392, 1975.
52. Haddad, F. S., and Risk, W. S. Isoprinosine treatment in 18 patients with subacute sclerosing panencephalitis: A controlled study. *Ann. Neurol.* 7:185, 1980.
53. Halsey, N. A., Modlin, J. F., Jabbour, J. T., et al. Risk factors in subacute sclerosing panencephalitis: A case-control study. *Am. J. Epidemiol.* 111:415, 1980.
54. Hanley, D. F., Johnson, R. T., Whitley, R. J. Yes, brain biopsy should be a prerequisite for herpes simplex encephalitis treatment. *Arch. Neurol.* 44:1289, 1987.
55. Harris, A. A., Segreti, J., and Levin, S. Central nervous system infections in patients with the acquired immune deficiency syndrome (AIDS). *Clin. Neuropharmacol.* 8:201, 1985.
56. Hart, M. N., and Earl, K. M. Hemmorhagic and perivenous encephalitis: A clinical-pathological review of 38 cases. *J. Neurol. Neurosurg. Psychiatry* 38:585, 1975.
57. Hawley, D. A., Schaefer, J. F., Schulz, D. M., and Muller, J. Cytomegalovirus encephalitis in acquired immunodeficiency syndrome. *Am. J. Clin. Pathol.* 80:874, 1983.
58. Hilt, D. C., Buchholz, D., Krumholz, A., et al. Herpes zoster and delayed contralateral hemiparesis due to cerebral angiitis: Diagnosis and management approaches. *Ann. Neurol.* 14:543, 1983.
59. Hirose, S., Uemura, Y., Fujishita, M., et al. Isolation of HTLV-I from cerebrospinal fluid of a patient with myelopathy. *Lancet* 2:397, 1986.
60. Hirsch, M. S. Azidothymidine. *J. Infect. Dis.* 157:427, 1988.
61. Ho, D. D., and Hirsch, M. S. Acute viral encephalitis. *Med. Clin. North Am.* 69:415, 1985.
62. Ho, D. D., Rota, T. R., Schooley, R. T., et al. Isolation of HTLV-III from cerebrospinal fluid and neural tissues of patients with neurologic syndromes related to the acquired immunodeficiency syndrome. *N. Engl. J. Med.* 313:1493, 1985.
63. Hoffman, P. M., Festoff, B. W., Giron, L. T., et al. Isolation of LAV/HTLV-III from a patient with amyotrophic lateral sclerosis. *N. Engl. J. Med.* 312:324, 1985.
64. Hollander, H., and Stringari, S. Human immunodeficiency virus-associated meningitis. *Am. J. Med.* 83:813, 1987.
65. Horton, B., Price, R. W., and Jimenz, D. Multifocal varicella-zoster virus leukoencephalitis temporally remote from herpes zoster. *Ann. Neurol.* 9:251, 1981.
66. Houff, S. A., Major, E. O., Katz, D. A., et al. Involvement of JC virus-infected mononuclear cells from the bone marrow and spleen in the pathogenesis of progressive multifocal leukoencephalopathy. *N. Engl. J. Med.* 318:301, 1988.
67. Hsiao, K. K., Scott, M., Foster, D., et al. Spon-

taneous neurodegeneration in transgenic mice with mutant prion protein. *Science* 250:1587, 1990.

68. Iwasaki, Y., Liu, D.-S., Yamamoto, T., and Konno, H. On the replication and spread of rabies virus in the human central nervous system. *J. Neuropathol. Exp. Neurol.* 44:185, 1985.
69. Jacobson, S., Raine, C. S., Mingioli, E. S., and McFarlin, D. E. Isolation of an HTLV-I-like retrovirus from patients with tropical spastic paraparesis. *Nature* 3311:540, 1988.
70. Johnson, K. P., and Johnson, R. T. California encephalitis: II. Studies of experimental infection in the mouse. *J. Neuropathol. Exp. Neurol.* 27:390, 1968.
71. Johnson, R. T. *Viral Infections of the Nervous System.* New York: Raven, 1982.
72. Johnson, R. T., and McArthur, J. C. Myelopathies and retroviral infections. *Ann. Neurol.* 21:113, 1987.
73. Jones, C. W., Dyken, P. R., and Huttenlocker, P. R. Inosiplex therapy in subacute sclerosing panencephalitis: A multicentre, nonrandomized study in 98 patients. *Lancet* 1:1034, 1982.
74. Kennard, C., and Swash, M. Acute viral encephalitis: Its diagnosis and outcome. *Brain* 104:129, 1981.
75. Kepes, J. J., Chou, S. M., and Price, L. W., Jr. Progressive multifocal leukoencephalopathy with 10-year survival in a patient with nontropical sprue. *Neurology* 25:1006, 1975.
76. Klatzmann, D., Barre-Sinoussi, F., Nugeyre, M. T., et al. Selective tropism of lymphadenopathy associated virus (LAV) for helper-inducer T-lymphocytes. *Science* 225:59, 1984.
77. Koenig, S., Gendelman, H. E., Orenstein, J. M., et al. Detection of AIDS virus in brain tissue from AIDS patients with encephalopathy. *Science* 233:1089, 1986.
78. Koskiniemi, M., Vaheri, A., and Taskinen, E. Cerebrospinal fluid alterations in herpes simplex virus encephalitis. *Rev. Infect. Dis.* 6:608, 1984.
79. Kristennson, K., Lycke, E., and Sjostrand, J. Spread of herpes simplex virus in peripheral nerves. *Acta Neuropathol.* 17:44, 1971.
80. Levine, D. P., Lauter, C. B., and Lerner, A. M. Simultaneous serum and CSF antibodies in herpes simplex virus encephalitis. *J.A.M.A.* 240:356, 1978.
81. Levy, J. A., Hollander, H., Shimabukuro, J., et al. Isolation of AIDS-associated retroviruses from the cerebrospinal fluid and brain of patients with neurological symptoms. *Lancet* 2:586, 1985.
82. Levy, R. M., Bredesen, D. E., and Rosenblum, M. L. Neurological manifestations of the acquired immunodeficiency syndrome (AIDS): Experience at UCSF and review of the literature. *J. Neurosurg.* 62:475, 1985.
83. Liberski, P. P., Rodgers-Johnson, P., Char, G., et al. HTLV-I-like viral particles in spinal cord cells in Jamaican tropical spastic paraparesis. *Ann. Neurol.* 23(Suppl.):S185, 1988.
84. Lin, H. F., and Thormar, H. Absence of M protein in a cell-associated subacute sclerosing panencephalitis virus. *Nature* 285:490, 1980.
85. Linneman, C. C., and Alvira, M. M. Pathogenesis of varicella-zoster angiitis in the CNS. *Arch. Neurol.* 37:329, 1980.
86. Maddon, P. J., Dalgleish, A. G., McDougal, J. S., et al. The T4 gene encodes the AIDS virus receptor and is expressed in the immune system and the brain. *Cell* 47:333, 1986.
87. Markand, O. N., and Panszi, J. G. The electroencephalogram in subacute sclerosing panencephalitis. *Arch. Neurol.* 32:719, 1975.
88. Masters, C. L., Gajdusek, D. C., and Gibbs, C. J. Creutzfeldt-Jakob disease virus isolations from the Gerstmann-Straussler syndrome. *Brain* 104:559, 1981.
89. Masters, C. L., Harris, J. O., Gajdusek, D. C., et al. Creutzfeldt-Jakob disease: Patterns of worldwide occurrence and the significance of familial and sporadic clustering. *Ann. Neurol.* 5:177, 1979.
90. McArthur, J. C. Neurologic manifestations of AIDS. *Medicine* 66:407, 1987.
91. McArthur, J. C., Cohen, B. A., Farzedegan, H., et al. Cerebrospinal fluid abnormalities in homosexual men with and without neuropsychiatric findings. *Ann. Neurol.* 32(Suppl.):S34, 1988.
92. McCormick, W. F., Rodnitzky, R. L., Schochet, S. S., and McKee, A. P. Varicella-zoster encephalomyelitis. *Arch. Neurol.* 21:559, 1969.
93. Miller, D. C. Creutzfeldt-Jakob disease in histopathology technicians. *N. Engl. J. Med.* 318:853, 1988.
94. Morrison, R. E., Shatsky, S. A., Holmes, G. E., et al. Herpes simplex virus type 1 from a patient with radiculoneuropathy. *J.A.M.A.* 241:393, 1979.
95. Moskowitz, L. B., Gregorios, J. B., Hensley, G. T., and Berger, J. R. Cytomegalovirus induced demyelination with acquired immune deficiency syndrome. *Arch. Pathol. Lab. Med.* 108:873, 1984.
96. Murphy, F. A., Bauer, S. P., Harrison, A. K., and Winn, W. C. Comparative pathogenesis of rabies and rabies-like viruses: Viral infection and transit from inoculation site to central nervous system. *Lab. Invest.* 28:361, 1973.
97. Murphy, F. A., Harrison, A. K., Winn, W. C., and Bauer, S. P. Comparative pathogenesis of rabies and rabies-like viruses: Infection of the central nervous system and centrifugal spread of vi-

rus to peripheral tissues. *Lab. Invest.* 29:1, 1973.

98. Murphy, J. V., and Yunis, E. J. Encephalopathy following measles infection in children with chronic illness. *J. Pediatr.* 88:937, 1976.

99. Nahmias, A. J., Whitley, R. J., Visintine, A. N., et al. Herpes simplex encephalitis: Laboratory evaluations and their diagnostic significance. *J. Infect. Dis.* 145:829, 1982.

100. Narang, H. K. Scrapie, an unconventional virus: The current views. *Proc. Soc. Exp. Biol. Med.* 184:375, 1987.

101. Nielsen, S. L., Petito, C. K., Urmacher, C. D., and Posner, J. B. Subacute encephalitis in acquired immune deficiency syndrome: A postmortem study. *Am. J. Clin. Pathol.* 82:678, 1984.

102. Osame, M., Matsumoto, M., Usuku, K., et al. Chronic progressive myelopathy associated with elevated antibodies to HTLV-I and adult T cell leukemialike cells. *Ann. Neurol.* 21:117, 1987.

103. Panitch, H. S., Gomez-Plascencia, J., Noris, F. H., et al. Subacute sclerosing panencephalitis: Remission after treatment with intraventricular interferon. *Neurology* 36:562, 1986.

104. Parry, G. J. Peripheral neuropathies associated with human immunodeficiency virus infection. *Ann. Neurol.* 32(Suppl.):S49, 1987.

105. Pert, C. B., Smith, C. C., Ruff, M. R., and Hill, J. M. AIDS and its dementia as a neuropeptide disorder: Role of VIP receptor blockade by human immunodeficiency virus envelope. *Ann. Neurol.* 32(Suppl.):S71, 1987.

106. Petito, C. K. Review of central nervous system pathology in human immunodeficiency virus infection. *Ann. Neurol.* 23(Suppl.): S54, 1987.

107. Petito, C. K., Cho, E.-S., Lemann, W., et al. Neuropathology of acquired immunodeficiency syndrome (AIDS): An autopsy review. *J. Neuropathol. Exp. Neurol.* 45:635, 1986.

108. Petito, C. K., Navia, B. A., Cho, E.-S., et al. Vacuolar myelopathy pathologically resembling subacute combined degeneration in patients with the acquired immunodeficiency syndrome. *N. Engl. J. Med.* 312:874, 1985.

109. Phillips, C. A., Aronson, M. D., Tomkow, J., and Phillips, M. E. Entero-viruses in Vermont 1969–1978: An important cause of illness throughout the year. *J. Infect. Dis.* 141:162, 1980.

110. Price, R., Chernick, N. L., Horta-Barbosa, L., and Posner, J. B. Herpes simplex encephalitis in an anergic patient. *Am. J. Med.* 54:222, 1973.

111. Price, R. W., Sidtis, J., and Rosenblum, M. The AIDS dementia complex: Some current questions. *Ann. Neurol.* 23(Suppl.):S27, 1987.

112. Prusiner, S. B. Molecular biology of prion diseases. *Science* 252:1515, 1991.

113. Puchhammer-Stockl,-E., Popow-Kraupp, T. Heinz, F. X., et al. Establishment of PCR for the early diagnosis of herpes simplex encephalitis. *J. Med. Virol.* 32:77, 1990.

114. Purvin, V., Herr, G. J., and De Meyer, W. Chiasmal neuritis as a complication of Epstein-Barr virus infection. *Arch. Neurol.* 45:458, 1988.

115. Rapidly progressive dementia in a patient who received a cadaveric dura mater graft. *M.M.W.R.* 36:49, 1987.

116. Ratzan, K. R. Viral meningitis. *Med. Clin. North Am.* 69:399, 1985.

117. Reshef, E., Greenberg, S. B., and Jankovic, J. Herpes zoster ophthalmicus followed by contralateral hemiparesis: Report of two cases and review of the literature. *J. Neurol. Neurosurg. Psychiatry* 48:122, 1985.

118. Rowley, A. H., Whitley, R. J., Lakeman, F. D., and Wolinsky, S. M. Rapid detection of herpes-simplex-virus DNA in cerebrospinal fluid of patients with herpes simplex encephalitis. *Lancet* 335:440, 1990.

119. Rupprecht, C. E., and Dietzschold, B. Perspectives on rabies virus pathogenesis. *Lab. Invest.* 57:603, 1987.

120. Samarasinghe, P. L., Oates, J. K., and MacLennan, I. P. B. Herpetic proctitis and sacral radiculomyelopathy: A hazard for homosexual men. *Br. Med. J.* 2:365, 1979.

121. Sarin, P. S., and Gallo, R. C. The involvement of human T-lymphotrophic retroviruses in T-cell leukemia and immune deficiency. *Cancer Rev.* 1:1, 1986.

122. Sarin, P. S., and Gallo, R. C. Leukemia, immune deficiency, and human T-lymphotrophic retroviruses. *J. Tumor Marker Oncol.* 1:13, 1986.

123. Schiff, J. A., Schaefer, J. A., and Robinson, J. E. Epstein-Barr virus in cerebrospinal fluid during infectious mononucleosis encephalitis. *Yale J. Biol. Med.* 55:59, 1982.

124. Schroth, G., Gawehn, J., Thron, A., et al. Early diagnosis of herpes simplex encephalitis by MRI. *Neurology* 37:179, 1987.

125. Sells, C. J., Carpenter, R. L., and Ray, C. G. Sequelae of central nervous system enterovirus infections. *N. Engl. J. Med.* 293:1, 1975.

126. Sergent, J. S., Lockshin, M. D., Christian, C. L., and Gocke, D. J. Vasculitis with hepatitis B antigenemia. *Medicine* 55:1, 1976.

127. Sharer, L. R., Epstein, L. G., Cho, E.-S., and Petito, C. K. HTLV-III and vacuolar myelopathy (letter). *N. Engl. J. Med.* 315:62, 1986.

128. Shaw, G. M., Harper, M. E., Hahn, B. H., et al. HTLV-III infection in brains of children and adults with AIDS encephalopathy. *Lancet* 1:177, 1985.

129. Silverstein, A. EB Virus Infections of the Nervous System. In P. J. Vinken and G. W. Bruyn (eds.), *Handbook of Clinical Neurology.* Amsterdam: North Holland, 1978. Vol. 34, pp. 185–192.

130. Snider, W. D., Simpson, D. M., Nielsen, S., et al.

Neurological complications of the acquired immune deficiency syndrome: Analysis of 50 patients. *Ann. Neurol.* 14:403, 1983.
131. Steel, J. G., Dix, R. D., and Baringer, J. R. Isolation of herpes simplex virus type 1 in recurrent (Mollaret) meningitis. *Ann. Neurol.* 11:17, 1982.
132. Stoler, M. H., Eskin, T. A., Benn, S., et al. Human T-cell lymphotrophic virus type III infection of the central nervous system: A preliminary in situ analysis. *J.A.M.A.* 256:2360, 1986.
133. Sweetser, M. T., Braciale, V. L., and Braciale, T. J. Class I major histocompatibility complex-restricted T lymphocyte recognition of the influenza hemagglutinin: Overlap between class I cytotoxic T lymphocytes and antibody sites. *J. Exp. Med.* 170:1357, 1989.
134. Timmons, G. D., and Johnson, K. P. Aqueductal stenosis and hydrocephalus after mumps encephalitis. *N. Engl. J. Med.* 283:1505, 1970.
135. Tsiang, H. Neuronal function impairment in rabies-infected rat brain. *J. Gen. Virol.* 61:277, 1982.
136. Usuku, K., Sonoda, S., Osame, M., et al. HLA haplotype-linked high immune responsiveness against HTLV-1 in HTLV-1-associated myelopathy: Comparison with adult T-cell leukemia/lymphoma. *Ann. Neurol.* 23(Suppl.):S143, 1988.
137. VanLandingham, K. E., Marsteller, H. B., Ross, G. W., and Hayden, F. G. Relapse of herpes simplex encephalitis after conventional acyclovir therapy. *J.A.M.A.* 259:1051, 1988.
138. Vernant, J. C., Maurs, L., Gessain, A., et al. Endemic tropical spastic paraparesis associated with human T-lymphotrophic virus type I: A clinical and seroepidemiological study of 25 cases. *Ann. Neurol.* 21:123, 1987.
139. Webster, A. D. B., Tripp, J. H., Hayward, A. R., et al. Echovirus encephalitis and myositis in primary immunoglobulin deficiency. *Arch. Dis. Child.* 53:33, 1978.
140. Whitley, R. J. Personal communications, 1989.
141. Whitley, R. J., Alford, C. A., Hirsch, M. S., et al. Vidarabine versus acyclovir therapy in herpes simplex encephalitis. *N. Engl. J. Med.* 314:144, 1986.
142. Whitley, R. J., Soong, S.-J., Dolin, R., et al. Adenine arabinoside therapy of biopsy-proved herpes simplex encephalitis. *N. Engl. J. Med.* 297:289, 1977.
143. Whitley, R. J., Soong, S.-J., Hirsch, M. S., et al. Herpes simplex encephalitis: Vidarabine therapy and diagnostic problems. *N. Engl. J. Med.* 304:313, 1981.
144. Whitley, R. J., Soong, S.-J., Linneman, C., et al. Herpes simplex encephalitis: Clinical assessment. *J.A.M.A.* 247:317, 1982.
145. Wiley, C. A., Schrier, R. D., Denaro, F. J., et al. Localization of cytomegalovirus proteins and genome during fulminant central nervous system infection in an AIDS patient. *J. Neuropathol. Exp. Neurol.* 45:127, 1986.
146. Wiley, C. A., Schrier, R. D., Nelson, J. A., et al. Cellular localization of the human immunodeficiency virus infection within brains of acquired immune deficiency syndrome patients. *Proc. Natl. Acad. Sci. U.S.A.* 83:7089, 1986.
147. Wilfert, C. M., Buckley, R. H., Mohanakumar, T., et al. Persistent and fatal central nervous system echovirus infections in patients with agammaglobulinemia. *N. Engl. J. Med.* 296:1485, 1977.
148. Wilfert, C. M., Thompson, R. J., Sunder, T. R., et al. Longitudinal assessment of children with enteroviral meningitis during the first three months of life. *Pediatrics* 67:811, 1981.
149. Wolinsky, J. S. Progressive Rubella Panencephalitis. In P. J. Vinken and G. W. Bruyn (eds.), *Handbook of Clinical Neurology.* Amsterdam: North Holland, 1978. Vol. 34, pp. 307–330.
150. Wolinsky, J. S., Swoveland, P., Johnson, K. P., Baringer, J. R. Subacute measles encephalitis complicating Hodgkin's disease in an adult. *Ann. Neurol.* 1:452, 1977.
151. Yanker, B. A., Skolnik, P. R., Shoukimas, G. A., et al. Cerebral granulomatous angiitis associated with isolation of human T-lymphotrophic virus type III from the central nervous system. *Ann. Neurol.* 20:362, 1986.
152. Yarchoan, R., Berg, G., Brouwers, P., et al. Response of human-immunodeficiency-virus-associated neurological disease to 3′-azido-3′-deoxythymidine. *Lancet* 1:132, 1987.
153. Yarchoan, R., Thomas, R. N., Grafman, J., et al. Long-term administration of 3′-azido-2′3′-deoxythymidine to patients with AIDS-related neurological disease. *Ann. Neurol.* 23(Suppl.):S82, 1988.
154. Zu Rhein, G. M. Association of papova-virions with a human demyelinating disease (progressive multifocal leukoencephalopathy). *Prog. Med. Virol.* 11:185, 1969.

20 Neurologic Paraneoplastic Syndromes

David A. Chad and Lawrence D. Recht

Cancer is associated with a wide variety of nervous system disorders. A useful classification separates these neurologic disorders into direct (i.e., metastatic) and indirect effects of cancer. Metastatic effects are well known. Indirect effects can be subgrouped into general categories (Table 20-1): (1) metabolic encephalopathies produced by tumor or treatment-associated organ failure or electrolyte imbalance; (2) central nervous system (CNS) infection caused by tumor-associated immunosuppression; (3) nervous system complications of tumor treatment; (4) so-called remote or paraneoplastic effects; and (5) cerebrovascular disease resulting from carcinoma-induced hypercoagulability [118].

In the broadest sense, all indirect effects of cancer can be considered paraneoplastic syndromes. However, neurologists have reserved this term for a number of rare, idiopathic syndromes associated with the presence or eventual appearance of a neoplasm. The recognition of these syndromes is important because they frequently herald the presence of a tumor and should prompt a careful tumor search. The paraneoplastic syndromes defy easy characterization because they cannot yet be defined according to pathogenesis. Furthermore, as we learn more about them, our classification changes. For example, progressive multifocal leukoencephalopathy (PML) was once routinely categorized as a paraneoplastic syndrome; however, with further study, it has become apparent that PML is in fact caused by the JC virus and as such is better characterized as an infectious complication of cancer.

The paraneoplastic syndromes can be separated into CNS and peripheral nervous system (PNS) disorders. The former include limbic encephalitis; brain stem encephalitis; subacute cerebellar degeneration, opsoclonus, myoclonus, and acute cerebellar encephalopathy; paraneoplastic retinopathy; and subacute necrotic myelopathy. PNS disorders include subacute sensory neuropathy; motor neuron disease, pe-

Table 20-1. Nonmetastatic neurologic complications of cancer

1. Metabolic encephalopathy
2. Infections
3. Vascular disorders
4. Side effects of therapy
5. "Remote effects"

Source: Posner [118].

ripheral neuropathy; disorders of the neuromuscular junction; and inflammatory myopathies. Because of their importance, we have also considered the indirect effects caused by the hypercoagulable state.

Before beginning our discussion, it should be stressed that direct or more readily defined indirect effects (e.g., infection, treatment complication) are much more commonly encountered than any of the paraneoplastic syndromes. The physician should, therefore, be skeptical of the diagnosis of a paraneoplastic syndrome until other more common conditions have been excluded.

CENTRAL NERVOUS SYSTEM SYNDROMES

Limbic Encephalitis

Limbic encephalitis is marked by progressive mental deterioration and rigidity that occurs in association with the eventual appearance of cancer in middle-aged patients [18,23, 32,48,61,62,143,150]. The onset of symptoms is often subacute and precedes the eventual diagnosis of cancer by as long as 2 years. The tumor most frequently associated with this syndrome is small-cell lung carcinoma [18,32,61,62,150], but there is also an association with tumors of the uroepithelial tract [23] and uterus [61]. One should suspect the diagnosis in middle-aged patients with rapid mental deterioration (especially severe impairment of memory) and evidence of cancer, in whom other causes such as viral and fungal infections, metabolic aberrations, and direct carcinomatous invasion of the CNS (i.e., intracerebral metastases, leptomeningeal carcinomatosis) have been ruled out. However, there is no pathognomonic sign or diagnostic test other than autopsy that will make the diagnosis with certainty. Examination of the cerebrospinal fluid (CSF) usually reveals a mild lymphocytic pleocytosis and a mildly elevated protein concentration, although the CSF may be normal. Computed tomography (CT) is uninformative. Neuropathologic examination reveals loss of hippocampal and amygdaloid neurons with microgliosis and perivascular lymphocytic cuffing (Fig. 20-1). In addition, autopsy studies reveal the frequent association between limbic encephalitis and brain stem encephalitis as well as dorsal root ganglioradiculitis (subacute sensory neuropathy) [61,62,143] (see later sections). It is important to note, however, that limbic encephalitis does not occur exclusively in association with cancer; clinically and pathologically typical examples have been reported in patients in whom no cancer can be detected even when extensive postmortem examinations are performed [37,48,89]. The etiology of this paraneoplastic syndrome is unknown. While the histologic appearance of limbic encephalitis (and, as we shall see, the brain stem and dorsal root ganglia syndromes) resembles that seen in viral-associated encephalitides, viral isolation has not been successful, and a rise in antibody titers to specific viruses has not been demonstrated [62,150].

Although limbic encephalitis has been reported to resolve with removal of primary lung tumors [17,96], it is unclear whether any treatment is efficacious in this disorder.

Brain Stem Encephalitis

Brain stem encephalitis presents with a multitude of symptoms and signs localizable to the pons and medulla including vertigo, nystagmus, dysphagia, ophthalmoplegia, and at times ataxia. Deafness [101], central hypoventilation [72], and internuclear ophthalmoplegia [116] have also been described. Occasionally, the midbrain is the main site affected [120]. This syndrome is frequently associated with limbic encephalitis and occasionally with subacute cerebellar degeneration (see next section). Neurologic symptoms often predate the diag-

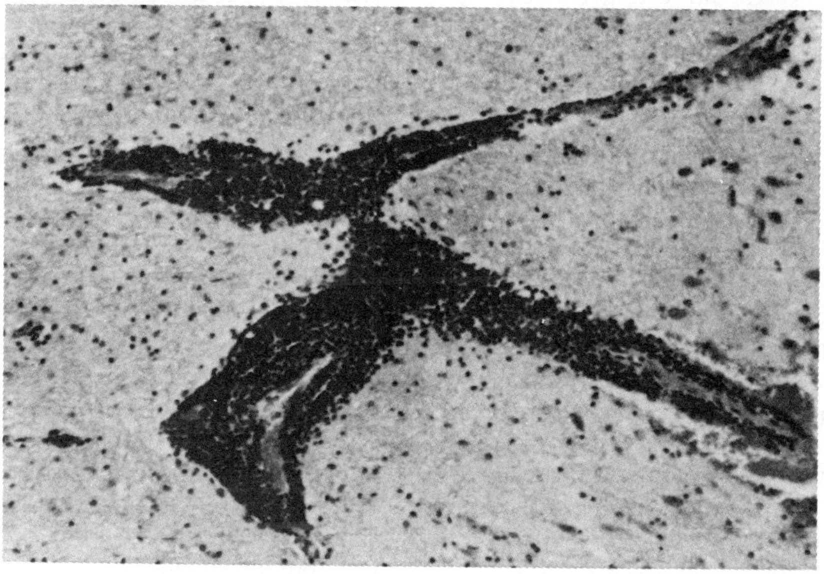

Fig. 20-1. Limbic encephalitis: lymphocytic cuffing in the amygdaloid nucleus. (From Henson and Urich [62].)

nosis of cancer, sometimes by several months [41,72,101,116,118,120,141,144]. It has been reported most frequently with small-cell lung carcinoma [72,101,116,141], but its association with other types of lung tumors [120], as well as breast [57] and uterine tumors [61], has also been described. Neurologic investigations are usually uninformative. The diagnosis usually rests on postmortem examination, although abnormalities may be detected on magnetic resonance imaging (MRI) [25]. Pathologic studies disclose signs of inflammation (perivascular cuffing, microgliosis, neuronophagia) in the brain stem; often, similar changes are found in hippocampus, amygdala, and dorsal root ganglia [41,57,62,116].

Subacute Cerebellar Degeneration

Subacute cerebellar degeneration is characterized by the subacute onset (over weeks to months) of progressive gait and limb ataxia. Walking is unsteady and broad-based with poorly coordinated finger-to-nose and heel-to-shin maneuvers. Dysarthria and nystagmus may also occur. The observed widespread incoordination (involving trunk, limb, head, and neck) reflects a pancerebellar disorder produced by few other conditions (for example, autosomal dominant cerebellar ataxias and rarely hypothyroidism can produce such a symptom complex). It is seen in association with certain cancers particularly small-cell lung carcinoma [13,25,110,128,129], ovarian cancer [99], breast cancer [25], and Hodgkin's disease [16,25,66,121,142].

Subacute cerebellar degeneration has been reported in association with other paraneoplastic syndromes such as the Lambert-Eaton myasthenic syndrome [12,129] (see later section). The syndrome can antedate the diagnosis of cancer by many months. CT may be normal, but eventually pancerebellar atrophy is noted [16]. The diagnosis should be entertained in any middle-aged person who presents with a syndrome of pancerebellar dysfunction; the picture is so dramatic when encountered that one can make the diagnosis on clinical grounds with reasonable assurance. Furthermore, recent work has demonstrated that over 25 percent of patients with bronchogenic cancer demonstrate cerebellar symptomatology that is not explainable by other causes, suggesting that this syndrome is not rare [148]. Definitive diagnosis of this syndrome requires histologic examination, which reveals widespread loss of Purkinje cells, neuronal loss and demyelination in the dentate nucleus, and thinning of the granular and molecular layers of the cerebellum [Fig. 20-2]. Inflammation is usually absent, but sometimes the cerebellar degeneration is part of a wider encephalomyelitis.

Immunologic mechanisms have been postulated to explain this syndrome [34,54,68]. To briefly summarize these findings (for a more in-depth review, see Anderson, Cunningham, and Posner [3]), Jaeckle and co-workers [68] found anti-Purkinje cell antibodies (APCA) in 6 of 12 patients with subacute cerebellar degeneration by indirect immunofluorescence on frozen sections of normal human cerebellum; these antibodies were only rarely found in neurologically normal patients with ovarian carcinoma [54,68]. The antigen has been partially characterized by Cunningham and associates [34], who found that APCA from 7 patients with the syndrome reacted with two groups of Purkinje cell antigens with molecular weights of 62/64 kD and 34 to 38 kD, respectively. The antigenic stimulus is not known, but possibilities include sharing of common antigens by both tumor and Purkinje cell, release of antigen by destruction of Purkinje cell, and opportunistic infection by an organism that shares antigenic similarities with Purkinje cells [68].

The development of subacute cerebellar degeneration in a woman who has APCA warrants intensive investigations for an underlying gynecologic neoplasm. Many workers are now favoring surgical exploration even when radiographic studies are negative; the yield of finding tumor is high, and these patients' tumors are often limited in extent at this point [64]. The syndrome responds only rarely to removal of the primary tumor, however [73,113]; plasmapheresis was reported to be successful in one case, but it is usually not helpful [28]. Treatment failure may in part be related to irreversible loss of or irreparable damage to Purkinje cells by the time treatment is instituted [3]. Failure to respond to treatment could also be related to the finding of autoantibody production within the CNS [47] and the observation that while plasmapheresis reduces the level of autoantibody in

Fig. 20-2. Subacute cerebellar degeneration: virtual absence of Purkinje cells in the cerebellar cortex. (×30.)

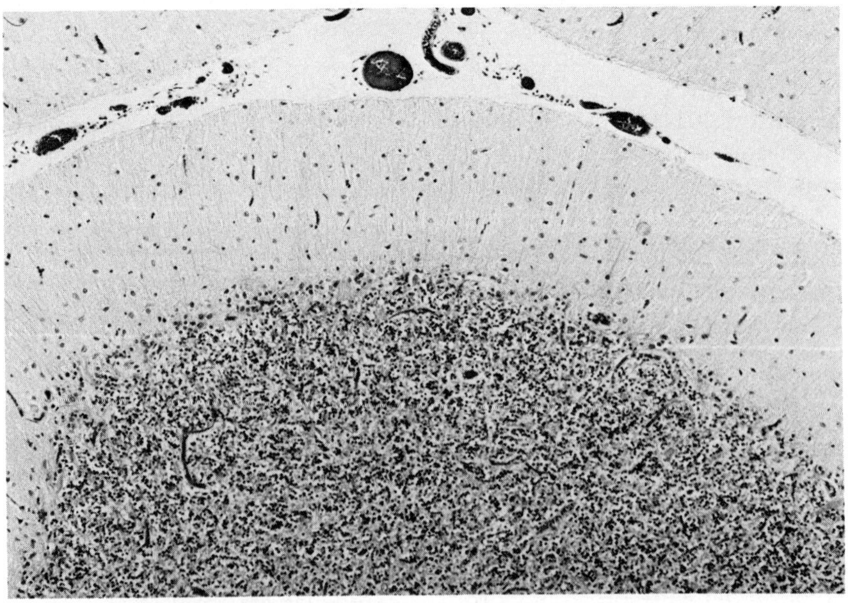

the serum, it does not cause significant removal of autoantibody from CSF [47,50].

Opsoclonus-Myoclonus (Acute Cerebellar Encephalopathy)

Opsoclonus-myoclonus is distinctive in its predilection for the pediatric population and its relationship to neuroblastoma. In 1962, Kinsbourne [81] described an acute, self-limited, presumably viral syndrome in children characterized by chaotic, irregular eye movements (opsoclonus) and shock-like myoclonic contractions that produced disorganization of willed movements. Soon after, reports appeared [1,14,15,70,97,104,135] noting the association of this syndrome ("dancing eyes, dancing feet") with neuroblastoma. This association is not rare; up to 50 percent or more of patients who develop the syndrome will subsequently prove to have neuroblastoma [70], an association so strong that investigators recommend that all children who present with opsoclonus-myoclonus be screened for neuroblastoma with vanillylmandelic acid (VMA) determinations. Interestingly, the outcome for patients with acute cerebellar encephalopathy and neuroblastoma is more favorable than for other patients with neuroblastoma [1,70]. In support of this interesting observation are recent preliminary data that demonstrate the favorable prognostic finding of single (as opposed to multiple) copies of the N-myc oncogene in four of four tumors from patients with this syndrome [31]. However, data indicate that up to 70 percent of patients with this syndrome have significant neurologic sequelae [70]. The few autopsy studies performed have shown no specific pathologic correlations.

Opsoclonus has also been described as a remote effect of carcinoma in adults in association with a variety of neurologic signs [10,44,125]; it is much rarer than subacute cerebellar degeneration but is distinguishable clinically from this syndrome by the predominance of truncal ataxia, the presence of myoclonus, and a tendency to follow a remitting and relapsing course [2]. In addition, in the few cases where postmortem material exists, Purkinje cells are preserved. Recently, a relatively specific antineuronal antibody was found in women with this syndrome; its presence was associated with breast and other gynecologic cancers [94]. Adrenocorticotropic hormone (ACTH) has been reported to be helpful in the childhood condition [10, 104,135] but is of no proven efficacy in the adult condition.

Paraneoplastic Retinopathy

A syndrome of progressive blindness secondary to retinal degeneration has been reported in association with carcinoma [79,82,85,130]. The blindness is often preceded by bizarre visual obscurations and night blindness. Narrowing of the retinal arterioles on funduscopic examination is noted. Electroretinograms are abnormal, although the visual evoked response latencies remain normal [20,130]. The syndrome may antedate or follow the diagnosis, which is usually small-cell lung carcinoma [20,84,85]. Pathologic examination of the eyes reveals loss of retinal photoreceptors and degeneration of the outer nuclear layer [79,130]. Retinal photoreceptor cell degeneration (with normal retinal bipolar and ganglion cells) is associated with accumulation of melanin in retinal pigmentary epithelium [20]. Immunohistochemically, high-titer immunoglobulins reactive with retinal ganglion cells are present in the sera of patients with small-cell lung carcinoma who have paraneoplastic retinopathy [84]. These immunoglobulins react with neurofilament protein antigen and can be detected at high serum dilution. They are specifically directed against retinal ganglion cells with no reaction detected against other retinal or CNS neurons [84]. The antigen against which these antibodies are directed is a 26 kD protein that is closely related to the cone-specific protein, visinin, a member of the calmodulin protein family [117]. Anecdotal reports suggest that corticosteroids may be beneficial in this condition [130].

Subacute Necrotic Myelopathy

Fewer than 30 cases of subacute necrotic myelopathy have been described, and in some the diagnosis is suspect because radiation myelopathy and involvement of the spinal cord by tumor could not be excluded [22,58,95,109]. A variety of both solid and hematologic tumors have been associated with subacute necrotizing myelopathy, including carcinoma of the prostate, lung, and lymphoma. The disorder is usually abrupt in onset and evolves rapidly, giving rise to flaccid paraplegia, loss of sphincter control, and profound sensory loss. The sensorimotor deficit ascends progressively, and it may result in death from respiratory failure. The CSF usually shows increased protein concentration. Myelographic examination may show slight widening of the involved segments of the spinal cord or serpiginous lucencies on the cord surface, but obstruction of dye is not seen. Pathologic studies disclose widespread spinal cord necrosis involving white and gray matter with little inflammation or blood vessel abnormality.

When a patient known to have cancer develops a rapidly progressive myelopathy, one should first consider a treatable lesion such as epidural spinal cord compression even if spine films are normal, since tumors, especially lymphomas, may gain access to the epidural space by spreading through intervertebral foramena from paravertebral sites. Myelography should be done immediately to rule out such lesions. Patients with cancer may also develop intramedullary spinal cord metastases, which clinically may resemble subacute necrotic myelopathy [24, 43]. We emphasize that only when a patient with cancer and rapidly progressive myelopathy has had an exhaustive work-up to exclude other possibilities should consideration be given to the diagnosis of paraneoplastic necrotizing myelopathy. The differential diagnosis of a noncompressive spinal cord lesion also includes multiple sclerosis, spinal cord infarction, viral myelitis, postinfectious myelitis, and the myelitis associated with collagen-vascular disorders [24].

PERIPHERAL NERVOUS SYSTEM SYNDROMES

Subacute Sensory Neuropathy

Subacute sensory neuropathy develops subacutely over a matter of weeks to months and is marked by pain, paresthesias, dysesthesias, and numbness in the limbs [39,62,67]. Symptoms and signs usually begin distally but spread to more proximal areas in a matter of weeks. The most dramatic components of the syndrome are severe unsteadiness of gait and poor limb coordination. Pseudoathetosis is observed because of the profound disturbance in proprioception. There is diminution or loss of sensory modalities (vibration and joint position sense) subserved by large myelinated fibers. Muscle strength tends to be relatively spared (for the motor system is only minimally affected or not involved), but many patients have limb hypotonia and some degree of muscle wasting. Stretch reflexes are generally absent. Bladder and bowel disturbances do not occur. In addition, many patients also demonstrate disturbances of brain stem and cognitive function, reflecting an associated encephalomyelitis [62].

In the majority of patients, symptoms of neuropathy antedate the discovery of cancer, sometimes by years. Therefore, the development of a relatively pure sensory neuropathy in a middle-aged adult should suggest the possibility of an underlying neoplasm. In a literature review of 29 patients [67], neuropathy preceded the discovery of the cancer in 24. In 12, the neoplasm was discovered only at autopsy. In the vast majority of cases the associated tumor is a small-cell lung carcinoma.

In most cases, there is a moderate elevation of the CSF protein (100–200 mg/dl) and a mild CSF lymphocytosis (5–30 cells/mm^3); oligoclonal bands may be present [3]. Nerve conduction studies disclose a widespread loss of sensory potentials with sparing of motor responses.

On neuropathologic examination (Fig. 20-3), there is neuronal degeneration of the sensory neurons of the dorsal root ganglia associated with inflammation and phagocytosis [67]. Inflammatory cells are prominent in the early stages of the syndrome, while Schwann cell proliferation and fibrosis are more common in later stages. Fibers of the posterior columns undergo wallerian degeneration, as do sensory axons in the peripheral nervous system. Inflammatory cell changes in spinal cord and brain occur in about 50 percent of the cases [62].

Subacute sensory neuropathy is associated with the presence of specific antineuronal anti-

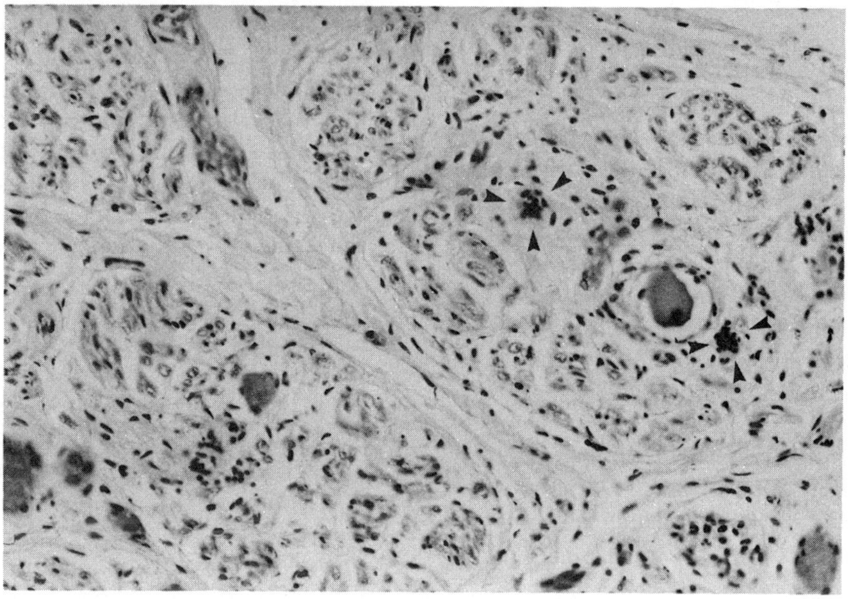

Fig. 20-3. Subacute sensory neuropathy: There is a drop out of neurons; nodules of Nageotte (*arrowheads*) occur at sites previously occupied by sensory neurons. (×60.)

bodies (anti-Hu antibodies) [51,52]. These are complement-fixing, polyclonal IgG antibodies that react with nuclei of CNS, dorsal root ganglia, and trigeminal ganglia neurons but not with non-neuronal nuclei [52]. The antigens recognized by the anti-Hu antibodies have been characterized as protein antigens with molecular weights 35 to 40 kD. They are present in most or all small-cell lung carcinomas but not in other normal tissues or most other tumors [36]. The presence of identical protein antigens in small-cell lung carcinoma cells and neuronal nuclei supports the view that the pathogenesis of subacute sensory neuropathy is immunologically mediated, with tumor antigens triggering the production of cross-reactive antibodies.

Patients with small-cell lung carcinoma and anti-Hu antibody may have other neurologic disorders in addition to subacute sensory neuropathy including motor neuron syndromes, autonomic neuropathy, cerebellar ataxia, myelopathy, and encephalomyelitis [4] as well as Lambert-Eaton myasthenic syndrome [66]. Therefore, anti-Hu antibody is a highly specific marker of small-cell lung carcinoma associated with neurologic dysfunction [4] and when present in high titer is almost always associated with paraneoplastic dysfunction [42].

There are some patients, however, with small-cell lung carcinoma and a low titer of anti-Hu antibodies who do not have a paraneoplastic disorder [36]. Because the small-cell lung carcinoma of these patients tends to be relatively limited, it has been suggested that the antitumor immune response protects against the spread of disease [36].

The differential diagnosis of the subacute sensory neuropathy syndrome includes a variety of different entities including hereditary, toxic, and immunologic neuropathies [6]. Hereditary sensory neuropathies are usually marked by their chronicity and occasional trophic ulcers, fractures, or osteomyelitis. Pyridoxine abuse and cisplatinum neurotoxicity are well-known causes of the syndrome. Sjögren's syndrome may be accompanied by a severe dorsal root ganglionitis leading to ataxia and kinesthetic loss [55]. Last and least well understood is a pure sensory syndrome that develops over hours to days and is immune mediated in some and possibly has a vascular pathogenesis in others [149].

Motor Neuron Disease

The nature of the relationship between motor neuron disease and neoplasia has not yet been completely defined. Some studies suggest that motor neuron disease might be a paraneoplastic syndrome because the incidence of this neurologic disorder was found to be increased in patients with cancer [107]. Indeed, paraneoplastic motor neuron disease mimicking amyotrophic lateral sclerosis may improve or stabilize with tumor treatment [45]. However, other authors have noted that the occurrence of motor neuron disease in patients with cancer is no greater than its occurrence in age-matched controls [8,27]. Henson and Urich [62] propose that paraneoplastic motor neuron disease is simply one manifestation of a generalized inflammatory disorder—encephalomyelitis.

Association with Plasma Cell Disorder

In one form of neoplasia, plasma cell dyscrasia, there is an intriguing if not yet fully understood relationship to motor neuron disease. Almost 10 percent of patients with motor neuron disease have paraproteinemias [151], suggesting that at least some motor neuron diseases may be immunologically mediated [136]. Sometimes the monoclonal protein has unique specificity to carbohydrate epitopes shared by gangliosides GM_1 [90,91]. In this regard, high titers of polyclonal autoantibodies to GM_1 and other glycolipids have been found in patients with motor neuron disorders that affect primarily the anterior horn cell. Several lower motor neuron syndromes have been defined [114], including multifocal motor neuropathy that may respond to intensive immunosuppressive therapy [115].

Association with Lymphoma

The presence of paraproteinemia in a patient with motor neuron disease increases the likelihood of there being an underlying lymphoma [152]. (Other laboratory features that suggest coexisting lymphoma are raised CSF protein and oligoclonal bands [152]). The syndrome of motor neuron disease associated with lymphoma, although rare, has been known for many years and has been designated subacute motor neuronopathy [126,132,147]. It has also been reported in association with thymoma [138]. It is generally characterized by subacute, progressive, painless, often patchy and asymmetric weakness of the lower motor neuron type (atrophy, fasciculation, reduced reflexes) with greater involvement of the legs than arms. However, some patients have prominent upper motor neuron signs (hyperreflexia, Babinski's sign, clonus) and qualify for the diagnosis of amyotrophic lateral sclerosis [152]. The neurologic disorder is an exclusively motor syndrome, and sensory symptoms and signs are minimal. The illness often progresses independently of the activity of the underlying neoplasm and tends to follow a relatively benign course; some patients demonstrate spontaneous improvement.

In the patient with lymphoma and subacute muscle weakness, it is important to exclude a variety of other disorders including leptomeningeal metastases, neoplastic plexopathy, and the Guillain-Barré syndrome before arriving at the diagnosis of paraneoplastic motor neuron disease.

Peripheral Neuropathies

It is difficult to ascertain the precise incidence of peripheral neuropathy associated with neoplasia. Overall it has been estimated to be on the order of 5 percent [33,102], but higher figures have been found. It probably depends on the nature of the study and the degree of vigor with which clinical examination and electrophysiologic study is pursued. For example, Walsh [146] found an 8 percent incidence of clinically evident neuropathy in lymphoma patients, but this figure increased to 35 percent when results of nerve conduction studies were taken into consideration. Similarly, clinical neuropathy occurs in about 13 percent of cases of multiple myeloma, but when detailed neurophysiologic studies are done the incidence increases to as high as 40 percent [76]. Tervainen and Larson [140] found an incidence of clinical polyneuropathy of 48 percent among 33 patients with carcinoma of the lung. Although the mechanism is unclear, Hawley and colleagues [59] made the observation that patients with cancer do not have an increased incidence of neuropathy if significant weight loss has not yet occurred. They noted that as soon as 15 percent of body weight is lost, a mild neuropathy becomes evident and as the disease progresses the severity of neuropathy correlates with increasing percentage of body weight loss. By the time 40 percent of weight is lost, all patients have moderate, symmetric polyneuropathy.

An understanding of the neuropathies associated with neoplasia can best be gained by recognizing that each component of the peripheral nervous system may be a target of a particular pathologic process [131]. We have already discussed the clinical syndromes resulting from damage to the dorsal root ganglia (subacute sensory neuropathy) and the anterior horn cells (subacute motor neuronopathy). We shall now describe other syndromes that result from disturbances in the function and structure of the components of peripheral nerve; the Schwann cell and its myelin sheath; and the axon. Disturbances in the former give rise to demyelinating neuropathies and in the latter to axonal neuropathies.

Demyelinating Neuropathies

There are two forms of demyelinating neuropathy: an acute, rapidly progressing disorder—the Guillain-Barré syndrome; and a chronic, inflammatory, demyelinating polyneuropathy known as the CIDP syndrome [7]. The former has been described as a paraneoplastic syndrome in patients with Hodgkin's disease [93]. The CIDP syndrome is generally a symmetric, predominantly motor neuropathy that affects distal and proximal muscle groups with hyporeflexia and mild sensory loss. However, in some patients this chronic syndrome is associated with prominent sensory loss [74]. The course of the chronic disorder may be steadily progressive, or relapsing and remitting. Laboratory features include a CSF profile of albuminocytologic dissociation and nerve conduction studies that disclose prolonged distal latencies, delayed late responses, severely slowed conduction velocities, and evidence for conduction block. This syndrome is associated with several types of plasma cell dyscrasia including an IgM monoclonal gammopathy of undetermined significance, osteosclerotic myeloma, and Waldenström's macroglobulinemia [74].

Monoclonal Gammopathy of Undetermined Significance Twenty-five to 50 percent of patients with this paraproteinemia have a peripheral neuropathy [74]. These patients usually have low levels of monoclonal protein and no definite evidence for a malignancy or amyloidosis, although studies show that in prolonged follow-up 17 percent develop a malignant gammopathy like Waldenström's macroglobulinemia or a lymphoma [74]. In patients with IgM monoclonal gammopathy that reacts with a myelin-associated glycoprotein, the CIDP syndrome is predominantly sensory [75]. Sustained lowering of the concentration of M protein by immunotherapy is associated with improvement in the peripheral neuropathy [75].

Osteosclerotic Myeloma Although osteosclerotic myeloma is a rare disorder occurring in less than 3 percent of patients with multiple myeloma [77], one-half of reported patients have peripheral neuropathy, usually a predominantly motor form of CIDP, and in many patients it is the presenting manifestation. Patients with osteosclerotic myeloma are younger and less ill than patients with the more commonly encountered osteolytic multiple myeloma. Many patients with osteosclerotic myeloma develop signs of multisystem involvement. Nonneurologic signs consist of organomegaly, endocrinopathy, and dermatologic abnormalities. The neuropathy may improve when radiation therapy to solitary bone lesions is administered; chemotherapy has been less effective [77].

Waldenström's Macroglobulinemia Peripheral neuropathy occurs in about 10 percent of patients with this plasma cell dyscrasia. The neuropathy is diverse in nature, but most authors report a CIDP syndrome [74]. In some cases, IgM can be demonstrated to bind to myelin sheaths [71,119]. In some cases, the neuropathy can be treated successfully with immunosuppressive therapy [35].

Axon-Loss Neuropathies

Axon-loss neuropathies have been associated with many different types of tumor, but they are perhaps most commonly associated with small-cell lung carcinoma. The most frequently encountered neuropathy is a distal, symmetric, sensorimotor polyneuropathy [131], although a mononeuritis multiplex has also been described [69,108]. The polyneuropathy affects both motor and sensory axons, producing weakness, sensory loss, and absent or diminished reflexes. Distal portions of the extremities are affected first, and as the disorder progresses weakness and sensory loss spread proximally. In most paraneoplastic axon-loss neuropathies, sensory loss involves large-fiber modalities such as touch, vibration, and joint position sense, while pain and temperature sensation are relatively spared. However, in amyloid neuropathy associated with primary systemic amyloidosis or multiple myeloma, there is prominent loss of pain and temperature sensation with lesser degrees of involvement of large proprioceptive fibers [78]. Associated features include lancinating and burning pain as well as autonomic dysfunction. With regard to the latter, a rare paraneoplastic neuropathy of the gastrointestinal tract has been described in association with small-cell lung carcinoma [30,133]. It manifests as intestinal pseudo-obstruction, a consequence of degeneration of the myenteric plexus.

The nerve conduction studies of the axon-loss neuropathies disclose reduced motor and sensory amplitudes, but in contrast to the demyelinating neuropathies, nerve conduction velocity is either normal or only mildly reduced, and there is minimal if any prolongation of distal latencies and little or no involvement of the late responses.

The pathogenesis of the paraneoplastic axon-loss polyneuropathies is uncertain. In some cases vasculitis may play a role [69], while in others immunologic mechanisms might be important [112].

Disorders of the Neuromuscular Junction

A number of conditions cause disturbed function of neuromuscular transmission by interfering either with the process of release of acetylcholine (a presynaptic disorder) or with the interaction of normally released acetylcholine with the acetylcholine receptor (a postsynaptic disorder). A number of different tumors may be associated with these disorders. We will consider the presynaptic disorder described in 1956, the Lambert-Eaton myasthenic syndrome (LEMS) [87], and the postsynaptic disorder myasthenia gravis.

Lambert-Eaton Myasthenic Syndrome

Most patients with LEMS are over the age of 40, and men outnumber women by a ratio of 5 : 1 [60,139]. Patients usually complain of weakness and fatigability, most notably in the musculature of the pelvic girdle and thighs. Muscle aching and limb pain are common. Symptoms of autonomic dysfunction occur in 80 percent of patients [111], the most common manifestations being dry mouth in 74 percent and impotence in 41 percent of men. Mild and transient cranial nerve symptoms such as diplopia and ptosis are common and may lead to the incorrect diagnosis of myasthenia gravis in almost half of the cases [111]. Physical examination discloses proximal muscle weakness and reduced deep tendon reflexes. The most remarkable aspect of this condition is the improvement in strength and potentiation of reflex activity that occurs after repeated muscle contraction [111]. Lung cancer, usually of the small-cell type, is found in 75 percent of patients. Other associated tumors include carcinoma of the rectum, kidney, breast, stomach, skin, and thymus gland and leukemia. Among women, by contrast, only 25 percent are found to have an underlying neoplasm [139]. Other diseases associated with LEMS include a variety of conditions thought to have an autoimmune basis, such as rheumatoid arthritis and Sjögren's syndrome [139].

Neurophysiologic studies help to confirm the diagnosis [87,111,139]. The amplitude of the compound muscle potential evoked by initial nerve stimulation is usually much lower than normal because of the severely reduced quantal content (number of individual quanta of acetylcholine released per nerve impulse) but increases after the muscle has been exercised for 10 to 15 seconds (strong isometric contraction); 3 to 5 seconds after exercise an increment of greater than 50 percent is considered abnormal, and patients with LEMS will usually demonstrate an increment of greater than 200 percent. O'Neill, Murray, and Newsom-Davis [111] noted a 75 percent reduction in initial mean amplitude, which increased by a mean increment of 890 percent after 15 seconds of maximum voluntary effort. Other conditions associated with smaller incremental responses, include botulism, magnesium toxicity, and myasthenia gravis [139].

It is well established that LEMS in both its cancer-associated and noncarcinomatous forms is an autoimmune disorder in which IgG reacts with voltage-gated calcium channels (VGCCs) on presynaptic cholinergic nerve terminals [145]. This insight was reached in a series of elegant experiments. When the IgG fraction from patients with LEMS is injected intraperitoneally into mice, the physiologic [88] and characteristic morphologic changes [46] of the disorder develop. Roberts and co-workers [123] showed that such IgG is capable of inhibiting K^+-simulated (voltage-gated) $^{45}Ca^{+2}$ flux in a small-cell carcinoma line. It is postulated that the VGCCs expressed on small-cell lung carcinoma cells trigger and sustain an autoantibody response in which IgG cross reacts with presynaptic VGCCs [145]. Loss of VGCCs results in reduced calcium entry during nerve terminal depolarization and a concomitant decrease in transmitter release [111]. The short-lived, beneficial effect of muscle contraction is due to an increase in calcium concentration in the axon terminal, temporarily enhancing acetylcholine release.

The syndrome historically has been treated with guanidine, which facilitates the release of acetylcholine. A dose of between 20 and 30 mg/kg/day often results in clinical and electrical improvement. Doses in excess of 30 mg/kg, however, may induce coarse tremor, confusion, and agitation. These side effects and other serious toxicity including hepatic dysfunction, bone marrow suppression, and renal insufficiency preclude treatment in many patients. Another agent, 3,4-diaminopyridine, is now available, which augments release of acetylcholine, improves weakness, and is the drug of choice for the short-term [100]. The autoimmune nature of LEMS suggests that it might respond to immunosuppressive treatment or plasmapheresis or both. Indeed, these modalities have a beneficial effect, albeit short-lived [38,106]. Sustained improvement in LEMS associated with small-cell lung carcinoma is much more likely to occur if successful antineoplastic treatment is administered [26].

Myasthenia Gravis

Myasthenia gravis is not usually considered among the paraneoplastic syndromes because the vast majority of patients with this condition do not have an underlying neoplasm. However, about 10 percent of patients with myasthenia gravis have an underlying thymoma, while about 30 percent of patients who present with thymoma turn out to have myasthenia gravis [105].

In most patients, myasthenia gravis is acquired, immunologically mediated, and noncarcinomatous. The diagnosis is supported by the presence of serum antibodies to the acetylcholine receptor and nerve conduction studies. In contrast to LEMS, the amplitude of the compound muscle action potential of the rested muscle is normal. The electrophysiologic hallmark of the disease is a decremental motor response at low rates of nerve stimulation.

Myasthenia gravis is found in all age groups, from childhood to the eighth decade, but thymoma is most commonly encountered in older patients, especially men. The antistriational antibody is found in 90 percent of patients with myasthenia gravis *complicated by* thymoma. All patients suspected of having myasthenia gravis should undergo CT of the mediastinum to search for thymoma [63]. If a thymoma is demonstrated, then thymectomy should be performed because of the tumor's propensity for local invasion. After thymoma removal, some recommend mediastinal radiation. Patients with myasthenia gravis secondary to thymoma tend to be more difficult to manage than patients with myasthenia gravis alone.

Patients with thymomas should be carefully evaluated for myasthenia gravis even if they do not complain of weakness, because even subclinical myasthenia gravis increases surgical morbidity. Myasthenia gravis patients tolerate surgery and general anesthesia poorly, and they may have serious intraoperative and postoperative difficulties if certain medications such as anesthetics or neuromuscular blocking agents, antibiotics, or antiarrhythmics are used [5].

Idiopathic Inflammatory Muscle Disease

The inflammatory myopathies are acquired, immunologically mediated disorders [98] that are sometimes associated with a neoplasm. Polymyositis is characterized by the subacute onset of weakness in a proximal distribution. About one-third of patients have dysphagia; other cranial-nerve innervated muscles are normal. A small percentage of patients develop cardiac conduction abnormalities and interstitial lung disease. When proximal muscle weakness is associated with skin rash (erythematous, pruritic, and scaly over sun-exposed areas), the myopathy is referred to as dermatomyositis. In both polymyositis and dermatomyositis, the serum creatine kinase (CK) level is usually increased, and electromyography discloses myopathic motor unit potentials and increased abnormal spontaneous activity. In both conditions, muscle biopsy discloses scattered muscle fiber necrosis, regeneration, and mononuclear inflammatory cell infiltration. Both conditions respond to corticosteroids and other immunosuppressive agents.

There has been considerable debate over whether an association exists between neoplasia and the inflammatory myopathies. Most investigators now think there is a higher incidence of neoplasms among older adult patients with these myopathies [21,40,92]. However, Lakhanpal and co-workers [86] questioned the association between polymyositis-dermatomyositis and malignancy. They proposed that the mild excess of cancer seen among patients at the Mayo Clinic with polymyositis-dermatomyositis could be explained by referral bias.

Our own impression is that there is probably an increased association of cancer with inflammatory myopathy, especially dermatomyositis in the older patient. Therefore, we recommend a search for malignancy in patients over 40 years who present with an inflammatory myopathy syndrome (proximal weakness, elevated CK, abnormal electromyelogram). This should include at least a careful and complete general physical examination, routine laboratory studies, chest roentgenogram, and stool analysis for occult blood. Further radiologic procedures such as CT and contrast studies of chest, abdomen, and pelvic structures do not appear to increase the tumor yield. There is little definite evidence that treatment of the underlying tumor is associated with the resolution of the myopathy.

CNS COMPLICATIONS OF THE HYPERCOAGULABLE STATE ASSOCIATED WITH CANCER

Patients with solid cancers seem particularly prone to develop symptomatic chronic disseminated intravascular coagulopathies [122,127], which produce migratory thrombophlebitis, bleeding, and arterial emboli. These are usually [103,124] but not always [19] due to mucin-secreting tumors. Otherwise known as the hypercoagulable state of cancer or Trousseau's syndrome, this disorder may produce neurologic symptoms by three mechanisms: (1) cerebral emboli from nonbacterial thrombotic endocarditis (NBTE), (2) small-vessel occlusions in disseminated intravascular coagulation (DIC), and (3) thrombosis of either cerebral veins or sinuses.

Forty percent of patients with NBTE are found to have cancer [11,53,124]. Furthermore, in one-third of patients with NBTE, cerebral emboli are noted at autopsy [11, 124]. Although usually occurring as a late phenomenon, cerebral emboli may herald the diagnosis of NBTE and systemic cancer [83].

The condition should be suspected in patients with known or suspected cancer who develop clinical syndromes compatible with single or multiple emboli, especially when there is coexistent migratory thrombophlebitis [9]. Since there is also often coexisting low-grade DIC [9], measurement of fibrin degradation products and fibrinogen levels may be helpful in suggesting the diagnosis; however, NBTE can occur in the absence of any clinical evidence of DIC. Despite

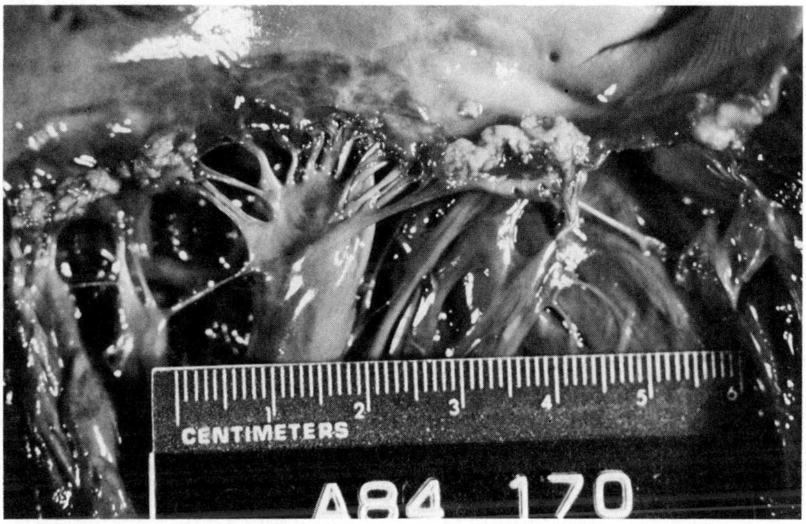

Fig. 20-4. Mitral valve with vegetations.

large valvular vegetations (Fig. 20-4), echocardiograms are usually normal; the diagnosis rests on a high index of suspicion in a patient who is clinically at risk. Although heparinization is advocated by most authors [53], it has been difficult to demonstrate a benefit. Since NBTE is difficult to diagnose and occurs relatively infrequently, it is unlikely that a controlled study to assess the effects of heparin will be possible. One potential method, however, in which the role of heparin may be assessed is by the study of measurable parameters of coagulation such as fibrinopeptide A, which is frequently elevated in hypercoagulable patients with cancer and may be partially normalized with anticoagulation [11]. Showing a reduction in embolic phenomenon with normalization of coagulation parameters would be strong inferential evidence of therapeutic benefit.

Unlike NBTE, DIC tends to be more strongly associated with hematologic malignancies [29]. It tends to produce generalized neurologic dysfunction, although focal signs may occur [29,134]. When large-vessel occlusions develop in the setting of DIC, it is often the result of coexisting NBTE [134]. Neuropathologic examination of patients with DIC reveals evidence of multifocal hemorrhagic or ischemic infarcts in the distribution of several cerebral vessels [29,53,80,134]. The role of heparinization in ameliorating CNS symptoms and signs of DIC, like that of NBTE, is uncertain [29,49,53].

When cerebral venous or sinus occlusions occur in the setting of cancer, they are usually secondary to carcinomatous invasion. However, occlusion of these vessels may also result from a hypercoagulable state [49,65]. Symptoms and signs of cerebral venous occlusion resemble those seen in other conditions; usually angiography is required for diagnosis [65,137]. The mortality of these conditions remains high; the value of heparinization remains uncertain [11,49,65].

REFERENCES

1. Altman, A. J., and Baehner, R. L. Favorable prognosis for survival in children with coincident opsomyoclonus and neuroblastoma. *Cancer* 37:846, 1976.
2. Anderson, N. E., Budde-Steffen, C., Rosenblum, M. K., et al. Opsoclonus, myoclonus, ataxia and encephalopathy in adults with cancer: A distinct paraneoplastic syndrome. *Medicine* 67: 100, 1988.
3. Anderson, N. E., Cunningham, J. M., and Posner, J. B. Autoimmune pathogenesis of

paraneoplastic neurological syndromes. *C.R.C. Crit. Rev. Neurol.* 3:245, 1987.

4. Anderson, N. E., Rosenblum, M. K., Graus, F., et al. Autoantibodies in paraneoplastic syndromes associated with small cell lung cancer. *Neurology* 38:1391, 1988.
5. Argov, Z., and Mastiglia, F. L. Disorders of neuromuscular transmission caused by drugs. *N. Engl. J. Med.* 301:409, 1979.
6. Asbury, A. K. Sensory neuronopathy. *Semin. Neurol.* 7:58, 1987.
7. Barohn, R. J., Kissel, J. T., Warmolts, J. R., and Mendell, J. R. Chronic inflammatory demyelinating polyradiculoneuropathy: Clinical characteristics course, and recommendations for diagnostic criteria. *Arch. Neurol.* 46:878, 1989.
8. Barron, K. D., and Rodichok, L. D. Cancer and Disorders of Motor Neurons. In L. P. Rowland (ed.), *Advances in Neurology.* New York: Raven, 1982. Vol. 36, pp. 267–272.
9. Barron, K. D., Siqueira, E., and Hirano, A. Cerebral embolism caused by non-bacterial thrombotic endocarditis. *Neurology* 10:391, 1960.
10. Bellur, S. Opsoclonus: Its clinical value. *Neurology* 25:502, 1975.
11. Biller, J., Challa, V. R., Toole, J. F., and Howard, V. J. Nonbacterial thrombotic endocarditis: A neurologic perspective of clinico-pathologic correlations of 99 patients. *Arch. Neurol.* 39:95, 1982.
12. Blumenfeld, A. M., Recht, L. D., Chad, D. A., et al. Coexistence of Lambert-Eaton myasthenic syndrome and subacute cerebellar degeneration: Differential effects of treatment. *Neurology* 41:1682, 1991.
13. Brain, L., and Wilkinson, M. Subacute cerebellar degeneration associated with neoplasms. *Brain* 88:465, 1965.
14. Brandt, S., Carlsen, N., Glenting, P., and Helweg-Larsen, J. Encephalopathia myoclonica infantalis (Kinsbourne) and neuroblastoma in children: A report of 3 cases. *Dev. Med. Child. Neurol.* 16:286, 1974.
15. Bray, P. F., Ziter, F. A., Lahey, M. E., and Myers, G. The coincidence of neuroblastoma and acute cerebellar encephalopathy. *Pediatrics* 75:983, 1969.
16. Brazis, P. W., Biller, J., Fine, M., et al. Cerebellar degeneration with Hodgkin's disease: Computed tomographic correlation and literature review. *Arch. Neurol.* 38:253, 1981.
17. Brennan, L. V., and Craddock, P. R. Limbic encephalopathy as a non-metastatic complication of oat cell lung cancer: Its reversal after treatment of the primary lung lesion. *Am. J. Med.* 75:518, 1983.
18. Brierly, J. B., Corsellis, J., and Nevin, R. Subacute encephalitis of later adult life: Mainly affecting the limbic areas. *Brain* 83:357, 1960.
19. Bryan, C. S. Nonbacterial thrombotic endocarditis with malignant tumors. *Am. J. Med.* 46:787, 1969.
20. Buchanan, T. A. S., Gardiner, T. A., and Archer, D. B. An ultrastructural study of retinal photoreceptor degeneration associated with bronchial carcinoma. *Am. J. Ophthalmol.* 97:277, 1984.
21. Callen, J. P., Hyla, J. F., Bole, G. G., Jr., et al. The relationship of dermatomyositis and polymyositis to internal malignancy. *Arch. Dermatol.* 116:295, 1980.
22. Case Records of the Massachusetts General Hospital. Case 26-1976. *N. Engl. J. Med.* 294: 1447, 1976.
23. Case Records of the Massachusetts General Hospital. Case 30-1985. *N. Engl. J. Med.* 313: 249, 1985.
24. Case Records of the Massachusetts General Hospital. Case 52-1985. *N. Engl. J. Med.* 313: 1646, 1985.
25. Case Records of the Massachusetts General Hospital. Case 9-1988. *N. Engl. J. Med.* 318: 563, 1988.
26. Chalk, C. H., Murray, N. M. F., Newsom-Davis, J., et al. Response of the Lambert-Eaton myasthenic syndrome to treatment of associated small-cell lung carcinoma. *Neurology* 40:1552, 1990.
27. Chio, A., Brignolio, F., Meineri, P., et al. Motor neuron disease and malignancies: Results of a population-based study. *J. Neurol.* 235:374, 1988.
28. Cocconi, G., Ceci, G., Juvarra, G., et al. Successful treatment of subacute cerebellar degeneration in ovarian carcinoma with plasmapheresis. *Cancer* 56:2318, 1985.
29. Collins, R. C., Mondhiry, H., Chernik, N. L., and Posner, J. B. Neurologic manifestations of intravascular coagulation in patients with cancer: A clinico-pathologic analysis of 12 cases. *Neurology* 25:795, 1975.
30. Colombel, J. F., Parent, M., Lescut, D., et al. Paraneoplastic intestinal pseudo-obstruction as the presenting features of small-cell lung cancer. *Gastroenterol. Clin. Biol.* 12:394, 1988.
31. Cohn, S. L., Salwen, H., Herst, C. V., et al. Single copies of the N-Myc oncogene in neuroblastomas from children presenting with the syndrome of opsoclonus-myoclonus. *Cancer* 62: 723, 1988.
32. Corsellis, J., Goldberg, G., and Norton, A. R. "Limbic encephalitis" and its association with carcinoma. *Brain* 91:481, 1968.
33. Croft, P. B., and Wilkinson, M. Carcinomatous neuromyopathy: Its incidence in patients with carcinoma of the lung and carcinoma of the breast. *Lancet* 1:184, 1963.
34. Cunningham, J., Graus, F., Anderson, N., and Posner, J. B. Partial characterization of the Pur-

kinje cell antigens in paraneoplastic cerebellar degeneration. *Neurology* 36:1163, 1986.

35. Dalakas, M. C., Flaum, M. A., Rick, M., et al. Treatment of polyneuropathy in Waldenström's macroglobulinemia: Role of paraproteinemia and immunologic studies. *Neurology* 33:1406, 1983.
36. Dalmau, J., Furneaux, H. F., Gralla, R. J., et al. Detection of anti-Hu antibody in the serum of patients with small cell lung cancer: A quantitative western blot analysis. *Ann. Neurol.* 27:544, 1990.
37. Daniel, S. E., Love, S., Scarvilli, F., and Harding, A. E. Encephalomyeloneuropathy in the absence of a detectable neoplasm: Clinical and postmortem findings in three cases. *Acta Neuropathol.* 66:311, 1985.
38. Dau, P. C., and Denys, E. H. Plasmapheresis and immunosuppressive drug therapy in the Eaton-Lambert syndrome. *Ann. Neurol.* 11:570, 1982.
39. Denny-Brown, D. E. Primary sensory neuropathy with muscular changes associated with cancer. *J. Neurol. Neurosurg. Psychiatry* 11:73, 1948.
40. DeVere, R., and Bradley, W. G. Polymyositis: Its presentation morbidity and mortality. *Brain* 98:637, 1975.
41. Dorfman, L. J., and Forno, L. S. Paraneoplastic encephalomyelitis. *Acta Neurol. Scand.* 48:556, 1972.
42. Dropcho, E. J., Stanton, C., and Oh, S. H. Neuronal antinuclear antibodies in a patient with Lambert Eaton myasthenic syndrome and small-cell lung carcinoma. *Neurology* 39:249, 1989.
43. Edelson, R. N., Deck, M. D. F., and Posner, J. B. Intramedullary spinal cord metastases: Clinical and radiographic findings in nine cases. *Neurology* 22:1222, 1972.
44. Ellenberger, C., Campa, J. F., and Netsky, M. G. Opsoclonus and parenchymatous degeneration of the cerebellum: The cerebellar origin of an abnormal ocular movement. *Neurology* 18:1041, 1968.
45. Evans, B. K., Fagan, C., Arnold, T., et al. Paraneoplastic motor neuron disease and renal cell carcinoma: Improvement after nephrectomy. *Neurology* 40:960, 1990.
46. Fukunoja, H., Engel, A. G., Osame, M., et al. Paucity and disorganization of presynaptic membrane active zones in the Lambert-Eaton syndrome. *Muscle Nerve* 5:686, 1982.
47. Furneaux, H. F., Reich, L., and Posner, J. B. Autoantibody synthesis in the central nervous system of patients with paraneoplastic syndromes. *Neurology* 40:1085, 1990.
48. Glaser, G. H., and Pincus, J. H. Limbic encephalitis. *J. Nerv. Ment. Dis.* 149:59, 1967.
49. Godal, H. C., and Abildgaard, A. The symptomatic effect of anticoagulant therapy in defibrination syndrome associated with demonstrable fibrin in plasma: A case report. *Acta Med. Scand.* 174:311, 1963.
50. Graus, F., Abos, J., Roquer, J., et al. Effect of plasmapheresis on serum and CSF autoantibody levels in CNS paraneoplastic syndrome. *Neurology* 40:1621, 1990.
51. Graus, F., Cordon-Cardo, C., and Posner, J. B. Neuronal antinuclear antibody in sensory neuropathy from lung cancer. *Neurology* 35:538, 1985.
52. Graus, F., Elkon, K. B., Cordon-Cardo, C., and Posner, J. B. Sensory neuropathy and small cell lung cancer: Antineuronal antibody that also reacts with the tumor. *Am. J. Med.* 80:45, 1986.
53. Graus, F., Rogers, L. R., and Posner, J. B. Cerebrovascular complications in patients with cancer. *Medicine* 64:16, 1985.
54. Greenlee, J. E., and Brashear, H. R. Antibodies to cerebellar Purkinje cells in patients with paraneoplastic cerebellar degeneration and ovarian carcinoma. *Ann. Neurol.* 14:609, 1983.
55. Griffin, J. W., Cornblath, D. R., Alexander, E., et al. Ataxic sensory neuropathy and dorsal root ganglionitis associated with Sjögren's syndrome. *Ann. Neurol.* 27:304, 1990.
56. Grunwald, G., Klein, R., Simmonds, M., and Kornguth, S. Autoimmune basis for visual paraneoplastic syndrome in patients with small cell lung carcinoma. *Lancet* i:658, 1985.
57. Halperin, J. J., Richardson, E. P., Ellis, J., et al. Paraneoplastic encephalomyelitis and neuropathy: Report of a case. *Arch. Neurol.* 38:773, 1981.
58. Handforth, A., Nag, S., Sharp, D., et al. Paraneoplastic subacute necrotic myelopathy. *Can. J. Neurol. Sci.* 10:204, 1983.
59. Hawley, R. J., Cohen, M. H., Saini, N., et al. The carcinomatous neuromyopathy of oat cell lung cancer. *Ann. Neurol.* 7:65, 1980.
60. Heinrikkson, K. G., Nilsson, O., Rosen, I., et al. Clinical, neurophysiological, and morphological findings in Eaton-Lambert syndrome. *Acta Neurol. Scand.* 56:117, 1977.
61. Henson, R. A., Hoffman, H. L., and Urich, H. Encephalomyelitis with carcinoma. *Brain* 88:449, 1965.
62. Henson, R. A., and Urich, H. The Neurological Manifestations of Systemic Malignant Disease. In *Cancer and the Nervous System.* London: Blackwell, 1982.
63. Hermann, C., Lindstrom, J. M., Keesey, J. C., et al. Myasthenia gravis: Current concepts. *West. J. Med.* 142:797, 1985.
64. Hetzel, D. J., Stanhope, R., O'Neill, B. P., and Lennon, V. A. Gynecologic cancer in patients with subacute cerebellar degeneration predicted by anti-Purkinje cell antibodies and lim-

ited in metastatic volume. *Mayo Clin. Proc.* 65:1558, 1990.

65. Hickey, W. F., Garnick, M. B., Henderson, I. C., and Dawson, D. M. Primary cerebral venous thrombosis in patients with cancer—a rarely diagnosed paraneoplastic syndrome: Report of 3 cases and review of the literature. *Am. J. Med.* 73:740, 1982.
66. Horwich, L., Buxton, P. H., and Ryan, M. S. Cerebellar degeneration with Hodgkin's disease. *J. Neurol. Neurosurg. Psychiatry* 29:45, 1966.
67. Horwich, M. S., Cho, L., Porro, R. S., et al. Subacute sensory neuropathy: A remote effect of carcinoma. *Ann. Neurol.* 2:7, 1977.
68. Jaeckle, K., Graus, F., Houghton, A., et al. Autoimmune response of patients with paraneoplastic degeneration to a Purkinje cell cytoplasmic protein antigen. *Ann. Neurol.* 18: 592, 1985.
69. Johnson, P. C., Roak, L. A., Hamilton, R. H., and Laguna, J. F. Paraneoplastic vasculitis of nerve, a remote effect of cancer. *Ann. Neurol.* 5:437, 1979.
70. Jones, A., Groover, R., and Smithson, W. Acute cerebellar encephalopathy: Its natural history and relationship to neuroblastoma. *Am. Soc. Clin. Onc. Proc.* 22:86, 1984.
71. Julien, J., Vital, C., Vallat, J.-M., Lagueny, A., et al. Polyneuropathy in Waldenström's macroglobulinemias deposition of M component in myelin sheaths. *Arch. Neurol.* 35:423, 1978.
72. Kaplan, A. M., and Itabashi, H. H. Encephalitis associated with carcinoma: Central hypoventilation syndrome with cytoplasmic inclusion bodies. *J. Neurol. Neurosurg. Psychiatry* 37:1166, 1974.
73. Kearsley, J. H., Johnson, P., and Halmagy, M. Paraneoplastic cerebellar disease: Remission with excision of the primary tumor. *Arch. Neurol.* 42:1208, 1985.
74. Kelly, J. J. Peripheral neuropathies associated with monoclonal proteins: A clinical review. *Muscle Nerve* 8:138, 1985.
75. Kelly, J. J., Adelman, L. S., Berkman, E., and Bhan, I. Polyneuropathies associated with IgM monoclonal gammopathies. *Arch. Neurol.* 45:1355, 1988.
76. Kelly, J. J., Kyle, R. A., Miles, J. M., et al. The spectrum of peripheral neuropathy in myeloma. *Neurology* 31:24, 1981.
77. Kelly, J. J., Kyle, R. A., Miles, J. M., et al. Osteosclerotic myeloma and peripheral neuropathy. *Neurology* 33:202, 1983.
78. Kelly, J. J., Kyle, R. A., O'Brien, P. C., and Dyck, P. J. The natural history of peripheral neuropathy in primary systemic amyloidosis. *Ann. Neurol.* 6:1, 1979.
79. Keltner, J. L., Roth, A. M., and Chang, R. S. Photoreceptor degeneration: Possible autoimmune disorder. *Arch. Ophthalmol.* 101:564, 1983.
80. Kim, H., Suzuki, M., Lie, J. T., and Titus, J. L. Nonbacterial thrombotic endocarditis (NBTE) and disseminated intravascular coagulation (DIC): Autopsy study of 36 patients. *Arch. Pathol. Lab. Med.* 101:65, 1977.
81. Kinsbourne, M. Myoclonic encephalopathy of infants. *J. Neurol. Neurosurg. Psychiatry* 25:271, 1962.
82. Klingele, T. G., Burde, R. M., Rappazzo, J. A., et al. Paraneoplastic retinopathy. *J. Clin. Neuro Ophthalmol.* 4:239, 1984.
83. Kooiker, J. C., MacLean, J. M., and Sumi, S. M. Cerebral embolism, marantic endocarditis and cancer. *Arch. Neurol.* 33:260, 1976.
84. Kornguth, S. E., Kalinke, T., and Grunwald, G. B., et al. Anti-neurofilament antibodies in the sera of patients with small cell carcinoma of the lung and with visual paraneoplastic syndrome. *Cancer Res.* 46:2588, 1986.
85. Kornguth, S. E., Llein, R., Appen, R., and Choate, J. Occurrence of anti-retinal ganglion cell antibodies in patients with small cell carcinoma of the lung. *Cancer* 50:1289, 1982.
86. Lakhanpal, S., Bunch, T. W., Ilstrup, D. M., and Melton, L. J. Polymyositis-dermatomyositis and malignant lesions: Does an association exist? *Mayo Clin. Proc.* 61:645, 1986.
87. Lambert, E. H., Eaton, L. M., and Rooke, E. D. Defect of neuromuscular conduction associated with malignant neoplasm. *Am. J. Physiol.* 187:612, 1956.
88. Lang, B., Newsom-Davis, J., Prior, C., and Wray, D. Antibodies to motor nerve terminals: An electrophysiological study of a human myasthenic syndrome transferred to mouse. *J. Physiol. (London)* 344:335, 1983.
89. Langston, J. W., Dorfman, L., and Forno, L. "Encephalomyeloneuritis" in the absence of cancer. *Neurology* 25:633, 1975.
90. Latov, N. Neuropathy and anti-GMl antibodies. *Ann. Neurol.* 27 (Suppl.):S41, 1990.
91. Latov, N., Hays, A. P., Donofrio, P. D., et al. Monoclonal IgM with unique specificity to gangliosides GM_1 and GD_1B and to lacto-*N*-tetraose associated with human motor neuron disease. *Neurology* 38:763, 1988.
92. Layzer, R. B. *Neuromuscular Manifestation of Systemic Disease.* Philadelphia: Davis, 1985. Pp. 265–267.
93. Lisak, R. P., Mitchell, M., Zweiman, B., et al. Guillain-Barré syndrome and Hodgkin's disease: 3 cases with immunological studies. *Ann. Neurol.* 1:72, 1977.
94. Lugue, F. A., Furneaux, H. F., Ferzinger, R., et al. Anti-Ri: An antibody associated with paraneoplastic opsoclonus and breast cancer. *Ann. Neurol.* 29:241, 1991.
95. Mancall, E. L., and Rosales, R. K. Necrotizing

myelopathy associated with visceral carcinoma. *Brain* 87:639, 1964.
96. Markham, M., and Abeloff, M. D. Small-cell lung cancer and limbic encephalitis. *Ann. Intern. Med.* 96:785, 1982.
97. Martin, E. S., and Griffith, J. F. Myoclonic encephalopathy and neuroblastoma: Report of a case with apparent recovery. *Am. J. Dis. Child.* 122:257, 1971.
98. Mastaglia, F. L., and Ojeda, V. J. Inflammatory myopathies. *Ann. Neurol.* 17:215, 1985.
99. McDonald, W. I. Cortical cerebellar degeneration with ovarian carcinoma. *Neurology* 11:328, 1961.
100. McEvoy, K. M., Windebank, A. J., Daube, J. R., Low, P. A. 3,4-Diaminopyridine in the treatment of Lambert-Eaton myasthenic syndrome. *N. Engl. J. Med.* 32:1567, 1989.
101. McGill, T. Carcinomatous encephalomyelitis with auditory and vestibular manifestations. *Ann. Otol.* 120, 1976.
102. McLeod, J. G., and Pollard, J. D. Neuropathies in Systemic Diseases: Hidden and overt. In A. K. Asbury and R. W. Gilliatt (eds.), *Peripheral Nerve Disorders.* Boston: Butterworth, 1984.
103. Min, K., Gyorkey, F., and Sato, C. Mucin-producing adenocarcinomas and non-bacterial thrombotic endocarditis: Pathogenetic role of tumor mucin. *Cancer* 45:2374, 1980.
104. Moe, P. G., and Nellhaus, G. Infantile polymyoclonia-opsoclonus syndrome and neural crest tumors. *Neurology* 20:756, 1970.
105. Namba, T., Brunner, N. G., and Grob, D. Myasthenia gravis in patients with thymoma with particular reference to onset after thymectomy. *Medicine* 57:411, 1978.
106. Newsom-Davis, J., and Murray, N. M. F. Plasma-exchange and immuno-suppressive drug treatment in the Lambert-Eaton myasthenic syndrome. *Neurology* 34:480, 1984.
107. Norris, F. H., and Engel, W. K. Carcinomatous Amyotrophic Lateral Sclerosis. In L. Brain and F. H. Norris (eds.), *The Remote Effects of Cancer on the Nervous System.* New York: Grune & Stratton, 1965.
108. Oh, S. J., Slaughter, R., and Harrell, L. Paraneoplastic vasculitis neuropathy: A treatable neuropathy. *Muscle Nerve* 14:152, 1991.
109. Ojeda, V. J. Necrotizing myelopathy associated with malignancy: A clinicopathologic study of two cases and literature review. *Cancer* 53:1115, 1984.
110. Olebaum, M. H., and Statham, R. Carcinoma of the bronchus presenting as a cerebellar neuropathy. *Postgrad. Med. J.* 37:546, 1961.
111. O'Neill, J. H., Murray, N. M. F., and Newsom-Davis, J. The Lambert-Eaton myasthenic syndrome: A review of 50 cases. *Brain* 111:577, 1988.
112. Ongerboer Devisser, B. W., Feltkamp-Vroom, T. M., Feltkamp, C. A. Sural nerve immune deposits in polyneuropathy as a remote effect of malignancy. *Ann. Neurol.* 14:261, 1983.
113. Paone, J. F., and Jeyasingham, K. Remission of cerebellar dysfunction after pneumonectomy for bronchogenic carcinoma. *N. Engl. J. Med.* 302:156, 1980.
114. Pestronk, A., Chaudrhy, V., Feldman, E. L., et al. Lower motor neuron syndromes defined by patterns of weakness, nerve conduction abnormalities, and high titers of anti-glycolipid antibodies. *Ann. Neurol.* 27:316, 1990.
115. Pestronk, A., Cornblath, D. R., Ilyas, A. A., et al. A treatable multi-focal motor neuropathy with antibodies to GM_1 ganglioside. *Ann. Neurol.* 24:73, 1988.
116. Pilay, N., Gilbert, J. J., Ebers, G. C., and Brown, J. D. Internuclear ophthalmoplegia and "optic neuritis": Paraneoplastic effects of bronchial carcinoma. *Neurology* 34:788, 1984.
117. Polans, A. S., Buczylko, J., Crabb, J., and Palczewski, K. A photo-receptor calcium binding protein is recognized by autoantibodies obtained from patients with cancer-associated retinopathy. *J. Cell Biol.* 112:981, 1991.
118. Posner, J. B. Neurological complications of systemic cancer. *D. M.* 25:3, 1978.
119. Propp, R. P., Means, E., Deibel, R., et al. Waldenström's macroglobulinemia and neuropathy. *Neurology* 25:980, 1975.
120. Reddy, R. V., and Vakili, S. T. Midbrain encephalitis as a remote effect of a malignant neoplasm. *Arch. Neurol.* 38:781, 1981.
121. Rewcastle, N. B. Subacute cerebellar degeneration with Hodgkin's disease. *Arch. Neurol.* 9:407, 1963.
122. Rickles, F. R., Edwards, R. L., Barb, C., and Cronland, M. Abnormalities of blood coagulation in patients with cancer: Fibrinopeptide A generation and tumor growth. *Cancer* 51:301, 1983.
123. Roberts, A., Perera, S., Lang, B., et al. Paraneoplastic myasthenic syndrome IgG inhibits $^{45}Ca^{2+}$ flux in a human small cell carcinoma line. *Nature* 317:737, 1985.
124. Rosen, P., and Armstrong, D. Non-bacterial thrombotic endocarditis in patients with malignant neoplastic diseases. *Am. J. Med.* 54:23, 1973.
125. Ross, A. T., and Zeman, W. Opsoclonus, occult carcinoma and chemical pathology in dentate nuclei. *Arch. Neurol.* 17:546, 1967.
126. Rowland, L. P., and Schneck, S. A. Neuromuscular disorders associated with malignant neoplastic disease. *J. Chronic Dis.* 16:777, 1963.
127. Sack, G. H., Levin, J., and Bell, W. Trousseau's syndrome and other manifestations of chronic disseminated coagulopathy in patients with neoplasms: Clinical, pathophysiologic and therapeutic results. *Medicine* 56:1, 1977.

128. Sarbach, B. Carcinomatous cerebellar degeneration with cortical atrophy and inflammatory reaction involving the dentate nucleus: Case report. *Acta Neurol. Belg.* 77:363, 1977.
129. Satoyoshi, E., Kowa, H., and Fukunaga, T. Subacute cerebellar degeneration and Eaton-Lambert syndrome with bronchial carcinoma: Case report. *Neurology* 23:764, 1973.
130. Sawyer, R. A., Selhorst, J. B., Zimmerman, L. E., and Hoyt, W. F. Blindness caused by photoreceptor degeneration as a remote effect of cancer. *Am. J. Ophthalmol.* 81:606, 1976.
131. Schaumburg, H. H., Spencer, P. S., and Thomas, P. K. *Disorders of Peripheral Nerves.* Davis: Philadelphia, 1983.
132. Schold, S. C., Cho, E. S., Somasundaram, M., et al. Subacute motor neuropathy: A remote effect of lymphoma. *Ann. Neurol.* 5:271, 1979.
133. Schuffler, M. D., Baird, H. W., Fleming, C. R., et al. Intestinal pseudo-obstruction as the presenting manifestation of small-cell carcinoma of the lung: A paraneoplastic neuropathy of the gastrointestinal tract. *Ann. Intern. Med.* 98:129, 1983.
134. Schwartzman, R. J., and Hill, J. B. Neurological complications of disseminated intravascular coagulation. *Neurology* 32:791, 1982.
135. Senelick, R. C., Bray, P., Lahey, M., et al. Neuroblastoma and myoclonic encephalopathy: 2 cases and a review of the literature. *J. Pediatr. Surg.* 8:623, 1973.
136. Shy, M. E., Rowland, L. P., Smith, T., et al. Motor neuron disease and plasma cell dyscrasia. *Neurology* 36:1429, 1986.
137. Sigsbee, B., Deck, M., and Posner, J. B. Nonmetastatic superior sagittal sinus thrombosis complicating systemic cancer. *Neurology* 29:139, 1979.
138. Stoll, D. B., Lublin, F., Brodovsky, H., et al. Association of subacute motor neuronopathy with thymoma. *Cancer* 54:770, 1984.
139. Swift, T. R. Disorders of neuromuscular transmission other than myasthenia gravis. *Muscle Nerve* 4:334, 1981.
140. Teravainen, H., and Larson, A. Some features of the neuromuscular complications of pulmonary carcinoma. *Ann. Neurol.* 2:495, 1977.
141. Tovik, A., and Slettebo, M. Encephalomyelitis with polyneuropathy. *Acta Neurol. Scand.* 61:287, 1980.
142. Trotter, J. L., Hendin, B. A., and Osterland, K. Cerebellar degeneration with Hodgkin's disease. *Arch. Neurol.* 33:660, 1976.
143. Verhaart, W. J. Grey matter degeneration of the CNS in carcinosis. *Acta Neuropathol.* 1:107, 1961.
144. Vick, N., Schulman, S., and Dau, P. Carcinomatous cerebellar degeneration, encephalomyelitis and sensory neuropathy (radiculitis): Report of a case incorporating both purely degenerative and intense inflammatory changes, with special prominence of the latter in the putamen. *Neurology* 19:425, 1969.
145. Vincent, A., Lang, B., and Newsom-Davis, J. Autoimmunity to the voltage-gated calcium channel underlies the Lambert-Eaton myasthenic syndrome, a paraneoplastic disorder. *T.I.N.S.* 12:496, 1989.
146. Walsh, J. C. Neuropathy associated with lymphoma. *J. Neurol. Neurosurg. Psychiatry* 34:42, 1971.
147. Walton, J. N., Tomlinson, B. E., and Pearce, G. W. Subacute "poliomyelitis" and Hodgkin's disease. *J. Neurol. Sci.* 6:435, 1968.
148. Wessel, K., Diener, H. C., Dichgans, J., and Thron, A. Cerebellar dysfunction in patients with bronchogenic carcinoma: Clinical and posturographic findings. *J. Neurol.* 235:290, 1988.
149. Windebank, A. J., Blexrud, M. D., Dyck, P. J., et al. The syndrome of acute sensory neuropathy: Clinical features and electrophysiologic and pathologic changes. *Neurology* 40:584, 1990.
150. Yahr, M., Duvoisin, R. C., and Cowen, D. Encephalopathy associated with carcinoma. *Trans. Am. Neurol. Assoc.* 90:80, 1965.
151. Younger, D. S., Rowland, L. P., Latov, N., et al. Motor neuron disease and amyotrophic lateral sclerosis: Relation of high CSF protein content to paraproteinemia and clinical syndromes. *Neurology* 40:595, 1990.
152. Younger, D. S., Rowland, L. P., Latov, N., et al. Lymphoma, motor neuron diseases, and amyotrophic lateral sclerosis. *Ann. Neurol.* 29:78, 1991.

21 Central Nervous System Manifestations of Radiotherapy

David A. Larson, William M. Wara, and John R. Fike

It is well known that irradiation of central nervous system structures can result in central nervous system injury. However, the actual risk of injury associated with any specific combination of clinical variables and radiation factors is poorly understood. Much of the literature on the tolerance of the central nervous system to therapeutic irradiation is fragmentary, anecdotal, incomplete, or conflicting. Nevertheless, several circumstances in which adverse reactions occur are known and allow clinicians to assess the possibility of injury following a particular course of radiotherapy.

Radiation delivered to structures beyond the brain and spinal cord rarely, if ever, causes central nervous system effects. For example, it has been suggested that neck irradiation may result in a slightly increased incidence of stroke [15]. However, statistically significant abscopal effects have not been demonstrated, and this chapter is therefore concerned with direct effects on the central nervous system following irradiation of central nervous system structures.

Adverse effects of irradiation of the human brain are usually categorized according to time of clinical manifestations: (1) *acute reactions*, which occur during the course of treatment; (2) *early delayed reactions*, which occur a few weeks to a few months following irradiation; and (3) *late delayed reactions*, which appear several months to years after treatment. Adverse effects of radiation to the human spinal cord, radiation myelopathies, are usually subdivided into (1) *transient radiation myelopathies*, which appear within the first year or so following treatment, and (2) *delayed radiation myelopathies*, usually appearing later. The risk for occurrence of these reactions and their severity depend both on technical factors, such as radiation fraction size, total radiation dose, number of elapsed days from start to completion of radiation, volume of central nervous system tissue irradiated, and number and distribution of beam ports, as well as on clinical factors, such as patient age, presence of central nervous system injury due to tumor or prior surgery, presence of infection or vascular disease, and treatment with chemotherapy in addition to radiation.

BRAIN INJURY

Acute Reactions

Acute reactions occur during a course of radiation treatment. Patients suffering acute reactions either develop an increase in preexisting neurologic deficits or demonstrate a clinical picture suggesting increased intracranial pressure. In most cases, reactions are mild and of little significance. They are commonly thought to be due to radiation-induced, vasogenic edema; although objective evidence that supports this view is limited. Computed tomography (CT) scans obtained during the course of treatment usually do not demonstrate increased peritumoral edema [10]. The old practice of commencing radiotherapy treatment to the brain with a few low-dose fractions to avoid edema is usually unnecessary [46], except for the occasional patient with a large or critically located brain tumor causing considerably elevated intracranial pressure despite high-dose dexamethasone [37].

Acute reactions are seen infrequently with conventional dose-fractionation schedules (180–200 cGy/day given 5 days/week to a total dose of 6000 cGy to a portion of the brain). Larger individual fractions of radiation, up to 600 cGy, are well tolerated acutely, provided the total dose is lowered appropriately. However, with larger fractions (2 fractions of 750 cGy each over 3 days, or 1000 cGy in a single fraction to the whole brain), up to 50 percent of patients develop acute complications including headache, nausea, vomiting, and pyrexia, and 10 percent of patients may develop cerebral herniation [17,51].

Historically, to avoid potential acute reactions, brain irradiation was initiated with small daily fractions, which were gradually increased up to 200 cGy during the first week of treatment. However, modern clinical experience indicates that constant daily radiation doses of 200 cGy are well tolerated acutely, even with large total doses. For occasional patients who develop acute reactions, and for patients with poor neurologic functions, concomitant corticosteroid administration usually leads to rapid resolution of signs and symptoms, even though survival is not significantly affected.

Early Delayed Reactions

Early delayed reactions occur a few weeks to a few months following irradiation but are not frequently recognized, although they are analogous to transient radiation myelopathies following spinal cord irradiation, seen more frequently (see Spinal Cord Injury). Clinically, most patients demonstrating early delayed reactions develop either exacerbations of preexisting signs and symptoms, or somnolence, seen mainly in children treated for acute lymphoblastic leukemia (ALL). Other patients may occasionally develop new neurologic abnormalities.

The somnolence syndrome occurs in up to 75 percent of children with ALL who undergo prophylactic irradiation of the central nervous system [16,26]. It is characterized by somnolence, anorexia, and irritability, without accompanying focal neurologic abnormalities. Symptoms develop 1 to 2 months following completion of radiation and resolve spontaneously within 2 to 5 weeks. They are more severe in children less than 3 years of age. Cerebrospinal fluid pleocytosis or mild protein elevation may be present, and diffuse slowing may be seen on EEG [3]. It is not entirely clear how radiation fraction size affects the incidence of somnolence. Parker and co-workers [35] reported somnolence in 40 percent of children receiving 125 cGy per fraction compared with 75 percent of children receiving 150 cGy per fraction to the same total dose (2400 cGy). Littman and colleagues [26] observed an equal incidence (58%) and severity of somnolence in children receiving either 100 cGy or 180 cGy per fraction to the same total dose (1800 cGy). In general, relapse and survival rates in children with ALL are not adversely affected by the somnolence syndrome. Further, the risk for development of cognitive dysfunction in children treated for ALL appears to be similar in those who do and those who do not develop the syndrome [2,48].

Early delayed reactions manifesting as new neurologic deficits are uncommon. Rider [40] described two patients who developed transient reactions approximately 10 weeks following radiation therapy for extracranial lesions. Both developed nausea, vomiting, dysarthria, dysphagia, ataxia, horizontal nystagmus, and a positive Romberg's sign. Recovery began after 1 month and was complete within 2. Boldrey and Sheline [4] described eight patients who developed transient reactions 10 weeks after radiation therapy for low-grade gliomas, meningiomas, and pituitary adenomas. None of the reactions could be attributed to tumor progression, since the symptoms resolved within 6 weeks. Hoffman, Levin, and Wilson [19] described 51 patients with malignant gliomas treated with radiation and BCNU. Neurologic changes suggesting tumor progression were seen in 25 patients within 18 weeks after radiation therapy. However, spontaneous improvement was seen in 7 of the 25 affected.

Early delayed reactions are usually transient and associated with an uneventful recovery. CT scans may show demyelination during the reaction period. It is thought that early delayed reactions, whether manifesting as the somnolence syndrome or otherwise, are a result of demyelination due to a temporary inhibition of myelin synthesis. The latency and recovery times of early delayed reactions correspond to the turnover time of myelin [14].

Late Delayed Reactions

Late delayed reactions are manifest several months to years following radiotherapy and are usually progressive and irreversible and sometimes fatal. Clinical signs and symptoms depend on the region of brain irradiated and may be related to the development of necrosis. Other late-occurring clinical sequelae include pituitary-hypothalamic dysfunction, decreased intellectual ability, necrotizing leukoencephalopathy or mineralizing microangiopathy, and radiation-induced malignant tumors.

The pathogenesis of the various manifestations of late delayed reactions is not completely understood. It is probable that multiple mechanisms are involved, including effects of radiation on brain vasculature or myelination, and their relative importance may depend on the latent interval. Vascular changes probably become more important with time.

Radiation Necrosis

The risk for the development of brain radionecrosis is difficult to establish for several reasons: Autopsies are not commonly performed, studies frequently fail to include the number of exposed patients who have survived at least as long as the latent period, and it is difficult to compare the results of various dose-fractionation schedules used. However, the data of Marks and associates [29] are frequently quoted. He reported 139 patients with various intracranial tumors treated with standard doses (180–200 cGy to a minimum total dose of 4500 cGy, with most patients receiving 5000–6000 cGy in 5–7 weeks), although only one of two parallel opposed fields was treated each day. Pathologically documented cerebral necrosis was seen in 7 of 139 patients (5%), and 2 additional patients developed clinically diagnosed radionecrosis. However, only 24 of the 139 patients underwent reoperation or autopsy, so this risk estimate may represent a lower limit. These data, representing patients treated during 1974 to 1976, were recently reviewed and compared to results in patients treated during 1976 to 1981, when dose was reduced an average of 7 percent [30]. No cases of radionecrosis were seen in 198 patients in the latter period. It was concluded that the risk of radionecrosis is extremely low for patients treated to 5400 cGy in 30 fractions over 42 days, but likely increases rapidly for higher doses. Recently, Lee and co-workers [23] reported on 9606 patients treated with radiation therapy for nasopharyngeal carcinoma. The patients were treated using unconventional, large fractions ranging from 250 to 420 cGy over 38 to 42 days, to a total dose of 4560 to 6000 cGy, using techniques that included the temporal lobes in the treatment fields. Late temporal lobe radionecrosis was diagnosed by correlating clinical features and CT scans rather than by brain biopsy. The incidence rate in this series was only 1 percent, and this too may represent an underestimate.

It is recognized that comparisons of the risk

for developing radionecrosis between various dose-fractionation schemes is difficult. As a result, several formulas have been developed to combine mathematically total dose (D), total number of radiation fractions (N), and elapsed time (T) from start to completion of radiotherapy, to produce a single number that can be related to outcome. An example is the nominal standard dose formula of Sheline, Wara, and Smith [46] to be applied to irradiation of the brain:

$$\text{NSD (neuret)} = D \times N^{-0.4} \times T^{-0.06}$$

The equivalent dose formula of Wara and colleagues [50] is usually applied to irradiation of the spinal cord:

$$\text{ED (ret)} = D \times N^{-0.377} \times T^{-0.058}$$

Although firm data are lacking, present evidence indicates that the threshold for brain necrosis is approximately 1000 to 1100 neuret or an equivalent dose of 1250 ret.

The diagnosis of radionecrosis in patients without intracranial tumors can be inferred from findings of CT or magnetic resonance imaging (MRI). However, it is difficult to make this diagnosis confidently in patients with intracranial neoplasms unless histologic samples are obtained [14]. At present, neither CT nor MRI can reliably distinguish radiation necrosis from recurrent tumor. Both may present similar, nonspecific, clinical and radiologic findings, and biopsy is required to confirm the diagnosis of radionecrosis if abnormalities are seen at the tumor site.

Surgical resection of focal areas of radiation necrosis frequently results in clinical improvement with occasional complete recovery. Resection is of little value in patients with diffuse lesions, lesions crossing midline, or lesions involving the brain stem or optic nerves. Little clinical benefit is seen following biopsy only. Corticosteroids frequently result in clinical improvement of neurologic deficits when surgery is not possible [14]. Anticoagulant agents have been reported to lead to dramatic clinical and CT improvement in a few patients [41].

Necrotizing Leukoencephalopathy and Mineralizing Microangiopathy

These reactions were first recognized as complications of treatment for childhood ALL. Necrotizing leukoencephalopathy, also called disseminating necrotizing leukoencephalopathy or subacute leukoencephalopathy, is manifest by the progressive development of personality changes, disorientation, memory loss, and frank dementia. It is seen in up to 15 percent of children receiving cranial radiation therapy and intrathecal or high-dose intravenous methotrexate [1,3]. The risk for its occurrence appears to be low in children who receive radiation therapy treatment following methotrexate administration, as opposed to those who receive methotrexate following irradiation or concomitant irradiation [3].

Children who develop leukoencephalopathy demonstrate nonenhancing periventricular hypodensities on CT scan. With time, ventricular dilatation and broadening of the sulci may occur. Similar abnormal CT findings have been reported in asymptomatic patients and probably represent subclinical leukoencephalopathy. Conversely, it has been noted that children in remission from ALL after receiving intrathecal methotrexate and less than 2500 cGy cranial irradiation may develop cognitive impairment suggestive of leukoencephalopathy, even though white matter changes are not seen on MRI [22].

The pathogenesis of this syndrome is thought to be demyelination of the cerebral hemispheric white matter. Histopathologically, lesions are characterized by demyelination, multifocal areas of coagulation necrosis, and gliosis. Most children who develop this syndrome survive with some degree of permanent neurologic deficit; in some the outcome is fatal, although a few may recover completely.

Although leukoencephalopathy is most frequently seen in children, it has also been described in adults treated for various cancers with either radiotherapy or chemotherapy, or both [24,47].

Mineralizing microangiopathy presents as headache, focal seizures, ataxia, behavior disorders, or perceptual motor disability. It is seen in approximately 25 percent of children who survive at least 9 months following central nervous system radiotherapy for ALL [3] and is seen more frequently in children less than 10 years of age at the time of treatment [38]. CT scans may show calcification of the basal ganglia. Histopathologically, small blood vessels are seen to be occluded by calcium deposits within their walls. Brain tissues surrounding these vessels may be mineralized and necrotic.

Radiologic Abnormalities

Late radiation injury may present radiologically as focal necrosis or as diffuse white matter injury. Both types of injury may appear together. On CT, focal necrosis produces a low-density region with surrounding edema and variable mass effect, with an irregular margin of contrast enhancement. This pattern is easily interpreted when seen following irradiation of an extracranial lesion but may be difficult to distinguish from that of tumor following irradiation of an intracranial lesion. MRI demonstrates edema, with increased signal on T2-weighted images, but is not specific for tumor or focal necrosis. In some cases, the distinction can be made by examining the blood-brain barrier and local glucose metabolism with positron emission tomography [12].

Diffuse white matter injury usually presents on CT as bilateral, diffuse, low-density lesions involving much of the hemispheric white matter but is more frequently appreciated on MRI, which is extremely sensitive to white matter edema. Such lesions are usually indistinguishable from white matter changes seen in nonirradiated, otherwise normal, older people or in persons with cerebral vascular disease. Depending on criteria used for defining injury following irradiation, diffuse white matter injury may be seen in a large percentage of patients following brain irradiation [8,49]. The incidence of such injury increases with volume of brain irradiated, radiation dose, interval between irradiation and imaging, and patient age. Although severe radiologic changes correlate with clinical neurologic findings, the clinical significance of mild and moderate radiologic abnormalities is not yet known [9].

Cerebral atrophy frequently accompanies diffuse white matter injury, although the clinical significance of this observation is also unknown; many patients with diffuse white matter injury and cerebral atrophy have no obvious intellectual compromise, especially those under 40 years of age [47]. It should be noted that diffuse white matter injury has also been observed following treatment with irradiation and chemotherapy and following chemotherapy only [24].

Diffuse white matter injury occurs at a somewhat lower dose and after a longer latent period than focal necrosis [33].

In exceptional circumstances, small-field, high-dose irradiation may damage major intracranial arteries, possibly resulting in brain necrosis at a site outside the radiation field; arteriography may demonstrate occluded or stenosed arteries within the radiation field [6,31].

Pituitary-Hypothalamic Dysfunction

Effects of brain irradiation on endocrine activity have long been recognized. For example, growth hormone deficiency, the most common deficiency, is noted in a large fraction of children receiving at least 2400 cGy to the hypothalamus during whole brain cranial irradiation and begins as early as 3 months following treatment [13]. Lustig and associates [28] demonstrated that such patients usually have functional pituitary somatotropes and a deficiency of endogenous hypothalamic growth hormone releasing factor (GRF), presumably reflecting the relative radioresistence of the pituitary and the relative radiosensitivity of the hypothalamus and higher neural centers, particularly that of the hypothalamic GRF-secretory mechanism. Other hypothalamic syndromes presenting as hypoadrenalism, hypogonadism, hypothyroidism, and hyperprolactinemia following brain irradiation have been described.

Mechanick, Hochberg, and LaRocque [32] identified 15 patients with clinically evident hypothalamic dysfunction 2 to 9 years following whole brain irradiation for extrahypothalamic astrocytoma or medulloblastoma. Hypothalamic endocrine dysfunction (hyperprolactinemia) or behavioral changes (anxiety, depression, lability, belligerence, thirst, and changes in sleep-wake cycle, appetite, and so on) were seen in all patients, without evidence on follow-up CT of a hypothalamic abnormality. Although the number of patients at risk was not precisely identified, it is likely that hypothalamic dysfunction in long-term survivors following whole brain irradiation is not rare. Younger children are at greater risk to develop hypothalamic dysfunction.

Impaired Intellectual Function

Cognitive dysfunction in children is a recognized sequela of radiation therapy for brain tumors and ALL. Less information exists on the relationship between cranial irradiation and subsequent intellectual impairment in adults. In either case, causes of such dysfunction may be difficult to determine, since surgery, chemotherapy, radiation therapy, psychological stress, and effectiveness of rehabilitation are often thought to be contributory.

Recently Mulhern and co-workers [34] studied 40 children in continuous complete remission from ALL to assess memory functioning 5 years after central nervous system prophylaxis. Initially, patients had been randomly assigned to receive CNS prophylaxis with either 1800 cGy cranial irradiation plus intrathecal methotrexate or intrathecal methotrexate plus intravenous high-dose methotrexate. No treatment- or age-related differences were seen on 16 standardized memory measures. However, scores of the combined groups of patients were significantly lower than age-corrected norms on tests of visual-spatial memory and verbal memory.

Peckham and colleagues [36] studied 23 long-term survivors of childhood ALL who had received 2400 cGy cranial irradiation and intrathecal methotrexate and standard chemotherapeutic agents 8 to 10 years previously. Cognitive function had been evaluated at the time of diagnosis and periodically thereafter. Long-term assessment of levels of school achievement demonstrated that children achieved less than expected levels in both reading and mathematics, in comparison to pre-treatment and most recent IQ scores. In addition, most children experienced difficulty with attention and concentration, memory, sequencing, and comprehension when performing school tasks. A small number of children performed better than expected, indicating that individualized tutoring and parental support may reduce some learning deficits.

Recently Bordeaux and associates [5] evaluated the effect of radiotherapy and surgery on neuropsychological function in two groups of children: seven who underwent surgery and seven who underwent radiotherapy. Treatment groups were composed of children ages 56 to 196 months at the time of evaluation who had heterogeneous tumor diagnoses and locations. Children underwent neuropsychological testing before and after therapy. Comparisons of pre-therapy findings with normative values indicated that both groups performed within the average range of most measures, although deficits at baseline were observed on test of fine-motor, psychomotor, and timed-language skills, all likely attributable to tumor-related effects. Comparisons of pre- versus post-therapy neuropsychological test findings demonstrated no significant interval changes for either group, possibly suggesting that surgery and radiotherapy are not associated with acute effects on neuropsychological functions. Testing in these children was performed at an average of 11 months, as opposed to testing done well beyond 1 year in many other studies.

Hochberg and Slotnick [18] studied 13 adult patients with high-grade astrocytomas who had survived at least 1 year after being treated with the combination of surgery, external beam irradiation to 6000 cGy, and CCNU chemotherapy. The 13 patients had failed to return to pre-morbid educational or vocational levels and were therefore examined with neuropsychological tests of specific and generalized higher cortical functions. All demonstrated diffuse cortical dysfunction. Their performance was unrelated to tumor type or location and could not be explained by existing focal deficits, psychotic or depressive thought disorders, metabolic difficulties, or hydrocephalus.

Looper and co-workers [27] and Johnson and colleagues [20] reported on patients who were survivors of small-cell lung carcinoma who had received prophylactic or therapeutic cranial irradiation in addition to chemotherapy. Three-fourths of patients in both studies had evidence of neurologic problems. In many cases this dysfunction was severe, either causing significant impairment of activity of daily living or requiring institutionalization. Onset typically occurred 2 to 3 weeks after treatment. Frequent problems included memory loss, confusion, dementia, ataxia, psychomotor retardation, and optic atrophy. CT scans were available in all patients at the time of initial evaluation in Johnson's series and were normal in 75 percent of patients. Of patients undergoing serial CT scans, progressive abnormalities were present in 61 percent.

These studies illustrate several points: Short-term follow-up after radiotherapy may fail to reveal dysfunction; long-term follow-up frequently demonstrates dysfunction, both in children and adults; and either chemotherapy or radiotherapy can lead to dysfunction.

Radiation-Induced Tumors

Radiation-induced brain tumors are rare, and the mechanism of radiation carcinogenesis is unknown. Before a histologically verified tumor can be attributed to prior irradiation, it must arise within the radiation field and it should be of a different cell type from any prior central nervous system tumor. Liwnicz and associates [25] reviewed 96 such cases in the literature and found 50 meningiomas, 24 gliomas, and 22 sarcomas. Most radiation-induced gliomas were found to occur in children and young adults, but there was no apparent correlation between dose and latency. However, a correlation was noted in radiation-induced meningiomas, with a latency of 31.3 years following low-dose irradiation and 20.8 years following high-dose irradiation.

More recently, Ron and co-workers [42] studied over 10,000 children treated for tinea capitis with low-dose orthovoltage irradiation between 1948 and 1960 and compared them to matched general-population controls and siblings who did not receive radiation treatment. The 30-year cumulative risk for the subsequent development of neural tumors in patients exposed as children was 0.8 percent. The estimated relative risk as compared with controls was 6.9 percent. Increased risks were found for meningiomas, gliomas, nerve-sheath tumors, and other neural tumors. A strong dose-response relationship was noted, with a relative risk of approximately 20 percent after doses of approximately 250 cGy. Tumors occurred between 6 and 29 years after radiation (mean, 17.6 years). Unfortunately, it is currently impossible to extrapolate these findings to obtain those expected in patients treated with modern high-energy linear accelerators, with different resultant dose distributions and higher prescribed doses (usually in the range 1800–6000 cGy).

Risk Factors

The incidence of late delayed reactions is increased in patients treated with methotrexate and radiotherapy for ALL. In addition, late delayed reactions are seen in long-term surviving patients with small-cell carcinoma of the lung who received prophylactic cranial irradiation of 3000 cGy in 10 fractions. Patients with underlying vascular disease secondary to diabetes mellitus, Cushing's disease, or acromegaly may be at increased risk for the development of radiation injury, as are patients with an underlying central nervous system infection or those who have received chemotherapy. It is generally thought that children under the age of 3 years are at increased risk to develop radiation injury, since myelination in young children is not complete.

SPINAL CORD INJURY

Transient Radiation Myelopathy

Patients with transient radiation myelopathy describe sudden, electric-like shocks radiating down the spine to the extremities on neck flexion (Lhermitte's sign). Symptoms are usually symmetric but are unrelated to a specific dermatome distribution, and neurologic examination is otherwise normal. Carmel and Kaplan [7] reported the finding in 15 percent of 377 patients treated with mantle field irradiation for Hodgkin's disease, with latent periods after radiotherapy of 1 to 29 months (median 4 months). The average duration of symptoms was 5.3 months.

It is believed that transient radiation myelopathy results from transient demyelination in the posterior columns and/or lateral spinothalamic tracts within the radiation field. Presumably, radiation inhibits the normal proliferation of myelin-producing oligoendroglial cells in the irradiated area. The latent period is consistent with temporary blockage in the synthesis of myelin. It is believed that symptoms result from stretching of the demyelinated, hypersensitive posterior fibers of the cord. In general, the clinical picture reverses spontaneously without specific therapy, although subsequent radiation myelitis has been reported occasionally, mostly in cases where commonly accepted spinal cord tolerance doses have been exceeded.

Delayed Radiation Myelopathy

Patients with delayed radiation myelopathy typically present with a several-month history of progressive neurologic signs and symptoms, such as paresthesias and decreased pain and temperature sensation. The latent period may range from several weeks to many years. A bimodal frequency distribution of latencies has been reported, with peaks at 13 and 26 months [43], possibly corresponding to white matter parenchymal damage and vascular damage, respectively [44]. A shorter latency period is associated with higher doses, lower age, and retreatment with radiation. Symptoms usually progress over 6 months to involve all spinal cord systems, although occasionally they develop acutely following infarction of the spinal cord as a result of radiation-induced vascular changes. Symptoms are usually irreversible, although occasional temporary remissions have been reported following treatment with corticosteroids or hyperbaric oxygen.

The diagnosis of radiation myelopathy is usually a diagnosis of exclusion and requires that the neurologic lesion lie within the radiation field and that local metastatic or primary spinal cord tumors be ruled out. Cerebrospinal fluid pressure is usually normal. Mild elevations in cerebrospinal fluid protein concentration may be seen. Myelography may be normal or may show an area of expansion or attenuation at the irradiated site. In general, CT and MRI are not useful in helping make the diagnosis, although midsagittal MRI of the spine can easily demonstrate fatty replacement of marrow in veretebral bodies, thus sharply delineating the upper and lower borders of the radiation field (even in patients receiving commonly accepted spinal cord radiation doses) [39]. Electrophysiologic measurements of spinal cord nerve conduction velocities are slowed following commonly accepted doses of radiation therapy to the spinal cord [11], but it is not yet known if such measurements can be used to monitor or predict the development of myelopathy.

Pathologic changes are seen in all cord elements, but particularly in white matter, and pathogenesis is usually attributed either to extensive demyelination progressing to white matter necrosis (white matter parenchymal lesion) or to intramedullary vascular damage progressing to hemorrhagic necrosis or infarct (vascular lesion) following irradiation. Histopathologic studies demonstrate varying degrees of endothelial swelling in small arteries and arterioles, endothelial proliferation, collagen and hyaline deposition, intimal and medial necrosis, and vascular occlusion, together with patchy demyelination and wallerian degeneration.

The relationship between various dose-fractionation schemes and risk for radiation myelitis is incompletely understood. However, for a given total dose, increased risk is associated with larger fractions, decreased number of treatments, and treatment of larger lengths of spinal cord. Larger total doses for a given daily fractionation are also associated with increased risk. Wara and colleagues [50] applied his equivalent dose formula

$$\mathrm{ED\ (ret)} = \mathrm{D} \times \mathrm{N}^{-0.377} \times \mathrm{T}^{-0.058}$$

to reported cases of spinal cord injury following radiation therapy and found a threshold dose of approximately 1000 ret. In general, a dose of 4500 cGy in 25 fractions is expected to lead to myelitis in no more than 5 percent of patients. However, this risk may be increased by predisposing factors. Preexisting hypertension is known to increase the likelihood of spinal cord damage in rats and may have a similar effect in humans. Some chemotherapeutic agents probably increase the risk. Younger patients may be at increased risk. The thoracic cord may be more radiosensitive than the cervical cord. It is sometimes thought that risk is increased in patients whose cords have suffered previous injury from tumor and surgery, although one study found no such increased risk [21].

There is no known effective treatment of delayed radiation myelopathy, although temporary remissions have been reported following administration of steroids or hyperbaric oxygen therapy. Although long-term survival is possible, the probability of dying of radiation myelopathy is approximately 30 percent for thoracic cord injuries and 70 percent for cervical cord injuries [45].

REFERENCES

1. Aur, J. A., Simone, J. V., Verzosa, M. S., et al. Leukoencephalopathy in children with lymphocytic leukemia receiving preventive central nervous system therapy. *Sangre (Barc.)* 23:1, 1978.
2. Berg, R. A., Chien, L. T., Lancaster, W., et al. Neuropsychological sequelae of postradiation somnolence syndrome. *J. Dev. Behav. Pediatr.* 4:103, 1983.
3. Bleyer, W. A., and Griffin, T. W. White Matter Necrosis, Microangiopathy and Intellectual Abilities in Survivors of Childhood Leukemia, Association with Central Nervous System Irradiation and Methotrexate Therapy. In H. A. Gilbert and R. Kagan (eds.), *Radiation Damage to the Central Nervous System: A Delayed Therapeutic Hazard.* New York: Raven, 1980. Pp. 155–174.
4. Boldrey, E., and Sheline, G. E. Delayed transitory clinical manifestations after radiation treatment of intracranial tumors. *Acta Radiol. Ther. Phys.* 5:5, 1966.
5. Bordeaux, J. D., Dowell, R. E., Copeland, D. R., et al. A prospective study of neuropsychologic sequelae in children with brain tumors. *J. Child. Neurol.* 3:63, 1988.
6. Brant-Zawadzki, M., Anderson, M., DeArmond, S. J., et al. Radiation-induced large intracranial vessel occlusive vasculopathy. *AJR.* 134:51, 1980.
7. Carmel, R. J., and Kaplan, H. S. Mantle irradiation in Hodgkin's disease: An analysis of technique, tumor eradication and complications. *Cancer* 37:2813, 1976.
8. Constine, L. S., Konski, A., Ekholm, S., et al. Adverse effects of brain irradiation correlated with MR and CT imaging. *Int. J. Radiat. Oncol. Biol. Phys.* 15:319, 1988.
9. Curran, W. J., Hecht-Leavitt, C., Schut, L., et al. Magnetic resonance imaging of cranial radiation lesions. *Int. J. Radiat. Oncol. Biol. Phys.* 13:1093, 1987.
10. Deck, M. D. F. Imaging Techniques in the Diagnosis of Radiation Damage to the Central Nervous System. In H. A. Gilbert and R. Kagan (eds.), *Radiation Damage to the Central Nervous System: A Delayed Therapeutic Hazard.* New York: Raven, 1980. Pp. 107–127.
11. Dorfman, L. J., Donaldson, S. S., Gupta, P. R., and Bosley, T. M. Electrophysiologic evidence of subclinical injury to the posterior columns of the human spinal cord after therapeutic radiation. *Cancer* 50:2815, 1982.
12. Doyle, W. K., Budinger, T. F., Valk, P. E., et al. Differentiation of cerebral radiation necrosis from tumor recurrence by [^{18}F]FDG and ^{82}Rb positron emission tomography. *J. Comput. Assist. Tomogr.* 11:563, 1987.
13. Duffner, P. K., Cohen, M. E., Voorhees, M. L., et al. Long-term effects of cranial irradiation on endocrine function in children with brain tumors. *Cancer* 56:2189, 1985.
14. Edwards, M. S. B., and Wilson, C. B. Treatment of Radiation Necrosis. In H. A. Gilbert and R. Kagan (eds.), *Radiation Damage to the Central-Nervous System: A Delayed Therapeutic Hazard.* New York: Raven, 1980. Pp. 129–144.
15. Elerding, S. C., Fernandez, R. N., Grotta, J. C., et al. Carotid artery disease following external cervical irradiation. *Ann. Surg.* 194:609, 1981.
16. Freeman, J. E., Johnston, P. G. G., and Voke, J. M. Somnolence syndrome after prophylactic cranial irradiation in children with acute lymphoblastic leukemia. *Br. Med. J.* 4:523, 1973.
17. Hindo, W. A., DeTrana, F. A., III, Lee, M.-S., and Hendrickson, F. R. Large dose increment irradiation in treatment of cerebral metastases. *Cancer* 26:138, 1970.
18. Hochberg, F. H., and Slotnick, B. Neuropsychologic impairment in astrocytoma survivors. *Neurology* 30:172, 1980.
19. Hoffman, W. F., Levin, V. A., and Wilson, C. B. Evaluation of malignant glioma patients during the postirradiation period. *J. Neurosurg.* 50:624, 1979.
20. Johnson, V. E., Becker, B., Goff, W. B., et al. Neurologic, neuropsychologic, and computed cranial tomography scan abnormalities in 2–10 year survivors of small cell lung cancer. *J. Clin. Oncol.* 3:1659, 1985.
21. Kopelson, G. Radiation tolerance of the spinal cord previously damaged by tumor and operation: Long term neurological improvement and time-dose-volume relationships after irradiation of intraspinal gliomas. *Int. J. Radiat. Oncol. Biol. Phys.* 8:925, 1982.
22. Kramer, J. H., Norman, D., Brant-Zawadzki, M., et al. Absence of white matter changes on mag-

netic resonance imaging in children treated with CNS prophylaxis therapy for leukemia. *Cancer* 61:928, 1988.

23. Lee, A. W. M., Ng, S. H., Ho, J. H. C., et al. Clinical diagnosis of late temporal lobe necrosis following radiation therapy for nasopharyngeal carcinoma. *Cancer* 61:1535, 1988.
24. Lee, Y., Nauert, C., and Glass, J. P. Treatment-related white matter changes in cancer patients. *Cancer* 57:1473, 1986.
25. Liwnicz, B. H., Berger, T. S., Liwnicz, R. G., and Aron, B. S. Radiation-associated gliomas: A report of four cases and analysis of postradiation tumors of the central nervous system. *Neurosurgery* 17:436, 1985.
26. Littman, P., Rosenstock, J., Gale, G., et al. The somnolence syndrome in leukemic children following reduced daily dose fractions of cranial radiation. *Int. J. Radiat. Oncol. Biol. Phys.* 10:1851, 1984.
27. Looper, J. D., Einhorn, L. H., Garcia, A., et al. Severe neurologic problems following successful therapy for small cell lung cancer (SCLC). *Proc. Ann. Meet. A.C.S.O.* 3:231, 1984.
28. Lustig, R. H., Schriock, E. A., Kaplan, S. L., and Grumbach, M. M. Effects of growth hormone-releasing factor on growth hormone release in children with radiation-induced growth hormone deficiency. *Pediatrics* 76:274, 1985.
29. Marks, J. E., Baglan, R. J., Prassad, S. C., and Blank, W. F. Cerebral radionecrosis: Incidence and risk in relation to dose, time, fractionation and volume. *Int. J. Radiat. Oncol. Biol. Phys.* 7:243, 1981.
30. Marks, J. E., and Wong, J. The risk of cerebral radionecrosis in relation to dose, time and fractionation. *Prog. Exp. Tumor Res.* 29:210, 1985.
31. Marks, M. P., Delapaz, R. L., Fabrikant, J. I., Intracranial vascular malformations: Imaging of charged-particle radiosurgery: Part II. Complications. *Radiology* 168:457, 1988.
32. Mechanick, J. I., Hochberg, F. H., and LaRocque, A. Hypothalamic dysfunction following whole-brain irradiation. *J. Neurosurg.* 65:490, 1986.
33. Mikhael, M. A. Dosimetric considerations in the diagnosis of radiation necrosis of the brain. In H. A. Gilbert and R. Kagan (eds.), *Radiation Damage to the Central Nervous System: A Delayed Therapeutic Hazard.* New York: Raven, 1980. Pp. 59–91.
34. Mulhern, R. K., Wasserman, A. L., Fairclough, D., and Ochs, J. Memory function in disease-free survivors of childhood acute lymphocytic leukemia given CNS prophylaxis with or without 1,800 cGy cranial radiation. *J. Clin. Oncol.* 6:315, 1988.
35. Parker, D., Malpas, J. S., Sandland, R., Outlook following "somnolence syndrome" after prophylactic cranial irradiation. *Br. J. Med.* 4:554, 1978.
36. Peckham, V. C., Meadows, A. T., Bartel, N., and Marrero, O. Educational late effects in long-term survivors of childhood acute lymphocytic leukemia. *Pediatrics* 81:127, 1988.
37. Plowman, P. N., Fuentos, J., and Harnett, A. N. Early radiation swelling remains a problem in the management of paediatric brain tumors. *Br. J. Radiol.* 60:931, 1987.
38. Price, R. A., and Birdwell, D. A. The central nervous system in childhood: Leukemia III. Mineralizing microangiopathy and dystrophic calcifications. *Cancer* 42:717, 1978.
39. Ramsey, R. G., and Zacharias, C. E. MR imaging of the spine after radiation therapy: Easily recognizable effects. *A.J.N.R.* 144:1131, 1985.
40. Rider, W. D. Radiation damage to the brain—a new syndrome. *J. Can. Assoc. Radiol.* 14:67, 1963.
41. Rizzoli, H. V., and Pagnanelli, D. M. Treatment of delayed radionecrosis. *J. Neurosurg.* 60:589, 1984.
42. Ron, E., Modan, B., Boice, J. D., et al. Tumors of the brain and nervous system after radiotherapy. *N. Engl. J. Med.* 319:1033, 1988.
43. Schultheiss, T. E., Higgins, E. M., and El-Mahdi, A. M. The latent period in clinical radiation myelopathy. *Int. J. Radiat. Oncol. Biol. Phys.* 10:1109, 1984.
44. Schultheiss, T. E., Stephens, L. C., and Maor, M. H. Analysis of the histopathology of radiation myelopathy. *Int. J. Radiat. Oncol. Biol. Phys.* 14:27, 1988.
45. Schultheiss, T. E., Stephens, L. C., and Peters, L. J. Survival in radiation myelopathy. *Int. J. Radiat. Oncol. Biol. Phys.* 12:1765, 1986.
46. Sheline, G. E., Wara, W. M., and Smith, V. Therapeutic irradiation and brain injury. *Int. J. Radiat. Oncol. Biol. Phys.* 6:1215, 1980.
47. Stylopoulos, L. A., George, A. E., de Leon, M. J., et al. Longitudinal CT study of parenchymal brain changes in glioma survivors. *A.J.N.R.* 9:517, 1988.
48. Trautman, P. D., Erickson, C., Shaffer, D., et al. Prediction of intellectual deficits in children with acute lymphoblastic leukemia. *J. Dev. Behav. Pediatr.* 9:122, 1988.
49. Tsuruda, J. S., Kortman, K., E., Bradley, W. G., et al. Radiation effects on cerebral white matter: MR evaluation. *A.J.N.R.* 8:431, 1987.
50. Wara, W. M., Phillips, T. L., Sheline, G. E., and Schwade, J. G. Radiation tolerance of the spinal cord. *Cancer* 35:1558, 1975.
51. Young, D. F., Posner, J. B., Chu, F., and Nisce L. Rapid-course radiation therapy of cerebral metastases: Results and complications. *Cancer* 34:1069, 1974.

22 Neurologic Toxicity of Chemotherapy

David M. Dawson

Neurologic signs and symptoms frequently appear during the course of treatment of patients with malignancies. These may reflect diffuse disorders of the nervous system, focal disorders of central nervous function, or peripheral nerve or nerve root damage. The commonest cause is metastasis either within the central nervous system or compressing the brain, spinal cord, or other structures. Patients may have metabolic changes with metabolic encephalopathy or confusional state, or vascular or infectious complications may occur. An infrequent but important source of neurologic disorder is toxicity of chemotherapy. Only a few of the many chemotherapeutic agents now in clinical use have serious neurotoxicity. In some instances, toxicity affects other tissues and limits the dose and duration of treatment. In other cases the chemotherapeutic agent does not enter the nervous system in adequate concentration to be toxic. As we will see, breakdown of the blood-brain barrier either experimentally or because of radiation damage may allow serious neurotoxicity that would not otherwise have occurred. In a few instances, such as the alkylating agent cyclophosphamide, the drug is known to enter the brain yet remains free of toxicity.

The overall neurotoxicity of commonly used antineoplastic drugs has been reviewed on several occasions [13,27,56]. Rather than list these drugs and their toxic reactions yet again, this review will focus on three major areas of clinical significance: diffuse necrotizing encephalopathy, acute cerebellar ataxia, and peripheral neuropathy.

It should be mentioned, however, that certain chemotherapeutic drugs do in fact cause diffuse metabolic changes that may be mistaken for those associated with hypercalcemia, hypoxia, or other common metabolic events. These include the agent procarbazine, which occasionally causes diffuse encephalopathy with confusional state or generalized seizures. Some patients have been reported to recover only very slowly from this encephalopathy, suggesting that there has been longer-term neuronal injury of some type. Nevertheless, complete recovery is normally the rule. Similarly, asparginase, which interferes with the Krebs' urea cycle, may cause confusion and mild stupor. These alterations are to be distinguised from those occurring with antimetabolites (especially with methotrexate) in which the milder confusional state is only one end of a spectrum of neurologic toxicity, ranging all the way to severe permanent brain damage.

NECROTIZING ENCEPHALOPATHY

The major agent in this category is methotrexate. Methotrexate is a cell-cycle-specific agent that blocks normal methyl group metabolism by competitive inhibition of dihydrofolate reductase. The activity of the drug can be reversed by citrovorum factor (folinic acid). Methotrexate is a widely used and effective agent used either orally, intravenously, or intrathecally to treat meningeal leukemia, lymphoma, or carcinoma and in children particularly in the prophylaxis of acute lymphatic leukemia. Its neurologic toxicity may be early or late and may reach a static phase or progress. It is the only chemotherapeutic agent now in widespread use that can cause severe structural brain damage.

The distribution of methotrexate has important clinical implications. The drug is negatively charged at neutral pH and therefore diffuses slowly across physiologic membranes. It enters the cerebrospinal fluid or other third space liquid collections poorly. At steady-state constant intravenous infusion, the drug levels in the spinal fluid are 3 percent of those in the plasma [26]. Methotrexate leaves the spinal fluid by two routes: passive reabsorption by bulk flow and active transport processes presumably involving choroid plexus and/or active tissues. The latter mechanism is sensitive to inhibition by probenecid and other competitive agents.

High-dose systemic administration of the drug (15–30 gm/m^2), followed by "rescue" with citrovorum factor, will give a more uniform distribution within the brain than will intrathecal administration. Lumbar intrathecal injection results in a concentration gradient of 1000 : 1 or higher between lumbar and ventricular fluid [26].

Severe Encephalopathy

Methotrexate leukoencephalopathy has been a well-known entity since the mid 1970s. As a result of work done at St. Jude Hospital in Memphis in the 1960s, intrathecal methotrexate and cranial-spinal radiation either separately or together were added to the treatment plan for children with acute leukemia. This important strategic step led to the eventual reduction in mortality and the current potential for cure in these patients. However, with this potential for cure came the potential for severe leukoencephalopathy.

In its most severe form the leukoencephalopathy produces a rapidly progressing necrosis of white matter of the brain with clinical signs of stupor, quadriplegia, seizures, and eventual death. The symptoms begin frequently some months following the administration of cranial irradiation. The motor symptoms may consist of ataxia, drooling, staring expression, or generalized rigidity. A few patients have shown a clear-cut cerebellar dysmetria or tremor. Both the motor deterioration and dementia progress over a matter of months. Children who have reached a severe level of disability rarely recover, although in a few instances moderate forms of the illness allow for some improvement.

The histologic changes were described in detail simultaneously by Price and Jamieson [44] and by Rubenstein and co-workers. [49]. The hallmark of the lesion is necrosis of focal areas of white matter. The lesions frequently have well-defined margins but may join with other lesions by confluence. When severe, the tissue may become severely necrotic, but in milder forms the lesion shows relative preservation of structure and of axons, with specific damage to myelin. However, conspicuous axonal retraction balls attest to damage to axons at all stages of the illness. The lack of any glial or inflammatory cellular response is a striking feature, and the macrophage response is often reduced compared to infarctions of comparable size and age.

This of course may reflect the antimetabolite and radiation treatment that has already been given.

Blood vessels may or may not show specific changes in patients who have received cranial radiation, usually over 2000 R. The proliferative and fibrinoid necrosis of blood vessels that is characteristic of radiation damage may be absent in patients who have received little or no radiation treatment.

The children treated with methotrexate and irradiation, extensive calcification of the putamen and the deep gray matter represents a variation of the primary lesion [43].

Periventricular necrosis has been recorded in patients who have received methotrexate by means of intraventricular catheter installation. Cerebellar white matter damage has been seen in a few patients. In rare patients, a spinal cord syndrome may develop due to white matter necrosis in the cervical region.

Computed tomography (CT) scans in patients with severe encephalopathy show a striking hypodensity of central white matter, accompanied in children by widespread deep calcification of gray and white structures. The changes on CT scan do not always parallel the clinical findings, and patients with severe dementia do not necessarily show the most severe changes on CT scan.

To summarize the distinctive features of the pathologic entity, they include (1) well-defined foci of necrosis, (2) paucity of cellular response, (3) predominant location in centrum semiovale and other deep white matter, and (4) fibrinoid necrosis of blood vessel walls when radiation therapy has accompanied the use of methotrexate.

Mild Encephalopathy, Chronic or Acute

The detection of the chronic severe form of methotrexate encephalopathy was naturally followed by a search by investigators for a milder version of this illness among survivors of childhood leukemia. A larger literature has grown up in this area, which has been well summarized by Bleyer and others [5–7,38].

In adults, the clinical aspects are those of a widespread disorder of cerebral function. This may consist of a confusional state with a failure of attention, disorientation, and difficulty in memory and concentration. Sometimes this state announces its presence by an unexpected seizure. The mild confusion is taken to be postictal but fails to clear, and a more permanent reduction in mental capacity may become apparent.

In children, the corresponding state is called somnolence syndrome and includes lethargy, nausea, and headache. In such children the electroencephalogram (EEG) will show some slowing [8].

Few long-term studies have been carried out in adults. In children, there is a clear association between the presence of somnolence syndrome at the time of treatment and later intellectual deficit. This may affect as many as one-third of patients who survive acute leukemia. These intellectual changes are not confined to children who have received methotrexate and are also observable in patients who have been treated with whole brain radiation, in whom neuropsychological test batteries have shown clear-cut changes.

According to Bleyer, [5] the risks are maximized in patients who receive radiation concomitantly with intrathecal methotrexate, or in whom the methotrexate is administered shortly after the completion of the course of x-ray. Protection is afforded by the reverse order of treatment, that is, methotrexate first followed by irradiation, or at least by separating the two modalities of treatment by many weeks of time. There is some risk from smaller doses given orally or intravenously, but less than that of intrathecal methotrexate. A few patients have been observed who have developed severe or moderate encephalopathy who have received no cranial radiation at all; usually these have been patients receiving high-dose methotrexate with rescue, although not invariably so.

With long experience with these agents [8], clinical oncologists now are usually able to avoid trouble, and the incidence of methotrexate encephalopathy seems to be steadily falling.

Alterations in spinal fluid dynamics may also increase the risk, and a limitation in total dosage of methotrexate has been recommended for patients receiving the drug by ventricular reservoir, which is now the standard method of treatment of meningeal malignancy in many centers. Patients who have increased methotrexate levels because of poor cerebrospinal fluid (CSF) dynamics were much more likely to develop acute toxicity. In one study the methotrexate levels ranged as high as 13 times those of patients without outlet obstruction or abnormalities of flow over the hemispheres [7].

The CT scan findings remain somewhat controversial. The scan usually demonstrates symmetric low density in the central white matter of the hemispheres. Enlargement of the ventricles or other signs of atrophy may develop (although these may also be due to steroid usage). In a study by Duffner and colleagues [15], hypodense white matter was found in 23 percent and calcification in 10 percent of 22 children at risk for encephalopathy.

Frequently the abnormality on CT scan is observed in patients who are completely asymptomatic [40]. Abnormalities of CT scan alone at this point in time do not appear to be an adequate reason to cease therapy if otherwise effective.

Insufficient experience has been gathered with the use of T2-weighted images on magnetic resonance imaging (MRI) [17] to indicate whether this technique, now standard in the assessment of patients with white matter disorders, will also be useful in this field.

The presence of leukoencephalopathy may also be detected by presence in the CSF of myelin basic protein, a constituent of normal white matter that is released into CSF after any type of white matter damage including cerebral infarction and multiple sclerosis. This test has not received widespread clinical acceptance, although values have been reported [21].

Transient Cerebral Dysfunction

The third and least common type of methotrexate encephalopathy may occur after high-dose intravenous use of the drug or rarely after intrathecal administration. Reports of its occurrence after high-dose usage have been more convincing [1,20,25,55]. In these instances patients have the sudden onset of a focal cerebral dysfunction, usually a hemiparesis, with or without aphasia or neglect syndrome. The clinical appearance is similar to that observed in patients with a large embolic stroke. Sometimes the hemiparesis has been accompanied by headache or by local seizures, suggesting a migrainous quality or element of vascular spasm.

The acute hemiplegic state has been seen most commonly after several courses of intrathecal methotrexate and usually 1 to 2 weeks after administration. One side may be involved and recover over several days, then the other side of the brain may be comparably affected.

In spite of its alarming appearance, acute hemiplegia in this setting has a better prognosis than does chronic confusional state, and most patients recover with little or no residual effects and in some instance have been successfully retreated without recurrence of the syndrome.

Mechanism of Damage

The primary chemotherapeutic effect of methotrexate is inhibition of dihydrofolate reductase. Reduced folic acid functions as a methyl group donor, and methyl groups are required for synthesis of purines and of thymidylate. Thymidylate synthesis ceases at about 10^{-8} M methotrexate concentration, while purine synthesis ceases at about 10^{-7} M concentration.

Both of these are well below concentrations of the drug achieved systemically in clinical circumstances [26]. The fact that leucovorin can reverse methotrexate-induced depression of regional cerebral metabolic rate in the rat is some evidence that the dihydrofolate reductase inhibition is significant. [41]. The reduced cerebral glucose metabolism and capillary permeability can also be observed in patients by the use of positron emission tomography (PET) scanning [42]. However, the active compounds in this metabolic sequence, folic acid, thymidylic acid, and adenine, all undergo active metabolism and transport in the brain, and local enzyme inhibition seems inherently unlikely to be the sole explanation.

Likewise, the pathologic alterations in methotrexate encephalopathy are to a degree nonspecific. Studies of the early changes following irradiation and intravenous methotrexate showed changes that lack specificity [33]. The changes in the blood vessels in the lesion closely resemble those changes seen in radiation encephalopathy in which there has been necrosis of tissue due to high-dosage local treatment [48]. The CT scan changes, which are frequently interpreted to indicate some long-lasting effect of the drug, in fact may be quite transient even when severe [57].

And finally, the changes seen in methotrexate encephalopathy are mimicked by those produced by cyclosporine, an immunosuppressive agent of antibiotic origin, when used for liver transplantation, particularly when serum cholesterol levels are low [12]. As will be discussed in subsequent paragraphs, other chemotherapeutic agents may cause encephalopathy that is clinically and histologically identical. These include the use of BCNU (a nitrosourea) and occasionally cisplatin and bleomycin. While far less frequent as a cause of difficulty than methotrexate, these agents do indicate that the condition is not necessarily a specific feature of that agent alone.

ENCEPHALOPATHY IN PATIENTS WITH BRAIN TUMOR OR FOLLOWING BLOOD-BRAIN BARRIER MODIFICATION

In ordinary clinical practice, dealing with systemic tumors, methotrexate is the only agent that is likely to cause widespread serious neurotoxicity. However, in specialized circumstances other agents may be neurotoxic. In the mid 1970s, intracarotid infusion of BCNU was introduced by several groups. The use of the technique has been limited by serious retinal toxicity and neurotoxicity, which has become apparent with further clinical trial. In a similar manner, very high-dose systemic cisplatin, used for advanced ovarian carcinoma, may cause both peripheral neuropathy and central nervous system toxicity. Experimental work employing modifications of the blood-brain barrier by mannitol or glycerol has demonstrated that many chemotherapeutic agents are highly neurotoxic once they enter the brain in sufficient concentration. These include methotrexate, nitrosoureas such as BCNU, and cisplatin, and the only agent appearing to be generally safe is cyclophosphamide.

In many instances the neuropathologic picture is not yet well defined but appears to be that of a widespread focal necrosis of brain. The mechanism by which BCNU could produce such a lesion is speculative. The mechanism of action of the nitrosoureas in general is not well defined. The agents have alkylating properties but also inhibit DNA repair. They are variably lipid soluble and pass through the blood-brain barrier to some extent. Schold [9,51] studied four patients who had developed multifocal areas of necrosis with fibrinoid change in blood vessels and calcification from high-dose BCNU treatment of systemic cancer. Supraophthalmic carotid artery infusion for glioma [10,19,28,29] has been followed by similar changes, demonstrable by CT or by neuropathologic study after death.

The changes seen in patients treated with high-dose cisplatin therapy (usually over 200 mg/m^2) have not been well studied as yet [39]. In several instances [14,18] the neurologic dysfunction has had a peculiar episodic quality, reminiscent of the stroke-like episodes seen rarely in patients treated with high-dose methotrexate. The nature of these disturbances remains unknown at this time. Recovery from such attacks certainly does not imply that long-term toxicity will not be observed.

Studies by Neuwelt and his group [37] indicate the widespread propensity of these agents for central nervous system toxicity.

CEREBELLAR DEGENERATION

The chemotherapeutic agent cytosine arabinoside in daily doses of 100 to 200 mg/m^2 has been used widely in the treatment of acute leukemia. The compound is an antimetabolite, which inhibits synthesis of pyrimidines. It has also been used extensively for intrathecal use, for control of meningeal leukemia.

Beginning in about 1979, doses 30 times the normal dose (called high-dose ARA-C, or HIDAC) have been introduced to induce remissions in malignant lymphoma. With this usage a specific cerebellar degeneration began to be observed [32,50,58]. In the study of Winkelman and Hines [58], 24 patients were treated with HIDAC at a dose of 3 gm/m^2 every 12 hours for 12 doses. Of the 24 patients, 4 developed cerebellar degeneration during treatment.

Classic cerebellar findings may appear. These include ataxia of gait, intention tremor of the hands, scanning speech, and nystagmus; the disorder of cerebellar function may be of any degree of severity. Milder patients seem to improve spontaneously after several weeks, while patients with more severe findings often have persistent deficit.

The specific lesions in the nervous system reported by Winkelman and Hines [58] include a striking loss of Purkinje cells, with little other damage to the nervous system.

With further experience with the drug, other syndromes have also been seen. These include ocular motor disturbances, confusion, and mild rigidity [16]. A patient has been reported who developed drug-induced parkinsonism following HIDAC [34].

The cerebellar toxicity is a well-recognized event and unfortunately appears to be a limitation on the usage of this drug in specific circumstances, particularly in adults.

The observations with HIDAC had been preceded by observations of comparable cerebellar toxicity with the drug 5-fluorouracil [45]. This agent was at one time commonly used in relatively high dose for colonic neoplasms and other solid tumors. The descriptions of the cerebellar toxicity are very reminiscent of those seen today with HIDAC, but the limited current usage of 5-fluorouracil prevents this from being seen frequently. Disorders of mentation, rigidity, and ophthalmoparesis have been observed in the past [4,31].

It may be significant that both of these agents interefere with pyrimidine synthesis within the body. Whether the cerebellum has a specific requirement or enzyme lack compared with other tissues is unknown.

PERIPHERAL NEUROPATHY

Patients with malignant disease are subject to peripheral neuropathy of many types. Nutritional neuropathy in those with advanced stage disease is probably the commonest form. Specific neoplastic neuropathy also occurs.

In this setting, the presence of a neuropathy due to toxic exposure to cancer therapeutic drugs is difficult to document. Two agents are, however, well-recognized as causes of symmetric mixed sensory motor neuropathy. These are vincristine, a vinca alkaloid, and cis-dichloraldiammine-platinum (cisplatin) [30]. In both instances, the neuropathy has the clinical and histologic characteristics of an axonal degeneration. It may be reversible if mild in degree.

Vincristine is one of several agents isolated from the periwinkle plant vinca. Other derivatives include vindesine and vinblastine, which do not commonly produce peripheral neuropathy, although it has been reported with vindesine. All vinca alkaloids cause mitotic arrest due to interaction with microtubules. Microtubules are likely also to participate in some processes of axonal transport, both peripherally and centrally. As the drugs are now used clinically, no central nervous system toxicity is observed, although the experience of Neuwelt and associates [37] indicates that severe central nervous system toxicity can be observed after breakdown of the blood-brain barrier in experimental animals.

Several efforts have been made to demonstrate experimentally that axonal transport is disturbed with vincristine. This requires special techniques, and the amount of reduction in axonal transport seems surprisingly small in view of the marked disturbance in function [22].

The mechanism of toxicity of cisplatin is not understood. The pathologic changes in the nervous system are those of a nonspecific axonal degeneration [11]. Likewise, the experimental version of the illness in experimental animals as well as in patients indicates electrophysiologic and morphologic findings of axonal degeneration [52]. Interestingly, a small peptide analogue of adrenocorticotropic hormone (ACTH) may be able to prevent development of cisplatin neuropathy [54].

The clinical aspects of neuropathy due to either cisplatin or vincristine are similar. Sensory symptoms predominate in the beginning, with tingling and numbness in the toes and feet. With more advanced disease, distal graded sensory loss is detectable. There may be some atrophy of small muscles of the feet, and when the sensory loss reaches above the ankles, then the fingers may also be affected [2,47]. Autonomic neuropathy is common.

A few scattered reports in the literature have suggested that unilateral facial palsy, diplopia, hoarseness, and other focal symptoms may be due to this agent, but such reports should be viewed with caution, since they are often observed in patients subject to malignant invasion of the leptomeninges.

Vincristine specifically may cause a marked aggravation of polyneuropathy in patients who already have peripheral nerve disease. This has been reported in hereditary motor neuropathy [24] and also in a patient who had the POEMS (polyneuropathy, organomegaly, endocrinopathy, M protein, and skin changes) [53].

The electrophysiologic assessment of axonal neuropathy does not differ in any significant way from the findings in other axonal neuropathies. Motor nerve conduction velocity is usually normal, and size of motor action potential is usually preserved except in the presence of severe disease. Distal motor latency may be prolonged. Distal sensory latencies are prolonged, and eventually the distal sensory action potentials become unrecordable [36,46,52].

REFERENCES

1. Allen, J. C., and Rosen, G. Transient cerebral dysfunction following chemotherapy for osteogenic sarcoma. *Ann. Neurol.* 3:441, 1978.
2. Bagley, C. M., Rudolph, R. H., Rivkin, S. E., et al. High dose cisplatin therapy for cancers of the ovary: Neurotoxicity. *Ann. Intern. Med.* 102:719, 1985.
3. Balis, F. M., and Poplack, D. G. Central nervous system pharmacology of anti leukemia drugs. *Am. J. Clin. Oncol.* 11:74, 1988.
4. Berman, I. J., and Mann M. P. Seizures and transient cortical blindness associated with cisplatinum (11) diamminedichloride (PDD) therapy in a thirty-year-old man. *Cancer* 45:764, 1980.
5. Bleyer, W. A. Methotrexate: Clinical pharmacology, current status, and therapeutic guidelines. *Cancer Treat. Rep.* 4:87, 1977.
6. Bleyer, W. A. Neurologic sequelae of methotrexate and ionizing radiation: A new classification. *Cancer Treat. Rep.* 65:89, 1981.
7. Bleyer, W. A., Drake, J. C., and Chabner, B. A. Neurotoxicity and elevated cerebrospinal fluid methotrexate concentration in meningeal leukemia. *N. Engl. J. Med.* 289:770, 1973.
8. Bleyer, W. A., and Griffin, T. W. White Matter Necrosis, Mineralizing Microangiopathy and Intellectual Abilities in Survivors of Childhood Leukemia: Associations with Central Nervous System Irradiation and Methotrexate Therapy. In H. A. Gilbert and A. R. Kagan (eds.), *Radiation Damage to the Nervous System.* New York: Raven, 1980. Pp. 155–174.
9. Burger, P. C., Kamenar, E., Schold, S. C., et al. Encephalomyelopathy following high dose BCNU therapy. *Cancer* 48:1318, 1981.
10. Casin, T. L. Intra-arterial BCNU in the treatment of metastatic brain tumors. *J. Neurooncol.* 1:211, 1981.
11. Clark, A. W., Parhad, I. M., Griffin, J. W., and Price, D. L. Neurotoxicity of cis-platinum: Pathology of the central and peripheral nervous systems. *Neurology* 30:429, 1980.
12. DeGroen, P. C., Aksamit, A. J., Rakela, J., et al. Central nervous system toxicity after liver transplantation: The role of cyclosporine and cholesterol. *N. Engl. J. Med.* 317:861, 1987.
13. Delattre, J. Y., and Posner, J. B. Neurological Complications of Chemotherapy and Radiation Therapy. In M. J. Aminoff *Neurology and General Medicine.* Philadelphia: Saunders, 1989. Pp. 365–88.
14. Doll, D. C., List, A. F., Greco, F. A., et al. Acute vascular ischemic events after cis-platin based combination chemotherapy for osteogenic sarcoma. *Ann. Intern. Med.* 105:48, 1986.
15. Duffner, P. K., Cohen, M. E., Brecher, M., et al. CT abnormalities and altered methotrexate clearance in children with CNS leukemia. *Neurology* 34:229, 1984.
16. Dwoskin, L. A., Goldman, R. D., Zivin, L. S., and Fuchs, P. C. Cerebellar toxicity following high dose cytosine arabinoside. *J. Clin. Oncol.* 3:613, 1985.
17. Ebner, F., Ranner, C., Slavc, I., et al. MR findings in methotrexate induced CNS abnormalities. *A.J.N.R.* 10:959, 1989.
18. Feldmann, E., and Posner, J. B. Episodic neurologic dysfunction in patients with Hodgkin's disease. *Arch. Neurol.* 43:1227, 1986.
19. Foo, S.-H., Choi, I. S., Bernstein, A., et al. Supraophthalmic intracarotid infusion of BCNU for malignant glioma. *Neurology* 36:1437, 1986.
20. Fritsch, G., and Urban, C. Transient encephalopathy during the late course of treatment with high-dose methotrexate. *Cancer* 53:1849, 1984.
21. Gangji, D., Reaman, G. H., and Cohen, S. R. Leukoencephalopathy and elevated levels of myelin basic protein in the cerebrospinal fluid of patients with acute lymphoblasic leukemia. *N. Engl. J. Med.* 303:19, 1980.

22. Green, L. S., Donos, J. A., Heller-Bettinger, I. E., et al. Axonal transport disturbances in vincristine-induced peripheral neuropathy. *Ann. Neurol.* 1:255, 1977.
23. Hadley, D., and Herr, H. W. Peripheral neuropathy associated with cis-dichlorodiammine-platinum treatment. *Cancer* 44:2026, 1979.
24. Hogan-Dann, C. M., Fellemeth, W. C., McGuire, S. A., and Kiley, Y. A. Polyneuropathy following vincristine therapy in two patients with Charcot-Marie-Tooth syndrome. *J.A.M.A.* 252: 2862, 1984.
25. Jaffe, N., Takaue, Y., Anzai, T., et al. Transient neurological disturbances induced by high-dose methotrexate treatment. *Cancer* 56:1356, 1985.
26. Jolivet, J., Cowan, K. H., Curt, G. A., and Chabner, B. A. The pharmacology and clinical use of methotrexate. *N. Engl. J. Med.* 309:1094, 1983.
27. Kaplan, S. K., and Wiernick, P. H. Neurotoxicity of antineoplastic drugs. *Semin. Oncol.* 9:103, 1982.
28. Kapp, J. P., and Sandord, R. A. Neurological deficit after carotid infusion of cisplatin and 1,3-bis(2-chloroethyl)-1-nitrosourea (BCNU) for malignant glioma: An analysis of risk factors. *Neurosurgery* 19:779, 1986.
29. Kapp, J. P., and Vance, R. B. Supraophthalmic carotid artery infusion for recurrent glioma: Rationale, technique, and preliminary results for cisplatin and BCNU. *J. Neurooncol.* 3:5, 1985.
30. Kedar, A., Cohen, M. E., and Freeman, A. I. Peripheral neuropathy as a complication of cis-dichlorodiammineplatinum (II) treatment: A case report. *Cancer Treat. Rep.* 62:819, 1978.
31. Koenig, H., and Patel, A. Biochemical basis for fluorouracil neurotoxicity. *Arch. Neurol.* 23:155, 1970.
32. Lazarus, H. M., Herzig, R. H., Herzig, G. P., et al. CNS toxicity of high-dose systemic cytosine arabinoside. *Cancer* 48:2577, 1981.
33. Ludwig, R., Calvo, W., Kober, B., and Brandeis, W. E. Effects of local irradiation and I.V. methotrexate on brain morphology in rabbits: Early changes. *J. Cancer Res. Clin. Oncol.* 113:235, 1987.
34. Lugue, F. A., Sclhorst, J. B., and Petruska, P. Parkinsonism induced by high-dose cytosine arabinoside. *Movement Disorders* 2:219, 1987.
35. Lynch, H. T., Droszcz, C. P., Albano, W. A., and Lynch, J. F. Organic brain syndrome: Secondary to 5-fluorouracil toxicity. *Dis. Colon Rectum* 24:130, 1981.
36. McLeod, J. G., and Penny, R. Vincristine neuropathy: An electrophysiological and histochemical study. *J. Neurol. Neurosurg. Psychiatry* 32:297, 1969.
37. Neuwelt, E. A., Glasberg, M., Frenkel, E., and Barnett, P. Neurotoxicity of chemotherapeutic agents after blood brain barrier modification: Neuropathological studies. *Ann. Neurol.* 14:316, 1983.
38. Ochs, J. J. Neurotoxicity due to central nervous system therapy for childhood leukemia. *Am. J. Pediatr. Hematol.* 11:93, 1989.
39. Parici, P. B., Greggi, S., Scanbia, G., et al. High dose (200 mg/M^2) cisplatin induced neurotoxicity in primary advanced ovarian cancer patients. *Cancer Treat. Rep.* 71:669, 1987.
40. Peylan-Ramu, N., Poplack, D. G., Pizo, P. A., et al. Abnormal CT scans of the brain in asymptomatic children with acute lymphocytic leukemia after prophylactic treatment of the CNS with radiation and intrathecal chemotherapy. *N. Engl. J. Med.* 298:815, 1978.
41. Phillips, P. C., Berger, C. A., Arnold, J. B., et al. High dose leukovorin reverses high-dose methotrexate-induced depression of regional cerebral metabolic rate for glucose in the rat. *Ann. Neurol.* 18:404, 1985.
42. Phillips, P. C., Dhawan, V., Strpother, S. C., et al. Reduced cerebral glucose metabolism and capillary permeability following methotrexate chemotherapy: A positron emission tomographic study. *Ann. Neurol.* 21:59, 1987.
43. Price, R. A., and Birdwell, D. A. The central nervous system in childhood leukemia: III. Mineralizing microangiopathy and dystrophic calcification. *Cancer* 42:717, 1978.
44. Price, R. A., and Jamieson, P. A. The central nervous system in childhood leukemia: II. Subacute leukoencephalopathy. *Cancer* 35:306, 1975.
45. Riehl, J. L, and Brown, W. J. Acute cerebellar syndrome secondary to 5-FU therapy. *Neurology (Minneap.)* 14:961, 1964.
46. Roeofs, R. I., Hrushesky, W., Rogin, J., and Rosenberg, L. Peripheral sensory neuropathy and cisplatin chemotherapy. *Neurology* 34:934, 1984.
47. Rosenthal, S. A., and Kaufman, S. Vincristine neurotoxicity. *Ann. Intern. Med.* 180:733, 1974.
48. Rottenberg, D. A., Chernik, N. L., Deck, M. D. F., et al. Cerebral necrosis following radiotherapy of extracranial neoplasms. *Ann. Neurol.* 1:339, 1977.
49. Rubinstein, L. J., Herman, M. M., Long, T. F., et al: Disseminated necrotizing leukoencephalopathy: A complication of treated central nervous system leukemia and lymphoma. *Cancer* 35:291, 1975.
50. Salinsky, M. C., Levine, R. L., Aubuchon, J. P., and Schutta, H. S. Acute cerebellar dysfunction with high-dose Ara-C therapy. *Cancer* 51:426, 1983.
51. Schold, S. C. Central nervous system toxicity from high-dose BCNU treatment of systemic cancer. *Neurology* 30:429, 1980.
52. Thompson, S. W., Davis, L. E., Kornfeld, M., et al. Cisplatin neuropathy, clinical electrophysiologic, morphologic and toxicologic studies. *Cancer* 54:1269, 1984.

53. Treves, R., Archambeaud-Moveroux, R., Tabaraud, F., et al. Aggravation brutale d'une neuropathic d'un POEMS syndrome aprés traitement a la vincristine. *Therapic* 42:63, 1987.
54. Van der Hoop, R. G., Vecht, C. J., Van der Burg, M. E. L., et al. Prevention of cisplatin neuropathy with an ACTH (4-9) analogue in patients with ovarian cancer. *N. Engl. J. Med.* 322:89, 1990.
55. Walker, R. W., Allen, J. C., Rosen, G., and Capairos, B. Transient cerebral dysfunction secondary to high-dose methotrexate. *J. Clin. Oncol.* 4:1845, 1986.
56. Weiss, H. D., Walker, M. E., and Wiernik, P. H. Neurotoxicity of commonly used antineoplastic agents. *N. Engl. J. Med.* 291:75, 1974.
57. Wendling, L. R., Bleyer, W. A., Dichiro, C. T., and McIlvanie, S. K. Transient severe periventricular hypodensity after leukemia prophylaxis with cranial irradiation and intrathecal methotrexate. *J. Comput. Assist. Tomogr.* 2:502, 1978.
58. Winkelman, M. D., and Hines, J. D. Cerebellar degeneration caused by high-dose cytosine arabinoside: A clinicopathologic study. *Ann. Neurol.* 14:520, 1983.

23 Central Nervous System Manifestations of Toxic Disorders

Neal L. Benowitz

Drugs and toxins represent a frequent cause of disordered central nervous system function. The clinical presentation may vary considerably, with a spectrum from altered personality or acute psychiatric disease to dementia or coma. This chapter will review the pathophysiology, clinical features, and management of the more common toxic disorders of the central nervous system.

CLINICAL SPECTRUM OF TOXIC DISORDERS

Intoxication with drugs commonly results in altered central nervous system functioning, either by direct action of the drug on the brain or via secondary systemic effects such as hypoxia, profound shock, or metabolic disturbances. Drug actions on the brain can be broadly categorized as stimulant or depressant. Stimulant drugs such as amphetamines or cocaine typically result in agitation, restlessness, muscular hyperactivity, seizures, sympathetic nervous hyperactivity, and hyperthermia. A similar clinical picture can result from withdrawal from habitual use of alcohol or sedative drugs.

Depressant drugs such as sedatives or narcotics typically result in ataxia and drowsiness, progressing to coma with respiratory depression and hypothermia. There is, however, considerable overlap, so that a stimulant abuser may present with depressed consciousness because he is postictal or has suffered brain injury due to vascular or infectious complications of drug abuse, while agitation, muscular hyperactivity, or toxic psychosis can be early manifestations of some types of depressant drug intoxication.

Specific syndromes of altered central nervous system function are presented along with drugs or toxins that induce these syndromes in Tables 23-1 through 23-4. Some of these disorders will be discussed in more detail later as individual drugs are discussed. It should be emphasized

Table 23-1. Drugs inducing agitation, psychosis, or delirium

Drug
Amantadine (A,D)
Amphetamines (A,P)
Anticholinergics (D,H)
Antihistamines (D,H)
Caffeine (P)
Cimetidine (H,P)
Cocaine (A,P)
Digitalis (D,P)
Disulfiram (D,P)
Ethanol and sedative drug withdrawal (A,H,P)
L-Dopa (D)
Lidocaine (A,D)
Lithium (D)
LSD (H,P)
Marijuana (H)
Phencyclidine (A,H)
Phenylpropanolamine (A,P,D)
Procaine (A,P)
Salicylates (A,D)
Theophylline (A)

Predominant manifestations: A = agitation; D = delirium; H = hallucinations; P = psychosis.
Source: Modified from Olson, Pentel, and Kelley [59].

Table 23-3. Drugs and chemicals commonly inducing seizures

Drug or chemical
Amoxapine
Amphetamines
Camphor
Carbon monoxide
Chlorinated hydrocarbon solvents
Cocaine
Cyanide
Dextropropoxyphene
Ethanol and sedative-hypnotic drug withdrawal
Fluoride (hypocalcemia)
Insulin
Isoniazid
Lead
Lidocaine
Lithium
Meperidine
Metaldehyde
Nicotine
Penicillins
Phenothiazines
Phenyclidine
Phenylpropanolamine
Salicylates
Strychnine*
Theophylline
Tricyclic antidepressants

* Rigidity and opisthotonos; not true seizures.
Source: Modified from Olson, Pentel, and Kelley [59].

Table 23-2. Drugs inducing a dementia-like picture

Drug
Alcohol
Anticholinergic drugs
Antihistamines
Antihypertensives
Antipsychotic drugs
Aspirin
Cimetidine
Corticosteroids
L-Dopa
Digitalis
Lithium
Narcotics
Phenytoin
Sedative-hypnotics

that drug toxicity must be considered in evaluating dementia in the elderly. There are many examples where dementia in the elderly has resulted from therapeutic use of psychotropic drugs or from unrecognized intoxication with drugs, such as aspirin. In elderly individuals, the glomerular filtration rate may be considerably below normal in individuals with a normal serum creatinine [13,62]. Thus, if drugs such as digitalis preparations and nephrotoxic antibiotics are normally excreted by the kidney, a therapeutic dose in the elderly may result in toxic blood levels. All drugs with potential effects on cognitive function should be discontinued in evaluating patients with dementia.

Table 23-4. Drugs inducing disturbance in temperature regulation

Hypothermia	*Hyperthermia*
Antipsychotic drugs	Amoxapine
Ethanol and other alcohols	Amphetamines
Sedative-hypnotic drugs	Anticholinergic drugs
Hypoglycemia	Antihistamines
Opiates	Antipsychotic agents
Tricyclic antidepressants	Cocaine
	Ethanol or sedative-hypnotic withdrawal
	Lithium
	LSD
	Monoamine oxidase inhibitors (MAOIs)
	Phencyclidine
	Salicylates
	Thyroid hormone
	Tricyclic antidepressants

Source: Modified from Olson, Pentel, and Kelley [59].

DRUG-INDUCED METABOLIC ENCEPHALOPATHY

Many drug intoxications produce a diffuse disorder of cerebral metabolism, resulting in a metabolic encephalopathy. Most drugs with sedative properties depress neuronal activity of the reticular activating system, thereby depressing cortical arousal and consciousness. Clinical features of metabolic encephalopathy are summarized in Table 23-5. Neurologic findings in drug-induced coma include reduced or absent motor activity, loss of oculocephalic and oculovestibular reflexes, and respiratory depression, a result of depressed brain stem function [69]. Pupillary reactivity is often maintained, even when all other brain stem functions are lost. An exception is intoxication with certain drugs, such as the tricyclic antidepressants or glutethimide, that have anticholinergic activity and may be associated with sluggishly reactive or unreactive pupils. A glutethimide-intoxicated comatose patient may be mistakenly diagnosed as being brain dead, even though the condition is generally reversible [5]. It is helpful to remember that fully dilated pupils are evidence of preserved sympathetic outflow and are not compatible with the diagnosis of brain death. In the brain dead patient, the pupils are not dilated but rather are fixed and midposition [81].

The differential diagnosis of drug-induced coma includes (1) mass lesions of the cerebral hemispheres causing herniation and brain stem compression (supratentorial lesions); (2) lesions of the posterior fossa that either directly destroy or compress the brain stem (infratentorial lesions); (3) seizures (including the postictal state); (4) infection (meningitis); (5) metabolic encephalopathy due to hypoglycemia or hypothermia or with brain edema due to hypoxia or hyponatremia (which can also occur in an individual who has also taken drugs that induce coma, such as barbiturates or narcotics). Key elements of the neurologic examination in the evaluation of coma are summarized in Table 23-6. Findings of asymmetric motor weakness or reflexes (or the Brudzinski's

Table 23-5. Clinical features of metabolic encephalopathy

Symmetric signs
Slow and/or incoherent thinking; impaired recent memory
Inattention
Irritability, excitability
Drowsiness
Disorientation
Delirium (toxic psychosis)
Akinetic state
Myoclonus, seizures
Coma

Table 23-6. Neurologic examination in coma

Level of consciousness
Eye opening
Verbal responses
Symmetry and character of motor responses to noxious stimulation
Neuro-ophthalmologic function
Pupillary size and response to light
Spontaneous eye movements
Oculocephalic reflex (doll's eyes)
Oculovestibular reflexes (ice-water calorics)
Vegetative function
Blood pressure
Respiratory pattern

sign), evidence of head trauma, fever or meningismus, or neurologic findings unusual for metabolic encephalopathy (such as loss of pupillary reactivity to light with persistence of oculomotor reflexes) should prompt a more detailed evaluation, including a computed tomography (CT) scan of the head and, if appropriate, lumbar puncture. It must be emphasized that drug intoxication not infrequently exists concurrently with head trauma, cerebrovascular accident, or meningitis, so a high degree of suspicion must be maintained.

DRUG-INDUCED SEIZURES AND HYPERTHERMIA

As noted in Table 23-3, many drug intoxications as well as withdrawal syndromes result in generalized convulsions [1,51]. The drugs most frequently causing seizures in poisoned patients are cylcic antidepressants, theophylline, cocaine, and isoniazid, whereas the most common drugs causing seizures during treatment in the hospital are penicillin (usually in patients with renal insufficiency), insulin, and lidocaine. Seizures from many drug intoxications and from alcohol withdrawal tend to be brief and self-limited, but others such as associated with theophylline or cyclic antidepressant poisoning may be protracted.

Status epilepticus that is sustained for more than an hour, particularly if associated with hyperthermia or hypotension, may produce permanent brain injury. Control of ventilation, oxygenation, temperature, and hemodynamic status are crucial in minimizing the likelihood of brain surgery, but neuronal injury has been observed (experimentally in baboons with drug-induced status epilepticus), even when systemic effects of seizures were eliminated by muscular paralysis and assisted ventilation [50]. Seizures of shorter duration do not appear to cause brain damage, and hypoxia does not appear to be present during and after the typical grand mal seizure [60].

Seizures increase the metabolic activity of the brain several-fold. Normally, seizures are associated with cerebral vasodilation and blood pressure elevation so that cerebral blood flow increases to match the increased metabolic demands of the brain. Cerebral metabolic activity and the cerebral blood flow needed to meet that metabolic activity increase further in the presence of fever. Hypotension, which is a common feature of drug intoxications, impairs the body's ability to increase cerebral blood flow. Thus the combination of seizures with hyperthermia or hypotension produces a situation where the metabolic demands of the brain exceed the supply, resulting in an extremely high risk for brain injury.

Hyperthermia may develop as a result of heat generated by increased muscular activity (due to seizures, myoclonus, or muscular rigidity), by a hypermetabolic state (such as with aspirin or dinitrophenol poisoning), impaired heat dissipation, or impaired sweating (as with anticholinergic drugs). Sustained hyperthermia (temperatures greater than 40.5°C) due to drug intoxication is associated with an extremely high morbidity and mortality due to brain injury and multiple organ damage [74]. Rapid control of seizures and hyperthermia and support of blood pressure are therefore critical elements in protecting the brain in drug-intoxicated patients.

GENERAL MANAGEMENT OF DRUG-INTOXICATED PATIENTS

A detailed discussion of decontamination and cardiopulmonary support in drug-intoxicated patients is beyond the scope of this chapter. The principles of emergency treatment of comatose patients are summarized in Table 23-7. Specific emergency medical therapies include glucose, thiamine, and naloxone. Glucose is administered to prevent hypoglycemic brain damage. Following the initial dose, the need for subsequent doses of glucose is judged by the clinical response to the first dose and by blood glucose measurements. Thiamine is administered because in chronic alcoholics or other malnourished patients, glucose administration may precipitate acute Wernicke's encephalopathy. Naloxone is routinely recommended, at least in urban hospitals, because narcotic abuse is common. Naloxone will reverse depressant effects of narcotics but may also precipitate acute nar-

Table 23-7. Emergency treatment of comatose patients

1. Protect/establish airway—assure oxygenation.
2. Intravenous access—maintain circulation.
3. Blood samples for measurement of glucose, electrolytes, calcium, liver and kidney function, arterial blood gases.
4. Intravenous glucose (25 gm).
5. Control seizures (diazepam, phenobarbital, phenytoin).
6. Thiamine, 100 mg IV.
7. Naloxone, 0.4–0.8 mg IV.
8. Restore acid-base and electrolyte balance.
9. If suspected head trauma or mass lesion—CT scan.
10. If suspected infection—lumbar puncture; antibiotic.
11. If suspected drug ingestion—lavage and charcoal.
12. Toxicology (blood, urine, gastric aspirate).

cotic withdrawal symptoms. The use of naloxone is discussed in more detail in the section on opiates. For some drug overdoses, specific antidotes or methods to accelerate drug removal may be useful. These are discussed in later sections.

DRUG INTOXICATION AND DETERMINATION OF BRAIN DEATH

The diagnosis of brain death is important in making decisions about termination of life support and in obtaining organs for transplantation. Several sets of criteria for brain death have been proposed [33,72]. All require that brain functions have ceased and that cessation of those functions is irreversible. In addition, the potential contribution of depressant drugs or other metabolic factors (i.e., hypothermia) must be excluded. Severe drug intoxications may result in cessation of neurologic function, producing an isoelectric electroencephalogram (EEG). In one series of sedative-hypnotic–intoxicated patients, 11 of 15 patients with a flat-line or isoelectric EEG subsequently had full recovery [74]. If there is any possibility that drug intoxication is contributing to depressed neurologic function, toxicologic screening for sedative drugs is required. If such intoxicants are found, confirmation of brain death by showing an absence of circulation to the brain (such as by cerebral arteriography or cerebral isotope angiography) is required.

ALCOHOL

Mechanisms and Site of Action

Recent research suggests a specific effect of ethanol on the excitatory (glutamate) receptor system [16,19]. Ethanol also acts on neuronal membrane lipids, resulting in "fluidization" of membranes. Ethanol, presumably by effects on the local lipid environment, affects some particular proteins that comprise receptors or enzyme systems at lower concentrations than others. Ethanol influences the responsiveness of the gamma-aminobutyric acid–benzodiazepine–barbiturate and delta-opiate receptor systems to their agonists. Ethanol inhibits monoamine oxidase B, sodium-potassium adenosine triphosphatase (ATPase) and adenyl cyclase.

Particular neural pathways seem to be essential for the reinforcing and neurologic effects of ethanol [42]. Noradrenergic, dopaminergic, endogenous opioid, and serotonergic systems have been implicated in mediating the pleasurable effects of ethanol. Of recent interest is evidence that serotonin uptake blockers such as fluoxetine may reduce ethanol intake and promote abstinence in alcoholics [56]. A role of purinergic mechanisms has been suggested by genetic studies that show a concordance between genetic differences in sedative- and ataxia-producing effects of ethanol and adenosine [35].

Tolerance develops rapidly to effects of ethanol. Mechanisms of tolerance include a theoretic "stiffening" of membranes, so that ethanol results in less fluidization. Chronic ethanol use may increase the number of excitatory postsynaptic receptors. While there is some neuropharmacologic and physical-chemical evidence to support these hypotheses, studies showing selective tolerance to some but not other effects of ethanol, and environmental influences on tolerance development, suggest that specific neural pathways are involved. That noradrenergic and serotonergic pathways are involved is suggested by findings that destroying or blocking these pathways inhibits the development of tolerance in rodents [42]. That vasopressin systems are involved is suggested by findings in rats that vasopressin administration can maintain ethanol tolerance even in the absence of further ethanol treatment and that animals lacking endogenous vasopressin systems do not become tolerant to ethanol [68]. In vitro studies of cultured neuronal cells suggest that changes in responsiveness to adenosine accompany the development of tolerance.

Physical dependence refers to the development of signs and symptoms that develop in the absence of the drug, under the influence of which the organism had previously been functioning normally. Homeostatic changes in numbers of receptors, membrane structure, and sensitivity of neural pathways that accompany the development of tolerance are thought to explain the development of abstinence syndromes.

However, at least in some systems, the development of tolerance can be blocked without affecting the development of an abstinence syndrome after ethanol withdrawal. Ethanol withdrawal is associated with a marked increase in noradrenergic activity, and adrenergic neural or receptor antagonists have been used to treat alcohol withdrawal in people.

Table 23-8. Blood concentrations of ethanol and clinical effects

Blood ethanol concentrations (mg/dl)	*Clinical effects*
30–100	Mild euphoria, talkativeness Decreased inhibitions Impaired attention, judgment Mild incoordination, nystagmus
100–200	Emotional instability (excitement; withdrawal) Impaired memory, impaired reaction time Loss of critical judgment Conjunctival hyperemia Ataxia, nystagmus, dysarthria Hypalgesia
200–300	Confusion, disorientation, dizziness Disturbed perception and sensation Diplopia, dilated pupils Marked ataxia, dysarthria
300–400	Apathy, stupor Decreased response to stimuli Vomiting; incontinence Inability to stand or walk
Over 400	Unconsciousness, coma Anesthesia Decreased or abolished reflexs Hypothermia Hypoventilation Hypotension Death (respiratory arrest)

Acute Intoxication

While specific neurotransmitter pathways may be involved in particular actions of ethanol, such as euphoria, the dose-dependent progression of intoxication may be viewed as a spectrum of neural depression, similar to that observed for anesthetics. At lower concentrations, inhibitory polysynaptic influences are inhibited, resulting in cortical disinhibition with the associated changes in mood and cognitive function (Table 23-8). At greater levels of intoxication, depression of excitatory presynaptic influences, potentiation of presynaptic inhibition, and/or direct depression of impulse propagation result in cerebellar dysfunction, delirium, or coma. Death may ensue from respiratory depression.

In general, blood alcohol concentrations correlate with the degree of intoxication (Table 23-8). There is a good general relationship between the quantity of ethanol ingested and the blood level [15], but other factors, such as the sex of the individual, also influence this relationship. For any given amount of ethanol ingested, blood levels will tend to be higher in women than in men [27]. There is in general a good correlation between blood levels of ethanol and brain levels [15].

The relationship between blood alcohol concentration and the degree of intoxication is influenced by the degree of tolerance that had been present and the rate of rise and duration of exposure to alcohol in the blood and brain. Thus a chronic alcoholic may function normally at a blood alcohol concentration of 350 mg/dl, whereas a nonalcoholic may be stuporous with the same blood level. Tolerance develops rapidly to effects of ethanol, even within the time course of a single drinking episode. Signs of intoxication diminish over hours in the face of unchanged blood alcohol concentrations. Ethanol may be lethal at concentrations of 450 to 500 mg/dl; however, the lethal concentration is variable due to different degrees of tolerance. Death has occurred at concentrations as low as 400 mg/dl, while survival has been observed at 700 mg/dl [55]. When coma is present at a blood alcohol concentration of less than 300 mg/dl, alternative causes of coma should be sought.

Hypoglycemia may contribute to alcohol-induced coma. Since alcohol blocks gluconeogenesis, the combination of alcohol consumption (even at moderate levels) plus fasting may lead to hypoglycemia and loss of consciousness. Children and people with chronic liver disease are particularly susceptible to alcohol-induced hypoglycemia.

The treatment of an alcohol-intoxicated patient is primarily supportive, with specific attention placed on maintaining a patent airway, assisting ventilation if necessary, correcting fluid and electrolyte disturbances, particularly hypokalemia and hypomagnesemia, and treatment of hypoglycemia. Intravenous fructose can increase the rate of ethanol metabolism by about 25 percent; however, since patients do quite well with supportive care and fructose is potentially toxic, such treatment is not recommended. The elimination of ethanol can also be accelerated by hemodialysis or peritoneal dialysis; however, this is rarely necessary.

Table 23-9. Clinical features of alcohol withdrawal

Minor (early withdrawal)	*Major (late withdrawal)*
Tremulousness	Delirium tremors
Coarse action tremor	Extreme agitation
Irritability, restlessness	Appears frightened, confused
Anxiety, agitation	Hallucinations
Insomnia	Disorientation
Anorexia, vomiting	Disordered sensory perception
Diaphoresis	Marked autonomic hyperactivity
Tachycardia	Dilated pupils
Mild hypertension	Tachycardia
Hallucinosis	Hypertension
Visual most common	Fever
Patient remains oriented	
Seizures	
Grand mal	
Multiple seizures common	

Alcohol Withdrawal

The severity of alcohol withdrawal symptoms is related to the level and the duration of prior alcohol consumption. Alcohol withdrawal symptoms not only occur after abrupt cessation of use, but also may be seen with reduction in the daily level of intake of alcohol.

The clinical manifestations of alcohol withdrawal are shown in Table 23-9. Minor or early symptoms are typically observed for up to 48 hours after cessation of alcohol consumption, with the peak intensity observed at 24 hours. Minor withdrawal typically presents with one or more of three syndromes: tremulousness, hallucinations, and seizures. Major or late withdrawal typically occurs from 1 to 6 days after the cessation of drinking and is characterized by agitation, hypertension, tachycardia, and hyperthermia. When disorientation and confusion are present, the syndrome is referred to as delirium tremens. The syndrome carries a significant morbidity and mortality owing primarily to concurrent infection, pancreatitis, trauma, or heart disease. Cardiac arrhythmias are common and may be the cause of sudden death.

Seizures generally occur from 6 to 48 hours after the cessation of drinking, with a peak occurrence from 13 to 24 hours. Of note is that seizures and other manifestations of alcohol withdrawal can be delayed in onset by the administration of sedative-hypnotic or anesthetic drugs, such as is often the case when alcoholics are admitted to the hospital for trauma or elective surgery. Usually, seizures are self-limited, but occasionally status epilepticus develops. One recent study suggests that seizures occur more commonly while drinking and that the probability of seizures is in proportion to the level of alcohol consumption and not to abstinence [58]. These authors suggest a direct effect of ethanol on the brain to cause seizures, although this is still controversial.

Management of alcohol withdrawal consists of supportive care and specific pharmacotherapy. Supportive care includes glucose, hydration, correction of electrolyte abnormalities, nutrition, and reassurance. Thiamine is routinely given to prevent the development of Wernicke's encephalopathy. For mild alcohol withdrawal, supportive care may be sufficient. For more severe withdrawal, pharmacotherapy is indicated.

Pharmacotherapy is designed to replace alcohol with a sedative drug, which can then be tapered in a controlled manner. A number of sedative drugs have been evaluated [79]. Benzodiazepines are the drugs of choice because they are as effective and less toxic than are the alternatives—phenothiazines, barbiturates, or paraldehyde. All benzodiazepines appear to be effective. A logical approach is to load a patient with a long-acting benzodiazepine such as diazepam or chlordiazepoxide until sedation is achieved, then to taper at 25 to 50 percent per day. Due to long half-lives of these drugs and their metabolites, the levels of drug in the body will decline gradually (even in the absence of tapering) to provide a gradual withdrawal with relatively few abstinence symptoms over many days.

A typical drug regimen is diazepam, 20 mg IV or PO, or chlordiazepoxide, 100 mg PO every hour until the patient is mildly sedated. Commonly, 40 to 80 mg of diazepam or equivalent doses of chlordiazepoxide are required. In some cases enormous doses (1000 mg or more of IV diazepam) may be required for sedation [85]. Following initial loading, no more diazepam may be needed to maintain sedation, as diazepam levels decline with a half-life of 40 to 50 hours or longer in patients with cirrhosis.

Alcohol-induced hallucinations may be better controlled with haloperidol, 0.5 to 2.0 mg IM every 2 hours, although benzodiazepines should also be administered to provide some anticonvulsant protection [40]. Seizures usually respond to diazepam. It has been common to follow this by a loading dose of phenytoin; however, a recent placebo-controlled trial found no benefit of phenytoin treatment after an alcohol withdrawal seizure on the risk of a later, recurrent seizure [2]. In alcoholics with their first seizure or presenting with focal seizures, a work-up for structural lesions should be performed. Seizures in alcoholics do not usually indicate epilepsy and do not require prolonged anticonvulsion therapy.

Beta blockers have been evaluated to reduce adrenergic manifestations of alcohol withdrawal, such as hypertension, tachycardia, and tremors. A recent study indicates that atenolol reduces alcohol withdrawal symptoms and slightly shortens hospital stay for patients with mild withdrawal [43]. However, beta blockers are potentially toxic; they may aggravate asthma or chronic lung disease or precipitate hypotension or cardiac failure, particularly in patients with more severe withdrawal. On balance, the modest benefits seem to be outweighed by the considerable and potentially life-threatening risks, so the routine use of beta blockers for treatment of alcohol withdrawal is not encouraged.

Central Nervous System Complications of Chronic Alcoholism

Chronic alcohol abuse may result in central nervous system dysfunction in association with nutritional deficiencies or direct alcohol-induced injury to the brain. These disorders include Wernicke-Korsakoff syndrome, alcoholic cerebellar degeneration, cerebral cortical atrophy, and other rarer disorders.

Wernicke-Korsakoff Syndrome

Wernicke-Korsakoff syndrome is caused by thiamine deficiency; its clinical features are described in Table 23-10. Wernicke's encephalopathy often has an abrupt onset, beginning with ataxia and progressing over days to weeks to confusion with ocular abnormalities such as nystagmus and ophthalmoplegia. Korsakoff's psychosis refers to the mental state in which short-term memory is disrupted out of proportion to changes in other cognitive functions. Korsakoff's psychosis is usually seen in association with Wernicke's encephalopathy, although

Table 23-10. Clinical features of Wernicke-Korsakoff syndrome

Ophthalmoplegia*
Horizontal and vertical nystagmus
Weakness or paralysis of extraocular muscles
Weakness or paralysis of conjugate gaze
Ataxia*
Disturbed mentation*
Confusional state (apathy, inattentiveness)
Drowsiness (stupor or coma may rarely develop if untreated)
Amnesic state (Korsakoff's psychosis)
Severely impaired short-term memory
Variable disturbance of remote memory
Confabulation
Peripheral neuropathy
Postural hypotension
Loss of odor discrimination

* Classic features of Wernicke's encephalopathy.

it can also be associated with other neurologic disorders.

Diagnostic studies include the measurement of blood transketolase, the activity of which is reduced in the presence of thiamine deficiency. The activity of the enzyme is augmented in vitro by adding thiamine pyrophosphate, which is a cofactor. It has been suggested that deficient binding of thiamine by transketolase may explain genetic differences in susceptibility to Wernicke-Korsakoff's syndrome, which develops in only a minority of chronic alcoholics [7]. Other findings include abnormal vestibular function with an impaired response to ice-water caloric testing, elevation of blood pyruvate concentration, and diffuse slow wave activity on EEG. The pathology in Wernicke's encephalopathy consists of symmetric degenerative or necrotic lesions involving the mammilary bodies, the paraventricular region of the thalamus and hypothalamus, the periaqueductal region of the midbrain, and the floor of the fourth ventricle. Lesions of the mammilary bodies may be observable by magnetic resonance imaging.

Wernicke-Korsakoff syndrome is treated with thiamine and other nutrients. Typically recovery begins within hours of treatment. The ocular palsies and confusion improve most rapidly, with subsequent improvement in other functions occurring over a few weeks. Horizontal nystagmus and ataxia may persist indefinitely. In contrast, complete recovery occurs in only a minority of patients with Korsakoff's psychosis. Recovery tends to be gradual, requiring a year or longer for maximal resolution. Many patients with Korsakoff's psychosis ultimately require chronic institutionalization. The dose of thiamine that is usually administered is 15 mg/day IM along with supplementation with other B vitamins.

Alcoholic Cerebellar Degeneration

Alcoholic cerebellar degeneration is characterized by truncal ataxia and incoordination, involving the lower extremities. This syndrome is more common than Wernicke's encephalopathy. Clinical features include a wide-based gait, instability of the trunk, and ataxia of the legs without nystagmus or dysarthria. The syndrome usually develops gradually over weeks or months.

The pathology includes degeneration of cells of the cerebellar cortex, with vermal atrophy, that can sometimes be identified by CT scan. Because of similarities in the pathology and clinical features to that of the ataxia component of Wernicke's encephalopathy, alcoholic cerebellar degeneration is believed to represent part of the spectrum of the former. In many patients, the syndrome responds to thiamine therapy, even if alcohol consumption continues, which is further support of the role of nutritional deficiency in the pathogenesis.

Cerebral Cortical Atrophy

Several studies have reported enlarged cerebral ventricles by CT scan or MRI in alcoholics compared to healthy controls [12,78]. However, abstinence from alcohol may result in partial reversal of ventricular enlargement, suggesting that there had been shrinkage, due to fluid shifts, rather than tissue loss or true atrophy. It is not clear whether ventricular enlargement represents a direct toxic effect of alcohol or whether it is a consequence of thiamine deficiency, metabolic disturbances, recurrent seizures, or head trauma.

Central Pontine Myelinolysis

Central pontine myelinolysis is an uncommon disorder characterized pathologically by selective demyelination in the pons and parts of the midbrain. The syndrome is invariably associated with serious illness including chronic alcoholism. Its etiology has not been defined but is believed to be related to nutritional or metabolic abnormalities. There is an association between Wernicke's syndrome and central pontine myelinolysis, although the pathology of the two disorders is distinctly different. The clinical presentation of central pontine myelinolysis includes quadriplegia and pseudobulbar palsy, with an inability to chew, talk, or swallow. Inability to talk and paralysis may result in pseudocoma, with intact sensation and comprehension. In the past, the diagnosis of central pontine myelinolysis was most often made at autopsy, but currently both CT and MRI can be used to diagnose pontine lesions antemortem [21,52].

Marchiafava-Bignami Disease

Marchiafava-Bignami disease is a very rare disorder with degeneration of myelin in the central portion of the corpus callosum. Most patients with this disorder are male chronic alcoholics. The etiology is unknown. The clinical picture is that of a frontal lobe syndrome with progressive dementia, often progressing over several years, and emotional disorders, including violent behavior or apathy. Frontal lobe release reflexes, dysarthria, and gait abnormalities have been described. Some patients make a remarkable recovery with nutritional therapy and cessation of alcohol consumption.

OPIATES

Mechanisms of Action

Opiates, either derived from the opium poppy or as synthetic drugs, are widely encountered both as analgesics and drugs of abuse. Opiates act on specific receptors in the nervous system and other parts of the body. Many of the actions of opiates mimic those of endogenous opioids (e.g., enkephalins, beta-endorphin, dynorphins). Stimulation of opiate receptors generally results in inhibition of cell firing, although inhibition of inhibitory neurons may result in increased cell firing in specific brain regions.

The major clinical actions of opiates are analgesia, respiratory depression, and slowed gastrointestinal transit. Other important pharmacologic effects include the release of prolactin and growth hormone, inhibition of vasopressin release, and increased turnover of dopamine and acetylcholine in specific regions of the brain. These actions are consequences of activation of one or more opiate receptor subtypes [63]. The pharmacology of opiates according to receptor subtype is summarized in Table 23-11. Opiate analgesia is believed to result from activation of both supraspinal (mu-1) and spinal (delta and kappa) receptors. Respiratory depression and constipation appear to be mediated primarily by mu-2 receptors. The psychotomimetic effect of certain opiate analgesics such as pentazocine, as well as drugs of abuse such as phencyclidine, may be mediated by sigma receptor activation.

Different opiate receptors are found in different concentrations in different regions of the nervous system. A well-studied neural pathway of endogenous opiate analgesia goes from the periaqueductal gray region via descending pathways to the spinal cord. Electrical stimulation or microinjections of morphine into the periaqueductal gray region of animals and humans result in analgesia that is antagonized by opiate antagonists [63]. The pleasurable or reinforcing effects of opiates that contribute to drug abuse appear to involve activation of mu receptors in the ventral tegmental area and nucleus acumbens. Reinforcement involves at least in part activation of dopaminergic neurons via disinhibition. The anatomic loci for physical dependence do not appear to be the same as those for reinforcement.

An extensively studied site of opiate action is the locus ceruleus, a nuclear structure in the pons that contains a large collection of noradrenergic neurons. The locus ceruleus is involved in the control of autonomic neural activity. Opiate receptor (mu) activation results in inhibition of locus ceruleus firing. Complete tolerance to the effects of morphine on such firing is observed experimentally during prolonged morphine treatment [42]. The mechanism of tolerance appears to be uncoupling of the re-

Table 23-11. Pharmacology of opiate receptor subtypes

Receptor subtype	*Prototype drugs*	*Major action*
μ		
μ_1	Opiates and most opioid peptides	Supraspinal analgesia Prolactin release Catalepsy
μ_2	Morphine	Respiratory depression Gastrointestinal transit Growth hormone release Most cardiovascular effects
δ	Enkephalins	Spinal analgesia Growth hormone release
κ	Ketocyclazocine and dynorphin	Spinal analgesia Inhibition of vasopressin release Sedation
ϵ	β-Endorphin	?
σ	*N*-Allylnormetazocine	Psychotomimetic effects

ceptors from the G-protein that increases potassium conductance to produce the pharmacologic action. Conversely, after the locus ceruleus has become tolerant to actions of morphine, removal of morphine exposure results in a marked increase in locus ceruleus firing, believed to be linked to the autonomic hyperactivity associated with opiate withdrawal. The opiate-induced increase in potassium conductance and resultant physiologic effects can also be produced by activation of alpha-2 receptors in the locus ceruleus. Centrally-acting alpha-2 agonists such as clonidine antagonize the increased firing of the locus ceruleus, thereby reducing autonomic discharge that accompanies opiate withdrawal.

Tolerance develops rapidly to effects of opiates, with cross tolerance generally developing across opiates. However, the rate and extent of development of tolerance to specific opiate effects may differ significantly. For example, in animals, tolerance to analgesia develops before tolerance to respiratory depression [63]. Differential development of tolerance may explain why patients requiring increasing doses of narcotics may develop respiratory depression despite inadequate pain relief. Tolerance to some effects such as constipation and pupillary constriction develop minimally or not at all.

Acute Intoxication

Many different opiates are used for analgesia or are abused. A detailed discussion of pharmacologic characteristics of the particular drugs in this class is beyond the scope of this chapter. Opiates will be discussed as a class, with reference to particular drugs when relevant to diagnosis or management.

Opiate intoxication occurs relatively frequently in drug abusers who either have misjudged the dose or are suicidal, but it also occurs with therapeutic use in patients with pain. Clinical features of opiate intoxication are summarized in Table 23-12. The usual cause of death is respiratory arrest. Respiratory arrest may occur within a minute of intravenous injection. After intramuscular or subcutaneous dosing with narcotics such as morphine, respiratory depression peaks 30 to 60 minutes after injection; the interval from dose to peak effect may even be larger after oral dosing. There appears to be a delay between peak plasma levels and peak respiratory depression, presumably due to a delay of entry of morphine into the brain [84]. After intramuscular, subcutaneous, or oral dosing, a progression of intoxication from sedation and slowing of respiratory rate to coma and respiratory arrest is expected. Respiratory depression from opiates may be enhanced when patients

Table 23-12. Clinical features of opiate intoxication and withdrawal

Intoxication	*Withdrawal*
Stupor or coma	Anxiety, restlessness
Symmetric, pinpoint, reactive pupils	Insomnia
Hypothermia	Chills, hot flashes
Bradycardia	Myalgias, arthralgias
Hypotension	Nausea, anorexia
Skin cool, moist	Abdominal cramping
Hypoventilation (respiratory slowing, irregular breathing, apnea)	Vomiting, diarrhea
Pulmonary edema	Yawning
Seizures (meperidine, propoxyphene, morphine)	Dilated pupils
Reversal with naloxone	Tachycardia, hypertension (mild)
	Hyperthermia (mild), diaphoresis, lacrimation, rhinorrhea
	Piloerection
	Spontaneous ejaculation

are receiving barbiturates or other sedative hypnotics, phenothiazines (including prochlorperazine), or drugs with neuromuscular blocking activity.

Particular opiates may produce specific manifestations in addition to those described in Table 23-12. Chronic therapy with meperidine, either in high doses or in patients with chronic renal failure, may result in neuromuscular excitability, believed to be due to accumulation of the metabolite normeperidine [6]. Propoxyphene intoxication can be associated with seizures, diabetes insipidus, and cardiovascular collapse due to myocardial depression, the last thought to be caused by the metabolite norpropoxyphene [45]. Methadone produces a typical picture of opiate intoxication, but because of its long half-life, intoxication may be prolonged for a day or longer. An unusual case of prolonged opiate intoxication seen at the San Francisco General Hospital resulted from a chunk of opium that was inserted into the rectum to escape police detection.

Most signs and symptoms of opiate intoxication are reversed by naloxone. This reversal is an important element in diagnosing opiate intoxication. Some intoxications, however, such as with propoxyphene may require extremely large doses (more than 10 mg) for reversal, and even then reversal may be incomplete. Some manifestations of intoxication such as seizures may respond poorly or not at all to naloxone. Naloxone in high doses (usually 5–10 mg or more) may also have a nonspecific arousing effect in patients with alcohol or benzodiazepine intoxication and in some patients with stroke.

Failure of a patient thought to be opiate-intoxicated to respond to naloxone should raise the suspicion of anoxic encephalopathy, head trauma, meningitis, or ingestion of drugs in addition to opiates. Failure to regain consciousness after a narcotic overdose, with or without evidence of recurrent seizure activity, particularly with a history of prolonged respiratory depression, suggests anoxic encephalopathy. However, when a postoperative patient who has been given narcotics for pain relief suddenly develops seizures and respiratory arrest, the syndrome of hyponatremia with respiratory depression (hyponatremic encephalopathy) must be considered [4]. As part of the differential, such patients will generally have a serum sodium level below 128 mM and there will be no response to naloxone [26].

Clonidine intoxication resembles opiate poisoning, and because clonidine is used to treat opiate withdrawal, it is not uncommonly seen in opiate addicts. As discussed in the mechanisms section, clonidine, a central alpha-2 agonist, acts on the locus ceruleus to mimic the actions of opiates. The typical picture of clonidine poisoning includes sedation, stupor, or coma with pinpoint pupils. In the early phase of clonidine poisoning, transient hypertension may be present due to direct vascular alpha-2-mediated vasoconstriction, but subsequently hypotension and bradycardia are the rule. Clonidine may be distinguished from opiate intoxication by relatively less respiratory depression for a given degree of sedation, although respiratory arrest has occasionally been observed after clonidine intoxication.

Management of opiate intoxication should be directed toward maintaining a patent airway and adequate ventilation. Naloxone, 0.4 to 2.0 mg IV, may be administered to reverse opiate intoxication. However, the patient must still be observed for several hours, as the effects of naloxone (2–3 hours) may be briefer than the effects of many narcotics, and late recurrent intoxication may ensue. In patients with intoxications by long-acting opiates such as methadone, continuous infusions or repeated bolus injections of naloxone may be administered. Pulmonary edema due to narcotic intoxication is probably a result of increased pulmonary capillary permeability and may take several days to resolve. Severe hypoxemia due to pulmonary edema may require positive-pressure mechanical ventilation.

Other neurologic complications of opiate abuse that should be part of the differential diagnosis of acute intoxication are described in a subsequent section.

Opiate Withdrawal

Prolonged use of opiates leads to development of tolerance and, after cessation of use, a withdrawal syndrome. Tolerance is selective, with development of a high level of tolerance to nausea, sedation, and respiratory depression but little tolerance to pupillary constriction or constipation. The severity of the withdrawal syndrome depends on the prior daily dose of opiates and is generally more severe in opiate abusers than in patients taking opiates for analgesia. Symptoms resembling opiate withdrawal can occur following administration of naloxone after even a single dose of morphine [38]. Opiate withdrawal is not life-threatening but is associated with severe psychological and moderate physical distress. The clinical features of the withdrawal syndrome range from a mild flu-like illness to a multisystem disorder as described in Table 23-12.

The onset of withdrawal symptoms is typically 8 to 16 hours after cessation of use of heroin or morphine. Autonomic disturbances and myalgias tend to appear first. By 36 hours, severe restlessness, piloerection, lacrimation, abdominal cramps, and diarrhea become more prominent. Symptoms reach peak intensity at 48 to 72 hours and then resolve over 7 to 10 days. Abstinence symptoms after cessation of methadone use develop more gradually, with an onset of 36 to 72 hours, peak at about 6 days, and also tend to be less severe.

Treatment of opiate withdrawal includes specific replacement with opiates and nonspecific or symptomatic care. The most commonly used replacement medication is methadone, doses usually at 20 to 40 mg/day PO as required to make the patient comfortable. After 2 or 3 days of stabilization, the dose can be gradually tapered over 1 to 3 weeks. Opiate abusers should be considered for methadone maintenance and, if interested, referred to a maintenance clinic. If narcotics are required for management of pain in an opiate addict, the usual doses of those narcotics may be administered above the baseline dose of methadone required to prevent withdrawal symptoms.

As discussed previously, clonidine produces opiate-like effects and has been used to manage opiate withdrawal symptoms. Typically, clonidine is initiated at 0.1 to 0.2 mg every 8 hours. The dose is increased as needed to a maxiumum of 0.8 to 1.2 mg/day. Subsequently clonidine is tapered over 10 to 14 days. Patients need to be observed for development of excessive hypotension. Nonspecific treatment for opiate withdrawal includes the use of benzodiazepines or chloral hydrate for sleep and anxiety and prochlorperazine for gastrointestinal symptoms. Propoxyphene and/or nonsteriodal anti-inflammatory drugs may be useful for treatment of myalgias.

Other Neurologic Complications of Opiate Abuse

Heroin abuse has been associated with a number of neurologic complications, most of which are related to injection of contaminated solutions or foreign material. Infectious complications include meningitis (often associated with endocarditis), mycotic aneurysm, brain abscess, subdural abscess, epidural abscess, tetanus, and cerebral malaria. Other complications of opiate abuse include postanoxic encephalopathy, stroke, toxic amblyopia (from quinine used as an adulterant), acute transverse myelitis, leukoencephalopathy, Horner's syndrome, and peripheral neuropathies.

1-Methyl-4-phenyl-1,2,3,6-tetrahydropyridine (MPTP), an impurity in the synthesis of meperidine analogues, produces a movement disorder resembling Parkinson's disease [10]. Typically parkinsonism develops within a few days of injecting an illicit narcotic contaminated with MPTP. In contrast to idiopathic parkinsonism, which may involve both dysaminergic and noradrenergic neurons, parkinsonism due to MPTP selectivity involves nigrostriatal dopaminergic neurons. Symptoms may improve with levodopa and carbidopa, although the parkinsonism is in most cases permanent. Animal studies suggest that treatment with the monoamine oxidase B inhibitor selegiline can prevent neuronal injury from MPTP [83].

SEDATIVE-HYPNOTIC DRUGS

Mechanisms of Action

Barbiturates and benzodiazepines potentiate the actions of the inhibitory neurotransmitter GABA [24]. GABA exerts its effects by increasing chloride ion conductance through the neuronal membrane chloride channel. Barbiturates may act by enhancing the binding of GABA to its receptor site on the membrance, possibly by decreasing the rate of dissociation of GABA from its receptor. In high concentrations, barbiturates may depress calcium-dependent action potentials and enhance chloride conduction in the absence of GABA. Barbiturates act throughout the brain but affect polysynaptic transmission and the reticular activating system at relatively low concentrations, so these sites are most sensitive to barbiturate action. The progression of signs and symptoms in the overdose has been discussed previously.

The action of benzodiazepines appears to be mediated by a receptor on the $GABA_A$-chloride ionophore complex that is distributed on postsynaptic neurons in the central nervous system. GABA, by increasing chloride flux, hyperpolarizes cell membranes and inhibits neuronal firing. Benzodiazapines potentiate the effects of GABA on the chloride flux and thereby enhance the inhibitory neurotransmitter effects of GABA.

Long-term treatment with benzodiazepines in animals is associated with downregulation of brain binding that is associated with the development of behavioral tolerance [53]. Conversely, discontinuation of benzodiazepines is associated with upregulation of receptor binding and function of the GABA receptor complex [54].

Intoxication

Sedative-hypnotic drugs are commonly involved in intentional drug intoxications. Barbiturates and benzodiazepines are the most important drugs in this class and will be the focus of discussion in this section. Less common are chloral hydrate, ethchlorvynol, glutethimide, meprobramate, methaqualone, and methprylon. For the most part, diagnostic and therapeutic considerations for the latter group resemble those for barbiturates.

Ingestion of excessive quantities of barbiturates results in a progressive metabolic encephalopathy and coma, as described earlier. The signs and symptoms of barbiturate intoxication are summarized in Table 23-13. Intoxication with other sedative-hypnotic drugs produces a similar picture with a few distinctions. Benzodiazepine intoxication is less likely to be associated with respiratory depression or hypotension, unless there is a co-ingestion of other sedative drugs or alcohol or the drug is absorbed extremely rapidly (as occurs with respiratory arrest following intravenous diazepam or midazolam or oral triazolam). Glutethimide, owing to its anticholinergic action, may pro-

Table 23-13. Sedative-hypnotic drug intoxication

Mild	Sedation Disorientation Slurred speech Ataxia Nystagmus
Moderate*	Coma; arousal by painful stimulation Depressed or absent deep tendon reflexes Slow respiration Absent oculocephalic reflexes Intact pupillary light reflex
Severe	Coma; unarousable Absent corneal, gag, and deep tendon reflexes Hypothermia Respiratory depression; apnea Hypotension, shock

* In the early phase of intoxication in occasional patients a state of neuromuscular hyperexcitability with increased muscle tone, hyperactive reflexes, ankle clonus, and/or decerebrate posturing may be observed.

duce dilated and unreactive pupils. Methaqualone tends to produce muscular hyperactivity with increased muscle tone, myoclonus, and/or seizures. Chloral hydrate intoxication is associated with cardiac arrhythmias, including ventricular tachycardia.

The time course of sedative-hypnotic drug intoxication depends on the pharmacokinetics of the particular drug. For intermediate-acting barbiturates such as pentobarbital, secobarbital, or amobarbital and many of the benzodiazepines, intoxication usually resolves within 48 hours. Long-acting barbiturates such as phenobarbital, benzodiazepines such as flurazepam, and ethchlorvynol (the last of which exhibits dose-dependent metabolism) are associated with prolonged coma, which may persist as long as 5 to 7 days. Glutethimide has been associated with waxing and waning of consciousness, due either to its anticholingeric effects producing intermittent bowel activity and absorption or to enterohepatic recirculation of an active metabolite, 4-hydroxyglutethimide.

The differential diagnosis of coma from drug overdose has already been discussed. Diagnosis is based on the history, toxicology results, and most importantly lack of evidence for either an infectious or a structural or metabolic cause for coma. EEG abnormalities in sedative-hypnotic drug intoxication have been extensively studied and tend to correlate with the depth of coma (Table 23-14). An isoelectric EEG has been observed for up to 28 hours in sedative-poisoned patients, with subsequent full recovery [34]. The primary importance of the EEG in evaluating poisoned patients is to distinguish status epilepticus from drug-induced central nervous system depression. Neurologic injury or death due to sedative-hypnotic overdose occurs primarily because of respiratory arrest or prolonged hypotension. Once the patient is in the hospital, the major morbidity and mortality are due to respiratory complications, primarily noncardiogenic pulmonary edema with or without infection. Predictors of a high risk for mortality

Table 23-14. Electroencephalographic changes in sedative-hypnotic drug poisoning

Grade	*EEG rhythm*
Grade I	Alpha rhythm or predominant alpha rhythm with beta or some rare theta waves
Grade II	Predominant theta rhythm with some alpha, beta, and low voltage delta activity
Grade III	Prominent low/high voltage delta activity mixed with some theta waves
Grade IV	Delta activity with or without brief isoelectric intervals
Grade V	Suppression-burst activity, where 3–10 c/sec activity of several seconds duration alternates with electrical silence
Grade VI	Near silence but with isolated and low voltage 3–7 c/sec waves occurring singly or in bursts of half a second
Grade VII	An isoelectric record, totally unresponsive to all stimuli

Source: Haider, Matthew, and Oswald [34].

include the presence of hypotension, metabolic acidosis, hypoxemia, aspiration, or abnormality of chest x-ray on admission [39].

The management of sedative drug overdoses centers on respiratory and cardiovascular support. Most patients supported with good intensive care will recover fully even in the face of prolonged coma. Occasionally, in a patient with pulmonary edema, respiratory tract infection, severe hypotension, or other life-threatening medical illness, it is desirable to shorten the course of coma. This may be done for certain drugs by hemodialysis (chloral hydrate, phenobarbital) or hemoperfusion (phenobarbital, short-acting barbiturates, ethchlorvynol). Repeated doses of oral charcoal (50 gm every 4 hours) accelerate the elimination of phenobarbital (by interrupting entero-enteric recirculation) but in one study did not shorten the duration of phenobarbital-induced coma [70]. In that study, patients awakened at a similar time after acute intoxication even though blood levels were lower in the group receiving charcoal treatment. Most likely this is because tolerance had developed to the high level of barbiturate in the untreated group.

A specific antagonist to benzodiazepines has been developed. Its role in the management of benzodiazepine intoxication is not yet defined. Flumazenil binds to benzodiazepine receptors and reverses sedation and coma caused by benzodiazepines. In higher doses flumazenil may have some agonist activity as well. Clinical trials in patients with mixed overdoses involving benzodiazepines showed significant improvement in coma scores in treated patients compared to placebo controls [61]. The dose was titrated in 0.2 to 0.3-mg increments to a total of 1 mg IV over approximately 5 minutes. The major hazard of flumazenil is precipitation of acute benzodiazepine withdrawal, including seizures. The duration of action of flumazenil is relatively short (half-life 60–90 minutes) compared with the duration of action of many of the benzodiazepines, so repeated doses may be necessary to maintain reversal of intoxication. Of concern is the possibility that a benzodiazepine intoxication will be reversed with flumazenil, then the patient left unattended. The flumazenil will be eliminated more quickly than the benzodiazepine, and the patient may decompensate and suffer respiratory arrest. For this reason, it is still necessary to manage benzodiazepine overdoses with careful observation and intensive care.

Sedative-Hypnotic Drug Withdrawal

Habitual use of sedative-hypnotic drugs is associated with the development of tolerance and, upon sudden cessation, a withdrawal syndrome similar to that of alcohol withdrawal. In general, there is a history of taking three or more times the usual sedative dose daily for longer than 1 month in patients with serious withdrawal syndromes. However, abstinence syndromes that are disruptive to the patient may occur after cessation of usual therapeutic doses, particularly when the drug has been consumed for several months or longer [11]. The concomitant use of alcohol on a prolonged basis may aggravate the severity of the sedative-hypnotic withdrawal syndrome.

The clinical manifestations are similar to those described for alcohol withdrawal (see Table 23-9), although the incidence of seizures may be higher after withdrawal from high doses of barbiturates. Most patients will experience anxiety, irritability, agitation, tremor, muscle twitching, insomnia, anorexia, and/or weakness during abstinence. Generalized seizures may occur with or without a subsequent state of delirium. Some patients develop an acute psychosis or delirium without seizures. The time course of withdrawal symptoms depends on the pharmacokinetics of the drug involved. Following cessation of pentobarbital, secobarbital, or amobarbital (half-lives 20–24 hours), symptoms usually begin within 8 to 12 hours, the time to peak is at 2 to 3 days, and symptoms persist for 6 to 7 days. For phenobarbital and diazepam, with half-lives of 50 to 100 hours or more, withdrawal symptoms tend to develop 5 to 7 days after cessation of drug use and may persist for several weeks. In general the severity of abstinence symptoms is greater after cessation of short versus long half-life drugs, consistent with the concept that the brain has more time to adapt to changing drug effects when the rate of decline of the concentration of the drug in the brain is gradual.

Severe withdrawal symptoms from barbiturates are most commonly seen in people who use many drugs simultaneously (polydrug abusers). In contrast, withdrawal symptoms from benzodiazepines are commonly seen in patients who are being treated for chronic psychiatric disturbances or anxiety. The anxiety and agitation seen during withdrawal from benzodiazepines may resemble the original condition for which the drug was taken, thereby reinforcing chronic use. Some patients develop considerable apprehension about the idea of withdrawing from benzodiazepines and may develop anxiety on that basis (pseudo-withdrawal) [75].

Treatment of sedative-hypnotic withdrawal signs and symptoms requires replacement with a sedative-hypnotic drug, followed by subsequent gradual tapering of the dose. Many approaches have been described [75]. It is most reasonable to select long-acting drugs such as phenobarbital for barbiturate and diazepam for benzodiazepine dependence to manage the withdrawal syndrome [36,73]. Typically such schedules involve loading with a long-acting sedative-hypnotic drug until the withdrawal symptoms are controlled, stabilizing the patient on this dose for a few days, then withdrawing the replacement drug at a rate of 10 percent of the dose every few days until totally discontinued.

STIMULANTS AND HALLUCINOGENS

Abuse of stimulants, particularly cocaine, is a common cause of neurologic morbidity and mortality. Hallucinogens are used less frequently than stimulants but may also present with acute neurologic syndromes. This section will review neurologic complications of some of the more common stimulants and hallucinogens.

Cocaine

Cocaine abuse is currently one of the most frequent causes of drug-induced central nervous system toxicity. Cocaine has become relatively inexpensive and is widely available for intravenous, intranasal (snorting), or inhalational (smoked) use. Crack cocaine (chunks of solid cocaine base) is the form most commonly smoked because cocaine base is more volatile than the hydrochloride salt, the latter of which decomposes with heating.

The mechanism of action of cocaine resembles that of amphetamines and related drugs. The major neurochemical actions include (1) a local anesthetic effect, (2) central nervous stimulation with release of dopamine and systemic activation of the sympathetic nervous system, (3) blockade of neuronal catecholamine uptake, and (4) release or blockade of neuronal reuptake of serotonin. The receptor for cocaine in the brain appears to be the catecholamine transporter in the neuronal membrane. Blockade of the dopamine transporter has been linked with the euphoric actions of cocaine [86]. Cocaine use produces euphoria, mental stimulation, and generalized sympathetic nervous system activation. The rewarding effects and many of the toxic effects of cocaine in animals can be blocked by dopamine antagonists, suggesting that dopamine release is critical to cocaine action. With chronic exposure in animals, there is depletion of brain catecholamines with an increased receptor sensitivity to their actions.

The clinical picture of cocaine intoxication is summarized in Table 23-15. Psychiatric disturbances are particularly common presentations of cocaine abusers to emergency departments. Acute cocaine intoxication often presents as an acute anxiety—panic attack or agitated delirium. Because cocaine has a short half-life (60–90 minutes), acute intoxication usually resolves within 6 hours. Chronic intoxication may present as a paranoid psychosis, indistinguishable from paranoid schizophrenia, and may last for many days. Neonatal intoxication has been reported immediately after birth and during breast-feeding by a cocaine-using mother [16, 17]. Typical features are irritability, tremulousness, tachycardia, and tachypnea, although seizures have also been reported.

Abstinence after habitual use of cocaine is also associated with neuropsychiatric symptoms [29]. A cocaine "crash," a state of profound exhaustion accompanied by anxiety, depres-

Table 23-15. Manifestations of intoxication with cocaine and other stimulant drugs

Behavioral/psychiatric	*Autonomic/ neuromuscular*
Euphoria	Tachycardia[b]
Hyperactivity, irritability[a]	Hypertension
Insomnia	Hyperthermia
Mood lability	Dilated pupils
Anorexia	Tremulousness[a]
Anxiety, agitation	Seizures
Suspiciousness, aggressiveness	Respiratory arrest
Psychosis (often paranoid)	Cardiovascular collapse
Delirium (agitated)	
Stupor	
Coma	

[a] Particularly neonatal intoxication.
[b] Except phenylpropanolamine and other primarily alpha-adrenergic agonists that produce reflex bradycardia.

Table 23-16. Neurologic complications of cocaine abuse

Headache
Seizures
Transient loss of consciousness
Transient focal signs and symptoms
Optic nerve infarction or neuritis
Toxic encephalopathy/coma
Stroke
Subarachnoid hemorrhage
Intracranial hemorrhage
Cerebral infarction
Embolic (endocarditis)

Source: Adapted from Lowenstein et al. [48].

sion, and a craving for cocaine is described. Decreased energy, anhedonia, and hypersomnolence ensue and may last for weeks or months. An intense desire for cocaine to ameliorate the severity of the abstinence syndrome commonly leads to relapse, thus sustaining addiction. Suicidal ideation is not uncommon in the cocaine abstinence state.

Numerous neurologic complications of cocaine abuse have been reported [48], as summarized in Table 23-16. Headaches are common and may be severe. Headaches may be the consequence of cocaine-induced hypertension or may be the first symptom of subarachnoid or intracranial hemorrhage. A patient who presents with severe headache and a normal blood pressure warrants brain imaging and lumbar puncture. On the other hand, severe headaches may be unrelated to hypertension or structural injury and may represent a migraine, precipitated by cocaine-incuded serotonin release. Seizures commonly occur in cocaine users, typically within minutes of administration. These are usually generalized tonic-clonic seizures and are brief, resolving by the time the patient reaches the emergency room. Occasionally, status epilepticus occurs that may be difficult to treat. Status epilepticus should raise concern about continued absorption of cocaine, such as from a ruptured packet in the gastrointestinal tract of a body packer or oral ingestion of crack cocaine.

Transient loss of consciousness may occur immediately after injection of cocaine in patients who upon later evaluation in the emergency department have no neurologic abnormalities or lesions. Presumably such loss of consciousness is due to nonsustained arrhythmias or unwitnessed seizures.

Transient focal neurologic signs and symptoms including sensory, motor, or visual changes, or a combination of these, have been seen. The pathophysiology of these disturbances has not been defined but may be related to spasm of small cerebral blood vessels. Sudden blindness in one eye due to retinal artery occlusion after use of cocaine and progressive bilateral loss of visual acuity due to optic nerve involvement by a chronic osteolytic sinusitis (in a chronic intranasal user) have been reported [20,57].

Toxic encephalopathy is relatively uncommon but may be the presentation of a massive intoxication, particularly with continued gastrointestinal absorption. In patients with a metabolic encephalopathy picture, causes other than cocaine, such as other drugs or infection, must be excluded.

There has been much recent interest in strokes caused by cocaine and other sympathomimetic drugs. Strokes have occurred following all routes of cocaine abuse [46,47]. Three pathologic processes have been evoked to explain cocaine-induced stroke. Subarachnoid hemorrhage may occur due to transient hypertension in patients with cerebral aneurysms (either congenital or mycotic) or arteriovenous malformations, the latter having been confirmed by angiography in some cases of subarachnoid hemorrhage. Intracerebral hemorrhage may occur in the cerebral cortices (most frequently frontoparietal) or in deep structures (putamen, thalamus) and resemble hemorrhages in hypertensive patients. Hypertension from cocaine is considered to be the cause of most cases of intracerebral hemmorrhage. Cerebral infarction may occur in any vascular territory, but middle cerebral artery occlusions have been most frequently reported. The pathophysiology of cerebral infarction is presumed to be vascular spasm, possibly associated with increased platelet aggregation and thrombosis induced by cocaine. Cerebral infarction may occur several hours following the use of cocaine, consistent with the role of thrombosis. There has been some discussion of cerebral vasculitis in cocaine abusers, based on findings of irregularities and narrowing (beading) on cerebral angiography. However, in some of these cases, there has also been intracranial hemorrhage, which also has angiographic findings similar to vasculitis. In intravenous drug abusers, embolic strokes related to bacterial endocarditis need always to be considered.

Hyperthermia may complicate cocaine intoxication, with or without seizures. As discussed in a previous section, sustained hyperthermia, particularly with seizures, may cause permanent brain injury. In experimental animals, preventing hyperthermia by either preventing seizures or body cooling reduced the mortality from cocaine intoxication [14].

Evaluation of neurologic abnormalities related to cocaine abuse should include urine toxicology for cocaine and its metabolites as well as other drugs, brain imaging (with CT or MRI), and a lumbar puncture. Further evaluation of such patients may include cerebral angiography and cardiac echocardiography, as well as chemistry studies such as antinuclear antibody, fluorescent treponemal antibody (FTA), and coagulation studies.

Treatment of neurologic complications of cocaine is largely supportive. Seizures are usually self-limited and do not need to be treated. For status epilepticus, diazepam and phenobarbital loading are indicated. Barbiturate anesthesia may be required to control status epilepticus in some cases of drug intoxication. Management of hyperthermia has been discussed previously.

Amphetamines and Related Hallucinogens

The mechanisms of action of amphetamines are similar to those of cocaine, with the addition of monoamine oxidase inhibiting activity for particular amphetamines. A number of amphetamine-like drugs are available either from licit or illicit sources.

The central nervous system toxicity of amphetamines is similar to that of cocaine, although the duration of effect may be longer. Amphetamines in general are eliminated from the body much more slowly than cocaine (e.g., the half-life of dextroamphetamine is 5–20 hours depending on urinary pH), and therefore the time course of intoxication with amphetamines is often prolonged. The most frequent causes of death in amphetamine abusers are strokes, sudden death (presumably due to arrhythmias), and hyperthermia. The most frequent psychiatric symptoms are acute anxiety or panic, psychosis or hallucinations, violent behavior (often a component of a paranoid psychosis), and a withdrawal syndrome producing depression, exhaustion, and somnolence. The somnolence may last several weeks and, as discussed for cocaine, may be associated with a risk of suicide.

The pathophysiology of stroke in stimulant abusers has been of considerable interest. Whereas many stimulant-induced strokes are believed to be a consequence of hypertension or vasospasm, as discussed for cocaine, case reports and an animal study have linked methamphetamine abuse with the development of cerebral vasculitis [76]. Findings on angiography include multiple occlusions with arterial beading in medium-sized vessels. The pathology of affected vessels shows a necrotizing angiitis, with fibrinoid degeneration and necrosis of the media and intima and a variable degree of leukocytic infiltration of vessel walls. The pathology resembles periarteritis nodosa, suggesting a possible hypersensitivity mechanism. It has been speculated that such a vasculitic process may lead to aneurysm formation, which then becomes the site of hemorrhage. As has been noted for cocaine, however, subarachnoid hemorrhage itself can cause vasculitis-like changes on angiography and may explain many cases of amphetamine-associated "vasculitis."

A number of chemical analogues of dextroamphetamine, sharing a common phenylethylamine structure, have been synthesized for recreational use. [8]. The most widely used at present are methamphetamine, 3,4-methylene dioxyamphetamine (MDA), and 3,4-methylene dioxymethamphetamine (MDMA). Mescaline is natural phenylethylamine, which is a component of the peyote cactus. The phenylethylamines have similar actions and toxicities to those of amphetamines, although some are more hallucinogenic [23,80].

Lysergic acid diethylamine (LSD) is a stimulant-hallucinogen that has been widely abused in the past but is less commonly used in the 1990s. Its central nervous system toxicity is primarily that of an acute psychosis (which has been associated with inadvertent or intentional suicide), convulsions, and violent behavior. Occasionally, prolonged psychosis or recurrent panic reactions have followed LSD intoxication. Rarely, massive intoxication with LSD has resulted in coma, associated with sympathomimetic signs, seizures, and hyperthermia, and in some cases requiring assisted ventilation. Cases of LSD intoxication with focal neurologic abnormalities, presumably due to cerebral vascular spasm or injury, have also been reported.

Monoamine Oxidase Inhibitors

Findings similar to those discussed for amphetamine may be observed after overdose of monoamine oxidase inhibitors (MAOIs) or following an interaction with certain drugs (meperidine or sympathomimetic drugs) or foods (tyramine-containing food). Typically agitation, delirium, neuromuscular excitability with seizures, sympathomimetic signs, and hyperthermia are observed. Combination therapy with MAOIs and tricyclic antidepressants, particularly clomipramine and fluoxetine, can produce a similar syndrome [25]. The onset of the syndrome may be delayed for 12 to 24 hours after an overdose of MAOIs. Death may be due to intracranial hemorrhage, hyperthermia, arrhythmias, or cardiovascular collapse.

Phencyclidine

Phencyclidine (PCP, angel dust, hog, crystal) is a dissociative anesthetic drug that has been abused since the 1960s. It is consumed by smoking, intravenous administration, snorting, or oral ingestion. Commonly it is added to marijuana and smoked. Historically, the peak period of use of PCP was in the early and middle 1970s, but in urban emergency departments PCP intoxication is still encountered on a regular basis. PCP is often misrepresented as LSD, mescaline, or THC (delta-9-tetrahydrocannabinol, the active chemical in marijuana), so its victims may not even know they have taken PCP.

The subjective effects of PCP are described as those of depersonalization and tranquilization. The clinical picture of PCP intoxication is summarized in Table 23-17. The most specific findings in PCP intoxication are abnormal motor activity, including spontaneous nystagmus and increased muscle tone. Intoxication may also be associated with cholinomimetic features such as sweating, salivation, and miosis. The most serious medical complications are similar to those seen with amphetamine intoxication. The toxic psychosis, which may wax and wane, may be protracted and is frequently associated with violent behavior and injuries. Coma from PCP may be prolonged, in some cases for weeks. Presumably this results from the slow release of PCP from tissues stores, maintaining high levels in the brain.

PCP-intoxicated people are sometimes described as having extraordinary physical strength, possibly due to the dissociative-anesthetic effect, which blocks pain as a restraint to extreme physical exertion. Several

Table 23-17. Phencyclidine intoxication

Confusion state (5 mg)*
Blank stare
Uncommunicative
Agitated, excited, combative, bizarre behavior
Horizontal and/or vertical nystagmus
Gait ataxia
Muscle rigidity or catalepsy
Hypertension
Coma (20 mg)*
Unresponsive, immobile
Eyes may remain open
Spontaneous nystagmus
Brain stem reflexes intact
Muscle rigidity
Opisthotonus, decorticate posturing
Increased deep tendon reflexes
Seizures
Hypertension
EEG—diffuse theta and delta slowing; periodic slow wave complexes
Massive overdose (500 mg)*
Hypoventilation, respiratory arrest
Seizures
Prolonged coma
Sustained hypertension
Prolonged and fluctuating confusional state following recovery from coma
Intoxication in children
Lethargy or coma
Strange behavior
Staring spells
Ataxia
Nystagmus
Miosis
Opisthotonus, hypertonia, rigidity
Increased salivation
Seizures

* Approximate dose producing these manifestations.
Source: Burns et al. [9].

deaths have occurred in PCP-intoxicated people while being forcefully restrained by police. These deaths are presumed to be due to ventricular arrhythmias induced by the sympathomimetic action of PCP in combination with catecholamine release from fear and physical struggle.

Phenylpropanolamine

Phenylpropanolamine is widely consumed as an over-the-counter decongestant and diet medication. The major central nervous system complication of phenylpropanolamine is stroke, with numerous case reports published in recent years [31,49]. Although a great number of strokes have been reported, in light of its tremendously widespread use, the risk of phenylpropanolamine-induced stroke in an individual is probably quite low.

Phenylpropanolamine is primarily an alpha-adrenergic agonist, that is, it causes vasoconstriction and hypertension. Unlike cocaine and amphetamines, phenylpropanolamine-induced hypertension is associated with reflex bradycardia. Strokes are felt to be primarily due to hypertension, as discussed for cocaine, although vasculitis has also been implicated [31]. Stroke has occurred in some patients after ingesting relatively low doses of phenylpropanolamine, possibly due to individual hypersensitivity to the pressor effects of phenylpropanolamine (such as has been documented in a patient with autonomic insufficiency with secondary denervation hypersensitivity) [65]. However, the most common cause of central nervous system injury is the acute consumption of excessive doses.

Headache is a common feature of phenylpropanolamine intoxication and is most likely related to hypertension. Headache with a neurologic deficit suggests that a stroke has already occurred and requires a detailed neurologic evaluation as described for cocaine. Behavioral toxicity (i.e., psychiatric disturbances) is less common with phenylpropanolamine than with other stimulant drugs; however, cases of agitation, acute mania, and paranoid or organic psychosis have been reported [44].

Management of Sympathomimetic Drug Intoxications

Psychiatric complications of sympathomimetic drugs should be treated by placing the patient in a nonthreatening environment, with use of benzodiazepines for sedation of agitated patients. Severe agitation or psychosis may require haloperidol or chlorpromazine. Hospitalization is recommended for patients with protracted paranoid behavior, suicidal tendencies, persistently impaired perceptual or cognitive function, or associated medical complications.

The medical problems of major concern are

hypertension, seizures, hyperthemia, and circulatory collapse. Acute drug-induced hypertension in a patient with a normal neurologic examination should be treated as soon as possible to prevent stroke. Since the hypertension is catecholamine-mediated, alpha-adrenergic blockers (such as phentolamine) or calcium channel blockers (such as nifedepine or verapamil) are usually effective, with the use of beta blockers as needed for associated tachycardia or tachyarrhythmias. The use of nonselective beta blockers alone may aggravate hypertension produced by sympathiomimetic drugs due to the blockade of beta-2-mediated vasodilation and unopposed alpha-adrenergic stimulation and should be avoided. Hypertension in the presence of a stroke is a more complicated issue, since hypertension may be a homeostatic response to maintain intracerebral blood flow in the presence of intracranial hypertension. In this case, blood pressure should not be lowered or, if there is ongoing evidence of sympathomimetic drug intoxication, lowered gradually to a diastolic blood pressure in the 100 to 110 mm Hg range. Seizures and hyperthermia may result in brain injury and should be treated vigorously, as discussed in previous sections.

OTHER COMMON INTOXICATIONS

A few other drugs or toxins present with neurologic signs and symptoms frequently enough to warrant brief discussion.

Salicylate

Salicylate intoxication is common and remains a significant cause of drug-induced mortality. The diagnosis is often missed, particularly when there has been chronic intoxication. The actions of salicylate include direct stimulation of the respiratory center of the brain, uncoupling of oxidative phosphorylation, and interference with the activity of enzymes of the cycle and enzymes involved in amino acid, lipid, and carbohydrate metabolism. Cerebral hypoglycemia is believed to contribute to the central nervous system manifestations of salicylate poisoning. Salicylates in high concentrations act on cell membranes to alter potassium and chloride conductance, thereby altering membrane potential.

Acute intoxication typically is associated with hyperventilation with respiratory alkalosis (in the early or mild stage) and metabolic acidosis (in the late or severe stage), accompanied by decreased auditory acuity, tinnitus, nausea and vomiting, lethargy, and irritability, progressing to disorientation, seizures, and coma. Asterixis has also been described in salicylate intoxication. Seizures or deep coma are uncommon and indicate a very severe intoxication with a guarded prognosis.

Chronic intoxication is more frequently associated with abnormal mental status than is acute intoxication, with encephalopathy of unknown etiology the diagnosis in many cases [3]. Neurologic abnormalities with chronic intoxication include confusion, agitation, slurred speech, hallucinations, seizures, and coma. Clues to chronic salicylate poisoning include hearing loss, tachypnea, unexplained metabolic acidosis, and a coagulopathy with an increased prothrombin time. Chronic salicylate intoxication is also associated with increased vascular permeability and the development of noncardiogenic pulmonary edema, proteinuria, and cerebral edema. Chronic salicylate poisoning is associated with a high morbidity and mortality, especially in the elderly, in whom mortality may be 25 percent or more [3]. Death is often due to sudden cardiac or respiratory arrest, possibly related to effects of salicylate on the brain. Serious salicylate toxicity is seen at much lower serum concentrations with chronic intoxications than with acute intoxications [28].

Cerebral edema has been described in patients after acute or chronic intoxications. Most of the cases are children or young adults. Cerebral edema may develop 2 or 3 days after presentation, at a time when salicylate levels have declined substantially [22]. Gross cerebral edema was noted at autopsy in 9 of 12 children who died from salicylate intoxication [82]. Vigorous hydration combined with increased cerebral permeability is believed to be the mechanism for cerebral edema.

Salicylate use has been implicated in the development of Reye's syndrome, a disease found primarily in children [67,82], which is characterized by acute encephalopathy and hepatic dysfunction. Most but not all cases follow a viral illness, particularly varicella and influenza. However, Reye's syndrome has also been reported in children receiving salicylate chronically for inflammatory arthritis in the absence of a viral syndrome [28].

Because salicylate intoxication produces coagulopathy, intracranial hemorrhage must be considered as a cause of disturbed mental status. We have seen two patients at San Francisco General Hospital felt to have salicylate-induced encephalopathy who in fact had intracranial hemorrhages.

The management of salicylate poisoning should focus on protecting vulnerable organs and accelerating the elimination of salicylate from the body. Salicylate, a weak acid, partitions favorably into the more alkaline side of a pH gradient. Development of acidemia is associated with movement of salicylate out of the blood into organs such as the brain, with increasing toxicity. Therefore, correction of acidosis and keeping the blood at a neutral or alkaline pH are essential. Alkalization of the urine is necessary to optimize the renal clearance of salicylate. Since life-threatening pulmonary and cerebral edema may complicate salicylate poisoning, fluids should be administered cautiously. Sodium bicarbonate can be administered in concentrated solutions (e.g., 150 mEq/liter) to minimize the volume of fluid needed while giving adequate doses of alkali [71]. Glucose should be administered to patients with even a normal serum glucose because cerebral hypoglycemia may contribute to encephalopathy.

The metabolism of salicylate is dose dependent and at high concentrations becomes saturated. Renal excretion becomes the primary route of elimination, the rate of which largely depends on the urine pH. At an alkaline pH renal clearance is facilitated, while at an acid pH excretion is minimal. In patients with chronic intoxication and abnormal mental status, especially the elderly, in patients with acidemia that cannot be corrected for fear of administering additional fluids in the face of pulmonary or cerebral edema, and in patients with impaired renal function who cannot themselves excrete salicylate, hemodialysis is indicated.

Lithium

Lithium intoxication commonly presents as a disorder of central nervous system function. Patients with lithium-induced neurotoxicity are frequently misdiagnosed, which may result in prolonged morbidity as well as mortality.

Lithium is a monovalent cation that can compete with other cations such as sodium and potassium in ion fluxes across cell membranes. The actions of lithium are extremely complex and include activation or inhibition of the sodium-potassium ATPase pump, inhibition of adenylate cyclase, and inhibition of calcium-dependent responses including the regulation of neurotransmitter release. Lithium blunts phasic changes in receptor sensitivity and is thought to stabilize neuronal activity, the latter presumed to be the basis for its efficacy in manic depressive illness.

Lithium is distributed in total body water but crosses cell membranes slowly. This is important because there is a time lag between peak levels of lithium in the blood and peak levels in the nervous system. As a result, the onset of neurotoxicity may be delayed after acute intoxication and neurotoxicity may persist for days (or even weeks in some cases) after blood levels have become quite low.

The manifestations of lithium toxicity depend on the serum level of lithium, the duration of intoxication, other drugs that have been coingested, and individual differences in susceptibility. Clinical features of lithium toxicity are listed in Table 23-18.

Toxicity is usually seen when serum lithium levels exceed the therapeutic range (up to 1.5 mEq/liter); however, there are many instances of toxicity at levels within the therapeutic range. Conversely, patients with extremely high levels (up to 7–8 mEq/liter) may be asymptomatic, particularly after acute poisoning. Acute poisoning is generally associated with much less severe intoxication for any given serum level than is chronic intoxication. Presumably this is because of slow penetration of lithium into the brain or a prolonged time course of neural response to the actions of lithium.

Tremor is a common feature of lithium toxic-

Table 23-18. Neurotoxicity of lithium

Common features with intoxication	*Less common features*
Tremor	Cognitive impairment; dementia-like syndrome
Weakness, fatigue	Creutzfeldt-Jacob-like syndrome
Nausea, vomiting	Dementia with mutism
Apathy, drowsiness	Myoclonic jerks, muscle rigidity
Hyperreflexia, muscle rigidity	Primitive reflexes
Muscular fasciculation	EEG slowing with runs of periodic sharp waves
Dysarthria, ataxia	Neuroleptic malignant syndrome
Confusion	Hyperpyrexia
Myoclonus	Muscle rigidity
Choreoathetoid movements	Autonomic lability
Akinesia, mutism	Confusional state
Seizures	Action myoclonus
Stupor	Generalized peripheral neuropathy
Coma	Mania
Circulatory collapse	

ity. Fine tremor is common even in patients receiving therapeutic doses. A coarse irregular tremor becomes more prominent with moderate toxicity. Several clinical presentations of lithium neurotoxicity deserve mention. A toxic-confusional state is well described in patients with both therapeutic and excessive levels of lithium [30]. This state often develops within a few weeks of initiation of therapy. It may be more common in patients who receive neuroleptic drugs, particularly haloperidol [18], and in patients with schizoaffective disorders, although these associations have not been strongly supported by research findings. The syndrome usually resolves within a week or two after discontinuation of treatment. Another toxic syndrome with rapidly progressive dementia, mutism, and motor abnormalities resembling Jacob-Creutzfeldt disease has been described in patients with lithium intoxication [41].

Lithium intoxication may present as a parkinsonian syndrome, with muscle rigidity (including cogwheeling), tremor, and in severe cases hypokinesia and akinesia [64]. Lithium may potentiate the effects of neuroleptics in causing parkinsonism, possibly because lithium blocks the development of supersensitivity to dopamine receptors, which usually follows chronic neuroleptic-induced dopamine receptor blockade. Lithium-induced parkinsonism tends not to responds very well to anticholinergic drugs.

Neuroleptic malignant syndrome has been described due to combination therapy with neuroleptics, particularly haloperidol, and lithium [37,77]. The syndrome consists of hyperpyrexia, muscle rigidity, autonomic disturbances (tachycardia, labile blood pressure, profuse sweating), and often a confusional state. It is fatal in 20 percent of patients. The incidence of neuroleptic malignant syndrome is quite low, probably less than 0.5 percent of patients receiving neuroleptics, but it has been suggested that the chronic use of lithium increases that risk.

In most patients, neurologic features of lithium intoxication resolve following discontinuation of lithium. However, there are reports of persistent neurologic dysfunction following acute or chronic intoxication despite discontinuation of lithium. [37,77]. The most frequently reported neurologic changes include dementia, cerebellar dysfunction (ataxia, dysarthria), tremor, nystagmus, and choreoathetoid movements. In some patients with permanent sequelae, their intoxications were complicated by hypotension and recurrent seizures, which could have caused or contributed to brain injury, but in other cases there appears to be no cause for neurologic injury other than lithium. The mechanism of brain injury from lithium is unknown.

Supportive management of lithium intoxication consists of rehydration to optimize renal function and to increase the excretion of lithium. Careful monitoring of the electrolyte status is essential because lithium often causes a nephrogenic diabetes insipidus syndrome. Administration of large volumes of isotonic sodium chloride may therefore result in hypernatremia, which may itself aggravate neurologic dysfunction. Therefore, once the patient is adequately hydrated, hypotonic (e.g., 0.45% saline) solutions are most appropriate. Hemodialysis may accelerate the elimination of lithium from the body, especially in patients with renal insufficiency. Hemodialysis is indicated in any patient with elevated levels of lithium and significant neurotoxicity or with impaired renal function and reduced endogenous clearance of the drug. As noted previously, acute intoxication rarely produces severe symptoms and signs, and hemodialysis is rarely indicated. After chronic intoxications, even when hemodialysis effectively lowers serum levels, central nervous system effects may persist up to 2 weeks, presumably due to slow exit of lithium out of brain cells.

Anticholinergic Drugs

A number of drugs and plants have anticholinergic activity that may present with central nervous system disturbances. Toxicity may occur following intentional overdose, therapeutic use of the drugs, abuse, or ingestion of plants. The drugs of most concern include antihistamines, tricylic antidepressants, antipsychotics, antiparkinsonian drugs (benztropine and trihexyphenidyl), spasmolytics (propantheline, belladonna), inhaled atropine (used for severe asthma), and scopolamine (used for motion sickness). Scopolamine is delivered in a transdermal system (patch), and serious intoxications have occurred in children who have accidentally applied the patch to the skin. A number of plants have anticholinergic activity. Some of those more widely known include jimsonweed and *Amanita muscaria* mushrooms.

The typical picture of anticholinergic drug toxicity includes sedation, confusion, agitation, and hallucination. Coma and respiratory depression may be present after a large ingestion. The presence of anticholinergic signs including tachycardia, mydriasis, fever, hot dry skin, urinary retention, and absence of bowel sounds confirms the diagnosis. Patients usually recover fully with supportive care. Administration of a centrally active cholinesterase inhibitor such as physostigmine will reverse coma, hallucination, and other anticholinergic manifestations and may assist in diagnosis. However, it should be used cautiously as physostigmine can cause excessive bradycardia and seizures. Physostigmine is *not* recommended in patients with anticholinergic syndrome due to cyclic antidepressant poisoning because the increase in cholinergic tone may aggravate the cardiac toxicity of the antidepressant and result in asystole [66]. Physostigmine is best reserved for patients with pure anticholinergic syndromes who have no evidence of cardiac toxicity other than sinus tachycardia on electrocardiogram.

REFERENCES

1. Alldredge, B. K., Lowenstein, D. H., and Simon, R. P. Seizures associated with recreational drug abuse. *Neurology* 39:1037, 1989
2. Alldredge, B. K., Lowenstein, D. H., and Simon, R. P. Placebo-controlled trial of intravenous diphenylhydantoin for short-term treatment of alcohol withdrawal seizures. *Am. J. Med.* 87:645, 1989.
3. Anderson, R. J., Potts, D. E., Gabow, P. A., et al Unrecognized adult salicylate intoxication. *Ann. Intern. Med.* 85:745, 1976.
4. Arieff, A. I. Hyponatremia, convulsions, respiratory arrest, and permanent brain damage after elective surgery in healthy women. *N. Engl. J. Med.* 314:1529, 1986.
5. Arieff, A. I., and Friedman, E. A. Coma following nonnarcotic drug overdosage: Management of 208 adult patients. *Am. J. Med. Sci.* 266:405, 1973.
6. Armstrong, P. J., and Bersten, A. Normeperidine toxicity. *Anesth. Analg.* 65:536, 1986.
7. Blass, J. P., and Gibson, G. E. Abnormality of a thiamine-requiring enzyme in patients with Wernicke-Korakoff syndrome. *N. Engl. J. Med.* 297:1367, 1977.
8. Buchanan, J. F., and Brown, J. F. "Designer

drugs": A problem in clinical toxicology. *Med. Toxicol.* 3:1, 1988.

9. Burns, R. S., Lerner, S. E., Corrado, R., et al. Phencyclidine: States of acute intoxication and fatalities. *West. J. Med.* 123:345, 1975.
10. Burns, R. S., LeWitt, P. A., Ebert, M. H., et al. The clinical syndrome of striatal dopamine deficiency: Parkinsonism induced by 1-methyl-4-phenyl-1,2,3,6-tetrahydropyridine (MPTP). *N. Engl. J. Med.* 312:1418, 1985.
11. Busto, U., Sellers, E. M., Naranjo, C. A., et al. Withdrawal reaction after long-term therapeutic use of benzodiazepines. *N. Engl. J. Med.* 315:854, 1986.
12. Carlen, P. L., Wortzman, G., Holgate, R. C., et al. Reversible cerebral atrophy in recently abstinent chronic alcoholics measured by computed tomography scans. *Science* 200:1076, 1978.
13. Carrie, B. J., Golbetz, H. V., Michaels, A. S., et al. Creatinine: An inadequate filtration marker in glomerular diseases. *Am. J. Med.* 69:177, 1980.
14. Catravas, J. D., and Waters, I. W. Acute cocaine intoxication in the conscious dog: Studies on the mechanism of lethality. *J. Pharmacol. Exp. Ther.* 217:350, 1981.
15. Charnes, M. E., Simon, R. P., and Greenberg, D. A. Ethanol and the nervous system. *N. Engl. J. Med.* 321:442, 1989.
16. Chasnoff, I. J., Lewis, D. E., and Squires, L. Cocaine intoxication in a breast-fed infant. *Pediatrics* 80:836, 1987.
17. Chasnoff, I. J., Burns, W. J., Schnoll, S. H., et al. Cocaine use in pregnancy. *N. Engl. J. Med.* 313:666, 1985.
18. Cohen, W. J., and Cohen, N. H. Lithium carbonate, haloperidol, and irreversible brain damage. *J.A.M.A.* 230:1283, 1974.
19. Deitrich, R. A., Dunwiddie, T. V., Harris, R. A., and Erwin, V. G. Mechanism of action of ethanol: Initial central nervous system actions. *Pharmacol. Rev.* 41:489, 1989.
20. Devenyi, P., Schneiderman, J. F., Devenyi, R. G., and Lawby L. Cocaine-induced central retinal artery occusion. *Can. Med. Assoc. J.* 138:129, 1988.
21. DeWitt, L. D., Buonanno, F. S., Kistler, J. P., et al. Central pontine myelinolysis: Demonstration by nuclear magnetic resonance. *Neurology* 34:570, 1984.
22. Dove, D. J., and Jones, T. Delayed coma associated with salicylate intoxication. *J. Pediatr.* 100:493, 1982.
23. Dowling, G. P., McDonough, E. T., and Bost, R. O. "Eve" and "Ecstasy": A report of five deaths associated with the use of MDEA and MDMA. *J.A.M.A.* 257:165, 1987.
24. Eldefrawi, A. T., and Eldefrawi, M. E. Receptors for γ-aminobutyric acid and voltage-dependent chloride channels as targets for drugs and toxicants. *F.A.S.E.B. J.* 1:262, 1987.
25. Feighner, J. P., Boyer, W. F., Tyler, D. L., and Neborsky, R. J. Adverse consequences of fluoxetine-MAO_1 combination therapy. *J. Clin. Psychiatry* 51:222, 1990.
26. Fraser, C. L., and Arieff, A. I. Fatal central diabetes mellitus and insipidus resulting from untreated hyponatremia: A new syndrome. *Ann. Intern. Med.* 112(2):113, 1990.
27. Frezza, M., de Padova, C., Pozzato, G., et al. High blood alcohol levels in woman. *N. Engl. J. Med.* 322:95, 1990.
28. Gaudreault, P., Temple, A. R., and Lovejoy, F. H. The relative severity of acute versus chronic salicylate poisoning in children: A clinical comparison. *Pediatrics* 70:566, 1982.
29. Gawin, F. H., and Ellinwood, E. H., Jr. Cocaine and other stimulants: Actions, abuse, and treatment. *N. Engl. J. Med.* 318:1173, 1988.
30. Ghadirian, A. M., and Lehmann, H. E. Neurological side effects of lithium: Organic brain syndrome, seizures, extrapyramidal side effects, and EEG changes. *Compr. Psychiatry* 21:327, 1980.
31. Glick, R., Hoying, J., Cerullo, L., and Perlman, S. Phenylpropanolamine: An over-the-counter drug causing central nervous system vasculitis and intracerebral hemorrhage. *Neurosurgery* 20:969, 1987.
32. Granoff, A. L., and David, J. M. Heat illness syndrome and lithium intoxication. *J. Clin. Psychiatry* 39:103, 1978.
33. Guidelines for the Determination of Death: Report of the Medical Consultants on the Diagnosis of Death to the President's Commission for the Study of Ethical Problems in Medicine and Biomedical and Behavioral Research. *J.A.M.A.* 246:2184, 1981.
34. Haider, I., Matthew, H., and Oswald, I. Electroencephalographic changes in acute drug poisoning. *Electroencephalogr. Clin. Neurophysiol.* 30:23, 1971.
35. Harris, R. A., and Allan, A. M. Alcohol intoxication: Ion channels and genetics. *F.A.S.E.B. J.* 3:1689, 1989.
36. Harrison, M., Busto, U., Naranjo, C. A., et al. Diazepam tapering in detoxification for high-dose benzodiazepine abuse. *Clin. Pharmacol. Ther.* 36:527, 1984.
37. Hartitasch, B., Hoenich, N. A., Leigh, R. J., et al. Permanent neurological sequelae despite haemodialysis for lithium intoxication. *Br. Med. J.* 4:757, 1972.
38. Heighmann, S. J., Stitzer, M. L., Bigelow, G. E., and Liebson I. A. Acute opioid physical dependence in postaddict humans: Naloxone effects after brief morphine exposure. *J. Pharmacol. Exp. Ther.* 248:127, 1989.
39. Jay, S. J., Johanson, W. G., and Pierce, A. K. Respiratory complications of overdose with sedative drugs. *Am. Rev. Respir. Dis.* 112:591, 1975.

40. Kaim, S. C., Klett, C. J., and Rothfeld, B. Treatment of the acute alcohol withdrawal state: A comparison of four drugs. *Am J. Psychiatry* 125:1640, 1969.
41. Kemperman, C. J. F., and Notermans, S. L. H. Creutzfeld-Jacob like syndrome due to lithium toxicity. *J. Neurol. Neurosurg. Psychiatry* 52:291, 1989.
42. Koob, G. F., and Bloom, F. E. Cellular and molecular mechanisms of drug dependence. *Science* 242:715, 1988.
43. Kraus, M. L, Gottlieb, L. D., Horwitz, R. I., and Anscher, M. Randomized chemical trial of atenolol in patients with alcohol withdrawal. *N. Engl. J. Med.* 313:905, 1985.
44. Lake, C. R., Masson, E. B., and Quirk, R. S. Psychiatric side effects attributed to phenylpropanolamine. *Pharmacopsychiatry* 21:171, 1988.
45. Lawson, A. A. H., and Northridge, D. B. Dextropropoxyphene overdose: Epidemiology, clinical presentation and management. *Med. Toxicol.* 2:430, 1987.
46. Levine, S. R., Brust, J. C. M., Futrell, N., et al. Cerebrovascular complications of the use of the "crack" form of alkaloidal cocaine. *N. Engl. J. Med.* 323:699, 1990.
47. Levine, S. R., and Welch, K. M. A. Cocaine and stroke. *Stroke* 19:779, 1988.
48. Lowenstein, D. H., Massa, S. M., Rowbotham, M. C., et al. Acute neurologic and psychiatric complications associated with cocaine abuse. *Am. J. Med.* 83:841, 1987.
49. McDowell, J. R., and LeBlanc, H. J. Phenylpropanolamine and cerebral hemorrhage. *West. J. Med.* 142:688, 1985.
50. Meldrum, B. S., Vigouroux, R. A., and Brierley, J. B. Systemic factors and epileptic brain damage. *Arch. Neurol.* 29:82, 1978.
51. Messing, R. O., Closson, R. G., and Simon, R. P. Drug-induced seizures: A 10-year experience. *Neurology* 34:1582, 1984.
52. Miller, G. M., Baker, H. L, and Okazaki, H., et al. Central pontine myelinolysis and its imitators: MR findings. *Radiology* 168:795, 1988.
53. Miller, L. G., Greenblatt, D. J., Barnhill, J. G., and Shader, R. I. Chronic benzodiazepine administration: I. Tolerance is associated with benzodiazepine receptor downregulation and decreased γ-aminobutyric acid$_A$ receptor function. *J. Pharmacol. Exp. Ther.* 246:170, 1987a.
54. Miller, L. G., Greenblatt, D. J., Roy, R. B., et al. Chronic benzodiazepine administration: II. Discontinuation syndrome is associated with up regulation of γ-aminobutyric acid$_A$ receptor complex binding and function. *J. Pharmacol. Exp. Ther.* 246:177, 1987b.
55. Minion, G. E., Solvis, C. M., and Boutiette, L. Severe alcohol intoxication: A study of 204 consecutive patients. *Clin. Toxicol.* 27:375, 1989.
56. Naranjo, C. A., Kadlec, K. E., Sanheuza, P., et al. Fluoxetine differentially alters alcohol intake and other consummatory behaviors in problem drinkers. *Clin. Pharmacol. Ther.* 47:490, 1990.
57. Newman, N. M., DiLoreto, D. A., Ho, J. T., et al. Bilateral optic neuropathy and osteolytic sinusitis: Complications of cocaine abuse. *J.A.M.A.* 259:72, 1988.
58. Ng, S. K. C., Hauser, W. A., Brust, J. C. M., and Susser, M. Alcohol consumption and withdrawal in new-onset seizures. *N. Engl. J. Med.* 319:666, 1988.
59. Olson, K. R., Pentel, P. R., and Kelley, M. T. Physical assessment and differential diagnosis of the poisoned patient. *Med. Toxicol.* 2:52, 1987.
60. Orringer, C. E., Eustace, J. C., Wunsch, C. D., et al. Natural history of lactic acidosis after grand-mal seizures: A model for the study of an anion-gap acidosis not associated with hyperkalemia. *N. Engl. J. Med.* 297:796, 1977.
61. O'Sullivan, G. F., and Wade, D. N. Flumazenil in the management of acute drug overdosage with benzodiazepines and other agents. *Clin. Pharmacol. Ther.* 42:254, 1987.
62. Papadakis, M. A., and Arieff, A. I. Unpredictability of clinical evaluation of renal function in cirrhosis. *Am. J. Med.* 82:945, 1987.
63. Pasternak, G. W. Multiple morphine and enkephalin receptors and the relief of pain. *J.A.M.A.* 259:1362, 1988.
64. Patterson, J. F. Lithium-induced akathisia. *J. Clin. Psychopharmacol.* 8:445, 1988.
65. Pentel, P., and Mikell, F. Reaction of phenylpropanolamine (chlorphenisamine) beladonna compound on a woman with unrecognized autonomic dysfunction. *Lancet* 2:274, 1984.
66. Pentel, P., and Peterson, C. D. Asystole complicating physostigmine treatment of tricyclic antidepressant overdose. *Ann. Emerg. Med.* 9:588, 1980.
67. Pinsky, P. F, Hurwitz, E. S., Schonberger, L. B., and Gunn, W. J. Reye's syndrome and aspirin: Evidence for a dose-response effect. *J.A.M.A.* 260:657, 1988.
68. Pittman, Q. J., Rogers, J., and Bloom, F. E. Arginine vasopressin deficient Brattleboro rats fail to develop tolerance to the hypothermic effects of ethanol. *Regul. Pept.* 4:33, 1982.
69. Plum, F., and Posner, J. B. *The Diagnosis of Stupor and Coma* (3rd ed.). Philadelphia: Davis, 1980.
70. Pond, S. M., Olson, K. R., Osterloh, J. O., and Tong, T. G. Randomized study of the treatment of phenobarbital overdose with repeated doses of activated charcoal. *J.A.M.A.* 251:3104, 1984.
71. Prescott, J. F., Balali-Mood, M., Critchley, J. A., et al. Diuresis or urinary alkalinisation for salicylate poisoning? *Br. Med. J.* 285:1383, 1982.
72. Report of the Ad Hoc Committee, Harvard Medical School. A definition of irreversible coma. *J.A.M.A.* 205:337, 1968.

73. Robinson, G. M, Sellers, E. M., and Janecek, E. Barbiturate and hypnosedative withdrawal by multiple oral phenobarbital loading dose technique. *Clin. Pharmacol. Ther.* 30:71, 1981.
74. Rosenberg, J., Pentel, P., Pond, S., et al. Hyperthermia associated with drug intoxication. *Crit. Care Med.* 14:964, 1986.
75. Roy-Byrne, P. P., and Hommer, D. Benzodiazepine withdrawal: Overview and implications for the treatment of anxiety. *Am. J. Med.* 84:1041, 1988.
76. Rumbaugh, C. L, Bergeron, T., Scanlan, R. L., et al. Cerebral vascular changes secondary to amphetamine abuse in the experimental animal. *Radiology* 101:345, 1971.
77. Saxena, S., and Mallikarjuna, P. Severe memory impairment with acute overdose lithium toxicity. *Br. J. Psychiatry* 152:835, 1988.
78. Schroth, G., Naegele, T., Klose, U., et al. Reversible brain shrinkage in abstinent alcoholics, measured by MRI. *Neuroradiology* 30:385, 1988.
79. Sellers, E. M., and Kalant, H. Alcohol intoxication and withdrawal. *N. Engl. J. Med.* 294:757, 1976.
80. Simpson, D. L., and Rumack, B. H. Methylenedioxyamphetamine: Clinical description of overdose, death and review of pharmacology. *Arch. Intern. Med.* 141:1507, 1981.
81. Smith, M. D., and Bleck, T. P. Techniques for determining brain death. *J. Crit. Illness* 4:67, 1988.
82. Starko, K. M., and Mullick, F. G. Hepatic and cerebral pathology findings in children with fatal salicylate intoxication: Further evidence for a causal relation between salicylate and Reye's syndrome. *Lancet* 1:326, 1983.
83. Tetrud, J. W., and Langston, J. W. The effect of deprenyl (selegiline) on the natural history of Parkinson's disease. *Science* 245:519, 1989.
84. Weil, J. V., McCullough, R. E., Kline, J. S., and Sodal, I. E. Diminished ventilatory response to hypoxia and hypercapnia after morphine in normal man. *N. Engl. J. Med.* 292:1103, 1975.
85. Woo, E., and Greenblatt, D. J. Massive benzodiazepine requirements during acute alcohol withdrawal. *Am. J. Psychiatry* 136:821, 1979.
86. Wyatt, R. J., Karoum, F., and Suddath, R. The role of dopamine in cocaine use and abuse. *Psychiat. Ann.* 18:531, 1988.

24 Metabolic Encephalopathy in Genetic Disease

Britt Anderson and Roger N. Rosenberg

In medicine, the term *metabolic* has a dual meaning. In a strict sense, it relates to the anabolic and catabolic reactions that sustain the individual. In a more colloquial sense, it is used to describe an individual with a diffuse dysfunction of higher cortical activities, an encephalopathy, in which the lesion is not believed structural, and where some amount of reversibility is anticipated. Both aspects of the term are relevant when considering neurogenetic illnesses. Since a mutated gene may express itself as the absence or increased amount of a protein, or even the production of an aberrant protein, all genetic illnesses are metabolic in the first sense. Within these genetic disorders there is a subset whose physical manifestations include an encephalopathy and cause a patient to present metabolic in the second sense.

This chapter will present a sample of neurogenetic illnesses that include an encephalopathy in their presentations. The pathophysiology will be emphasize in an attempt to show the variety by which an abnormal segment of DNA may produce a clinical syndrome. The restricted nature of the primary defect in these neurogenetic illnesses makes them excellent windows through which to observe the mechanisms producing higher cortical activities. Unfortunately, we still see through this glass but darkly.

PHENYLKETONURIA

Folling's report [75] of phenylpyruvic acid in the urine of a subset of patients with mental retardation was the first description of the disorder that would be called phenylketonuria (PKU). The location of the metabolic block at the conversion step between phenylalanine and tyrosine was made by Jervis [29,30] about 15 years later (Fig. 24-1). Classic PKU is associated with a loss of phenylalanine hydroxylase activity, the enzyme that catalyzes the conversion of phenylalanine to tyrosine [30]. The disorder has

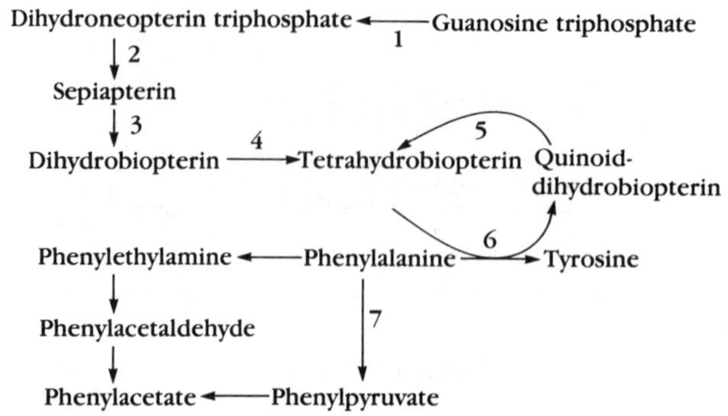

Fig. 24-1. Phenylalanine and pterin metabolism: (1) guanosine triphosphate cyclohydrolase; (2) "dihydrobiopterin synthetase"; (3) sepiapterin reductase; (4) dihydrofolate reductase; (5) dihydropteridine reductase; (6) phenylalanine hydroxylase; (7) phenylalanine-alanine aminotransferase.

a frequency of somewhat less than 1 : 10,000, with regional variations, and is inherited as an autosomal recessive trait [89]. Hyperphenylalaninemia may be due to other than an absence of phenylalanine hydroxylase activity. Most interesting are those variants where hyperphenylalaninemia results from a deficiency of tetrahydrobiopterin, an essential cofactor for phenylalanine hydroxylase. Tetrahydrobiopterin is produced by de novo and salvage pathways. Dihydrobiopterin synthetase is involved in the catalysis of dihydroneopterin triphosphate to sepiapterin, intermediates in the de novo pathway. Tetrahydrobiopterin is reclaimed from quinoid dihydrobiopterin, to which it is converted in its role as cofactor, by dihydrobiopterin reductase. Deficiencies of these two enzymes, dihydrobiopterin reductase and dihydrobiopterin synthetase, are the most common causes of tetrahydrobiopterin deficiency [2,14,84]. Tetrahydrobiopterin also serves as a cofactor for the additional enzymes tyrosine hydroxylase and tryptophan hydroxylase. Therefore disorders of this variety show all the effects of hyperphenylalaninemia with additional signs attributed to deficiences of neurotransmitters dopamine, norepinephrine, epinephrine, and serotonin. These additional signs consist of dystonia, choreoathetosis, and oculogyric crises.

The classic clinical syndrome for phenylalanine hydroxylase deficiency involves a normal child at birth. Mental retardation becomes noticeable at 4 to 9 months with developmental delay. A mousy odor may be reported. Seizures are frequent by 18 months of age, and many of the children have eczema. Intellectual compromise may be severe enough to preclude speech or toilet training. Hyperactivity with repetitive gestures may be noticed in the older afflicted individual [75].

The basis for the encephalopathy may be considered at the anatomic, physiologic, and biochemical levels. Further, distinctions should be made between the untreated phenylketonuric, the treated phenylketonuric coming off dietary control, and the normal child born of the phenylketonuric mother where the child has been exposed to high levels of phenylalanine in utero. The last syndrome will not be discussed here.

Both white matter and synaptic abnormalities have been reported as the cause of the mental retardation. The white matter changes are impressive, with spongy degeneration of white matter and hypomyelination composing the major pathologic changes seen in untreated adults at post-mortem examination [54,72]. The mechanism of the hypomyelination has been argued to result from the inhibition of transport of essential amino acids across the blood-brain barrier by high serum levels of phenylalanine. The paucity of amino acids within the central nervous system would yield decreased proteolipid synthesis and, secondarily, hypomyelination.

Supporting this logic, the proteolipid content in the brains of two untreated phenylketonurics was found to be 60 percent of age-matched controls [72].

Golgi studies have revealed a disturbance in the number and morphology of dendritic spines [4]. A rat model of PKU, in which disease is produced by administration of phenylacetate, suggests a maturational arrest in dendritic spine development [39,40]. With abnormal dendritic spine morphology, defective synaptogenesis and function seem a logical contributor to the encephalopathy. This possibility is supported by the work of Loo [47,48], who reports decreased high-affinity uptake of tritiated choline by 27 to 35 percent and of ^{14}C-labeled gamma-aminobutyric acid (GABA) by 23 to 45 percent in hippocampal, frontal, and occipital cortices using a synaptosomal preparation from the phenylacetate animal model of PKU. Loo [47,48] also reports normal glutaminergic, serotonergic, and noradrenergic junctions as assessed by high-affinity uptake studies, suggesting some neuronal specificity for the dysfunction. The most likely biochemical cause for similar changes in human PKU is an elevated amount of phenylacetate. This compound is produced from the metabolism of phenylpyruvate by an enzyme related to P-hydroxyphenylpyruvic acid oxidase. The contention that phenylacetate is the primary biochemical lesion is supported by the fact that administration of phenylpyruvate to rats fails to produce the characteristic clinical syndrome [47], and administration of phenylacetate, 0.75 to 1.25 μmol/gm twice a day 7 hours apart beginning at 2 days of age and continuing to day 21, with 0.25-μmol dosage increments on days 11 and 16, induces characteristics of phenylketonuria in animals with normal brain levels of phenylalanine [48]. Further, phenylacetate is produced in increased amounts during sustained hyperphenylalaninemia [51] and readily enters brain [49]. Brain converts phenylacetate to phenylacetyl coenzyme A (CoA), which reacts with acetyl CoA to form phenylbutyric acid. Interference with the normal metabolism of acetyl CoA by phenylacetyl CoA has been shown in the rat model [50] and suggests a basis for the delay in brain maturation. ^{14}C-labeled 3-hydroxybutyrate was converted to acetyl CoA in normal amounts in both PKU rats and normals, but a decreased percentage of radioactivity was recovered as sterol (13.05 ± 1.56 for experimental animals versus 16.41 ± 1.64 for animals) and fatty acids (for experimental animals 19.92 ± 1.71 and for control animals 25.19 ± 2.29). Additionally, the amount of radioactivity recovered as *n*-acetylneuraminic acid was significantly decreased from 11.93 ± 1.10 in the control animals to 8.63 ± 0.97 in the PKU rats [50]. In the biosynthetic pathway of *n*-acetylneuraminic acid, *n*-acetylation of glucosamine requires acetyl CoA.

Further support for the role of phenylacetate comes from two human illnesses, transient tyrosinemia of infancy and tyrosinosis, where phenylalanine and phenylpyruvate are elevated in serum but phenylacetate is not, and the children have at worst mild mental retardation [62,81].

In treated children who have undergone normal development, poorer scores on tests measuring higher integrative capacities (e.g., forced choice reaction time) have been observed in association with hyperphenylalaninemia [36]. A correlation between higher reaction times and phenylalanine levels was documented. Due to early therapy, brain structure is believed normal in these children, and the late brain dysfunction here appears to correlate with transient decreased brain neuronal dopamine and serotonin [22,36,57]. The decrease in brain dopamine and serotonin seems to relate less to competition for amino acid transport systems by phenylalanine [36] and more to phenylalanine-dependent inhibition of tyrosine and tryptophan hydroxylases in brain. These enzymes are rate-limiting steps in the production of dopamine and serotonin. A decrease in the rates of these enzymes would lead directly to decreased levels of these neurotransmitters [57,88].

The hallmark of therapy for PKU is a diet low in phenylalanine with tyrosine supplementation. Treatment of those patients with defects of tetrahydrobiopterin synthesis includes supplements of catecholamine and indoleamine precursors. The former is usually given as L-dopa, the latter as 5-hydroxytryptophan. Further, analogues of tetrahydrobiopterin may be given with some success [33]. However the general outlook for children with these defects is poor.

UREA CYCLE ENZYMOPATHIES

The urea cycle, described in 1932, was the first metabolic cycle discovered [37]. Its function is to take ammonia produced from the degradation of amino acids and purines, combine it with a carbon derived from carbon dioxide, and yield urea that may be excreted from the body [85]. The cycle contains five enzymatic steps (Fig. 24-2). Defects of each have been discovered and are associated with clinical disease. The disorders are carbamyl phosphate synthetase deficiency, ornithine transcarbamylase deficiency (OTC), citrullinemia, argininosuccinase deficiency, and arginase deficiency. Inheritance is autosomal recessive, except for OTC deficiency where it is X-linked dominant [61].

Although some of the urea cycle enzymes are found in the brain, the cycle is basically hepatic, and the cerebral dysfunction is secondary to the systemic hyperammonemia. The degree of hyperammonemia may vary with the completeness of the enzymatic defect as well as with external factors such as the presence of a systemic illness or the protein content of the diet. Because these factors may vary over time, it follows that the exacerbations of the illness may be cyclic.

The clinical characteristics of the disorders vary more with the degree of enzyme dysfunction than with the specific enzyme affected. Neonatal, infantile, childhood, and adult presentations are all recorded. The generally reported symptoms include irritability, vomiting, changes in muscle tone, failure to thrive, mental retardation, seizures, coma, and death [75].

The pathology of fatal cases varies but frequently reveals Alzheimer type II astrocytosis [9].

Hyperammonemia is the laboratory hallmark of the diagnosis but is not sufficient for diagnosis. Other disorders with similar presentations

Fig. 24-2. Urea cycle: (1) malate dehydrogenase; (2) aspartate aminotransferase; (3) glutamate acetyltransferase; (4) carbamyl phosphate synthetase; (5) ornithine carbamyltransferase; (6) argininosuccinate synthetase; (7) argininosuccinase; (8) arginase. NAD = nicotinamide-adenine dinucleotide; ATP = adenosine triphosphate; AMP = adenosine monophosphate; P_i = orthophosphate; ADP = adenosine diphosphate; CoA-SH = coenzyme A.

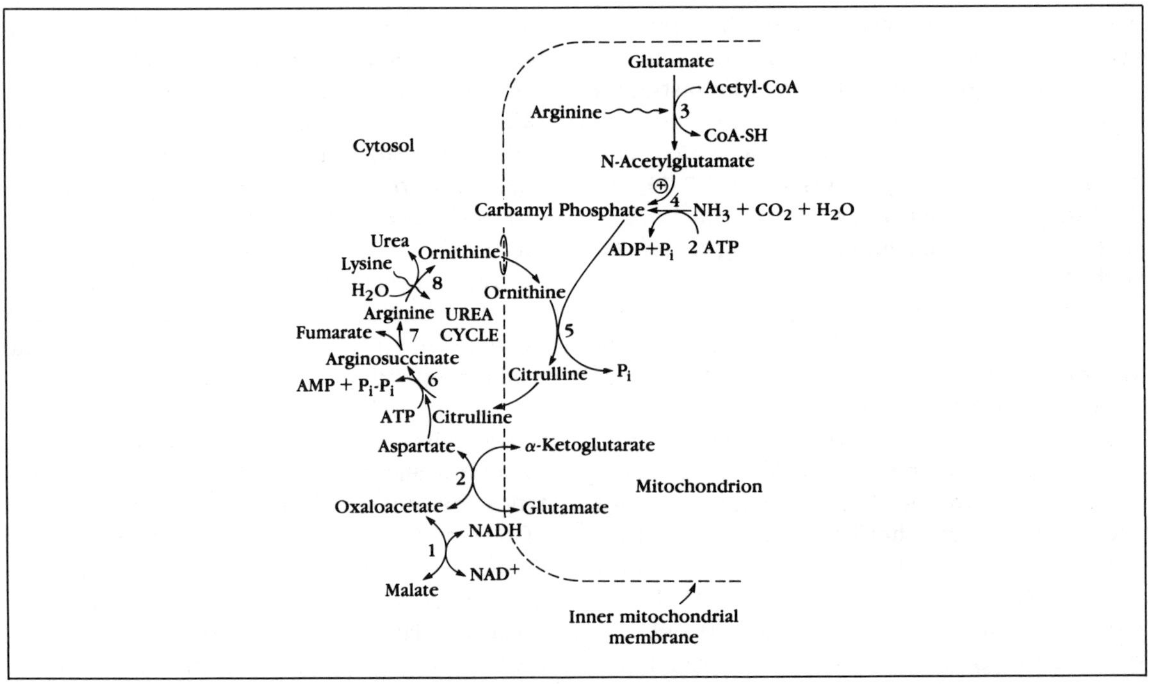

such as methylmalonic aciduria and Reye's syndrome may also show hyperammonemia in a clinically similar setting. Specific diagnosis requires the measurement of the metabolic intermediaries with demonstration of the enzymatic block.

Pathogenesis of the disorders relates to the ammonia, and the toxicity is probably mediated through astrocytes. When exposed to excessive levels of ammonia, the brain absorbs it by combining it with glutamate and forming glutamine [11] (Fig. 24-3). Catalyzed by glutamine synthetase, this reaction takes place primarily in glial cells [55,69]. Astrocytes possess a high-affinity receptor for glutamate, and astrocytes are probably the primary locus for the sequestration of glutamate after neuronal release at the synapse [79]. The synthesized glutamine is then released by astrocytes, where it is available for uptake by neurons and conversion to GABA or glutamate [23].

Evaluation of L-glutamate uptake assessing the capacity of crude synaptosomal fractions of brain to incorporate tritiated L-glutamate showed potassium-dependent and independent components. In the presence of 4 mM potassium, uptake increased from 6 pmol/minute/mg of protein to 9 pmol/minute/mg of protein. Ammonia at a concentration of 10 mM returned uptake of L-glutamate back to the basal value of 6 pmol/minute/mg of protein [60]. Ammonia may, therefore, produce toxicity by blocking the uptake of L-glutamate and thereby increase the extracellular pool of this excitotoxic amino acid neurotransmitter. Support for the concept of abnormal glial function comes from Norenberg's research. Astrocytes grown in culture and exposed to 2, 5, and 10 mM NH_4Cl for 1 or 4 days showed dose- and time-dependent evidence of toxicity [21]. One manifestation of this toxicity was a decreased capacity for astrocytes to produce cyclic adenosine monophosphate (AMP) when stimulated with beta-adrenergic agonists. In the group treated with 10 mM NH_4Cl for 4 days, cyclic AMP production in response to 1 μM isoproteronol was only 40 percent of control values [43]. The role of astrocytes as direct respondents to neurotransmitters is being increasingly recognized [66]. Astrocyte responses mediated by beta-adrenergic stimulation and increased cyclic AMP levels include accelerated glycogen turnover and taurine release [66]. Other authors have suggested a potential interference of ammonia with brain protein synthesis [68]. The incorporation of tritiated lysine into the brains of portocaval shunted rats was 0.83 nmol/hour/mg of protein, while in sham operated controls it was 1.6 nmol/hour/mg of protein [91]. In an animal model of extrahepatic cholestasis, incorporation of tritiated leucine was decreased in the treatment group, and when the results were broken down by cell type, the only significant decrement occurred in the glial fraction, which was 83 percent of controls [53].

Fig. 24-3. Glial-neuronal interaction for glutamate metabolism. Glutamate is taken up into glia by a high-affinity uptake system and metabolized to glutamine, which is then available for conversion to glutamate or GABA by neurons.

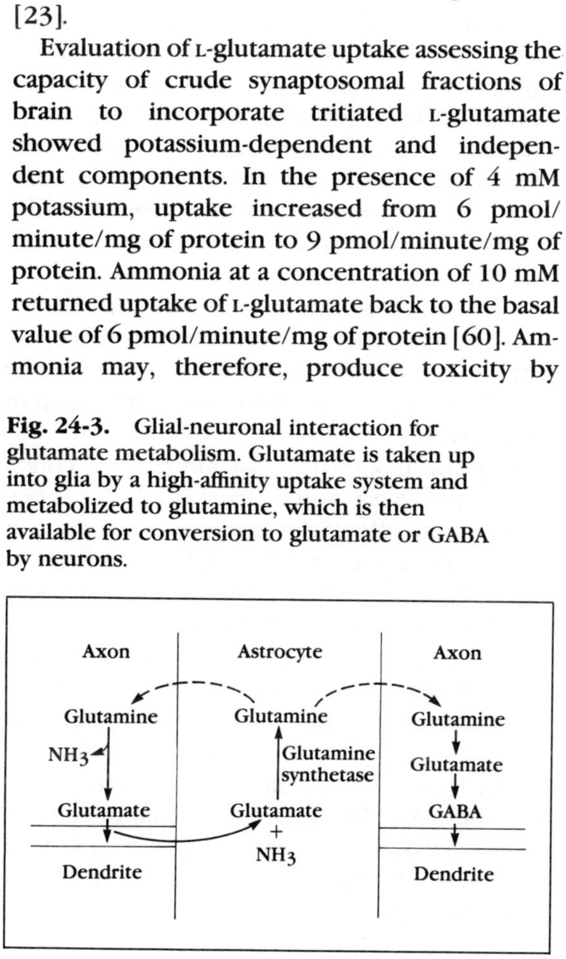

Treatment currently depends on protein restriction and the administration of the alpha-keto acid derivatives of the essential amino acids to act as an ammonia sink. By giving substrates that will react with ammonia and that are not harmful, a route for the drainage of excess ammonia is provided. If ammonia can be thus consumed, then levels should drop and toxic effects be blunted. A case in point is an 8-month-old infant with citruillinemia who was treated with alpha-keto acid derivatives of the essential amino acids. Ammonia levels fell from greater than 500 μM to 25 to 60 μM [87]. A similar approach is to give sodium benzoate, which can conjugate the nitrogen in glycine to form hippurate, and provide a nonurea nitrogen compound for excretion. Four children, ages 6 months to

17 years, were treated with sodium benzoate as sole therapy and had a significant improvement in ammonia levels. In one child, the fall in serum ammonia was from 207 μM to 55 μM. In very severe cases, peritoneal dialysis may be useful as an adjuvant to a lower ammonia levels [3].

ACUTE PORPHYRIAS

Porphyrins are intermediates in the production of heme. Heme is a component of several cytochromes as well as the oxygen-carrying pigments (e.g., hemoglobin). Succinyl CoA, from the citric acid cycle, is combined with glycine to form delta-aminolevulinic acid (delta-ALA) by the action of delta-ALA synthetase. Delta-ALA synthetase is the rate-limiting step for this cytosolic-mitochondrial pathway, which ends with the production of heme (Fig. 24-4). Heme exerts significant negative feedback on delta-ALA synthetase, thereby regulating its own production. A decrease of delta-ALA synthetase inhibition by heme is felt crucial to the development of the acute prophyrias. The three acute porphyrias are all inherited as autosomal dominant traits. Acute intermittent porphyria results from a 50 percent deficiency of porphobilinogen deaminase. Hereditary coproporphyria results from a 50 percent deficiency of coproporphyrinogen oxidase. Variegate porphyria is a partial deficiency of protoporphyrinogen oxidase. All result in decreased production of heme. This reduction in heme production leads to a secondary increase in the activity of delta-ALA synthetase. Delta-ALA and the product of the next step of the pathway, porphobilinogen, accumulate to excess as a result. Measurement of these intermediates in serum or urine is a staple of diagnosis [75,85].

Fig. 24-4. The heme biosynthetic pathway: (1) aminolevulinic acid (ALA) synthetase; (2) ALA dehydratase; (3) *porphobilinogen deaminase;* (4) uroporphyrinogen III cosynthase; (5) uroporphyrinogen decarboxylase; (6) *coproporphyrinogen oxidase;* (7) *protoporphyrinogen oxidase;* (8) ferrochetalase. The italics mark the defective enzymes in acute intermittent porphyria, hereditary coproporphyria, and variegate porphyria, respectively.

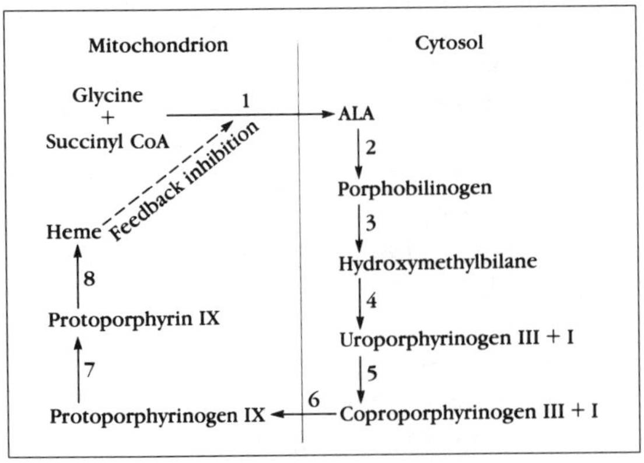

The symptoms and signs include abdominal pain, neuropathy, psychosis, and seizures. The typical first symptom is abdominal pain, which is thought to result from autonomic neuropathy with consequent gastrointestinal dysmotility and spasm.

The acute peripheral neuropathy is predominantly motor, but sensory components can be seen. Cranial nerves may be affected with long-lasting deficits. Quadriplegia with respiratory failure may result. Severe distal extremity weakness with a wrist- or footdrop, similar to that seen in lead toxicity, another disease where heme metabolism is disordered, is also encountered.

A history of photosensitive rash may be elicited from patients with hereditary coproporphyria but more usually is seen in variegate porphyria and is not seen in acute intermittent porphyria.

The encephalopathy can range from confusion to psychosis, stupor, coma, and death. Seizures frequently supervene and pose difficult therapeutic issues. Seizures occur despite elevated delta-ALA levels. Delta-ALA has a GABA mimetic effect and induces hyperpolarization of frog spinal motor neurons. This effect is blocked by the administration of picrotoxin, a GABA receptor antagonist, but not strychnine, a glycine receptor antagonist [67]. In common with other GABA agonist drugs, such as valproate, delta-ALA increases the seizure threshold of animals. Administration of 1.5 mmol/kg of delta-ALA intraperitoneally to C3H mice increased the latency to seizures induced by flurothyl from 30 to 70 seconds [93].

Depletion of heme is the general method of inducing an acute porphyric attack. This event occurs by either inhibition of heme synthetic enzymes or, more commonly, induction of enzymes producing heme-containing products. As free heme decreases, delta-ALA synthetase activity increases and symptoms result. Stress, fasting, infection, or a legion of drugs may precipitate an attack. Phenobarbitol is the prototypic agent. As cytochrome P450 synthesis is increased by phenobarbital administration, heme is consumed and the scenario begins. Classes of drugs that precipitate attacks include tricyclic antidepressants, other anticonvulsants (excluding bromides), several antihypertensives, oral contraceptives, and many antibiotics. Indeed a published list of "safe" drugs [63] is significantly shorter than a published list of unsafe drugs [56].

The pathology of this disorder in peripheral nerve is one of axonal degeneration and demyelination. Demyelination, chromatolysis, and vacuolation are seen in brain and spinal cord [17].

The pathogenesis of the central nervous system dysfunction remains obscure. Classically, two lines have been favored. One holds that delta-ALA or another precursor produced in abundance is directly toxic to nervous tissue. Unfortunately, infusions of these materials have not been observed to have clear toxic effects in animals or humans in vivo, and the levels to produce toxic effects in vitro are greater than seen in porphyric patients during attacks. In studies of frog spinal cord and frog muscle, the lowest dose of delta-ALA to affect these symptoms was 0.1 mg/ml and 0.1 mM, respectively [7,52]. In the cerebrospinal fluid (CSF) of porphyric patients during an attack, the maximum delta-ALA was 0.035 mg/ml (0.0003 mM) [70]. The second line of evidence is that a deficient production of heme interferes with neuronal energy metabolism, involving heme incorporation into cytochromes as part of the electron transport system. Against this latter hypothesis is the fact that activity of the heme biosynthetic pathway in brain is only 12.5 to 0.002 percent of liver, and starvation, phenobarbitone, or allyisopropylacetamide have no effect on induction of brain heme biosynthetic enzymes, although they effect liver heme biosynthesis and are known to induce porphyric attacks [71]. If depletion of brain heme occurred, increased brain delta-ALA synthetase activity should have resulted. Since the latter event does not occur, the former hypothesis is then doubted. Also inconsistent is the fact that heme infusions ameliorate some neurologic signs but heme does not cross the blood-brain barrier and therefore could not serve as a substrate for neuronal cytochromes [41].

More recently another suggestion has been made regarding pathogenesis. The basic thesis is that liver heme deficiency leads to enzymatic alterations, which exert distant effects on brain. Tryptophan pyrrolase, a hepatic enzyme, is the major catabolizer of circulating tryptophan. In rats made porphyric by administration of phenobarbital and 3,5-dicarbethoxy-2,6-dimethyl-4-ethyl-1,4-dihydropyridine, the latter being a heme depletor by destroying cytochrome P450 and inhibiting ferrochetalase, tryptophan pyrrolase activity falls to less than 25 percent of the initial value. As a result, brain tryptophan levels increased from 3 to 5 μg/gm of tissue, and circulating 5-hydroxytryptamine increased to 150 percent of basal values. These effects were reversible. Five hours after administration of heme (11 mg/kg), brain tryptophan returned to normal values. These effects of increased brain tryptophan were assessed by analyzing latency to tail flick in the presence of morphine and a noxious stimulus. After 2 mg/kg of morphine subcutaneously, the latency to tail flick increased from 4 seconds to 8 seconds in control rats, but increased to 12 seconds in porphyric rats. This augmentation of analgesia was not seen if valine, 250 mg/kg, or *p*-chlorophenylalanine was first given. Valine competes with tryptophan for transport across the blood-brain barrier, and *p*-chlorophenylalanine inhibits tryptophan hydroxylase, and enzyme in the tryptophan to serotonin pathway [44,45].

The summation of this evidence is that dysfunction of a hepatic enzyme, tryptophan pyrrolase, may lead to abnormally increased levels of a specific neurotransmitter, serotonin, which can be shown indirectly to affect brain function. Further, the effect of heme on this system is to increase tryptophan pyrrolase, and therefore tryptophan catabolism, and thus provide a possible explanation for the ameliorative effect of heme in this disorder. It is not yet clear, however, if these experimental animal models provide a realistic insight into the pathogenesis of the human disorder.

Despite these suggestions, treatment remains prophylactic by avoiding precipitating drugs and, at the time of an attack, administration of glucose and heme. Glucose may be given as a D10 solution in a dosage of 300 to 500 gm/day. The rationale is that carbohydrate blocks the induction of delta-ALA synthetase [90]. Hematin, ferric heme, is given as a maximal dosage of 4 mg/kg. It is infused over at least 15 minutes and frequently for several hours. The clinical response and improvement may be delayed. Hematin serves as a substrate in place of heme to inhibit delta-ALA synthetase.

LESCH-NYHAN SYNDROME

Lesch-Nyhan syndrome was first clinically described in 1964 by Lesch and Nyhan [42]. The enzyme defect is hypoxanthine-phosphoribosyltransferase (HPRT). HPRT levels in affected patients are less than 0.01 percent of control subjects as reported by Seegmiller, Rosenbloom, and Kelley in 1967 [82].

This X-linked recessive disorder is clinically characterized by hyperuricemia, choreoathetosis, dystonia, mental retardation, and self-mutilating behavior. It becomes manifest in infancy with irritability, feeding problems, and developmental delay apparent by 3 to 5 months.

Genetically it is a heterogenous disorder with different defects in the HPRT gene or its regulation in different patients. These different defects include production of a present but abnormal HPRT protein, absence of HPRT mRNA production, and most usually an apparently normal HPRT mRNA without immunologically detectable HPRT protein. Restriction enzyme digests of lymphocyte DNA examined on Southern blots were "normal" for 23 out of 28 patients [96]. This fact suggests that the degree of altered DNA must be very small and is likely a single base substitution or small deletion. A single base substitution in DNA could result in insertion of an inappropriate amino acid into the HPRT protein. The abnormal protein might then be susceptible to rapid degradation, as suggested by Wilson and Kelley [94].

Neuropathologic studies have failed to demonstrate consistent, significant structural abnormalities [92], implying that the pathogenesis is entirely biochemical without accompanying morphologic alterations.

A dissection of the abnormal biochemistry begins with a review of purine metabolism (Fig. 24-5). Purines for nucleic acid synthesis are derived from both de novo and salvage or alternative pathways. In the de novo pathway, ribose-5-phosphate, the product of the pentose monophosphate shunt, goes through a series of enzymatic steps to yield phosphoribosylpyrophosphate (PRPP) and ultimately inosine monophosphate (IMP). Adenylic and guanylic acids are both produced from IMP. IMP is degraded to hypoxanthine and guanine, which is converted to uric acid by xanthine oxidase and then excreted. The salvage pathway using HPRT transfers a phosphoribosyl moiety to guanine and hypoxanthine to yield guanosine monophosphate or inosine monophosphate. Patients with Lesch-Nyhan lack HPRT and cannot synthesize purine nucleotides by this alternative pathway. As a result of decreased negative feedback from guanosine and inosine monophosphates on the rate-limiting step of PRPP to 5-phosphoribosyl-1-amine, the activity of the de novo pathway is increased. As the brain lacks xanthine oxidase, it cannot convert the excessive hypoxanthine to uric acid. Therefore, levels of hypoxanthine, as the final product, are greatly increased in the brain and cerebrospinal fluid of these patients.

Some have suggested that the abnormal brain function is directly related to the abundance of purines seen in patients with Lesch-Nyhan syndrome and that these metabolites are directly toxic. Arguments against this premise have recently been reviewed [5]. Most convincing is that patients with partial defects of HPRT may have hypoxanthine levels as high as Lesch-Nyhan patients but do not develop any of the neurologic signs characteristic of Lesch-Nyhan patients [34].

It appears that a more direct relationship exists between an early neonatal lesion of the nigrostriatal dopamine projections and the presence of self-mutilatory behavior. Lesions of

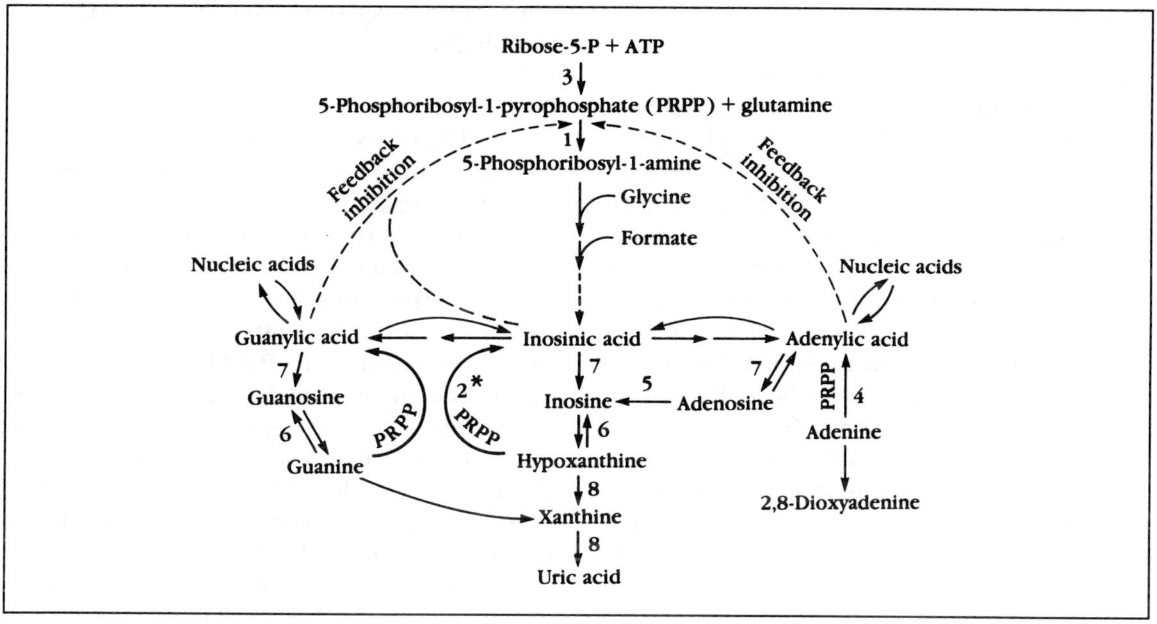

Fig. 24-5. Purine metabolism: (1) amidophosphoribosyltransferase; (2) HPRT; (3) PRPP synthetase; (4) adenine phosphoribosyltransferase; (5) adenosine deaminase; (6) purine nucleoside phosphorylase; (7) 5′-nucleotidase; (8) xanthine oxidase.

the ventral tegmental midbrain of young monkeys involving dopaminergic neurons permit the induction of self-mutilation at an older age when the animals are given dopamine agonists. Administrations of L-dopa, apomorphine, and abeorphine 201-678, mixed D_1 and D_2 dopamine receptor agonists, induced self-mutilation. Subsequent administration of fluphenazine, a mixed D_1 and D_2 receptor antagonist, or selective D_1 receptor antagonist SCH 23390 abolished the behavior, but selective D_2 antagonist sulpiride did not, suggesting the primacy of the adenylate cyclase linked D_1 receptor in the production of the self-mutilating behavior [20]. Further dissection of this model in rats demonstrates that the critical time for placement of the lesion is during the neonatal period. If the dopamine pathway lesion is placed in an adult animal, later administration of dopamine agonists L-dopa or apomorphine, 10 to 100 mg/kg as a single dose, does not induce self-mutilation [8]. High-dose caffeine, 250 mg/day for 10 to 15 days, another animal model of self-mutilatory behavior, works with greater effectiveness in dopamine-lesioned animals [10]. It appears that these models may relate to Lesch-Nyhan on more than a behavioral level. Evidence suggests a decrease in the function of dopamine terminals in Lesch-Nyhan subjects. Flurometric measurement of dopamine in the basal ganglia structures of Lesch-Nyhan subjects showed values 25 percent of controls, and dopamine synthetic enzymes were decreased to 10 to 30 percent of control values in the caudate, putamen, external pallidum, and nucleus accumbens [46]. Homovanillic acid, the major dopamine metabolite, was measured in CSF by high-performance liquid chromatography and found decreased below the mean of age-matched control values in 18 of 19 Lesch-Nyhan subjects [83]. Goldstein and co-workers [19] have used this information with some effectiveness to treat a patient with a D_1 dopamine receptor antagonist. A 20-month-old child was given 0.5 mg of fluphenazine twice a day in a double-blind fashion with placebo. During the fluphenazine period, biting decreased and motor behavior was "somewhat better." Within 12 hours of switching to placebo, biting increased markedly and continued to increase until fluphenazine was restarted.

Although it appears the self-mutilation relates to an early life hypodopaminergic state, it is still not entirely clear how this follows from the HPRT deficiency, but there are some clues. Brain seems more dependent on the salvage pathway for the production of nucleotides than is extraneural tissue. This statement derives from evidence showing high levels of HPRT in normal brain and low levels of amidophosphoribosyltransferase, a de novo pathway enzyme, in brain. Amidophosphoribosyltransferase activity was assessed by measuring the incorporation of ^{14}C-labeled glycine into alpha-*N*-formylgycinamide by rat brain and liver slices. Incorporation was 113 pmol/hour/100 mg in liver and 31 pmol/hour/100 mg in brain [28]. HPRT activity in basal ganglia is 170 percent of frontal lobe values, the next highest brain region, and 2000 percent of liver values [76]. At a time when demand for purine nucleotides is high, the brain in general, and the basal ganglia in particular, will be unable to provide required purine substrates in Lesch-Nyhan patients. This state is due to a low capacity of brain to use the de novo pathway and because Lesch-Nyhan patients lacking HPRT activity will not be able to use the salvage pathway. Since brain levels of DNA and RNA peak in late pregnancy and early postnatal life, this is the time period when the decreased brain purine production capacity of Lesch-Nyhan patients might be felt most acutely. This is also the time when the brain will be establishing dendritic contacts and forming synapses. It follows that these processes might primarily suffer, but this line of reasoning currently remains a hypothesis.

Somatic gene therapy in this disorder has been proposed [64]. However, if the above pathogenesis is correct, the reintroduction of HPRT by somatic gene therapy techniques using hematopoietic cell precursors several months after birth may be too late and may not be effective.

Recently a mouse model of this disease has been reported. Embryonal stem cells mutant for HPRT deficiency were injected into mouse blastocysts, and chimeric mice were produced. Some of these animals had incorporation of the mutant cells into their germ cells, and male animals negative for HPRT were produced by appropriate matings. At age 11 weeks, these mice had not yet shown behavioral abnormalities [26,38].

In summary, Lesch-Nyhan is an X-linked recessive disorder that presents in infancy with pyramidal and extrapyramidal signs, mental retardation, and later, self-mutilation. The last behavior may result from defective arborization of dendritic trees related to a shortage of purines in areas of brain dependent on the salvage pathway for the primary production of purine nucleotides. Dopamine terminals in the basal ganglia may be principally affected. Self-mutilation may be dependent on stimulation of D_1 receptors. Somatic cell gene therapy has been proposed but may not be effective particularly because of the need to provide enzyme early in brain development and the problem of extraneurally located enzyme being able to pass the blood-brain barrier. The chimeric animal model may offer an excellent system for study of these issues.

METACHROMATIC LEUKODYSTROPHY

Metachromatic leukodystrophy (MLD) is an autosomal recessive disorder with clinical and genetic heterogeneity. In all forms (late infantile, juvenile, and adult), the enzymatic defect is a deficiency of arylsulfatase A. The clinical course is consistent within families, suggesting distinct mutations give rise to the three forms [35]. Arylsulfatase A hydrolyzes the sulfate group from cerebroside sulfate [15], and a deficiency of this enzyme results in the accumulation of 3′-sulfo-galactocerebroside in the lysosomal compartment of cells. The predominant clinical signs relate to white matter disease. In the adult form, a patient may present with psychotic or encephalopathic features including depression, hallucinations, and emotion lability. Dementia may occur in some patients. Ataxia, spasticity, and a mixed neuropathy may also be present [35].

Diagnosis may be conveniently determined by measurement of arylsulfatase A levels in peripheral leukocytes or measurement of catabolism of labeled cerebroside sulfate. The latter test allows differentiation of heterozygotes with low arylsulfatase A levels from homozygous MLD patients. In MLD patients, the enzyme activity is totally absent. Inspection of cells in the urinary sediment, or of sural nerve, for the presence of metachromasia after staining with 1% acidified cresyl violet may allow diagnosis in a clinically suggestive case.

The characteristic pathologic finding in the brain is demyelination, frequently with sparing of nerve fibers and the "U" fiber layer. Metachromatic granules are easily found occurring in macrophages, oligodendrocytes, neurons of the dentate nucleus, brain stem nuclei, and the extracellular space.

The pathogenesis of the disorder is unknown, but several reasonable suggestions exist. Two myelin compartments exist in nerve [12]. Resorption of the fast turnover compartment, which corresponds to the innermost layer of myelin, is necessary for neuronal growth [1]. It has been suggested that defective arylsulfatase A activity may interfere with this normal degradative process of normal myelin metabolism. An abnormality of myelin as the direct cause of demyelination has also been suggested [35].

Another proposal that may be common to all the sphingolipidoses is an extension of the psychosine hypothesis [65]. It has been noted in Krabbe's globoid cell leukodystrophy that, despite the defect in galactocerebrosidase, galactocerebroside does not accumulate, but rather galactosylsphingosine does [86]. This substance is known to be highly cytotoxic. Sulfogalactosylsphingosine has not been identified in brains of MLD patients, but the possibility of its presence is supported by the presence of galactosylsphingosine and its sulfotransferases in normal brain [16]. This compound would be highly reactive, and due to a free amino group it could bind to proteins and interfere with normal cellular metabolism. Recently, lysosphingolipids including galactosylsphingosine and sulfogalactosylsphingosine have been shown to be potent inhibitors of protein kinase C [24]. This kinase is important for neural function [31], as it is part of the effector mechanism of the polyphosphoinositide second messenger system. This second messenger is diffusely present in brain and may serve to regulate calcium, chloride, and potassium channel conductances. This potential defect in channel conductance could affect transmitter release [31]. Thus in summary, the encephalopathy of adult MLD may be related to the accumulation of sulfo-galactosylsphingosine, which inhibits neuronal protein kinase C and interferes with neurotransmitters by an effect on calcium, potassium, and chloride channels.

Therapy for this disorder is supportive. A preliminary report suggests some benefit secondary to bone marrow transplantation [6]. In this case, a boy received a bone marrow transplant from his HLA-identical sister. Six months after the graft, all CSF leukocytes were confirmed to be of female origin by the presence of Barr bodies. This child followed a course that compared very favorably to two older siblings who are both deceased from complications of MLD. Thus, lymphocytes from a donor containing normal arylsulfatase A activity may enter brain and favorably affect disease progression.

TAY-SACHS DISEASE

Tay-Sachs disease is an autosomal recessive disorder of higher gene frequency in the Ashkenazi Jewish population. It presents in early infancy as a failure to obtain normal motor milestones. Regression of motor skills, blindness, and very frequently seizures occur. Children usually die of secondary infectious complications in their first few years.

The enzymatic defect is in hexosaminidase A [77]. Ganglioside GM_2 is solubilized by an activator complex that permits hexosaminidase A to catalyze removal of the terminal *N*-acetylgalactosamine. The alpha subunit of the hexosaminidase A gene maps to chromosome 15, and the beta subunit maps to chromosome 5. Mutations affecting the alpha subunit of hexosaminidase A are characteristic of Tay-Sachs disease [78]. In fibroblasts from infants with this disorder, no immunochemically cross-reacting material directed against the alpha subunit of hexosaminidase A can be detected.

Despite the extensive categorization of the enzymatic defect, the mechanism leading to neurologic dysfunction remains unclear. It is clear that a prominent accumulation of ganglioside GM_2 in the lysosomal compartment of neurons does take place [18].

Pathologically a ballooning of the neuronal cell bodies with meganeurite formation is also seen [73]. These meganeurites may form synapses, and this aberrant synaptogenesis may account for some of the neuronal dysfunction. Further, Purpura [73] has reported abnormalities of dendritic spine morphology that may also alter normal synaptic communication. A purely mechanical effect of excessive storage material on the Golgi apparatus and endoplasmic reticulum interfering with protein synthesis has been proposed [80].

At present there is no therapy.

In summary, the encephalopathy of this disorder appears to relate to ganglioside accumulation mechanically interfering with normal cell protein synthesis and biochemically inducing abnormal synaptic contacts.

MUCOPOLYSACCHARIDOSES I-H, I-S, and II

These three disorders provide some insight into the idiosyncrasies of genetic encephalopathies. Two of these disorders involve the same enzyme and yet differ phenotypically. Two of the disorders involve different enzymes and resemble each other phenotypically.

Mucopolysaccharides are complex polyglycosaminoglycans with a protein core with attached carbohydrate moieties [74] (Fig. 24-6). The enzyme defects fall into categories separable on the basis of which combination of the following three components of glycosoaminoglycans they fail to adequately metabolize: keratan sulfate, dermatan sulfate, or heparan sulfate. Mucopolysaccharides are components of many tissues. The defects of these syndromes relate to the defective degration of mucopolysaccharides and their subsequent accumulation.

In both Hurler's (I-H) and Scheie's (I-S) syndromes, the inheritance is autosomal recessive and the enzyme defect is alpha-*L*-iduronidase [75]. Alpha-*L*-iduronidase cleaves alpha-*L*-iduronidate residues from both heparan sulfate and dermatan sulfate, so both of these polymers accumulate in Hurler's and Scheie's syndromes. Hurler's children show organomegaly with increased liver and spleen size. They are severely mentally retarded. Corneal clouding and severe skeletal deformities are present. Death in the first decade of life is most commonly due to respiratory infections and heart failure. Heart failure is related to involvement by mucopolysaccharide accumulation of the heart valves and coronary arteries. Scheie's syndrome, on the other hand, while having corneal clouding, lacks most of the other Hurler's components [61]. Scheie's patients are adults, slightly hirsute with mild muculoskeletal changes and are mentally normal. McKusick and associates [58] suggested Hurler's and Scheie's disorders to be allelic and predicted an intermediate, compound form possessing both alleles. In the case of these compound patients, one allele is of the Hurler's variety and one is of the Scheie's variety. Their disease is more severe than Scheie's syndrome since they possess one Hurler's gene, and it is less severe than Hurler's syndrome since they possess one Scheie's allele. Such compound patients have been reported [95]. The patient of Winters and colleagues is interesting because she presented with acute paranoia and without previous suspicion of a neurogenetic disorder [95]. Allelism has been confirmed by the inability of fibroblasts of patients with each of the two disorders to cross correct each other in cell culture [27]. Activity of the different mutant enzymes seems to account for the different syndromes and affects pathogenesis. Hopwood and Muller [27] examined enzyme from Hurler's and Scheie's patients' fibroblasts by assessing hydrolysis of iduronysl-anhydro-mannitol-6-sulfate. In both syndromes, the V_{max}, or maximum velocity of alpha-*L*-iduronidase activity, was severely but equivalently reduced, being 11 and 12 pmol/minute of product formed in Hurler's and Scheie's syndromes patients and 822 pmol/minute of product formed in controls. However, the Km values, essentially a measure of affinity between substrate and enzyme, as measured by the substrate concentration that produces one-half maximum enzyme velocity, showed that Scheie's patients and controls were approximately equal at 50 and 53 μmol/liter, while the

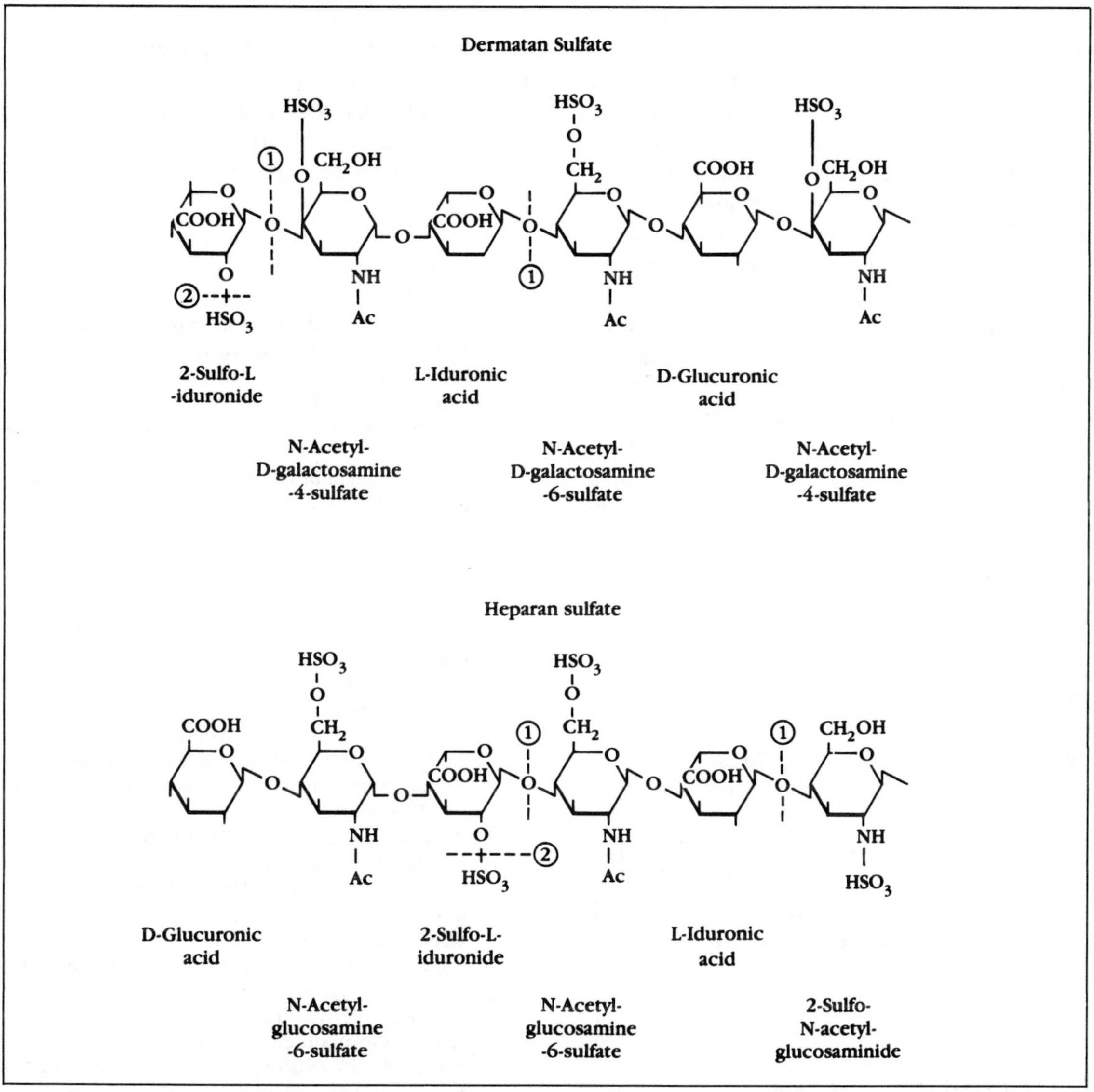

Fig. 24-6. Location of enzyme action for Hurler's (I-H), Scheie's (I-S), and Hunter's (II) syndromes: (1) alpha-*L*-iduronidase (I-H and I-S); (2) iduronidate sulfatase (II).

value of 650 μmol/liter from Hurler's patients' fibroblasts showed a greatly reduced capacity for substrate metabolism at usual substrate concentrations. Different CSF levels of glycosaminoglycans in Hurler's and Scheie's syndromes have been reported to correlate with mental retardation. This point is supported by the finding that acid mucopolysaccharide levels in CSF were 21 to 123 μg/dl in Scheie's syndromes (control value 15–45), and 855 to 1200 μg/dl in Hurler's syndromes [13].

Hunter's syndrome is an X-linked recessive disorder characterized by a deficiency of iduronate sulfatase. Iduronate sulfatase is also required for degradation of both dermatan sulfate and heparan sulfate. A single sulfated residue can prevent degradation of the polymer of the other degradative enzymes. Although Hunter's patients are said to be more placid and somewhat easier to care for than Hurler's patients, in general they share all other features—mental retardation, organomegaly, skeletal deformities, and deafness, with the exception of corneal clouding. This last feature may relate to undersulfation of the glycosaminoglycan in the corneal stroma, making degradation of the mucopolysaccharide of this organ less dependent on iduronate sulfatase [59].

The pathologic abnormality is deposition of mucopolysaccharide that is only partially degraded.

Diagnosis is based on the measurement of specific mucopolysaccharides in the urine, including heparan sulfate and dermatan sulfate. Normal mucopolysaccharide excretion in the urine is in the range of 5 to 25 mg/liter. Levels in Hurler's and Scheie's syndromes were a mean of 131 mg/liter and in Hunter's syndrome a mean of 168 mg/liter [32]. An assay of iduronate sulfatase or alpha-*L*-iduronidase may be done on fibroblasts in tissue culture. Hurler's and Scheie's syndromes patients cannot be consistently differentiated on enzyme levels but require reference to phenotypic characteristics.

There is no effective therapy. Bone marrow transplantation has been partially effective [25].

It is of considerable interest that Hurler's and Scheie's syndromes, which are allelic for the same gene, can produce widely different clinical syndromes.

CONCLUSIONS

The disorders discussed serve as a primer for the mechanisms of encephalopathy in neurogenetic illnesses. Mental functions can be altered quantitatively and differentially in disorders affecting the same enzymes, as seen in the variants of MLD and the Hurler's and Scheie's mucopolysaccharidoses. Altered cognition can result from altered metabolism in brain secondary to defective systemic metabolism, as seen in the porphyrias and urea cycle diseases. Brain function can also be impaired from primary brain enzyme defects, as in Lesch-Nyhan syndrome.

In summary, there is no common mechanism for the production of encephalopathies in neurogenetic disorders. For the patient there is frequently no specific therapy. Although we have traveled far in understanding the biochemical basis of these encephalopathies, the road is yet long and largely unexplored.

REFERENCES

1. Austin, J. Metachromatic Leukodystrophy (Sulfatide Lipidosis). In H. G. Hers and F. Van Hoof (eds.), *Lysosomes and Lysosomal Storage Diseases.* New York: Academic Press, 1973.
2. Bartholone, K., Byrd, D. J., Kaufman, S., and Milstien, S. Atypical phenylketonuria with normal phenylalanine hydroxylase and dihydropteridine reductase activity in vitro. *Pediatrics* 59:757, 1977.
3. Batshaw, M. L., and Brusilow, S. W. Treatment of hyperammonemic coma caused by inborn errors of urea synthesis. *J. Pediatr.* 97:893, 1980.
4. Bauman, M. L., and Kemper, T. L. Morphologic and histoanatomic observations of the brain in untreated human phenylketonuria. *Acta Neuropathol. (Berl.)* 58:55, 1982.
5. Baumeister, A. A., and Frye, G. D. The biochemical basis of the behavioral disorder in the Lesch-Nyhan syndrome. *Neurosci. Biobehav. Rev.* 9:169, 1985.
6. Bayever, E., Ladisch, S., Philippart, M., et al. Bone marrow transplantation for metachromatic leukodystrophy. *Lancet* 2:471, 1985.
7. Becker, D. M., Goldstuck, N., and Kramer, S. Effects of delta-aminolevulinic acid on the resting membrane potential of frog sartorius muscle. *South African Med. J.* 49:1790, 1975.
8. Breese, G. R., Baumeister, A. A., McCown, T. J., et al. Behavioral differences between neonatal and adult 6-hydroxydopamine treated rats to dopamine agonists: Relevance to clinical syndromes with reduced brain dopamine. *J. Pharmacol. Exp. Ther.* 231:343, 1984.
9. Brutton, C., Corsellis, J., and Russel, A. Hereditary hyperammonemia. *Brain* 93:423, 1970.
10. Casas-Bruge, M., Alemar, C., Grau, I. M., et al. Dopaminergic receptor supersensitivity in self mutilatory behavior of Lesch-Nyhan disease. *Lancet* 1:991, 1985.
11. Copper, A. J. L., Mora, S. N., Cruz, N. F., and Gelbard, A. S. Cerebral ammonia metabolism in hyperammonemic rats. *J. Neurochem.* 44:1716, 1985.
12. Davidson, A. N., and Gregson, N. A. Metabolism of cellular membrane sulfolipids in the rat brain. *Biochem. J.* 98:915, 1966.
13. Dekaban, A. S., and Constantopolous, G. Muco-

polysaccharidoses: Relation of elevated cerebral spinal fluid glycosaminoglycans and mental retardation. *Arch. Neurol.* 28:385, 1973.

14. Dhondt, J. L. Tetrahydrobiopterin deficiency: Preliminary analysis from an international survey. *J. Pediatr.* 104:501, 1984.
15. Farooqui, A. A. Purification and properties of human placenta arylsulfatase A. *Arch. Int. Physiol. Biochim.* 84:479, 1976.
16. Farooqui, A. A., and Horrocks, L. A. Biochemical aspects of globoid and metachromatic leukodystrophies. *Neurochem. Pathol.* 2:189, 1984.
17. Gibson, J. B., and Goldberg, A. The neuropathology of acute porphyria. *J. Pathol. Bacteriol.* 71:495, 1956.
18. Goebel, H. H. Morphology of the gangliosidoses. *Neuropediatrics* 15(Suppl.):97, 1984.
19. Goldstein, M., Anderson, L. T., Reuben, R., and Dancis, J. Self-mutilation in Lesch-Nyhan disease is caused by dopaminergic denervation. *Lancet* 1:338, 1985.
20. Goldstein, M., Kuga, S., Kusano, N., et al. Dopamine agonist induced self-mutilative biting behavior in monkeys with unilateral ventral tegmental lesion of the brainstem: Possible pharmacologic model for Lesch-Nyhan syndrome. *Brain Res.* 367:114, 1986.
21. Gregorios, J. B., Mozes, L. W., Norenberg, L.-O. B., and Norenberg, M. D. Morphologic effects of ammonia on primary astroctye cultures: 1. Light microscopic studies. *J. Neuropathol. Exp. Neurol.* 44:397, 1985.
22. Gutter, F., and Lou, H. Dietary problems of phenylketonuria: Effect on CNS transmitters and their possible role in behavioral and neuropsychological function. *J. Inherited Metab. Dis.* 9(Suppl. 2):169, 1986.
23. Hamberger, A., Nystrom, B., Salstrom, A., and Woiler, U. Amino acid transport in isolated neurons and glia. *Adv. Exp. Med. Biol.* 69:221, 1976.
24. Hannun, Y. A., and Bell, R. M. Lysosphingolipids inhibit protein kinase C: Implications for the sphingolipidoses. *Science* 235:670, 1987.
25. Hobbs, J. R., Hugh-Jones, K., Barrett, A. J., et al. Reversal of clinical features of Hurler's disease and biochemical improvement after treatment by bone marrow transplantation. *Lancet* 2: 709, 1981.
26. Hooper, M., Hardy, K., Handyside, A., et al. HPRT-deficient (Lesch-Nyhan) mouse embryos derived from germline colonization by cultured cells. *Nature* 326:292, 1987.
27. Hopwood, J. J., and Muller, V. Biochemical discrimination of Hurler and Scheie syndromes. *Clin. Sci.* 57:265, 1979.
28. Howard, W. J., Kerson, L. A., and Appel, S. H. Synthesis de novo of purines in slices of rat brain and liver. *J. Neurochem.* 17:121, 1970.
29. Jervis, G. A. Studies on phenylpyruvic oligophrenia: The position of the metabolic error. *J. Biol. Chem.* 169:651, 1947.
30. Jervis, G. A. Phenylpyruvic oligophrenia deficiency of phenylalanine-oxidizing system. *Proc. Soc. Exp. Biol. Med.* 82:514, 1953.
31. Kaczmarek, L. K. The role of protein kinase C in the regulation of ion channels and neurotransmitter release. *Trends Neurosci.* 10:30, 1987
32. Kaplan, D. Classification of the mucopolysaccharidoses based on the pattern of mucopolysacchariduria. *Am. J. Med.* 47:721-9, 1969.
33. Kaufman, S., Kapatos, G., Rizzo, W. B., et al. Tetrahydrobiopterin therapy for hyperphenylalaninemia caused by defective synthesis of tetrahydrobiopterin. *Ann. Neurol.* 14:308, 1985.
34. Kelley, W. N., Greene, M. L., Rosenbloom, F. M., et al. Hypoxanthine-guanine phosphoribosyl transferase deficiency in gout. *Ann. Intern. Med.* 70:155, 1969.
35. Kolodny, E. H., and Moser, H. W. Sulfatide Lipidoses: Metachromatic Leukodystrophy. In J. B. Stanbury, J. B. Wyngaarden, D. S. Fredrickson, et al. (eds.), *The Metabolic Basis of Inherited Disease* (3rd. ed.). New York: McGraw-Hill, 1982.
36. Krause, W., Halminski, U., McDonald, L., et al. Biochemical and neuropsychological effects of elevated plasma phenylalanine in patients with treated phenylketonuria. *J. Clin. Invest.* 75:40, 1985.
37. Krebs, H. Urea Synthesis. In J. B. Sumner and K. Myrback (eds.), *The Enzymes,* vol. 2, part 2. New York: Academic, 1951.
38. Kuehn, M. R., Bradley, A., Robertson, E. J., and Evans, M. J. A potential animal model for Lesch-Nyhan syndrome through placement of HPRT mutations into mice. *Nature* 326:295, 1987.
39. Lacey, D. J. Hippocampal dendritic abnormalities in a rat model of phenylketonuria. *Ann. Neurol.* 16:577, 1984.
40. Lacey, D. J. Normalization of dendritic spine numbers in rat hippocampus after termination of phenylacetate injections (PKU model). *Brain Res.* 329:354, 1985.
41. Lamon, J. M., Fryholm, B. E., Hess, B. A., and Tschudy, D. P. Hematin therapy for acute porphyria. *Medicine (Baltimore)* 58:252, 1979.
42. Lesch, M., and Nyhan, W. A familial disorder or uric acid metabolism and central nervous system function. *Am. J. Med.* 36:561, 1964.
43. Liskowsky, D. R., Norenberg, L.-O. B., and Norenberg, M. D. Effects of ammonia on cyclic AMP production in primary astrocyte cultures. *Brain Res.* 386:386, 1986.
44. Litman, D. A., Correia, M. A. L-Tryptophan: A common denominator of biochemical and neurological events of acute hepatic porphyria. *Science* 222:1031, 1983.
45. Litman, D. A., and Correia, M. A. Elevated brain

tryptophan and enhanced 5-hydroxytryptamine turnover in acute hepatic heme deficiency: Clinical implications. *J. Pharmacol. Exp. Ther.* 232:337, 1985.

46. Lloyd, K. G., Hornykiewicz, O., Davidson, S., et al. Biochemical evidence of dysfunction of brain neurotransmitters in the Lesch-Nyhan syndrome. *N. Engl. J. Med.* 305:1106, 1981.
47. Loo, Y. H., Fulton, T. R., Hyde, K. R., and Wisniewski, H. M. Biochemical indices of neuronal development in experimental phenylketonuria: High affinity transport systems and gangliosides. *Dev. Neurosci.* 6:235, 1983/84.
48. Loo, Y. H., Fulton, T. R., Miller, K. A., and Wisniewski, H. M. Phenylacetate and brain dysfunction in experimental phenylketonuria: Synaptic development. *Life Sci.* 27:1283, 1980.
49. Loo, Y. H., Fulton, T. R., and Wisniewski, H. M. Vulnerability of the immature brain to phenylacetate intoxication: Tissue permeability to phenylacetate. *J. Neurochem.* 32:1697, 1979.
50. Loo, Y. H., Potenspska, A., and Wisniewski, H. M. A biochemical explanation of phenylacetate neurotoxicity in experimental phenylketonuria. *J. Neurochem.* 45:1596, 1985.
51. Loo, Y. H., Scotto, H., and Horning, M. G. Aromatic acid metabolites of phenylalanine in the hyperphenylalaninemic rat. *J. Neurochem.* 29:411, 1977.
52. Loots, J. M., Becker, D. M., Meyer, B. J., et al. The effect of porphyrin precursors on monosynaptic reflex activity in the isolated hemisected frog spinal cord. *J. Neural Trans.* 36:71, 1975.
53. Lundborg, H., and Blomstrand, C. Protein synthesis in neurons and glial cells by extrahepatic cholestasis in rats. *Exp. Neurol.* 44:274, 1974.
54. Malamud, N. Neuropathology of phenylketonuria. *J. Neuropathol. Exp. Neurol.* 25:254, 1966.
55. Martinez-Hernandez, A., Bell, K. P., Norenberg, M. D. Glutamine synthetase: Glial localization in brain. *Science* 195:1356, 1977.
56. McColl, K. E. L., Moore, M. R., and Goldberg, A. The Acute Porphyrias. In F. C. Rose (ed.), *Metabolic Disorders of the Nervous System.* London: Pitman, 1980.
57. McKean, C. M. The effects of high phenylalanine concentration on serotonin and catecholamine metabolism in human brain. *Brain Res.* 47:469, 1972.
58. McKusik, V. A., Howell, R. R., Hussels, I. E., et al. Allelism, non-allelism, and genetic compounds among the mucopolysaccharidoses. *Lancet* 1:993, 1972.
59. McKusik, V. A., and Neufeld, E. F. The Mucopolysaccharide Storage Diseases. In J. B. Stanbury, J. B. Wyngaarden, D. S. Fredrickson, et al. (eds.), *The Metabolic Basis of Inherited Disease.* New York: McGraw-Hill, 1982.
60. Mena, E. E., and Cotman, C. W. Pathologic concentrations of ammonium ions block L-glutamate uptake. *Exp. Neurol.* 89:259, 1985.
61. Menkes, J. H. *Textbook of Child Neurology,* (3rd ed.). Philadelphia: Lea & Feberger, 1985.
62. Menkes, J. H., and Avery, M. E. The metabolism of phenylalanine and tyrosine in the premature infant. *Bull. Johns Hopkins Hosp.* 113:301, 1963.
63. Meyer, V. A. Porphyrias. In K. J. Isselbacher, R. D. Adams, E. Braunwald, et al. (eds.), *Harrison's Principles of Internal Medicine* (9th ed.) New York: McGraw-Hill, 1980.
64. Milenski, E. A. Discussions on human gene therapy. *Recomb. DNA* 9:88, 1986.
65. Miyatake, T., and Suzuki, K. Globoid cell leukodystrophy: Additional deficiency of psychosine galactosidase. *Biochem. Biophys. Res. Comm.* 48:538, 1972.
66. Murphy, S., and Pearce, B. Functional receptors for neurotransmitters on astroglial cells. *Neurosci.* 22:381, 1987.
67. Nicoll, R. A. The interaction of porphyrin precursors with GABA receptors in the isolated frog spinal cord. *Life Sci.* 19:521, 1976.
68. Norenberg, M. D. The Astrocyte in Liver Disease. In S. Fedoroff and S. Hertz (eds.), *Advances in Cellular Neurobiology.* New York: Academic, 1981. Vol. 2, pp. 303–352.
69. Norenberg, M. D., and Martinez-Hernandez, A. Fine structural localization of glutamine synthetase in rat brain. *Brain Res.* 161:303, 1979.
70. Percy, V. A., and Shanley, B. C. Porphyrin precursors in blood, urine, and cerebrospinal fluid in acute porphyria. *South Aftrican Med. J.* 52:219, 1977.
71. Percy, V. A., and Shanley, B. C. Studies on haem biosynthesis in rat brain. *J. Neurochem.* 33:1267, 1979.
72. Prensky, A. L., Carr, S., and Moser, H. W. Development of myelin in inherited disorders of amino acid metabolism: A biochemical investigation. *Arch. Neurol.* 19:552, 1968.
73. Purpura, D. P. Pathobiology of Cortical Neurons in Metabolic and Unclassified Amentias. In R. Katzman (ed.), *Congenital and Acquired Cognitive Disorders.* New York: Raven, 1979.
74. Roder, L. Structure and Metabolism of Connective Tissue Proteoglycans. In W. J. Lennarz (ed.), *The Biochemistry of Glycoproteins and Proteoglycans.* New York: Plenum, 1980.
75. Rosenberg, R. N. *Neurogenetics: Principles and Practice.* New York: Raven, 1986.
76. Rosenbloom, F. M., Kelley, W. N., Miller, J., et al. Inherited disorder of purine metabolism: Correlation between central nervous system dysfunction and biochemical defects. *J.A.M.A.* 202:175, 1967.
77. Sandoff, K., Andrease, V., and Jatzkewitz, H. Deficient hexosaminidase activity in an exceptional case of Tay-Sachs disease with additional

storage of kidney globoside in visceral organs. *Life Sci.* 7:283, 1968.
78. Sandoff, K., and Conzelmann, E. The biochemical basis of gangliosidoses. *Neuropediatrics* 15(Suppl.):85, 1984.
79. Schousbol, A. Transport and metabolism of glutamate and GABA in neurons and glial cells. *Int. Rev. Neurobiol.* 22:1, 1981.
80. Schulte, F. J. Clinical course of GM_2 gangliosidoses: A correlative attempt. *Neuropediatrics* 15(Suppl.):66, 1984.
81. Scriver, C. R., Larochelle, J., and Silverberg, M. Hereditary tyrosinemia and tyrosyduria in a French Canadian geographic isolate. *Am. J. Dis. Child.* 113:416, 1967.
82. Seegmiller, J., Rosenbloom, F., and Kelley, W. An enzyme defect associated with a sex linked human neurological disorder and excessive purine synthesis. *Science* 155:1682, 1967.
83. Silverstein, F. S., Johnston, M. V., Hutchinson, R. J., and Edwards, N. L. Lesch-Nyhan syndrome: CSF neurotransmitter abnormalities. *Neurology* 35:907, 1985.
84. Smith, L., Clayton, B. E., and Wolff, O. H. New variant of phenylketonuria with progressive neurological illness unresponsive to phenylalanine restriction. *Lanct* 1:1108, 1975.
85. Stryer, L. *Biochemistry.* San Francisco: Freeman, 1975.
86. Svennerholm, L., Vanier, M., and Mansson, J., Krabbe's disease: A galactosylsphingosine (psychosine) lipidosis. *J. Lipid Res.* 21:53, 1980.
87. Thoene, J., Batshaw, M., Spector, E., et al. Neonatal citruillinemia: Treatment with keto-analogues of essential amino acids. *J. Pediatr.* 90:218, 1977.
88. Tong, J. H., and Kaufman, S. Tryptophan hydroxylase: Purification and some properties of the enzyme from rabbit hindbrain. *J. Biol. Chem.* 250:4152, 1975.
89. Tourian, A., and Sidbury, J. B., Phenylketonuria and Hyperphenylalaninemia. In J. B. Stanbury, J. B. Wyngaarden, D. S. Fredrickson, et al. (eds.), The *Metabolic Basis of Inherited Disease* (5th ed.). New York: McGraw-Hill, 1982.
90. Tschudy, D. P., Welland, F. H., Collins, A., and Hutner, G., Jr. The effect of carbohydrate feeding on the induction of L-amino-levulinic synthetase. *Metabolism* 13:396, 1964.
91. Wasterlain, C. G., Lockwood, A., and Conn, M. Chronic inhibition of protein synthesis after portocaval shunting. *Neurology* 28:233, 1978.
92. Watts, R. W. E., Spellacy, E., Gibbs, D. A., et al. Clinical, post-mortem, biochemical, and therapeutic observations on the Lesch-Nyhan syndrome with particular reference to the neurological manifestations. *Q. J. Med.* 201:43, 1982.
93. Wehner, J. M., and Marley, R. J. Genetic differences in the effects of delta-aminolevulinic acid on seizure latency in mice. *Exp. Neurol.* 94:280, 1986.
94. Wilson, J. M., and Kelley, W. N. Molecular genetics of hypoxanthine-guanine phosphoribosyl-transferase deficiency in man. *Arch. Intern. Med.* 145:1895, 1985.
95. Winters, P. R., Harrod, M. J., Molenick-Heetred, S. A., et al. Alpha-L-iduronidase deficiency and possible Hurler-Scheie genetic compound: Clinical, pathologic and biochemical findings. *Neurology* 26:1003, 1976.
96. Yang, T. P., Patel, P. I., Chinau, H. A. C., et al. Molecular evidence for new mutation at the HPRT locus in Lesch-Nyhan patients. *Nature* 310:412, 1984.

Index

Page numbers followed by f *indicate figures; page numbers followed by* t *indicate tables.*